Birthsong
Midwifery Workbook with Coloring Pages

Basic Level Study Guide for Midwives

7th Edition

Daphne Singingtree and Dana Moore, BSM, CPM, LM

Birthsong Midwifery Workbook with Coloring Pages, 7th Edition

© 2026 All rights reserved.

No part of this publication may be reproduced, distributed, transmitted, or stored in a retrieval system in any form or by any means, including photocopying, recording, or other electronic or mechanical methods, without the prior written permission of the publisher, except for brief quotations used in reviews.

This work is intended for human learning and teaching and may not be used for training artificial intelligence systems without permission. Permission inquiries should be directed to:

daphnesingingtree@gmail.com

ISBN 979-8-9940224-0-5

This workbook is intended for educational purposes only. It does not provide medical advice, diagnosis, or treatment, and it is not a substitute for professional medical or midwifery care. The information presented is designed to support learning and should be used alongside formal education, clinical training, and appropriate supervision. Readers are responsible for practicing within their scope of training, licensure, and local regulations.

First edition, 1984

Second edition, 1993

Third edition, 2000

Fourth edition, 2005

Fifth edition, 2007

Sixth edition, 2010

Seventh edition, 2026

All proceeds from this workbook support Zaníyan Center, a 501 c (3) nonprofit dedicated to promoting health through plants and a connection to the earth. www.zaniyan.org

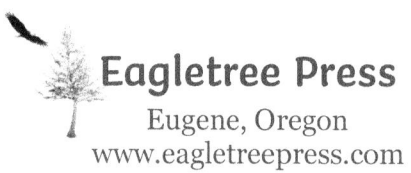

Eagletree Press
Eugene, Oregon
www.eagletreepress.com

Dedication

To all midwifery students, those who carry this calling with courage and tenderness, and to the families who invite us into their most sacred moments:
you are the heart of this work.

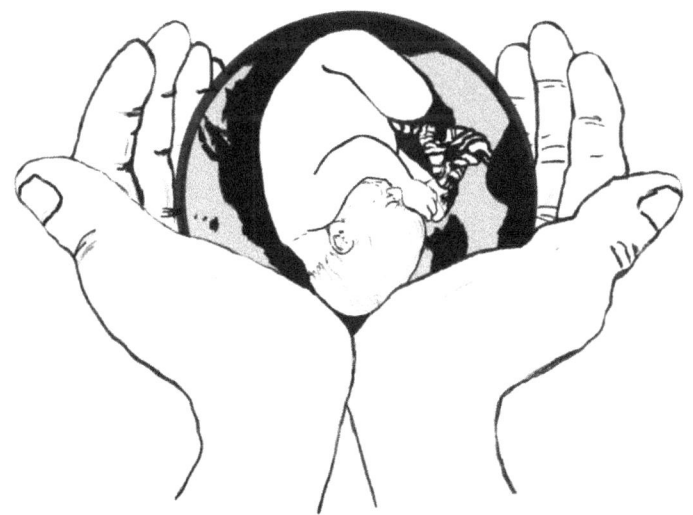

Introduction

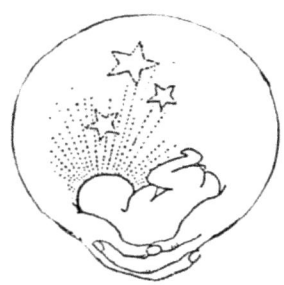

I wrote the first edition of this book in 1984. My youngest daughter, Trillium, was a year old, and I dedicated it to her "for taking long naps." I had just begun teaching midwifery and had founded the Birthsong School of Midwifery, which grew out of an informal study group and evolved over time. One of my students recorded all my classes, transcribed them, and presented the notes to me at the end of the term. Those transcripts, combined with the many photocopied materials I had been gathering, became the foundation for this book.

I was inspired by the anatomy coloring books that had recently been published and wanted to create a similar resource specifically for student midwives. In 1984, personal computers were just beginning to appear, but I did not have one. I typed everything on a typewriter. A couple of my students created the artwork, and using a light table, waxer, and X-Acto knife, I assembled the first edition by hand.

The first four editions were photocopied and comb-bound. By the third edition, I had acquired a computer and taught myself desktop publishing. As the print runs slowly grew, I was eventually able to produce a perfect-bound edition. Print-on-demand was not yet common, which meant storing boxes of books and selling them gradually over time.

Those early editions were filled with spelling and grammatical errors. At that stage of my life, I had no formal education. I left home at age twelve and followed what would now be called an unschooling path, studying what interested me, particularly herbs and midwifery. I earned a GED at seventeen, but it was not until much later, after I retired from midwifery, that I began college. In my fifties, I completed a master's degree in education with a focus on learning technologies from Ashford University.

I learned midwifery through apprenticeship, working alongside my first husband, a physician who attended home births. Teaching classes and writing books became central to how I learned in those early years. Over time, I founded and participated in several midwifery schools, helped establish the Midwifery Education and Accreditation Council, contributed to writing Oregon's direct-entry midwifery licensing legislation, and remained active in midwifery education for many years.

Eventually, I stepped away from midwifery and turned my attention to building an herbal product business. In 2023, I closed that business to focus on writing a series of speculative fiction novels. Meanwhile, the sixth edition of the *Birthsong Midwifery Workbook* remained in circulation, increasingly outdated and in need of substantial revision. Because I had been out of midwifery practice and education for over a decade, I did not feel it would be responsible to revise the book on my own. Midwifery, like all medical professions, requires ongoing education and active engagement.

After posting a request on Facebook seeking a co-author, I was fortunate to connect with J. Dana Moore (formerly Davis), BSM, CPM, LM. Dana brought current clinical experience, updated evidence, and deep practical insight to the project. Her contributions strengthened the book in every chapter. She also created many of the new illustrations and took the lead on revising and expanding the material. Working together allowed this edition to honor the original intent of the workbook while bringing it fully into the present.

Dana began practicing midwifery in 2006. In 2015, she became both a Certified Professional Midwife and a Licensed Midwife. She earned her Bachelor of Science in Midwifery from the Midwives College of Utah. Dana currently works as a licensed midwife at Harmony Health Medical Clinic and Family Resource Center in Marysville, California. Her scope includes birth center deliveries, prenatal and postpartum care, comprehensive women's health services, and community outreach.

Together, Daphne and Dana bring over fifty years of combined experience serving families and educating future midwives. This edition reflects that shared commitment to skilled, grounded, and compassionate care, and it is offered in support of those who are learning the art and science of midwifery and preparing to carry it forward.

How to Use This Workbook

This workbook is designed as a companion to your primary midwifery textbooks, not as a stand-alone resource. You may already be studying with classic texts such as *Varney's Midwifery* or *Myles Textbook for Midwives*. Many other excellent books exist, and each chapter in this workbook ends with a recommended reading list that highlights additional resources to deepen your understanding.

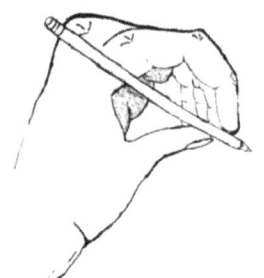

This book is also meant to be used as a coloring book. Fine-tipped colored pencils or felt markers work best. Color the HOLLOW letters for each anatomical structure, then color the structure itself. Doing this strengthens the connection between a part's name and its location in the body. Your brain uses different pathways when you engage with information by hand rather than simply reading. For readers using the digital edition, plan to print any pages you wish to color. There are quite a few of them.

Color with intention. Begin with the hollow letters and say the name of the structure as you fill them in. Then color the matching anatomy. This simple pairing of sound and motion boosts memory in surprising ways.

The exercises throughout the chapters provide another layer of active learning. Space is sometimes limited because of page constraints. You are welcome to write small, use a separate notebook, or complete exercises on your computer. The goal is flexibility, not perfect penmanship. Work through the exercises gradually. These questions are meant to help you think, not simply to test you. Spread them out over several study sessions if needed.

Many illustrations are included simply because learning is sweeter with art. These pieces are formatted for coloring. Although they do not teach anatomy in the same way the labeled structures do, they offer benefits in relaxation, artistic expression, and pure enjoyment.

We have made every effort to use inclusive and respectful language throughout the workbook. Birthing families come in many forms and from many cultural and racial backgrounds. Family structures, relationships, and gender identities vary. We use the words woman and mother in this workbook, while understanding that not every reader identifies with those terms and that gender experiences are diverse.

By design, this is a basic-level workbook that focuses on normal childbearing. Complications are mentioned only when necessary for context and are not explored in detail. We hope to create a companion workbook on birth complications in the future. For now, our attention remains on foundational knowledge and on supporting students as they enter the world of midwifery.

Use this book for group study. Many students find it helpful to compare answers, discuss differences, and quiz one another using the diagrams. Keep it visible. A workbook within reach gets used more often than one that lives on a shelf. Midwifery is hands-on, and your study tools should be too.

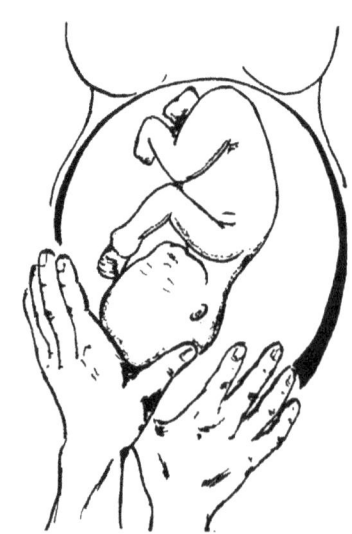

This workbook is meant to be as interactive as possible. Our hope is that it becomes more than a study tool. As you color, write, question, and reflect, may these pages help ideas take root and confidence grow. Midwifery is a calling of both hands and heart. Let this book walk beside you as you learn, practice, and step into the work that awaits you. May it support you, challenge you, and accompany you throughout your midwifery journey.

Acknowledgments

In the forty-two years since the first edition of this workbook was published, many people have contributed to its growth and evolution, far too many to name individually. Each edition has built upon the past, shaped by practice, teaching, and lived experience. The seventh edition is the most substantial to date and reflects an unprecedented level of revision, expansion, and clinical refinement.

This edition was made possible through the invaluable collaboration of my brilliant co-author, Dana Moore. Dana brought deep clinical knowledge, clarity of thought, and a strong educational lens to this work. Her contributions strengthened the clinical accuracy, organization, and accessibility of the material throughout the book. The seventh edition is richer, clearer, and more grounded because of her partnership.

I would like to acknowledge the thousands of students I have had the privilege to teach over the decades. I have learned as much from my students as they have from me. Their questions, insights, challenges, and experiences have continually shaped how I think, teach, and practice midwifery. This workbook exists because of them.

I am deeply grateful to my midwifery teachers and mentors, whose guidance continues to inform my work. I especially honor Marion Toepke-McLean, CNM, my midwifery teacher and enduring guiding light. Now well into her eighties, she continues to teach midwives in Ghana, embodying a lifelong commitment to service, skill, and integrity. Her influence is woven throughout these pages.

I also wish to acknowledge my first husband, Russell Nickels, MD, who passed this year. His support during my early years of practice and teaching was foundational, and his presence remains part of the history that shaped this work.

Special thanks to Feyo Edo Ambia, MD, an OB/GYN resident at Asela Referral and Teaching Hospital in the Oromia Region of Ethiopia, who reviewed and edited many technical details and offered essential insights on low-resource and cultural perspectives. Deep gratitude to my editor, Elian Wren, who helped keep commas in place, Chicago Manual of Style conventions in check, and offered thoughtful support with clarity, structure, and consistency throughout the manuscript. My sincere thanks also to my publishing assistant, Mary Glo Cuda, who designed the cover and provided extensive support with marketing materials. Thank you to peer editors Tammy Robinson and Emily Moore for their feedback.

I would like to extend a special thank-you to my home helpers. Since my car accident, everyday tasks have become difficult and time-consuming. Their assistance makes it possible for me to continue writing. They are my friends and support system, always there when needed. Thank you, Shari Arthur, Sharon Cohen, Cindy Herzog, and Brita Pastor.

My children, Alder, Aradia, Terran, and Trillium, grew up with a practicing midwife who missed many key events. Despite this each of them has become an incredible person. Their love sustains me.

Image Credits and Permissions

All images and illustrations in this workbook are used for educational purposes. Copyright remains with the original creators. Images are credited to the best of our knowledge, and every effort has been made to acknowledge original sources and comply with fair-use and permission standards. If any credit has been inadvertently omitted, please notify the publisher so the record may be corrected in future printings.

Illustrations by Blissborn Education, World Health Organization, Jennifer Buccilli, Patricia Edmonds, Amanda Greavette, Wahaba Heartsun, Bonnie Gruenberg, Andrea Roos, Amani Omejer, Cameron Scales, Ruth Simer, and YoSayam Sun.

Contents

Introduction i
How to Use This Workbook.. ii
Acknowledgments iii
Image Credits and Permissions... iii

CHAPTER ONE MIDWIFERY YESTERDAY & TODAY 1
The History and Legacy of Midwifery... 4
The Certified Nurse Midwife (Cnm) Credential 17
CPM Credential: Expertise in Community Birth 18
ICM and Midwifery Regulation 21
A Unified Framework for Core Competencies 22
Midwifery Education 26
Chapter One Self-Assessment 29
Chapter One Reading & References 31

CHAPTER TWO: LEARNING TO LEARN 32
Midwifery Education: A Balance of Science and Art 33
Pedagogy vs. Andragogy: Adaptations for Adult Learners 35
The Spiral Method of Learning 36
Asynchronous and Competency-Based Learning 39
Cognitive Domain: Understanding the Science of Clinical Midwifery Practice 39
Affective Domain: Building Emotional Intelligence 40
Psychomotor Domain: Clinical Competency and Technical Skills Development 40
Practical Application of Study Skills 42
The 5-P Reading System and SQ4R Method for Active Reading and Comprehension 44
Integrating Didactic Material with Clinical Experience 45
Tips for Studying Midwifery-Specific Materials 46
Using Grading Rubrics as a Learning Tool 47
Identifying and Mitigating Distractions 48
Integrating Clinical Placements into the Study Process 48
Integrating the Eisenhower Matrix into Task Management 54
Tips for Integrating Educational Tools 58
The Role of Self-Assessment in Mastering Content 58
Strategies for Preparing for Exams and Certifications 59
A Holistic Approach to Learning... 59
Chapter Two Self-Assessment 62
Chapter Two Reading & References 64

CHAPTER THREE TERMINOLOGY FOR MIDWIVES 66
Common Root Words in Medical Terminology 68
Common Prefixes in Medical Terminology 69
Common Suffixes in Medical Terminology 70
Common General Abbreviations 71
Antepartum (AP)–Prenatal Abbreviations.. 72
Intrapartum (IP)–Labor & Birth Abbreviations 72
Postpartum (PP) – After Birth Abbreviations 73
Newborn (NB) Abbreviations 73
Definitions of Pregnancy 74
Gestational Age Terms.. 74
The Use of Mnemonics in Midwifery Practice 76
Anatomical Directions 77
Chapter Three Self-Assessment 83
Chapter Three Reading & References 85

CHAPTER FOUR REPRODUCTIVE ANATOMY & PHYSIOLOGY 86
Bony Pelvis 87
Uterus 95
Cervix: Structure and Function 96
Vagina 97
Vulva 98
The Clitoris 99
Muscles of the Perineum 101
The Ovaries 105
Ovarian and Related Hormones 106
Hormonal Regulation of the Menstrual and Ovulation Cycle 108
Ovulation 112
The Male Reproductive System 114
Chapter Four Self-Assessment 118
Chapter Four Reading & References 120

CHAPTER FIVE BIOLOGY FOR MIDWIVES 122
Foundations of Biology for Student Midwives 123
Cellular Transport and Energy 124
Organelle 125
Stem Cells in Early Development 130
The Human Microbiome 131
Genetics for Midwives 133
Chapter Five Self-Assessment 139
Chapter Five Reading & References 141

CHAPTER SIX HOW LIFE BEGINS 142
How Life Begins 143
Conception: The Beginning of Pregnancy 143
The Process of Early Development 146
Early Placental Development 151
Functions of Amniotic Fluid 152
Umbilical Cord Circulation 153
Transition at Birth 155
Embryonic Period (Weeks 2 to 8) 156
The Fetal Period (Week 9 to Birth) 157
Third Trimester 160
Fetal Readiness for Labor 160
Post-Term 160
Teratogens and Critical Windows of Susceptibility 162
Sensory Development 163
Fetal Awareness and Learning 163
Chapter Six Self-Assessment 165
Chapter Six Reading & References 167

CHAPTER SEVEN: PHYSIOLOGY OF PREGNANCY 168
Physiology of Normal Pregnancy 169
The Midwife's Role in Normal Pregnancy 169
Holistic Midwifery Care 169
Length of Gestation and Estimated Due Date (EDD) 171
Signs of Pregnancy 173
Changes in System Physiology During Pregnancy 175
Weight Gain During Pregnancy 193
Common Discomforts of Pregnancy 195
Pregnancy Emotional Journey and Psychosocial Adaptation 201
Sexuality During Pregnancy 203
Chapter Seven: Self-Assessment 205
Chapter Seven Reading & References 208

CHAPTER EIGHT: HEALTH PROMOTION FOR MIDWIVES 209
- Introduction to Health Promotion in Pregnancy 210
- The Midwife's Role 210
- Stress Management 211
- Self-Esteem and Body Image 212
- Self-Care Behaviors 212
- Healthy Relationships and Social Support 212
- Intimate Partner Violence Screening 213
- Lifestyle Safety Considerations 213
- Environmental Exposures in Pregnancy 214
- Harm Reduction: Tobacco, Alcohol, Cannabis, and Substance Use 215
- Nutrition in Pregnancy 217
- Herbs in Pregnancy 231
- Herbs for Threatened Miscarriage 236
- Herbs as Uterine Stimulants 236
- Herbs During Active Labor 236
- Herbs for Postpartum 237
- Herbs for Lacation: 238
- Herbs for Infants 239
- Herbs to Avoid 241
- Principles of Herbal Midwifery Practice 244
- Chapter Eight Self-Assessment 247
- Chapter Eight: Reading & References 250

CHAPTER NINE INFECTION, IMMUNITY, & MIDWIFERY PRACTICE 251
- Pregnancy, Immunity & Infection Prevention 252
- The Maternal Immune System in Pregnancy 253
- Blood Types 254
- The Rh Factor 254
- Common Infections in Pregnancy 257
- Practical Tips for Supporting the Microbiome 260
- How Infection Spreads 263
- Standard Precautions 263
- 10 Steps for Proper Handwashing 265
- Glove Use and Safety 266
- Home Birth Infection Control 267
- Instrument Cleaning, Disinfection, and Sterilization 268
- What Needs Disinfection and What Needs Sterilization 268
- Low-Resource Sterilization 271
- Chapter Nine: Self-Assessment 272
- Chapter Nine Reading & References 275

CHAPTER TEN PRENATAL CARE 276
- The Five Questions of History Taking 278
- Risk and Responsibility in Out-of-Hospital Birth 282
- Vital Signs and Measurements 286
- Prenatal Laboratory Testing 289
- Informed Consent and Client Communication 289
- Public Health Reporting and Mandatory Action Reports (MARs) 289
- Noninvasive Prenatal Testing (NIPT) 291
- Ultrasound in Prenatal Care 292
- Physical Exam 294
- Pelvimetry 297
- Prenatal Skills and Fetal Assessment 298
- Subsequent Prenatal Visits 304
- Charting and Documentation 306
- Chapter Ten: Self-Assessment 312
- Chapter Ten Reading & References 315

CHAPTER ELEVEN LABOR & BIRTH ... 316
Mechanics of Normal Labor ... 317
The Passenger ... 318
The Passage ... 323
The Powers ... 326
The Psyche ... 329
Stages of Labor ... 332
Before Labor Begins ... 332
Prodromal Labor ... 333
When to Consider Induction ... 334
The Uterus and Cervix During Labor ... 336
Formation amd Rupture of the Membranes of Waters ... 338
Maternal Response to Labor ... 339
The Midwife's Role in Labor and Delivery ... 342
The Partner in Labor and Birth ... 342
The Power of Natural Birth ... 342
Latent Phase ... 343
Active Phase ... 343
Monitering Fetal Well-Being ... 346
Transition ... 348
Clinical Assessment in Second Stage ... 349
Communication and Emotional Grounding ... 350
Birth Positions ... 350
Preventing Perineal Trauma ... 351
Normal Vaginal Birth: Step-by-Step ... 352
Immediate Newborn Care ... 353
Umbilical Cord Clamping ... 353
Benefits of Skin-to-Skin Contact ... 353
Third Stage Management ... 354
Chapter Eleven Self-Assessment ... 355
Chapter Eleven Reading & References ... 358

CHAPTER TWELVE PLACENTA & POSTPARTUM ... 359
Placental Variations ... 361
Signs of Placental Separation ... 362
Mechanisms of Placental Delivery ... 363
Cord Blood Collection and Banking: ... 364
Blood Loss Assessment) ... 365
Maternal Comfort and the Golden Hour ... 365
Placenta ... 366
Umbilical Cord ... 366
Cultural and Traditional Practices ... 367
Postpartum Physiology ... 368
Uterine and Reproductive Recovery ... 370
Postpartum Discomforts and Comfort Measures ... 372
Genital and Perineal Assessment and Care ... 374
Postpartum Emotional Health and Adjustment ... 376
Risk Factors for Postpartum Emotional Distress ... 377
Perinatal Mood and Anxiety Disorders (PMADs) ... 377
Core Elements of Postpartum Preparation ... 380
Feeding and Infant Care ... 381
Emotional and Mental Well-Being ... 381
Postpartum Assessment ... 382
The 24-hour Visit ... 383
The Three-day Visit ... 383
The Two-week Visit ... 383
The Six-week Postpartum Exam ... 384
Chapter Twelve Self-Assessment ... 386
Chapter Twelve Recommended Reading & References ... 389

CHAPTER THIRTEEN: MIDWIFERY CARE OF THE NEWBORN 390
Midwifery Care of the Newborn 391
Antenatal Risk Factors 392
Intrapartum Risk Factors 392
Observation and Preparedness 392
Documentation and Communication 392
Airway and Ventilation 393
Immediate Care of the Newborn 394
The Newborn's First Breath 395
Cord Care After Birth 396
APGAR Scoring System 397
Monitoring Temperature 399
The Newborn's Experience of Birth and the Golden Hour 400
The Newborn Examination 402
Newborn Screenings and Procedures 410
Male Circumcision 413
Female Circumcision (Female Genital Mutilation) 413
Weight and Feeding 414
Jaundice 416
Referral and Collaborative Care 416
Parent Education and Discharge Observation 417
Transition of Care 420
Chapter Thirteen: Self-Assessment 422
Chapter Thirteen: Recommended Reading & References 425

CHAPTER FOURTEEN: BREASTFEEDING PHYSIOLOGY & PRACTICE 426
Midwifery Support of Breastfeeding 427
Anatomy and Physiology of Lactation 428
Integration 433
Positioning for Comfort and Effectiveness 433
Breastfeeding Challenges and Midwifery Management 435
Pumping Methods 439
Milk Collection and Storage 440
Maintaining Supply and Returning to Work 440
Understanding Weaning 441
Maternal Health and Recovery 442
Medications and Breastfeeding 442
Breastfeeding After Complicated Births 443
Special Feeding Situations 443
Supporting Emotional Health 443
Holistic Midwifery Perspective 443
Cultural Beliefs and Practices 444
Global Perspectives and Lactation Equity 444
Inclusive Language and Family Structures 444
Integrating Cultural Competence into Practice 445
Chapter Fourteen Self-Assessment 447
Chapter Fourteen: Recommended Reading & References 450

ANSWER KEY 451
About Zaníyan Center 457

Birthsong

Round bellied woman
beautiful, radiant
Inner light shining
with the power
Of creation
Laboring, with the new life emerging
focusing, breathing and centering.
Deep strength within,
showing without
Dancing the dance,
singing the
Song of Birth

D.S. 1984

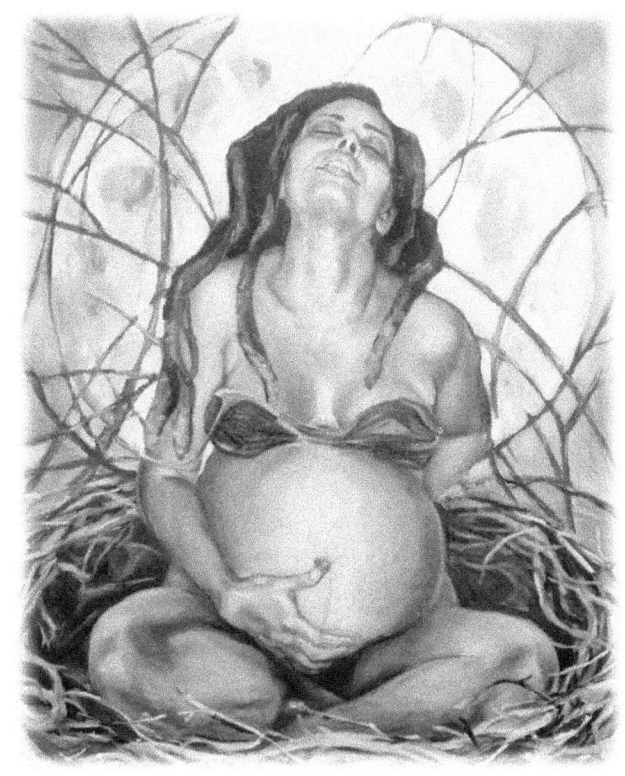

Chapter One
Midwifery Yesterday & Today

Objectives
After completing this chapter, the student should be able to:
1. **Describe** the core philosophy of midwifery as a holistic, person-centered model of care.
2. **Compare** the Midwifery Model of Care with the Medical Model of Care, including philosophy, interventions, outcomes, and integration.
3. **Explain** how midwives support autonomy, informed decision-making, and culturally competent care.
4. **Identify** how midwives have attended births across cultures and historical periods.
5. **Explain** how midwifery was shaped by cultural, political, and religious forces throughout history.
6. **Discuss** the persecution of midwives during witch trials and its impact on the profession.
7. **Describe** the apprenticeship model and its role in traditional midwifery education.
8. **Match** influential historical midwives and physicians with their contributions to childbirth and midwifery education.
9. **Summarize** the contributions of key figures such as Louise Bourgeois Boursier, Madame du Coudray, Catharina Schrader, Ina May Gaskin, and Mary Breckenridge.
10. **Trace** the development and decline of midwifery in the US during the 19th and 20th centuries.
11. **Describe** the impact of systemic racism, professional regulation, and medicalization on midwifery access and outcomes.
12. **Recognize** the roles of "granny midwives" and their importance in Black and rural communities.
13. **Define** the roles and scopes of CPMs, CNMs, CMs, LMs, and DEMs.
14. **Explain** the functions of professional organizations: NARM, NACPM, MEAC, ICM, and others.
15. **Understand** the impact of regulation, credentialing, and licensure on access to midwifery care.
16. **Identify** the benefits and challenges of various midwifery pathways (e.g., MEAC, PEP, community colleges, hybrid programs).
17. **Explain** how midwifery addresses racial disparities in maternal health outcomes.
18. **Describe** the midwife's role in public health, advocacy, and community care.
19. **Evaluate** how regulation and integration into healthcare systems affect safety and access to midwifery care.
20. **Summarize** the International Confederation of Midwives (ICM) core competencies and how they align with the NACPM Job Analysis.
21. **Define** the Midwifery Student Bill of Rights and its importance for equitable and supportive education.
22. **Recognize** the importance of lifelong learning, cultural humility, and client advocacy in modern midwifery.

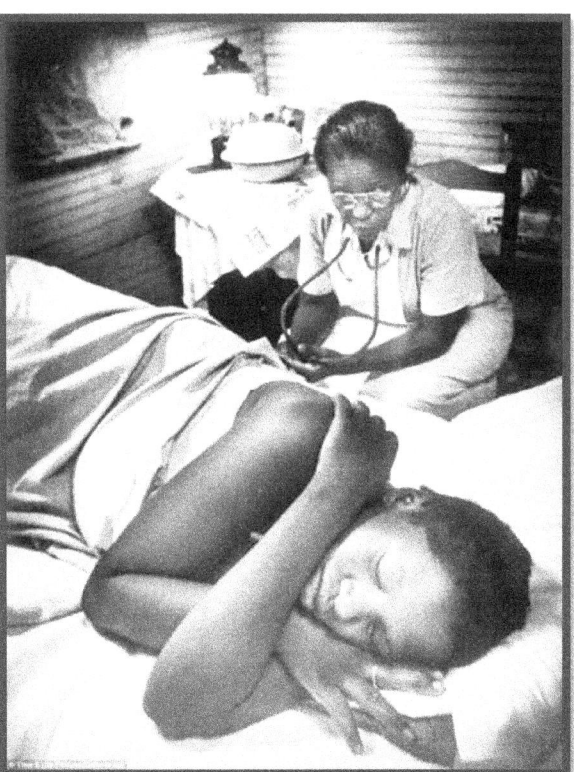

Maude Callen, public health nurse and midwife, attending a woman in labor in 1951.

Why Midwifery?

Midwifery is both an art and a science, deeply rooted in the philosophy that childbirth is a natural, physiological process and a profound life event. This philosophy respects the autonomy, cultural context, and lived experiences of birthing individuals, viewing them as active participants in their care. Midwifery has evolved from an apprenticeship model outside of the hospital into a critical component of modern health care, integrating evidence-based practices into collaborative, interdisciplinary care models. This integration reflects a growing recognition of midwifery as a bridge between holistic traditions and advanced medical science. Regardless of practice setting, all midwives share a common goal: to listen, support, and care for the people they serve.

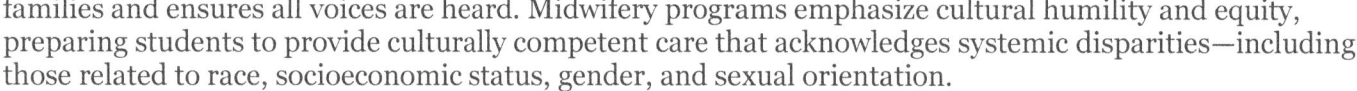

Central to midwifery is the belief that birthing individuals are the primary decision-makers in their care. Midwives act as advocates and educators, fostering informed choices and tailoring care to meet each person's unique needs. This inclusive, personalized approach empowers families and ensures all voices are heard. Midwifery programs emphasize cultural humility and equity, preparing students to provide culturally competent care that acknowledges systemic disparities—including those related to race, socioeconomic status, gender, and sexual orientation.

As health care systems respond to the complexities of modern maternal care, midwives have become vital contributors across a range of environments—including hospitals, birth centers, and home births. They collaborate with obstetricians, nurses, mental health professionals, and others, contributing their unique expertise to interdisciplinary teams. This integration ensures care is comprehensive and person-centered, balancing medical innovation with the wisdom of physiological birth.

The science of midwifery complements its philosophical roots through clinical expertise and evidence-based practice. Midwives learn advanced techniques, including fetal monitoring, pharmacology, and emergency response, while also prioritizing support for natural birth. This blend of clinical skill and relational care allows midwives to manage complications effectively while preserving dignity and autonomy.

Midwives are also key players in addressing public health challenges such as maternal mortality, perinatal mental health, and disparities in care for underserved populations. Their ability to build trust, provide continuity, and offer compassionate support positions them at the forefront of efforts to improve maternal health outcomes. Learners gain both technical and interpersonal skills; learning to be inclusive, empathetic, and adaptable. This ensures midwifery continues to honor its roots while embracing modern scientific advancements, thus creating a future where every birth is supported with dignity, respect, and excellence. The role of midwives has expanded significantly in recent years as health care systems adapt to meet the diverse needs of childbearing families. Midwives are no longer confined to traditional home births or community settings; they are now integral players in hospitals, birth centers, and even digital spaces through telehealth services. This evolution reflects a growing recognition of the midwife's unique ability to provide comprehensive, personalized care that bridges the gap between traditional and medicalized childbirth approaches.

Hospitals increasingly recognize midwives as essential members of interdisciplinary health care teams. They work collaboratively with obstetricians, nurses, and pediatricians to ensure safe and positive birth experiences, often leading efforts to reduce cesarean section rates and promote physiological births. This collaboration not only enhances outcomes but also fosters an environment of mutual respect and shared expertise.

Birth centers have also become a focal point for midwifery care, offering an alternative to hospital or home birth. These centers combine the comfort and personalization of home-like settings with access to essential medical resources, empowering midwives to provide family-centered care in a supportive environment. The rise in the popularity of birth centers underscores the demand for midwife-led care models that emphasize safety, autonomy, and individualized attention.

Telehealth has further expanded the midwife's reach, enabling them to provide care across geographic and logistical barriers. Virtual consultations for prenatal education, postpartum support, and even lactation counseling have become standard offerings in many practices. This digital transformation ensures continuity of care and expands access to midwifery services for individuals in underserved areas.

The evolving role of midwives reflects a broader societal shift toward valuing compassionate, evidence-based, and inclusive care. By integrating midwifery's historical roots with modern practices, midwives continue to be pivotal in shaping the future of maternal and neonatal health care. Understanding why midwifery holds such importance today requires looking back at its origins and the role midwives have played throughout history.

Exercise 1.1: Why Midwifery?

Fill out

1. Why do you want to be a midwife?

2. What life experiences do you have that you feel will be assets to you in midwifery?

3. Explain how a specific person, philosophy, or author has influenced your ideas in midwifery.

4. What are the qualities you possess that will be assets to you as a midwife?

MIDWIFERY MODEL OF CARE VS. MEDICAL MODEL OF CARE

Childbirth care in the United States typically follows two primary approaches: the midwifery model and the medical model. While both aim to ensure the health of birthing individuals and their babies, they differ in philosophy, focus, and method.

The **midwifery model** treats pregnancy and birth as natural processes, emphasizing individualized, holistic care with minimal intervention. Midwives build trust-based relationships and support birth in homes, birth centers, and hospitals.

The **medical model** views childbirth as potentially risky, relying on protocols, diagnostics, and technology to manage complications. Care is physician-led and hospital-based, ideal for high-risk pregnancies.

Each model plays a vital role. Midwifery suits low-risk pregnancies seeking personalized care, while medical care is essential for complex needs. Increasingly, collaborative models blend the strengths of both.

Comparison Chart: Midwifery Model vs. Medical Model of Care		
Aspect	Midwifery Model of Care	Medical Model of Care
Philosophy	- Views pregnancy and childbirth as normal physiological processes. - Emphasizes holistic, individualized care.	- Views pregnancy and childbirth as potentially risky medical events. - Emphasizes risk management and technological solutions.
Core Principles	– Empowerment and informed decision-making. – Continuity of care and trust-based relationships. – Minimally invasive practices.	– Risk mitigation through diagnostics and interventions. – Standardized protocols led by physicians. – Emphasis on physician authority in clinical decision-making.
Focus of Care	– Physiological birth with minimal intervention. – Support for physical, emotional, and cultural needs. – Care provided in homes, birth centers, and hospitals.	– Focus on potential pathology and continuous monitoring. – Technology-driven safety measures. – Primarily hospital-based care.
Interventions	– Low rates of interventions (e.g., cesareans, inductions). – Natural pain relief options – Encourages delayed cord clamping and immediate skin-to-skin contact.	– Higher rates of intervention for proactive risk management. – Pharmacological pain relief (e.g., epidurals). – Protocol-driven practices, often emphasizing efficiency.
Patient Autonomy	– Prioritizes informed consent and shared decision-making. – Builds personalized care plans and long-term relationships.	– Often emphasizes institutional protocol over individual preference. – Care may feel more transactional due to time and system constraints.
Outcomes	– Lower cesarean rates and faster postpartum recovery. – Higher rates of breastfeeding initiation and satisfaction.	– Higher intervention rates; essential for managing complications. – Critical for high-risk pregnancies requiring advanced care.
Best For	– Low-risk pregnancies seeking non-interventive, personalized care.	– High-risk pregnancies or individuals with complex medical needs.
Integration Potential	– Strengthens team-based care when integrated with medical systems.	– Provides vital emergency, surgical, and diagnostic resources.

Exercise 1.2: Comparing Models of Childbirth Care

Write your responses in the space provided.

Aspect	Guiding Question	Response
1. Philosophy	How does each model view pregnancy and childbirth?	
2. Core Principles	What principles guide decision-making and care in each model?	
3. Focus of Care	What are the priorities in each model during prenatal care and labor?	
4. Interventions	How are pain and complications typically managed?	
5. Patient Autonomy	How involved is the birthing person in their care decisions?	
6. Outcomes	What outcomes are typically associated with each model?	
7. Best For	What types of pregnancies or individuals are best served by each model?	
8. Integration Potential	How can the two models complement each other in collaborative care?	

The History and Legacy of Midwifery

The word "midwife" translates to "with woman," encapsulating the essence of midwifery as a practice rooted in companionship and support during childbirth. Midwifery evolved from the simple yet profound act of women attending to one another during birth. Experienced women, often those who had borne many children or witnessed many births, became trusted figures within their communities. These "wise women" were sought after for their knowledge and guidance, serving as pillars of support and wisdom. Around the world, almost every society includes midwifery in its cultural practices.

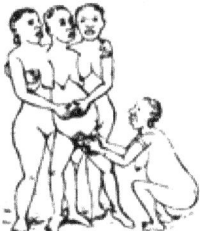 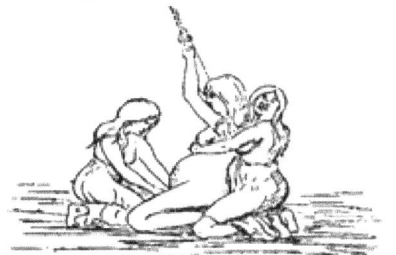

While birth is a natural process, it has not always been without peril. Historically, high rates of infant and maternal mortality were an unfortunate reality. The principle of "survival of the fittest" shaped early human populations. For instance, women with small pelvises or those prone to severe obstetric complications rarely survived childbirth, nor did their babies. Likewise, premature and fragile newborns frequently perished. It was within this challenging context that midwives emerged as pivotal figures, working tirelessly to improve survival rates and alter the course of what was once inevitable. Their skills and determination have always sought to save lives, shifting the odds in favor of both mothers and babies.

Historical records show the central role of midwives across cultures. Egyptian hieroglyphics, early Chinese and Hindu texts, and biblical accounts all highlight the significance of midwifery. **Peseshet**, an ancient Egyptian physician is often cited as was known as the *Overseer of Female Physicians*. The Book of Exodus (Exodus 1:15–21) recounts the story of two Hebrew midwives, **Shiphrah** and **Puah**, who defied the Pharaoh's order to kill all male Hebrew infants. In the first recorded act of civil disobedience, the midwives protected the newborns, cleverly explaining that the Hebrew women birthed their children too quickly for them to arrive and to kill them.

In early societies, midwives were deeply respected and revered. Birth was considered a sacred mystery, and people honored women for their unique ability to bring forth life. This reverence is visible in ancient art and mythology, where goddesses often appeared pregnant or giving birth. Midwifery has thus always stood at the intersection of the practical and the spiritual, a testament to the profound power and resilience of women.

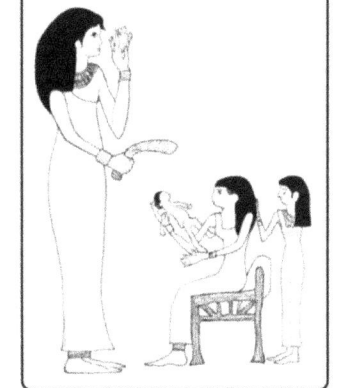
Peseshet (c. 2400 BCE)

As civilizations advanced, midwifery grew into a respected and esteemed profession. Hippocrates wrote male physicians were summoned only for difficult births, while midwives firmly handled normal labor care and management. Socrates' mother practiced as a midwife, and Aristotle praised the wisdom and intelligence of Greek midwives, highlighting their vital role in society.

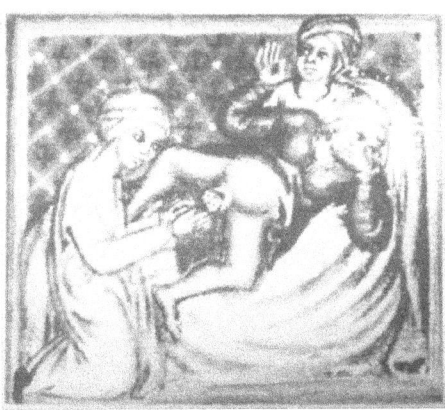
Twelfth Century tapestry showing midwives attending a birth.

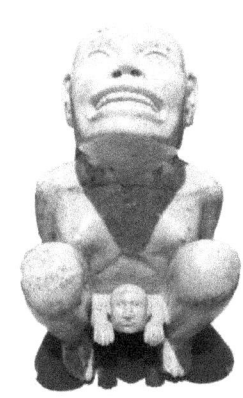
The Aztec Goddess of Childbirth Tlazolteotl

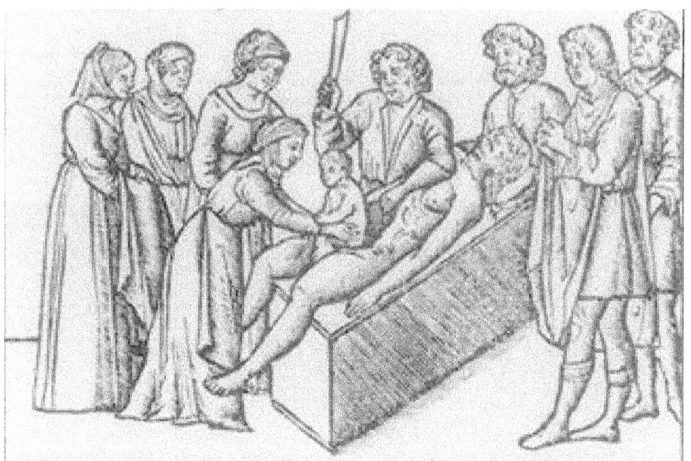

From Suetonius' Lives of the Twelve Caesars, 1506 woodcut. Purportedly the birth of Julius Caesar. A live infant being surgically removed from a dead woman.

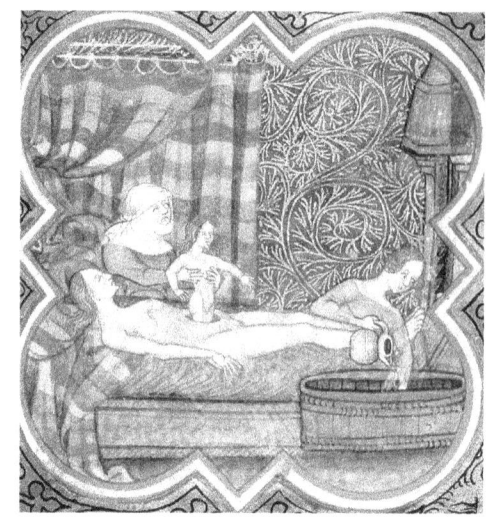

A woman surgeon performs a Cesarean in this medieval tapestry.

Before the 1600s, midwives were central figures in their communities, serving not only as birth attendants but also as primary health care providers. Midwives, who possessed extensive knowledge of herbs and natural remedies, oversaw nearly all deliveries. This expertise allowed them to support not only childbirth but also a wide range of health needs, often acting as the sole health care providers in their villages.

Midwives were trusted for their ability to aid the sick and provide care during times of illness, offering remedies, guidance, and emotional support to individuals and families alike. Their role extended far beyond childbirth; they were present at life's end and its beginning. Midwives frequently attended the dying, providing comfort to both the individual and their family during the final stages of life. They were also responsible for the ritualized care of the deceased, often referred to as "laying out" the dead, which involved preparing the body for burial in accordance with cultural or religious practices.

Birth oThis multifaceted role made midwives indispensable to their communities. They bridged the gap between health, healing, and spirituality, serving as caregivers who accompanied individuals and families through all of life's major transitions—birth, illness, and death. Their deep connection to the cycles of life and their reliance on natural, holistic practices cemented their position as vital contributors to the health and well-being of society during this period.

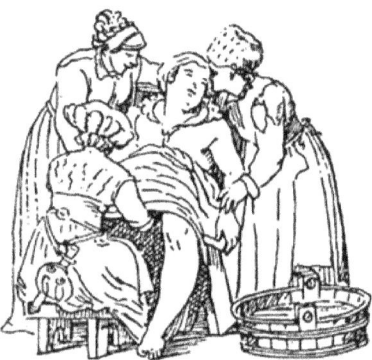

During the Middle Ages, midwives often found themselves at the center of persecution because of their deep knowledge of healing and their role in the enigmatic process of childbirth. Fear and superstition held great sway, and the mystery surrounding birth, combined with the midwife's expertise in herbs and natural remedies, made them frequent targets of accusations of witchcraft. The Inquisition, which wielded immense political and religious power, led widespread efforts to prosecute midwives and other perceived heretics.

Midwives, by nature and necessity, were often strong-minded, independent women. They were respected within their communities for their skills and their essential contributions to health care, yet their autonomy and influence also made them threatening to the patriarchal structures of the time. Those who dared to speak out against injustices perpetrated by the ruling class or the church risked being branded as witches. Midwives who used herbs for birth control or abortions were especially vulnerable, because the church considered these practices heretical and unnatural.

The general hysteria of the period conflated any deviation from strict religious orthodoxy with being in league with the devil. The term "Good Christian" became a flexible label used to silence dissenters and marginalize anyone who posed a challenge to established authority. For midwives, who often operated outside the male-dominated medical field and within spaces of personal autonomy and intimacy, this paranoia was especially dangerous.

Accusations of witchcraft had devastating consequences. Thousands of midwives were discredited and publicly disgraced, stripped of their standing and livelihoods. Many were subjected to brutal torture designed to extract confessions. Those found guilty—on little more than suspicion or hearsay—faced horrifying punishments, including being burned at the stake, hanged, or drowned. Entire communities lost skilled midwives to these purges, leaving vulnerable populations without their only access to health care.

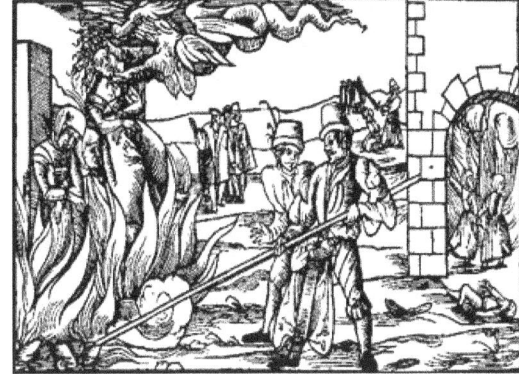
Witch burning in the Middle Ages

This dark period in history not only marked a tragedy for countless midwives but also for the practice of midwifery itself. The persecution of these women silenced voices of wisdom and care and created a lingering shadow over the role of midwives in society. Despite this, midwifery survived, a testament to the resilience of those who continued to dedicate their lives to supporting birthing individuals and their communities. The story of this persecution is a reminder of the strength and courage midwives have historically demonstrated in the face of immense adversity.

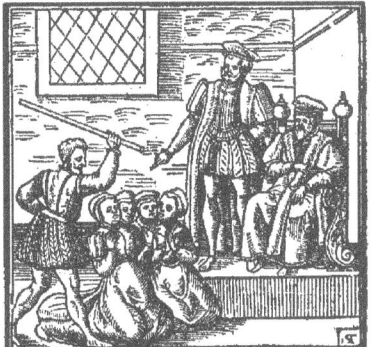
1591 Suspected witches from North Berwick are beaten as they appear before two Scottish magistrates.

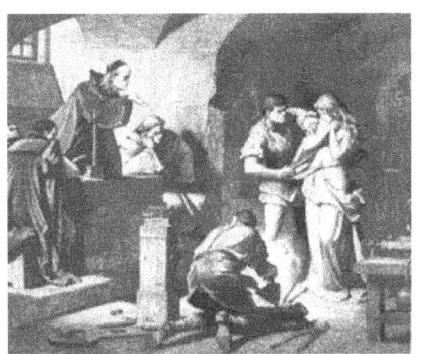
Midwives were put on trial for witchcraft for their knowledge of herbs and healing

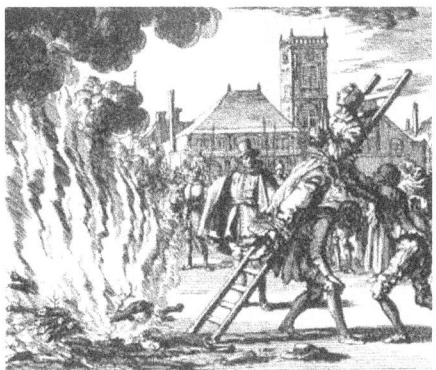
Witch burning in Amsterdam, 1571

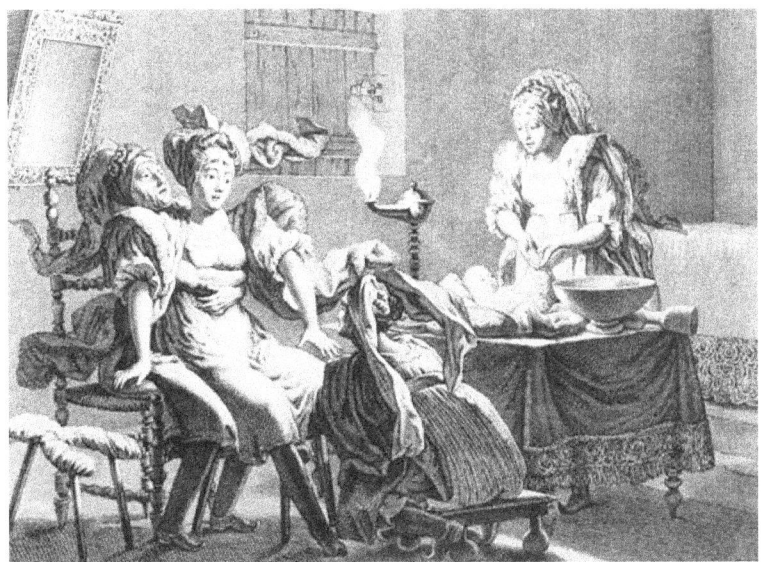
1801 painting shows three midwives supporting a new mother.

Until the 17th century, midwives played a central role in childbirth, delivering the vast majority of babies. Male physicians were called upon only in rare, life-threatening situations. However, because women, especially those from lower socioeconomic backgrounds, had limited access to formal education, they were excluded from the emerging scientific knowledge of obstetrics and anatomy. Despite this, midwives continued to master their craft through the traditional apprenticeship model, where experienced midwives passed their knowledge, skills, and wisdom on to younger generations. For centuries, midwifery was one of the few medical professions available to women, and many midwives made groundbreaking contributions to the field.

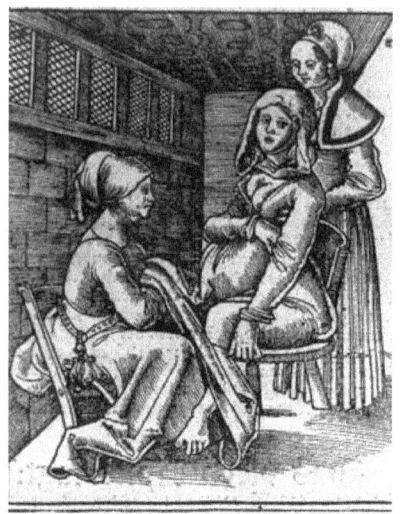
From one of the first textbooks for midwives, published in Germany in 1513, *The Pregnant Woman's and Midwife's Rosegarden* by Eucharius Roslin

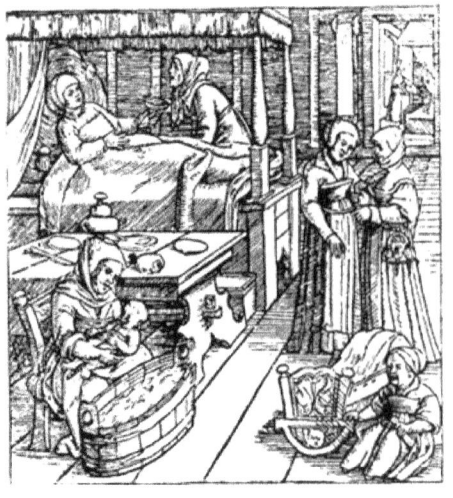
Three midwives assist a woman in labor, from the textbook *The Birth of Mankind* by Jakob Rueff, 1544

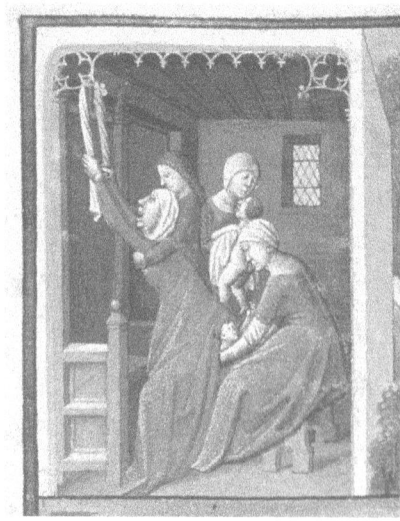
Birth of Esau and Jacob 1475-1480

THE RISE OF FORMAL MIDWIFERY EDUCATION

Midwifery education has been documented in the earliest writings found in parts of Egypt, Greece and Sumeria. In the early modern era, in 1609, Louise Bourgeois Boursier published the first of three successive volumes on obstetrics. These publications include observation-based, innovative obstetrical protocols to manage difficult births as well as advice for pregnant and postpartum mothers and newborns. Bourgeois also offered recipes for various kinds of medications that would have been easy for a woman to make herself. The three volumes include over four dozen detailed case histories that made a substantial contribution to the emerging empiricism of seventeenth-century European science and medicine.

Louise Bourgeois Boursier (1563-1636)

Boursier served as the Royal Court's midwife for 27 years, attending the births of King Henry IV's children, including the future Louis XIII. She is credited with promoting the use of the podalic version, a procedure that significantly advanced the safety of childbirth by aiding in difficult deliveries.

Another prominent French midwife, Madame Le Boursier du Coudray, was instrumental in advancing midwifery education. With the approval of Louis XV, she traveled throughout the provinces of France, providing free instruction to midwives. She also invented a life-size mannequin, enabling her to demonstrate fetal positioning and delivery techniques effectively. Her innovation became a key tool for midwifery education, bridging the gap between theory and practice.

Angélique Marguerite Le Boursier du Coudray (1712 –1794)

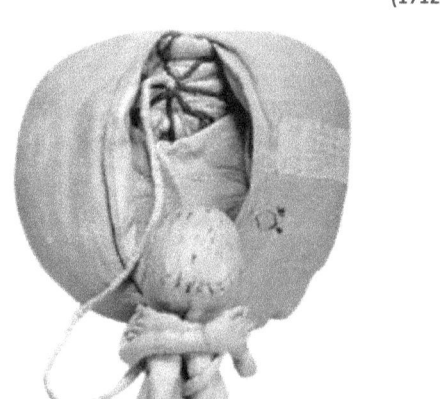
Du Coudray invented obstetrical mannequins in 1760

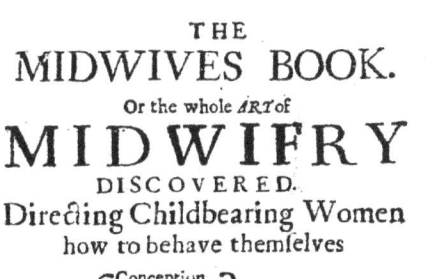

In England, **Jane Sharp** became the first midwife to publish a comprehensive book on midwifery, The Midwives Book or the Whole Art of Midwifery Discovered, in 1671. Her work aimed to empower midwives with knowledge, offering a detailed guide to the art and science of childbirth.

In the late 16th and early 17th-century England, the **Chamberlen** family significantly impacted the field of obstetrics. Peter Chamberlen, the elder, invented the obstetric forceps, a groundbreaking tool that allowed women with contracted pelvises to give birth vaginally without resorting to cesarean sections, which were almost always fatal at the time. Rather than sharing this innovation widely, the Chamberlen family guarded the forceps as a closely held secret, using them to advance their professional status and personal gain. The forceps were hidden away and only discovered years later in the floor of a closet after the death of a Chamberlen descendant. While lifesaving in some cases, the introduction of such instruments contributed to the growing influence of male physicians in childbirth.

By the 17th century, obstetrics had become recognized as a specialized branch of medicine. Although midwives continued to attend most births for lower-income families, the wealthier classes increasingly sought "accoucheurs," the new male obstetricians. These early practitioners often lacked formal training, with many entering the field from unrelated professions, such as barbers or butchers, to supplement their income. The rising presence of male physicians in childbirth marked a shift in societal perceptions of birth and care, paving the way for the medicalization of childbirth while marginalizing the contributions of midwives.

In 1765, Dr. William Shippen Jr. opened the first formal midwifery school in Philadelphia, was limited to men because of prevalent illiteracy and financial barriers preventing women from receiving formal education. This era reflects both the resilience of midwives and the challenges they faced as their profession navigated the pressures of emerging medical science and shifting social dynamics.

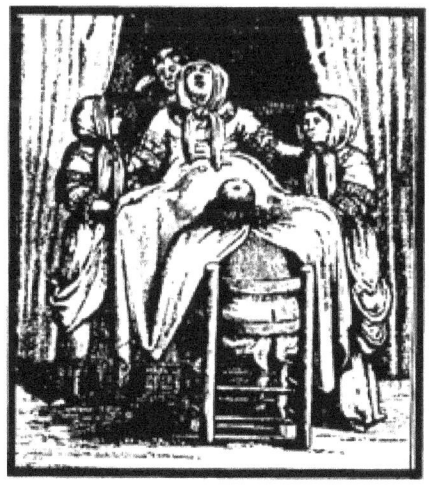
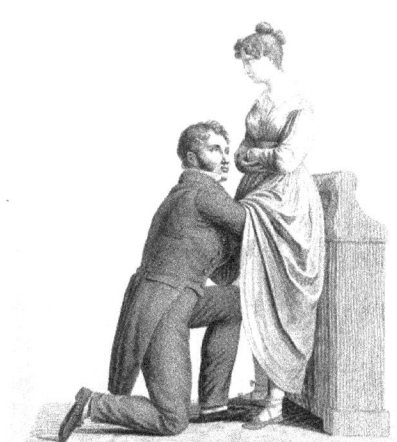

As men entered obstetrics, the modesty mores were extreme, which could impact negatively care.

Throughout history, midwives have been vital figures in childbirth and community health, adapting their practices and philosophies to changing cultural and medical landscapes. Women, especially in lower socioeconomic classes, lacked access to formal education, leaving midwives to learn their craft through the apprenticeship model, where knowledge, skills, and wisdom were passed from experienced midwives to the next generation. Despite these limitations, midwives made significant contributions to medicine and maternal care.

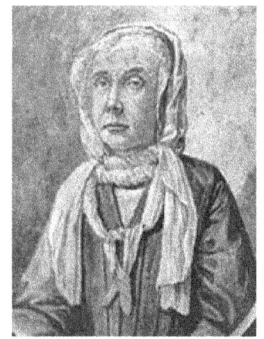

Catharina Geertruida Schrader
(1656–1746)

Catharina Schader was a Dutch midwife who, when she retired in 1745, had delivered over 3000 babies. She left a diary detailing her experiences which provides us an insightful and rare look at the midwifery techniques used during that time. She delivered her last baby at age 88.

During the seventeenth century, midwifery began to be recognized as a profession, and midwifery schools were established in Europe. In the "New World", the colonists continued using professional midwives. **Brigit Lee Fuller** was the midwife who attended three births on the Mayflower, and she continued to have a well-respected practice in colonial America. **Martha Ballard** (1785-1812) was a colonial midwife whose diary detailed her everyday activities delivering babies and caring for the sick. In 1989, historian Laurel Thatcher Ulrich excerpted her diary entries into a book, *Diary of a Midwife*. It earned a Pulitzer Prize for the and became the subject of a PBS movie.

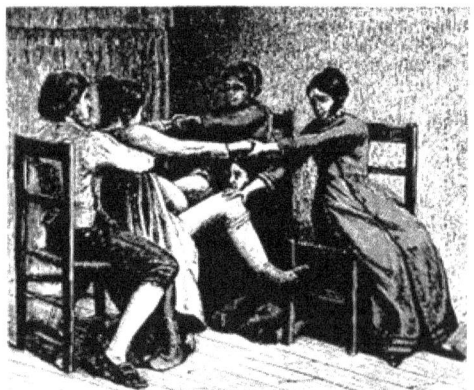

Birth in Colonial America

In 1765, Americas first midwifery school was opened in Philadelphia by Dr. William Shippen Jr. Most midwives still practiced at home and in rural areas, but some now began to work independently in maternity hospitals, calling upon obstetricians only in cases with serious complications.

Shifts in Childbirth Settings and Practices

The 17th and 18th centuries saw the emergence of "lying-in" hospitals for childbirth, which were initially fashionable among upper-class women seeking the care of male physicians. However, these hospitals often had poor sanitary conditions, leading to maternal mortality rates as high as 20%. Midwives, still attending the majority of births for lower-class women, consistently achieved lower mortality rates due to their non-invasive practices. The widespread issue of puerperal fever (childbed fever) plagued hospitals during this period, with little understanding of its cause.

Key discoveries eventually reshaped maternal care. In 1855, **Oliver Wendell Holmes** proposed that puerperal fever was contagious, suggesting that physicians themselves were spreading the disease. Though ridiculed, his ideas laid the groundwork for **Ignaz Semmelweis**'s groundbreaking work. In 1861, Semmelweis demonstrated the life-saving impact of handwashing with chloride of lime, reducing mortality rates from 12% to less than 3% in his Viennese hospital. Despite initial resistance, his findings, later supported by Pasteur and Lister, revolutionized hospital practices and introduced asepsis, leading to significant drops in maternal mortality.

Professionalization and Regulation of Midwifery

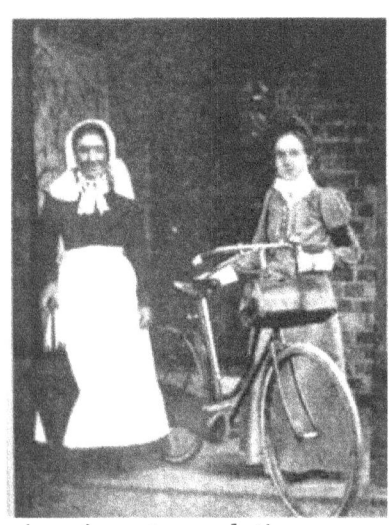

By the late 19th century, midwifery began to gain formal recognition in Europe. The 1902 Midwives' Act in England established licensing boards and professional standards for midwives. This marked a transition from traditional "handywomen," who provided a range of community services like laying out the dead, to formally trained midwives. However, tension arose between these traditional attendants and the emerging professional class, much like the modern-day divide between direct-entry midwives and Certified Nurse-Midwives.

In America, the rise of obstetrics during the early 20th century marginalized midwifery. Hospitals became more accessible to middle- and lower-class women, driven by a perception that doctors provided safer care. Midwifery schools were closed, and legislative restrictions severely limited midwives' practice. By 1935, only 10.7% of US births were attended by midwives, with 54% of those involving nonwhite populations. Despite these challenges, midwives remained essential caregivers in rural and underserved communities, particularly among Black and immigrant populations.

An English "handywoman" and a professional midwife

In 1925, the **Manhattan Midwifery School** opened in 1925 in New York City to educate graduate nurses in midwifery. This began the trend of the only formal education for midwives in the US being for nurses. Also in 1925, **Mary Breckenridge**, after researching different models, opened the Frontier Nursing Service in Hyden, Kentucky, a school for the training of nurse-midwives. Her clinic treated the poor in the hills of Appalachia, often traveling by horseback. After its service opened, the infant and maternal mortality rates dropped dramatically for the rural population it served. Praised by some for creating a pathway for midwifery education and certification, Breckenridge's beliefs reflected racist values and did not allow African American women to be educated as midwives. The formalization of education and certification ultimately delegitimized apprentice-trained midwives in every community.

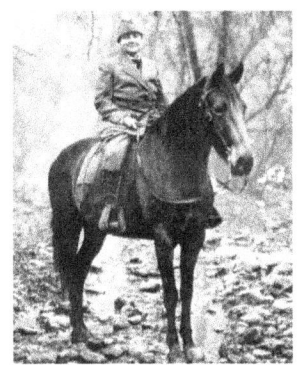

Mary Breckenridge
(1881-1965)

MIDWIFERY'S ROLE IN COMMUNITY HEALTH

In the rural South, "granny midwives" continued the tradition of apprenticeship-based training, often serving as the only health care providers for Black communities excluded from segregated hospitals. Health departments attempted to educate and support these midwives, but by the 1930s, medical lobbies had largely outlawed midwifery in most states. Exceptions existed in isolated areas where midwives were indispensable due to a lack of access to doctors or hospitals.

Onnie Lee Logan was an Alabama midwife and Civil rights activist, who relied on traditional knowledge and who trained lay midwives and served the needs of birthing women in an era when black women were not served equally in the era when hospitals emerged. In 1984 her autobiography *Motherwit: An Alabama Midwife's Story* was published, an important work in the history of Black Midwifery.

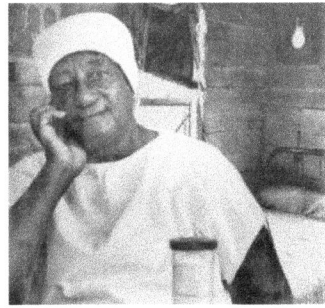

Onnie Lee Logan
(1910 – 1995)

Other Black "granny" midwives of note include **Mary Francis Coley**, a midwife in Georgia for over three decades, known for her advocacy for healthy babies and her role as a bridge between the health care system and her community. She starred in a documentary film, *All My Babies*, that followed her on her home visits, and two births she attended. This film became an important teaching tool for both midwives and medical students.

Margaret Charles Smith who attended nearly 3,000 births during her 30-year career in rural Alabama, with a remarkable record of no maternal deaths and very few infant deaths. She co-authored a book about her experiences, *"Listen to Me Good: The Life Story of an Alabama Midwife"*.

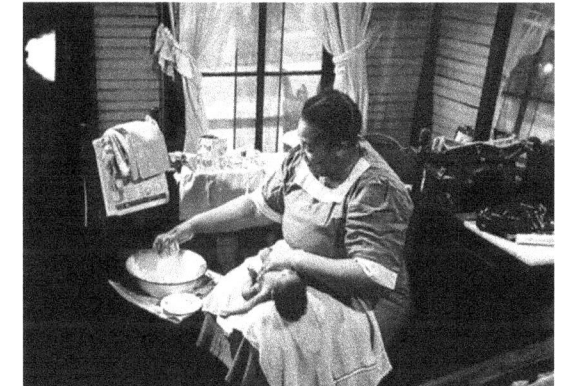

Mary Francis Hill Coley
(1900–66)

Gladys Milton, a midwife who practiced for 35 years in the tiny community of Flowersview, Florida. She delivered thousands of babies and was well respected in her community. Arsonists targeted her clinic and home, because she advocated for the legalization of midwifery. A book written about her life, *Why Not Me* by Wendy Bovard & Gladys Milton, describes her life and her struggles to continue to practice midwifery.

There were many other Granny midwives who preserved the art of midwifery through apprenticeships over many years, especially serving rural Black communities.

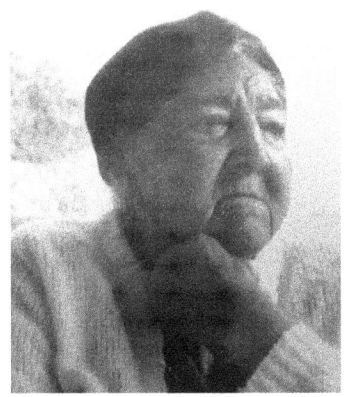

Margaret Charles Smith
(1901-2004)

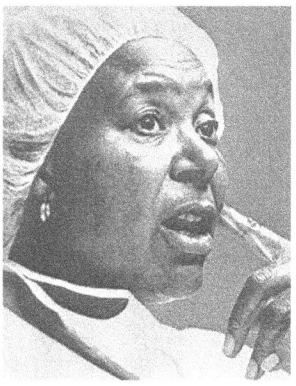

Gladys Nichols Milton
(1924 – 1999)

Path to Modern Midwifery in the United States

By the 1940's, fewer babies were born at home; independent midwives all but ceased to exist in the US, except in very rural areas, mainly in the South. People saw hospitals as the only safe place to give birth, and they considered midwives a relic of the past. The medical community condemned home birth, based on a few studies that showed that the practice resulted in high infant mortality rates. Omitted from these studies of mortality rates were the effects of poverty, poor nutrition, and harsh living conditions, as well as the fact that, with few midwifery training programs left, many of the granny midwives had little or no access to education, training, or equipment.

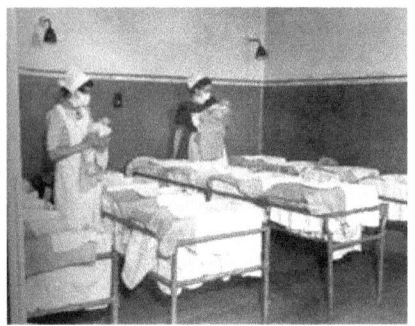

Infant Nursery in the 1940s, babies were routinely separated from their mothers

By the mid-20th century, the US medical system largely shifted childbirth into hospitals, often at the expense of personal care. Women were subjected to impersonal and sometimes harmful practices, including excessive use of forceps, episiotomies, and drugs that left them disconnected from the birthing process. This environment sparked a growing movement in the 1960s and 1970s to reclaim natural childbirth.

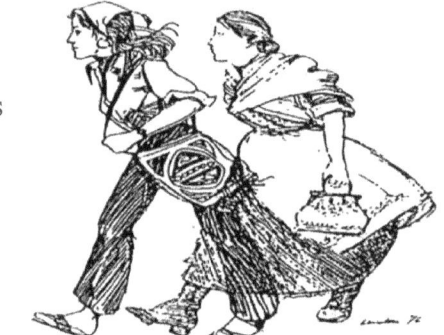

"Midwives Old & New" depicts a '70's era midwife going to a birth with her 19th century counterpart in her shadow.

The home birth movement emerged during this period, driven by families seeking alternatives to the highly medicalized model of care. Lay midwives, many of whom were self-taught, began attending home births. Books like **Ina May Gaskin's** *Spiritual Midwifery* inspired a resurgence of interest in midwifery and helped shape the modern home birth movement. Gaskin also contributed to clinical practice with the development of the *Gaskin Maneuver* for shoulder dystocia, marking the first obstetric technique named for a midwife. Considered the mother of modern midwifery in the US, Ina May Gaskin continues to be a leader in midwifery. *Immaculate Deception* by Suzanne Arms exposed some abuses in the childbearing system of the time. *The Birth Book* by Raven Lang was one of the first books that showed how a group of self-taught midwives delivered babies at home.

The **Midwives Alliance of North America (MANA)** was founded in 1982 to foster collaboration among midwives and to promote midwifery as a path to improving maternal and child health. Before it closed in 2023, MANA played a critical role in the professionalization of midwifery and in establishing a national credential. It laid the groundwork for the **North American Registry of Midwives (NARM)**, which now administers the competency-based **Certified Professional Midwife (CPM)** credential. The **Midwifery Education Accreditation Council (MEAC)** was launched in 1991 during a meeting of the National Coalition of Midwifery Educators. Recognized by the US Department of Education, MEAC accredits midwifery education programs, including those that incorporate apprenticeship-based training through the **Portfolio Evaluation Process (PEP)**.

These organizations were founded by women deeply committed to midwifery excellence. For years, they worked without pay, covering their own travel expenses to attend meetings across the country. Long before the era of Zoom, their efforts to organize and build a professional movement were extraordinary. **Hillary Schlinger** documented many of their stories in her 1992 book *Circle of Midwives: Organized Midwifery in North America*. A second edition was published twenty years later and, while not commercially available, it can still be found through online searches. The history of the modern midwifery movement in the United States is both fascinating and inspiring—a testament to grassroots determination and collaborative vision.

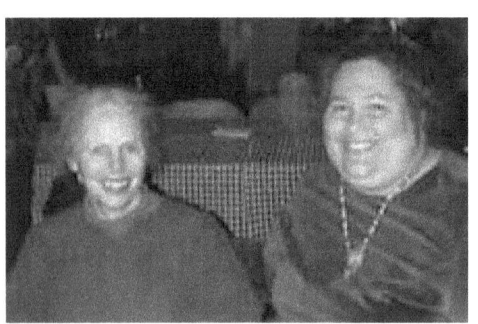

Ina May Gaskin (l) and Daphne Singingtree (r) March 1998 at MEAC/MANA/NARM meeting

Color Timeline of Midwifery History

Period	Key Developments
Ancient Civilizations	Midwives appear in Egyptian, Chinese, and Hindu texts. The biblical account of Shiphrah and Puah (Exodus 1:15–21) shows early midwifery roles.
Classical Antiquity	Greek philosophers praised midwives. Socrates' mother was a midwife; Aristotle and Hippocrates acknowledged their importance.
Medieval Europe	Midwives provided care during birth, illness, and death. Persecuted as witches during the Inquisition because of healing knowledge and independence.
Renaissance & Reformation	Books like *The Rosegarden* (1513) and *The Birth of Mankind* (1544) published. Formal education began for midwives.
1600s–1700s	Louise Bourgeois Boursier and Jane Sharp published groundbreaking texts. Madame du Coudray taught midwives using anatomical mannequins.
18th Century	Male obstetricians ('accoucheurs') gained prominence. Forceps were invented and closely guarded by the Chamberlen family.
Colonial America	Midwives like Bridget Lee Fuller and Martha Ballard practiced widely. Ballard's *Diary of a Midwife* documented everyday midwifery.
19th Century	Puerperal fever reduced by Holmes and Semmelweis with handwashing. Shift toward hospital births among upper classes.
20th Century	Midwifery marginalized, then revived through home birth movement. MANA and CPM credential established.
21st Century	Midwifery being integrated into health care systems. Focus on equity, collaborative care, and licensure across states.

Exercise 1.3: Historical Figures in Midwifery

Match answers:

1.	____Ina May Gaskin	A.	Colonial midwife whose diary later became a Pulitzer Prize winner
2.	____Jane Sharp	B.	Used life-size mannequin to teach midwifery
3.	____Mary Breckenridge	C.	Royal midwife; published three obstetrics volumes
4.	____Mary Francis Coley	D.	First English midwife to publish a midwifery book
5.	____Onnie Lee Logan	E.	Dutch midwife whose diary documented over 3,000 deliveries
6.	____Martha Ballard	F.	Invented forceps and then kept them a secret for generations
7.	____Madame du Coudray	G.	Showed how handwashing prevented postpartum infections
8.	____Louise Bourgeois Boursier	H.	Invented obstetrical mannikins
9.	____Peter Chamberlen	I.	Founded the first Nurse Midwifery school in Kentucky.
10.	____Catharina Schader	J.	Starred in an influential documentary about Black midwives in the South.
11.	____Ignaz Semmelweis	K.	Wrote MotherWit
12.	____ Angélique du Coudray	L.	Wrote Spiritual Midwifery

Exercise 1.4: History Critical Thinking Questions

Fill out the following:

1.	Why were midwives often targeted during periods of religious and political upheaval?	
2.	How did the invention of obstetric forceps both help and harm the role of midwives?	
3.	What role did midwives play beyond childbirth, and how did that affect their status?	
4.	How did class and gender influence who had access to obstetric knowledge?	

Modern Recognition and Challenges

In recent decades, midwifery has seen significant advancements in professional recognition, with **Certified Nurse-Midwives (CNMs)** and **Certified Professional Midwives (CPMs)** becoming integral to maternal health care. However, challenges remain regarding regulatory consistency, the limited recognition of certain credentials like the **Certified Midwife (CM)**, and the lack of regulation in some states.

While CNM credential is recognized in all fifty states, direct-entry midwifery regulation in the United States is highly fragmented, with each state setting its own laws governing midwifery practice. This patchwork system creates substantial variability in how midwives are licensed, what services they can provide, and where they can practice.

Whenever midwives cannot obtain licensure or legal recognition, it creates numerous problems:

1. **Lack of oversight**: Without regulation, there are no standardized training requirements, making it difficult for consumers to assess the qualifications of midwives.
2. **Access barriers**: Families in these states often struggle to find legally practicing midwives, particularly for home births, leading to reduced maternal care options. Lack of Medicaid reimbursement severely limits access to care.
3. **Criminalization of practice**: In some states, midwives may face legal penalties for practicing without licensure, even if they are highly trained and certified elsewhere.
4. **No integration with health care systems**: Unregulated states lack mechanisms to integrate midwives into broader health care systems, which hinders collaboration and referrals in emergencies.

State Certification or Licensure for Direct-Entry Midwives

State laws governing direct-entry midwifery vary widely. Some states offer licensure and allow for Medicaid reimbursement. The scope of practice varies from state to state. The CPM credential often provides a path for licensing. Others provide only certification or registration pathways, while several operate in a legal gray area with no specific statutory framework. In a few states, the practice of direct-entry midwifery is explicitly prohibited and may be prosecuted as practicing medicine without a license, which can carry felony charges. Ongoing advocacy efforts aim to clarify and improve midwifery laws, particularly in states where the practice is outlawed or undefined. For the most current legal status, consult your state midwifery organization or the narm.org website.

Currently, **37 states** and the District of Columbia provide a pathway for licensure or regulation of Certified Professional Midwives (CPMs) and other direct-entry midwives (DMs). These jurisdictions establish practice standards and oversight, enabling CPMs to legally attend home births and provide care. Regulation typically includes training and certification requirements through the North American Registry of Midwives (NARM).

Licensed states include: Alabama, Alaska, Arizona, Arkansas, California, Colorado, Delaware, District of Columbia, Florida, Hawaii, Idaho, Illinois, Indiana, Iowa, Kentucky, Louisiana, Kentucky, Maine, Maryland, Massachusetts, Michigan, Minnesota, Montana, New Hampshire, New Jersey, New Mexico, Oklahoma, Oregon, Rhode Island, South Carolina, South Dakota, Tennessee, Texas, Utah, Vermont, Virginia, Washington, Wisconsin, and Wyoming.

States where direct-entry midwifery is illegal: Alabama, Illinois, Iowa, Nebraska, North Carolina, and South Dakota.

States where midwifery is not legally defined: Connecticut, Georgia (has a statute but a license unobtainable), Connecticut, Georgia, Kansas, Massachusetts, Mississippi, Missouri, Nevada, North Dakota, Ohio, Pennsylvania, and West Virginia.

By contrast, CPM practice remains **explicitly prohibited** in two states: North Carolina and Nebraska.

Addressing Racial Disparities in Maternal Health

One of the most urgent issues in maternal health is the severe racial disparity in outcomes—especially for Black birthing individuals, who are three to four times more likely to die from pregnancy-related complications than their white counterparts. These disparities persist even when controlling for income, education, and insurance status, driven by systemic racism, implicit bias, and the chronic stress of navigating inequities.

Midwives play a vital role in addressing these challenges. In states with strong midwifery regulation and integration, midwife-led care has been linked to improved outcomes in marginalized communities, including lower rates of preterm birth and low birthweight, and higher satisfaction with care. Midwives are often strong advocates within the system, helping to counteract implicit bias and increase trust.

Expanding midwifery education—especially for providers from diverse racial and cultural backgrounds—and integrating midwives into public health systems can help reduce barriers to care. This is particularly important in underserved urban and rural communities with high maternal mortality rates.

The Certified Nurse Midwife (CNM) Credential

The CNM credential represents a highly trained professional in midwifery care, blending nursing and advanced midwifery education. CNMs must first complete a nursing degree and achieve licensure as a **Registered Nurse (RN)** before pursuing graduate-level midwifery education accredited by the **Accreditation Commission for Midwifery Education (ACME)**. This rigorous program combines academic coursework in obstetrics, gynecology, and primary care with extensive clinical training in diverse settings, preparing CNMs to provide holistic, evidence-based maternity care. Upon graduation, CNMs must pass the certification examination administered by the **American Midwifery Certification Board (AMCB)**, ensuring they meet the highest standards for safe and effective practice.

Building on the robust framework of the CNM credential, the **Certified Midwife (CM)** offers an alternative pathway for individuals who aspire to midwifery but do not hold a nursing background. While the CM education and certification process parallels that of CNMs in rigor and scope, it attracts candidates from various educational disciplines, emphasizing accessibility and inclusivity within the profession. This parallel pathway shows the versatility of midwifery credentials in meeting the diverse needs of birthing populations. Despite the credential's equivalency to CNMs in education and competencies, only thirteen states currently recognize CMs. This limited recognition creates significant barriers for CMs. In states without CM licensure, these midwives often cannot practice, limiting their ability to serve communities and advance their careers. This also restricts access to midwifery care in areas where CNMs and CPMs are already scarce.

Regulatory inconsistencies and limited credentialing remain significant barriers to equitable access to care. Expanding the recognition of the CM credential, introducing universal standards aligned with ICM guidelines, and addressing the lack of regulation in unlicensed states are critical steps toward ensuring that midwives can contribute to improving maternal and infant outcomes nationwide. These efforts will not only support midwives but also enhance care for the diverse populations they serve.

This recognition allows CMs to practice midwifery in these jurisdictions. However, in other states, the CM credential may not be recognized, which can limit the ability of Certified Midwives to practice. This lack of uniform recognition poses challenges for midwives seeking licensure and for individuals seeking midwifery care across different states.

The controversy surrounding the CM credential reflects broader tensions within midwifery regulation. Critics of the nursing requirement for CNMs argue it marginalizes non-nursing pathways, particularly for individuals seeking direct-entry midwifery education. Proponents of broader CM recognition contend that the credential aligns with international standards, such as those set by the **International Confederation of Midwives (ICM)**, and that its limited acceptance reduces access to qualified care providers.

DISTINCTIONS BETWEEN THE CPM AND CNM/CM CREDENTIALS

The **Certified Professional Midwife (CPM)** credential reflects a focus on holistic, community-based maternity care, especially in out-of-hospital settings like home births and birth centers. CPMs emphasize physiological birth and client-centered care that honors the natural process of childbirth. In contrast, **Certified Nurse-Midwives (CNMs)** and **Certified Midwives (CMs)** are typically trained within the medical model and more often practice in hospitals, although both also serve in birth centers. Together, these midwives offer a spectrum of expertise that enhances maternal health care.

CPM Credential: Expertise in Community Birth

CPMs follow direct-entry training pathways that prioritize hands-on experience in out-of-hospital settings. Their scope of practice includes:

- **Holistic Practices:** Incorporating evidence-based natural approaches such as herbal remedies, nutrition, and lifestyle counseling.
- **Support for Physiological Birth:** Emphasizes minimal intervention and continuous, individualized care.
- **Cultural and Community Connection:** Serving rural and underserved populations with culturally competent care.
- **Emergency Management:** Skillfully handling complications in low-resource environments where hospital support is not immediately available.

Emergency Skills in Low-Resource Settings

CPMs are uniquely prepared to manage emergencies in environments with limited resources. They apply preventive strategies, early detection, and manual techniques to ensure safety:

- **Prevention and Detection:** Early identification of complications during prenatal care and labor.
- **Managing Postpartum Hemorrhage:** Using uterotonics, manual techniques, and rapid decision-making when advanced interventions are not available.
- **Neonatal Resuscitation:** Proficiency in bag-and-mask ventilation for newborns needing assistance.

Challenges for Clinicians in Community Settings

Clinicians trained in hospital environments may face challenges in adapting to low-resource settings:

- **Technology Dependence:** Reliance on tools like continuous monitoring and advanced imaging.
- **Limited Experience:** Lack of practice managing emergencies without surgical or pharmacological backup.
- **Transfer Complexities:** Unfamiliarity with emergency transfer protocols from home or birth center settings.

CNM/CM Credential: Expertise in Hospital and Birth Center Care

CNMs and CMs are trained in midwifery philosophy combined with clinical expertise. Their scope of practice includes:

- **Hospital-Based Care:** Managing labor and delivery with access to advanced medical technology.
- **Collaborative Care Models:** Working within interdisciplinary teams to support complex or high-risk pregnancies.
- **Expanded Services:** Providing family planning, gynecologic care, and primary care services.

Shared Practice in Birth Centers

Birth centers often bring together CPMs and CNMs/CMs, offering families both personalized and clinically supported care:

- CPMs: Provide holistic, non-interventionist care and strong community ties.
- CNMs/CMs: Bring clinical training and the ability to use medical tools when needed.

Complementary Strengths and Future Directions

CPMs and CNMs/CMs fulfill essential but distinct roles in maternal health care. CPMs offer low-intervention, community-based care and are equipped to manage emergencies outside hospital settings. CNMs and CMs contribute hospital-based expertise and broader clinical services.

Despite different training models, all midwives are united by a shared goal: to improve maternal outcomes. By leveraging their complementary strengths, the midwifery profession can meet the diverse needs of families—whether at home, in birth centers, or in hospitals.

The Role of Regulation in Maternal Outcomes

States with strong midwifery regulation and integration across all credential types consistently report better maternal and neonatal outcomes, especially for home births. Licensing and oversight help ensure midwives meet high standards and are integrated into health care systems for timely emergency referrals. These systems promote not only safety but also trust and collaboration between midwives and other health care providers.

In contrast, states without regulation may face greater risks. A lack of standardized pathways can push even highly skilled midwives underground, increasing the likelihood of poor outcomes during emergencies. In regulated environments, midwives are better supported, resulting in lower cesarean rates, fewer complications, and higher rates of breastfeeding initiation.

Balancing Safety and Autonomy

The debate over regulation often hinges on how to balance safety with the autonomy of birthing individuals. Supporters of regulation emphasize the need for standardized training, licensing, and accountability to ensure quality care. Critics contend that strict regulation can shift control away from birthing individuals and limit midwives' ability to offer personalized, culturally sensitive care over personal choice, limiting the scope of midwifery and undermining culturally sensitive, individualized care.

For example, in states where regulations closely mirror hospital-based models, midwives may face restrictions on home births and non-interventionist approaches. Many families seek midwifery care precisely for these alternatives. When regulation disregards such values, it risks eroding the very qualities that draw people to midwifery in the first place.

Risks of Non-Regulation

In states without regulation, consumers often lack clear ways to assess a midwife's qualifications. This absence of transparency can endanger families and isolate midwives from the broader health care system. Criminalization of unlicensed midwives further discourages collaboration, leaving families without access to safe, integrated care.

Thoughtful regulation can mitigate these risks by setting competency benchmarks and protecting families from unqualified providers—without eliminating choice or undermining midwifery's holistic strengths.

A Collaborative Model

Rather than viewing regulation as a constraint, it can be designed to empower midwives and their clients. When developed collaboratively—with input from midwives, birthing people, and policymakers—regulatory frameworks can uphold safety while supporting autonomy. Culturally competent, evidence-based models can preserve the heart of midwifery care while improving systemic support and accountability.

Contrasting Perspectives

Supporters of autonomy-driven models emphasize the importance of preserving care that aligns with cultural and personal values. Advocates for regulation focus on establishing consistent standards to improve safety and outcomes. Bridging these perspectives requires flexible policy frameworks that support midwifery expertise, promote integration into health care systems, and protect the rights and preferences of birthing individuals.

The Path Forward

Creating inclusive, equitable regulation for CNMs, CMs, and CPMs is key to improving outcomes across the board. Universal standards for education, certification, and practice can ensure that all birthing individuals—regardless of race, income, or geography—have access to safe, culturally competent midwifery care, without compromising their autonomy or values.

Lasting change will require collaboration among midwifery organizations, health care providers, and policymakers. Together, they can build a system that honors both the safety and the autonomy of birthing individuals, reduces racial disparities, and strengthens maternal health for generations to come.

Exercise 1.5: Licensing & Credentialing

Fill out the following:

1. In what ways do consumers benefit from programs or legislations that licenses and/or regulates midwives?

2. In what ways do midwives benefit from licensing and/or regulations?

3. What potential problems may emerge when licensing and/or regulations are required?

The International Confederation of Midwives (ICM)

The **International Confederation of Midwives (ICM)** is a global organization r currently representing over 136 midwives' associations in 117 countries, more than one million midwives globally. ICM is an accredited non-governmental organization registered in The Netherlands. The ICM mission is to strengthen midwives' associations and to advance the profession of midwifery globally by promoting autonomous midwives as the most appropriate caregivers for childbearing women and in keeping birth normal, to enhance the reproductive health of women, their newborns and their families.

Founded in 1922, the ICM's mission is to strengthen midwifery worldwide, ensuring high-quality, evidence-based, and culturally sensitive care for individuals during pregnancy, birth, and the postpartum period. The ICM plays a pivotal role in establishing international standards for midwifery education, regulation, and practice, providing a framework that promotes consistency and excellence across the profession.

ICM and Midwifery Regulation

ICM's Global Standards for Midwifery Regulation ensure that midwives are licensed and regulated in ways that safeguard the public while supporting professional autonomy. These standards encourage governments to implement consistent frameworks for midwifery practice, including licensing processes, continuing professional development, and mechanisms for public accountability.

In the United States, midwifery regulation varies by state, but the ICM standards provide a model for unifying the profession. The CPM, CM, and CNM credentials reflect aspects of ICM's approach, such as requiring demonstrated clinical competencies and ongoing professional education. However, the lack of universal credentialing and state-to-state variability in regulation creates challenges in aligning fully with ICM recommendations.

ICM and Midwifery Credentialing

The ICM advocates for standardized midwifery education and credentialing globally. Its Essential Competencies for Midwifery Practice outline the knowledge, skills, and behaviors that midwives must show to provide safe and effective care. In the US, these competencies influence the education and certification processes for CPMs, CMs, and CNMs.

- **CPMs:** Focus on community birth and out-of-hospital settings, aligning with ICM's emphasis on physiological birth and holistic care.
- **CNMs and CMs:** Meet ICM-aligned standards through accredited graduate programs, reflecting the ICM's focus on advanced education and interprofessional collaboration.

The ICM's framework underscores the need for a universal midwifery credential, a concept that could unify the diverse pathways in the US and improve consistency in training and practice.

The **ICM's Global Standards for Midwifery Practice** define a broad scope that includes prenatal, intrapartum, postpartum, and newborn care, as well as health promotion, education, and family planning. These guidelines emphasize midwifery autonomy while encouraging integration into multidisciplinary health care systems.

In the US, the scope of practice for midwives often depends on state laws and credentialing. While CNMs typically have a broader scope within hospital systems, CPMs and CMs align closely with ICM's emphasis on physiological birth and community-based care. Efforts to incorporate ICM principles into US midwifery practice could help bridge gaps between different credentials and foster greater collaboration across settings.

Integrating Core Competencies: A Modern Framework for Midwifery Practice

With the dissolution of the Midwives Alliance of North America (MANA), a cohesive and forward-thinking standard for midwifery core competencies is essential. Drawing from the globally recognized International Confederation of Midwives (ICM) Essential Competencies and the National Association of Certified Professional Midwives (NACPM) Job Analysis Model, this framework defines the core competencies for midwifery practice, establishing a clear foundation for education, certification, and clinical care. By aligning these established models, this standard ensures midwifery education and practice reflect the needs of diverse birthing populations while adhering to rigorous global and national benchmarks.

A Unified Framework for Core Competencies

The ICM Essential Competencies outline the knowledge, skills, and behaviors required for midwives to provide safe, effective, and respectful care. These competencies equip midwives to meet international standards of care and are categorized into four domains:
1. **General Competencies:** Foundational knowledge in anatomy, physiology, and public health.
2. **Pre-pregnancy and Antenatal Care:** Screening for risks, health promotion, and education.
3. **Care During Labor and Birth:** Supporting physiological birth and managing complications.
4. **Ongoing Care:** Postpartum, newborn, and family support, as well as reproductive health services.

NACPM Job Analysis Model

The **National Association of Certified Professional Midwives (NACPM)** is a professional organization that represents and advocates for Certified Professional Midwives (CPMs) in the United States. It created the NACPM Job Analysis Model to provide a US-specific perspective, detailing the critical tasks and responsibilities of CPMs in community and out-of-hospital birth settings. It focuses on:
- **Individualized Care Plans:** Tailored to the physical, emotional, and cultural needs of clients.
- **Holistic Health Practices:** Incorporating nutritional counseling, natural remedies, and lifestyle support.
- **Emergency Skills:** Preparedness for urgent situations, such as postpartum hemorrhage and neonatal resuscitation.
- **Community Engagement**: Addressing social determinants of health and fostering equitable care access.

Exercise 1.6: Alphabet Soup	
What do these midwifery initials mean?	
1. CNM	
2. CPM	
3. CM	
4. DM or DEM	
5. LM or LDEM	
6. NARM	
7. NACPM	
8. MEAC	
9. ICM	
10. ACME	
11. PEP	
12. AMCB	
13. MANA	

Core Competencies for Midwifery Practice

By integrating ICM competencies with the NACPM job model, it establishes a unified standard for midwifery practice. By combining the global insights of ICM with the US-specific focus of NACPM, it ensures midwives are equipped to deliver equitable, effective, and culturally competent care across all practice settings, advancing the health and well-being of individuals and families worldwide.

The following comprehensive standard defines the core competencies for midwifery practice:
- Foundational Knowledge and Clinical Skills.
- Mastery of anatomy, physiology, pharmacology, and evidence-based practices.
- Proficiency in health promotion, risk assessment, and public health initiatives.
- Culturally Competent, Person-Centered Care.
- Respect for individual autonomy and cultural practices.
- Capacity to provide care that reflects the diverse needs of communities.
- Comprehensive reproductive and maternal health services.
- Preconception care, fertility guidance, reproductive health education, and family planning.
- Prenatal care with an emphasis on health optimization and client education.
- Safe management of labor and birth, focusing on physiological processes and minimizing unnecessary interventions.
- Postpartum care addressing maternal recovery, newborn health, and family adjustment up to six weeks.
- Emergency Preparedness and Response.
- Expertise in managing complications such as shoulder dystocia, hemorrhage, and neonatal resuscitation.
- Knowledge of transfer protocols and collaboration with medical teams for high-risk cases.
- Advocacy and Education.
- Promoting informed decision-making and empowering clients with knowledge about their care.
- Engagement in community education and initiatives addressing health disparities.
- Professional Integration and Development.
- Commitment to lifelong learning and adherence to professional standards.
- Collaboration with interdisciplinary teams and contribution to health care system integration.

Implementation and Accountability
1. **Education and Certification:** Midwifery programs must adopt this integrated competency model to ensure graduates are prepared for diverse practice environments. Certification should rigorously assess these competencies.
2. **Evaluation and Development:** Licensure should include robust assessments and feedback to support ongoing professional growth.
3. **Collaborative Practice Models:** Midwives must work within integrated health care teams to ensure continuity of care and access to multidisciplinary resources, especially for high-risk cases.
4. **Regulatory Oversight:** States and national organizations must adopt these standards as the basis for licensure, creating consistency across midwifery practice and ensuring accountability.

Towards a Universal Credential
The push for a universal midwifery credential that meets ICM standards is gaining momentum. A unified credential would encompass CNMs, CMs, and CPMs under one regulatory framework, ensuring consistency in education, competencies, and practice. Such a system would also allow midwives to practice across state lines, improving mobility and addressing maternal health gaps, particularly in rural and underserved areas.

Achieving this goal requires bridging divides between nursing-based and direct-entry pathways. Medical lobbying groups and some physician organizations continue to oppose expanded practice, while advocates for direct-entry and independent midwifery emphasize inclusive systems that protect consumer choice and recognize diverse training.

INFORMED CONSENT AND SHARED DECISION-MAKING

Informed consent is both an ethical duty and a legal requirement in midwifery care. It means a client voluntarily agrees to a care plan after receiving clear, evidence-based information about procedures, risks, benefits, and alternatives. More than a signature on a form, it is an ongoing conversation throughout pregnancy, birth, and postpartum.

Shared decision-making builds on informed consent by emphasizing partnership. The midwife brings professional knowledge, clinical expertise, and awareness of community standards; the client brings her personal values, beliefs, and preferences. Together, they create a plan of care that can be revisited and revised as circumstances change.

Key Components

1. **Disclosure:** The midwife explains procedures, options, risks, benefits, and alternatives.
2. **Capacity and Voluntariness:** The client must understand the information and decide freely, without pressure.
3. **Documentation:** Consent or refusal is signed by both client and midwife, especially when care differs from standard guidelines.
4. **Ongoing Dialogue:** Consent is revisited as new information or conditions arise.

Midwives provide an **informed disclosure** at the start of care, including:

- Education, training, and philosophy of practice.
- Scope of care and emergency transfer plans.
- Services provided, current credentials, and legal status.
- Practice guidelines, consultation/referral options, and HIPAA disclosures.

> ### Why It Matters
> - **Client Autonomy:** Informed consent empowers women to be co-authors of their care, fostering confidence in their choices.
> - **Ethical Practice:** It is central to the midwifery model, which emphasizes respect, trust, and collaboration.
> - **Legal Protection:** Midwives have a legal responsibility to obtain informed consent, and proper documentation protects both client and midwife.
> - **Risk Management:** A well-documented process shows that the client understood the implications of her care plan and helps prevent misunderstandings.

When a client chooses care outside the midwife's routine plan, the midwife must document that she gave evidence-based information, discussed risks and benefits, and offered consultation or referral. The midwife may then continue or transfer care, depending on what best supports client safety and professional standards.

The Role of Education and Counseling

Information should be presented in language the client understands, avoiding medical jargon. Written materials should be accessible and clear, supporting the ongoing conversation. The process integrates evidence, clinical judgment, and the client's values to arrive at a care plan that belongs to both midwife and client.

Bottom Line

Informed consent and shared decision-making protect the client's right to choose while enabling the midwife to provide safe, ethical care. Practiced consistently, they build trust, reduce stress, and strengthen the midwife–client partnership.

Exercise 1.7: Informed Consent in Action			
Place a check mark on which part of the informed consent process is missing, incomplete or present.			
Scenario	Incomplete	Missing	Present
1. A midwife explains the risks and benefits of a lab test, but doesn't mention that the client has the option to decline.			
2. A client is asked to sign a consent form, but the midwife never checks whether she understands the information.			
3. A client agrees to a procedure after feeling pressured by her partner.			
4. A midwife provides clear information, answers questions, and the client signs a consent form that is placed in the chart.			
5. A midwife updates the client about new test results, discusses options, and revises the care plan together with her.			
6. A client declines a recommended test. The midwife documents the refusal, explains risks, and has the client sign the form.			

THE CURRENT STATE OF MIDWIFERY

Midwifery today is recognized as a vital component of maternity care, addressing systemic gaps in maternal health and improving outcomes, particularly among marginalized communities. With rising maternal mortality rates in the United States, especially among Black and Indigenous populations, midwifery offers a solution through its holistic, culturally sensitive, and client-centered approach. Midwifery is also evolving within the broader health care system. In many states, Certified Professional Midwives (CPMs), Certified Nurse-Midwives (CNMs), and traditional or Indigenous midwives collaborate with physicians, doulas, and community health workers to create integrated care networks. These partnerships improve continuity of care, expand options for families, and reduce unnecessary interventions. The profession emphasizes physiological birth, person-centered care, and advocacy, fostering trust and equity in maternity care. At the same time, differing state laws and fragmented regulations continue to create barriers, leaving some midwives vulnerable to legal challenges and limiting families' access to safe out-of-hospital birth.

Globally, midwifery is recognized by the World Health Organization as an essential strategy to improve maternal and newborn outcomes. Research consistently shows that expanding access to midwives could prevent a significant portion of maternal and neonatal deaths worldwide. In the United States, growing recognition of this evidence has spurred legislative efforts, grassroots advocacy, and community organizing to expand midwifery services. These movements emphasize reproductive justice, cultural humility, and the right of all families to choose the setting and provider that best fits their needs.

> **Key Fact**
> Studies show that universal access to midwifery care could prevent up to 80% of maternal deaths, stillbirths, and newborn deaths worldwide (WHO, 2021).

Public demand for midwifery services has grown, driven by concerns over medicalized childbirth and an interest in personalized, non-invasive care options. Midwives also play a crucial role in addressing social determinants of health, offering community-based care in underserved areas, and advocating for equitable access to maternal health services. Despite these advancements, challenges such as inconsistent regulation, scope of practice limitations, and access to midwifery education persist.

Mechanisms for Midwifery Education

CPMs are uniquely trained to provide care in out-of-hospital settings, emphasizing community-based and person-centered care. Pathways to the CPM credential include MEAC-accredited programs, the Portfolio Evaluation Process (PEP), and emerging community college programs. These pathways are designed to meet the varying needs of students and align with rigorous national and international standards.

A critical element of midwifery education is the **Midwifery Student Bill of Rights**, which ensures students have equitable, respectful, and supportive learning environments. It addresses the rights of students to quality education, fair treatment, and mentorship, while also setting expectations for institutions and preceptors to uphold ethical and inclusive standards.

Midwifery Student Bill of Rights

The **Midwifery Student Bill of Rights** establishes essential standards to ensure that students in all educational pathways are treated fairly, respectfully, and equitably. *Key principles include:*

- **Equitable Access to Education:** Students have the right to access high-quality midwifery education, regardless of race, gender, socioeconomic status, or geographic location.
- **Fair Assessment and Feedback:** Students are entitled to transparent grading, constructive feedback, and timely evaluations of their progress.
- **Supportive Learning Environments:** Institutions and preceptors must provide safe, respectful, and inclusive spaces for learning, free from discrimination or harassment.
- **Mentorship and Resources:** Students must have access to qualified mentors, learning resources, and opportunities to achieve competency in all required skills.
- **Advocacy and Accountability:** Students have the right to advocate for their educational needs and expect accountability from their programs and preceptors.

Currently, in the United States, there are several routes to becoming a direct-entry midwife. Some choose the path of traditional midwifery, often rooted in apprenticeship, spiritual practice, or community-based teaching without formal education or licensure. Others pursue structured pathways such as accredited programs, portfolio evaluation, or college-based training. Having multiple routes into midwifery helps honor diverse traditions while also providing accessible options that meet community needs.

1. MEAC-Accredited Schools and Programs

- The **Midwifery Education Accreditation Council (MEAC)** accredits midwifery programs that meet national standards for the CPM credential. MEAC-accredited programs offer:
- **Comprehensive Coursework:** Covering anatomy, physiology, pharmacology, and evidence-based practices.
- **Clinical Training:** Hands-on experience in prenatal care, labor, delivery, postpartum care, and newborn care under qualified preceptors.
- **Certification Alignment:** Graduates are prepared to sit for the North American Registry of Midwives (NARM) exam, which certifies CPMs.

2. Portfolio Evaluation Process (PEP)

The PEP apprenticeship model emphasizes experiential learning and mentorship with experienced midwives. Features include:

- **Individualized Training:** Students gain practical skills through direct supervision in real-world settings.
- **Flexibility:** This model is accessible for students in rural or underserved areas where formal programs may not exist.
- **Competency Documentation:** Students compile a portfolio of their skills and clinical experiences, which is evaluated by NARM to determine eligibility for certification.

3. Community College Integration

Community colleges represent an emerging model of midwifery education, particularly in states like Wisconsin, Florida, and potentially California. These programs offer an accessible and affordable route to the CPM credential. Examples include:

Wisconsin: Southwest Wisconsin Technical College
- Offers an Associate Degree in Direct Entry Midwifery.
- Combines academic coursework with clinical placements under MEAC accreditation.
- Accommodates both local and distance learners.

Florida: Florida School of Traditional Midwifery
- Combines classroom instruction with clinical training in birth centers, hospitals, and home birth settings.
- Prepares students for the Florida Midwifery Licensing Exam, with reciprocity for CPMs in states like California.

California: Emerging Models
- There is speculation about community colleges in California offering courses for CPM credentialed midwives.
- These programs could provide affordable, regionally tailored training to meet the demand for midwives in underserved areas.

4. Hybrid and Online Programs

Hybrid midwifery programs combine online coursework with in-person clinical training, offering flexibility for students balancing education with personal and professional responsibilities.

These programs often include:
- **Interactive Virtual Learning:** Online lectures, simulations, and discussions.
- **Regional Clinical Placements:** Hands-on training through local partnerships.
- **Global Accessibility:** Allowing students in remote areas to access high-quality midwifery education.

Considerations for Midwifery Education

- **Accessibility and Affordability:** Community college and hybrid models provide affordable pathways, making midwifery education accessible to a broader range of students.
- **Diversity and Inclusion:** Programs must actively recruit and support students from underrepresented backgrounds, ensuring a workforce reflective of the communities it serves.
- **Standardization and Accountability:** All pathways must adhere to rigorous standards to ensure consistency in midwifery education and certification.
- **Preceptor Support:** Apprenticeship-based pathways rely on the availability and expertise of preceptors, who must be adequately supported and compensated.
- **Advocacy and Public Awareness:** Public education campaigns should raise awareness about midwifery's role in improving maternal and neonatal outcomes.

Midwifery education today is not just about clinical competency; it also reflects the values of equity, accessibility, and respect for diverse traditions. By offering multiple educational routes, the profession welcomes students with different backgrounds, learning styles, and life experiences. Whether through formal programs, apprenticeship, or hybrid pathways, each route contributes to a stronger and more inclusive workforce.

At the same time, midwifery education carries a responsibility to prepare students for the realities of practice—balancing evidence-based care, cultural humility, and advocacy. The sustainability of the profession depends on strong mentorship, adequate support for preceptors, and systems that protect both students and families. Investing in midwifery education is therefore an investment in the future of safe, respectful, and equitable birth.

Exercise 1.8: Exploring Educational Pathways
Match each description to the correct educational pathway

Descriptions	Pathways
1. _____Students compile a portfolio of supervised clinical experiences for review by NARM. 2. _____Combines online coursework with local clinical placements to increase accessibility. 3. _____Accredited by MEAC, these programs include coursework in anatomy, pharmacology, and evidence-based practice. 4. _____Offers affordable, regionally tailored programs through institutions like Southwest Wisconsin Technical College. 5. _____Rooted in apprenticeship or community-based learning, often outside formal licensure systems.	A. MEAC-Accredited Schools and Programs B. Portfolio Evaluation Process (PEP) C. Community College Integration D. Hybrid and Online Programs E. Traditional Midwifery

MIDWIFERY YESTERDAY & TODAY ESSENTIAL TAKEAWAYS

Midwifery has endured for millennia because it speaks to something timeless and essential: the human experience of birth. From ancient traditions to professional evolution, its history tells a story of courage, wisdom, and care. Today's midwives carry that legacy forward, grounding their practice in cultural respect, clinical skill, and deep connection.

Community has always been the foundation of midwifery. Midwives have served as healers, counselors, and advocates, linking families with knowledge and support that extends far beyond the birth itself. Their work has promoted health across generations, strengthening not only mothers and babies but also the fabric of community life.

Midwifery today balances this heritage with the demands of professionalism. Out-of-hospital midwives, in particular, stand at the intersection of tradition and innovation, offering care that is both deeply personal and grounded in evidence. As midwives advance into the future, their role is not only to safeguard birth but also to model respect, equity, and resilience in health care.

Understanding the past is not only about honoring history but also about shaping a future in which every birthing family is supported and heard. The future of safe, respectful, and equitable birth begins with how we teach, how we listen, and how we care—starting from the very first moments of life.

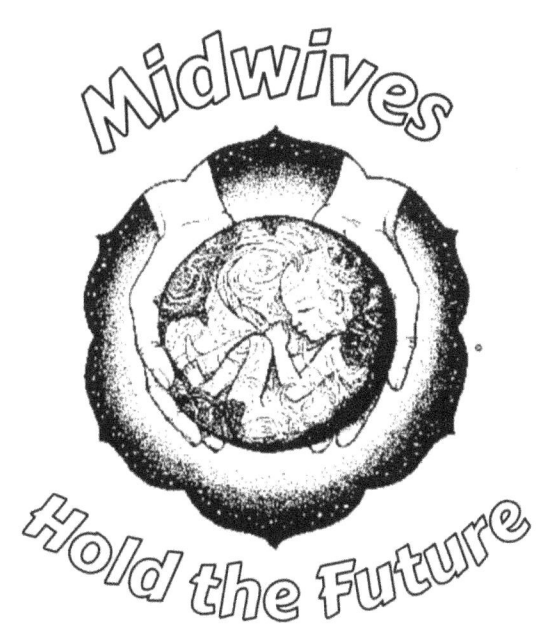

Chapter One Self-Assessment

Multiple Choice
1. Which of the following best describes the philosophy of midwifery?
   a) Birth is a medical event requiring intervention.
   b) Birth is a natural, physiological process, and midwifery emphasizes autonomy.
   c) Midwifery focuses solely on emergency interventions.
   d) Midwifery promotes institutionalized care over individual care.

2. Midwifery care is characterized by which of the following?
   a) Reliance on standardized procedures.
   b) A focus on individual autonomy and cultural competence.
   c) Limited prenatal visits.
   d) Use of advanced medical technology as a primary focus.

3. A key principle of midwifery advocacy is:
   a) Limiting client involvement in decisions.
   b) Standardizing all birth plans.
   c) Promoting informed decision-making and respecting client preferences.
   d) Reducing access to alternative birth settings.

4. Historically, midwives were primarily responsible for:
   a) Delivering babies only in hospitals.
   b) Replacing physicians during the 20th century.
   c) Community-based support for pregnancy, labor, and postpartum care.
   d) Providing care exclusively to wealthy families.

5. The decline of midwifery in the early modern era was due to:
   a) A lack of community-based models.
   b) The rise of medicalized childbirth practices.
   c) Improved acceptance of holistic approaches.
   d) Increasing maternal mortality rates under midwifery care.

6. Which of the following contributed to the shift from midwifery to physician-led birth care?
   a) Advances in surgical techniques and hospitals.
   b) The widespread acceptance of cultural traditions.
   c) A lack of interest in medical interventions.
   d) Improved access to midwives in rural areas.

7. Midwives play a critical role in reducing maternal health disparities by:
   a) Limiting their care to affluent urban areas.
   b) Addressing systemic barriers and improving access for underserved populations.
   c) Operating exclusively within hospital systems.
   d) Relying on standardized institutional protocols.

8. Which of the following trends is shaping modern midwifery care?
   a) A shift away from community-based care.
   b) Declining emphasis on cultural competence in practice.
   c) Decreasing access to midwifery-led care.
   d) Increasing integration with health care systems while maintaining holistic approaches.

9. Midwifery is associated with which of the following outcomes?
   a) Higher cesarean rates in low-risk pregnancies.
   b) Increased maternal satisfaction and lower intervention rates.
   c) More reliance on fetal monitoring technology.
   d) Decreased accessibility in underserved communities.

10. The International Confederation of Midwives (ICM) Essential Competencies focus on:
    a) Outlining knowledge, skills, and behaviors required for effective, safe midwifery practice.
    b) Restricting midwifery practice to home births.
    c) Replacing national competency models.
    d) Limiting cultural competence in care.

11. The Midwifery Student Bill of Rights ensures:
    a) Reduced opportunities for practical experience.
    b) Exclusive rights for rural students.
    c) Equitable access to education and respectful mentorship for students.
    d) The removal of client-centered care from student training.

12. Which competency aligns with the NACPM job model?
    a) Tailoring care plans to the individual needs of clients.
    b) Focusing exclusively on technological interventions.
    c) Requiring universal, standardized approaches.
    d) Limiting collaboration with interdisciplinary teams.

Fill in the blank

13. Midwifery care often involves _____ support for the physical, emotional, and cultural needs of clients.

14. The introduction of _____ as the primary attendants in childbirth shifted the focus from community to institutionalized care.

15. The Midwifery Model of Care emphasizes _____ and culturally competent care while reducing unnecessary interventions.

16. Midwifery care emphasizes _____ decision-making, allowing clients to actively participate in their care.

True/False

17. Midwifery is a profession that has only existed since the 19th century.

18. Male physicians began to participate in births in Europe primarily after the invention and use of forceps.

19. In the United States, midwives were more common in rural, immigrant, and marginalized communities.

20. The decline of midwifery in the 20th century was due in part to the medicalization of childbirth.

21. The midwifery model of care emphasizes quick intervention and routine surgical procedures.

Chapter One Reading & References

Recommended Reading: History of Midwifery
- Borst, C. G. (1995). ***Catching Babies: The Professionalization of Childbirth, 1870–1920***. Harvard University Press. Examines the professionalization of childbirth in the US and the shift from midwives to physicians.
- Burst, Helen Varney. (2015) ***A History of Midwifery in the United States: The Midwife Said "Fear Not."*** Springer Publishing. An overview of US midwifery from community traditions to professionalization, licensing debates, and the modern resurgence.
- Ehrenreich, B., & English, D. (2010). ***Witches, Midwives, and Nurses: A History of Women Healers*** The Feminist Press. A brief, influential text linking midwifery history to women's health activism and feminist struggles.
- Loudon, I. (1992). ***Death in Childbirth: An International Study of Maternal Care and Maternal Mortality, 1800–1950***. Oxford University Press. Provides a global historical view of maternal mortality and the evolution of maternity care systems.
- Marland, H. (1993). ***The Art of Midwifery: Early Modern Midwives in Europe***. Routledge. Discusses European midwives' practices and roles from the 17th to 19th centuries.
- Rooks, J. P. (1997). ***Midwifery and Childbirth in America***. Temple University Press. Comprehensive overview of the American midwifery model, its history, and its modern challenges.
- Logan, O. L. (1989). ***Motherwit: An Alabama Midwife's Story***. New American Library. Autobiography of Onnie Lee Logan, a traditional African American midwife, offering a rich oral history of community practice.
- Worth, J. (2002). ***Call the Midwife: A True Story of the East End in the 1950s***. Penguin. Memoir that inspired the popular television series, providing vivid insight into midwifery in postwar London.
- Ulrich, L. T. (1990). ***A Midwife's Tale: The Life of Martha Ballard, Based on Her Diary, 1785–1812***. Vintage Books. Brings to life the work of an 18th-century midwife through her personal diary and contextual analysis.
- Wertz, R. W., & Wertz, D. C. (1989). ***Lying-In: A History of Childbirth in America*** Yale University Press. Explores childbirth practices and professional tensions in American history.

References

Borst, C. G. (1995). Catching babies: The professionalization of childbirth, 1870–1920. Harvard University Press.

Davis-Floyd, R. E. (2003). Birth as an American rite of passage (2nd ed.). University of California Press.

Donnison, J. (1988). Midwives and medical men: A history of inter-professional rivalries and women's rights. Heinemann.

Ehrenreich, B., & English, D. (2010). Witches, midwives, and nurses: A history of women healers (2nd ed.). The Feminist Press.

Evenden, D. (2000). The midwives of seventeenth-century London. Cambridge University Press.

Hobby, E. (1999). Virtue of necessity: English women's writing 1649–88. University of Michigan Press.

Marland, H. (1993). The art of midwifery: Early modern midwives in Europe. Routledge.

Marland, H., & Rafferty, A. M. (Eds.). (1997). Midwives, society, and childbirth: Debates and controversies in the modern period. Routledge.

McGregor, D. (1998). From midwives to medicine: The birth of modern obstetrics. Harvard University Press.

Morton, C. H., & Clift, E. G. (2014). *Birth ambassadors: Reflections on midwifery and birth activism*. Praeclarus Press.

Rooks, J. P. (1997). Midwifery and childbirth in America. Temple University Press.

Schlinger, H. (2009). Circle of midwives. [Publisher name if available].

Skowronski, G. A. (2002). The midwife's tale: An oral history from Handywoman to professional midwife. Routledge.

Towler, J., & Bramall, J. (1997). Midwives in history and society. Croom Helm.

Ulrich, L. T. (1990). A midwife's tale: The life of Martha Ballard, based on her diary, 1785–1812. Vintage Books.

Walsh, D., & Newburn, M. (2002). Birth centres: A social model for maternity care. Books for Midwives Press.

Wertz, R. W., & Wertz, D. C. (1989). Lying-in: A history of childbirth in America (Expanded ed.). Yale University Press.

Wilson, A. (1995). The making of man-midwifery: Childbirth in England, 1660–1770. Harvard University Press.

Chapter Two
Learning to Learn

Objectives
After completing this chapter, the student should be able to:
1. **Describe** the unique challenges and rewards of midwifery education.
2. **Explain** the concept of lifelong learning as it applies to the midwifery profession.
3. **Identify** key characteristics of adult learners.
4. **Compare** asynchronous and competency-based learning models.
5. **Explore** various learning styles and determine personal learning preferences.
6. **Apply** strategies to support effective learning based on individual needs.
7. **Differentiate** between the cognitive, affective, and psychomotor domains of learning.
8. **Summarize** Howard Gardner's theory of multiple intelligences and its relevance to midwifery education.
9. **Describe** hemispheric dominance (left-brain vs. right-brain) and how it influences learning styles.
10. **Apply** memory-enhancement techniques including loci, chunking, mnemonics, and directed visualization.
11. **Use** the 5-P Reading System for improved comprehension.
12. **Implement** the SQ4R method for active reading and retention.
13. **Use** study techniques specific to midwifery content (e.g., terminology, protocols, charts).
14. **Organize** and participate in study groups to promote collaborative learning.
15. **Use** flashcards, diagrams, and models to support anatomical and physiological understanding.
16. **Set** SMART goals to enhance academic focus and direction.
17. **Develop** a balanced study schedule that accommodates academic, clinical, and personal responsibilities.
18. **Identify** common distractions and implement strategies to reduce them.
19. **Explain** the role of self-care in sustaining learning and performance.
20. **Identify** and use technology tools that enhance learning, including medical terminology apps and online simulations.
21. **Use** textbooks and supplementary resources efficiently.
22. **Interpret** and create charts, graphs, and videos to support diverse learning needs.
23. **Conduct** self-assessment to monitor learning progress and mastery.
24. **Seek** and utilize peer and instructor feedback to improve performance.
25. **Apply** strategies to prepare effectively for exams and certifications.

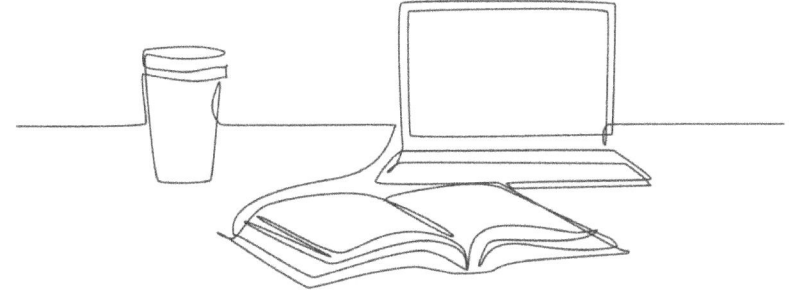

Midwifery Education: A Balance of Science and Art

Midwifery education weaves together the **scientific training** including mastering diagnostic tools, interpreting lab results, and applying evidence-based protocols with the **art of midwifery**—the ability to build trust, communicate with empathy, and honor each client's cultural values and personal preferences. Midwives offer emotional presence alongside medical skill, supporting families through the transformational process of birth. At its best, midwifery integrates science and art seamlessly. This balanced approach shapes students not just as providers, but as advocates for respectful, dignified birth experiences.

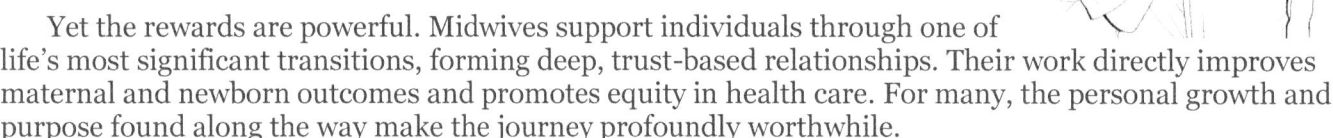

Midwifery education is both demanding and deeply meaningful. It requires students to balance rigorous academic study with hands-on clinical training—often while juggling work, family, and personal responsibilities. Time management and emotional resilience are essential, as students face high expectations and occasionally intense experiences in clinical care.

Yet the rewards are powerful. Midwives support individuals through one of life's most significant transitions, forming deep, trust-based relationships. Their work directly improves maternal and newborn outcomes and promotes equity in health care. For many, the personal growth and purpose found along the way make the journey profoundly worthwhile.

Midwifery as a Lifelong Journey

Midwifery education extends beyond initial training to encompass a lifelong journey of self-exploration and professional growth. To stay at the forefront of evidence-based care, midwives must commit to ongoing education through professional development workshops, continuing education, and engagement with current research. This dedication to lifelong learning ensures that midwives can adapt to new challenges and continue to provide the highest quality of care.

By encouraging a balance of science and art, head and heart, and logic and intuition, midwifery education prepares students to become not only competent practitioners but also advocates for equitable, respectful care. It is this holistic approach that makes midwifery an essential and transformative profession.

Self-Care as a Foundation

A central theme in midwifery is learning to "midwife self so that you may midwife others." Midwifery is an emotionally and physically demanding profession. To sustain their ability to serve others, midwives must cultivate resilience and balance in their own lives. Intentional self-care mentally, emotionally, and physically is not just a personal necessity but a professional responsibility. By caring for themselves, midwives ensure they can provide the compassionate, effective care their clients deserve.

Holistic Growth

The path of midwifery is as much about personal development as it is about professional mastery. Students are challenged to cultivate empathy, resilience, and reflective thinking alongside clinical excellence. Engaging in self-reflection, seeking mentorship, and participating in peer support networks are vital tools for navigating the demands of midwifery education and practice. This holistic growth ensures that midwives are not only skilled practitioners but also well-rounded individuals.

The Challenges

Midwifery education requires a rigorous commitment to both academic study and clinical practice. Students delve deeply into subjects such as anatomy, physiology, pharmacology, and obstetrics, while simultaneously gaining hands-on experience through clinical placements. This dual focus demands intellectual stamina and dedication.

For many students, managing time effectively is a significant hurdle. The need to balance coursework, clinical placements, and personal responsibilities can feel overwhelming, particularly for adult learners who may also be caring for families or working part-time jobs. Developing strong organizational skills is essential to navigating these competing demands successfully.

Emotionally, midwifery students face intense experiences that can test their resilience. From dealing with emergencies to witnessing loss, the emotional weight of the profession requires students to develop coping mechanisms and seek support when needed. Learning to process these challenges is an integral part of becoming a compassionate and effective midwife.

The Rewards

Despite its challenges, the rewards of midwifery education are profound. Midwives have the privilege of supporting individuals during some of the most pivotal moments of their lives. Witnessing the strength and resilience of birthing individuals, and being part of their journey, provides a deep sense of fulfillment and purpose.

Building meaningful relationships with clients is another significant reward. The trust and connection fostered during prenatal care, childbirth, and postpartum support create lasting bonds that enrich the midwifery experience. These relationships are central to empowering clients and ensuring positive outcomes.

Finally, midwifery plays a critical role in improving maternal and neonatal health outcomes. By advocating for equitable and compassionate care, midwives contribute to reducing mortality and morbidity rates, fostering healthier families and communities. The impact of this work resonates far beyond the individual, shaping the broader landscape of maternal healthcare.

Understanding Learning Styles in Adult Education

Midwifery students are predominantly adult learners who bring diverse experiences and backgrounds to their studies. Unlike traditional students, adult learners often balance education with significant responsibilities, including families, jobs, and other commitments. Recognizing and addressing their unique learning styles is crucial in creating a supportive educational environment, particularly in asynchronous and competency-based programs. By understanding different learning styles and applying tailored learning strategies, students can optimize their study habits to better retain information and best succeed in their educational endeavors.

Adult learners approach education with distinct traits:
- **Self-Direction:** Adult learners are naturally inclined to take ownership of their education. They often set personal goals, seek out additional resources, and actively engage with the material to align their studies with their individual aspirations and career objectives. This self-motivation makes them well-suited to asynchronous learning environments, where flexibility and autonomy are key.
- **Experience as a Resource:** The life experiences of adult learners serve as a valuable asset in their education. These experiences provide context for new knowledge, allowing learners to connect theoretical concepts to real-world applications. For example, a midwifery student who has previously worked in health care might find it easier to grasp clinical protocols or understand patient-centered care.
- **Pragmatic Orientation:** Adult learners prioritize learning that is immediately applicable. They are driven by the desire to acquire practical skills and knowledge that they can use in their professional roles. This pragmatic approach ensures that their education feels relevant and impactful, enhancing their engagement and commitment.
- **Intrinsic Motivation:** Personal growth and professional advancement are powerful motivators for adult learners. Unlike younger students, who may be influenced by external pressures, adult learners often pursue education out of a deep-seated desire to improve themselves and contribute meaningfully to their fields.

Pedagogy vs. Andragogy: Adaptations for Adult Learners

As an adult learner in midwifery, it's important to understand the difference between pedagogy and andragogy, as it influences how you engage with your education. Pedagogy, often associated with teaching children, focuses on a structured, teacher-directed approach where the learner depends heavily on the instructor for guidance. Andragogy emphasizes self-directed learning, a hallmark of adult education, where you take an active role in your educational journey.

In the andragogical model, you bring your life experiences into the learning process, using them to contextualize new knowledge. This approach values your ability to set goals, manage your time effectively, and integrate learning into real-world applications. For example, instead of passively listening to lectures, you might engage in collaborative discussions, tackle problem-solving activities, or reflect on how classroom concepts apply to clinical practice. Understanding this distinction empowers you to tailor your study methods and seek opportunities that align with your strengths as an adult learner.

Educational Theories in Adult Learning

Midwifery education is supported by numerous key theories of adult learning:

- **Andragogy** (Malcolm Knowles): Andragogy emphasizes the self-directed nature of adult learners and the importance of relevance in education. It highlights the need for problem-solving and the application of learning to real-life situations, making it particularly suited to competency-based programs.

- **Experiential Learning** (David Kolb): Kolb's model underscores the importance of learning through experience. His cycle of concrete experience, reflective observation, abstract conceptualization, and active experimentation aligns seamlessly with the practical nature of midwifery training.

- **Transformative Learning** (Jack Mezirow): This theory encourages learners to challenge existing beliefs and perspectives through critical reflection. It fosters adaptability and deeper understanding, preparing midwifery students to navigate the complexities of their profession.

- **Constructionism (Seymour Papert):** Constructionism expands on the idea of experiential learning by emphasizing that learners build their understanding most effectively through active creation. It focuses on the concept that knowledge is constructed when learners are engaged in creating tangible products or projects that reflect their learning.

- **Howard Gardner's Theory of Multiple Intelligences** Howard Gardner's theory proposes that individuals possess different types of intelligence, which influence how they learn and engage with material. In midwifery education, recognizing these diverse intelligences allows educators to tailor learning experiences that resonate with students' strengths, enhancing their ability to grasp complex concepts and apply them effectively.

- **Linguistic Intelligence:** Students with strong language skills benefit from reading, writing, and verbal discussions. They may excel in creating detailed care plans or informed consent documents.

- **Logical-Mathematical Intelligence:** These learners thrive on problem-solving and analytical tasks, such as interpreting lab results or creating evidence-based policies.

- **Visual-Spatial Intelligence:** Visual learners excel when information is presented through diagrams, charts, or anatomical models, making this intelligence crucial for mastering clinical skills.

- **Bodily-Kinesthetic Intelligence:** Hands-on learners flourish in practical environments like clinical rotations or simulations, where they can physically engage with the material.

- **Interpersonal Intelligence:** These students shine in collaborative settings, such as study groups or peer-led discussions, where they can explore concepts through interaction.

- **Intrapersonal Intelligence:** Reflective learners benefit from journaling and self-assessment, which allow them to connect personal growth with professional development.

The Spiral Method of Learning

The spiral method is a teaching approach in which topics are revisited at increasing levels of depth and complexity over time. Rather than mastering a concept in a single lesson, students return to it again and again—each time building on prior understanding. This approach reflects how knowledge deepens through experience: a student first learns the theory, then applies it in simulation, and finally integrates it through real-life clinical practice. By circling back to foundational ideas in new contexts, learners strengthen memory, develop critical thinking, and connect physiology, skills, and intuition into a cohesive whole.

Exploring Learning Styles

Understanding individual learning styles is essential for success in midwifery education. Common styles include:

- **Visual learners** process information best through images, diagrams, and spatial representations. Tools like flowcharts, anatomical illustrations, and video demonstrations are invaluable. They may also benefit from color-coded notes and apps that help visualize complex processes.
- **Auditory learners** thrive on spoken language and auditory input. They excel when listening to lectures, engaging in discussions, or using audio-based resources. Strategies include recording lectures, participating in group discussions, and using mnemonic devices that can be spoken or sung.
- **Kinesthetic learners** absorb information through movement and physical interaction. They benefit from clinical rotations, skills labs, and using physical models to study anatomy. Incorporating movement—such as pacing while reviewing material—can enhance retention.
- **Read/write learners** prefer textual information and written expression. They excel with textbooks, detailed note-taking, and written summaries. Writing essays, analyzing case studies, and organizing ideas in written form strengthens their understanding.
- **Multimodal Learning:** Many students use a blend of learning styles. For example, a student might read about a procedure, watch a demonstration, discuss it in a group, and then practice it hands-on. This multimodal approach creates an inclusive learning environment ensuring all students are supported, regardless of their dominant style.

Exercise 2.1: Matching Learning Styles to Strategies	
Write the correct letter next to each learning style.	
_____ Visual Learner	A. Use color-coded notes and diagrams
_____ Auditory Learner	B. Record and replay lectures
_____ Kinesthetic Learner	C. Practice with hands-on models
_____ Read/Write Learner	D. Write summaries and outlines

Exercise 2.2: What's Your Learning Style? Self-Assessment		
Rate how the statement applies to you (1 = Never, 5 = Always). Then, total the scores under each category.		
Statement	Score (1–5)	Learning Style
I remember best when I draw or visualize information.		Visual
I talk things through or say them out loud to understand.		Auditory
I learn best when I move or engage physically with the material.		Kinesthetic
I like to read and rewrite notes to learn.		Read/Write
Total Your Scores: Visual: _____ Auditory: _____ Kinesthetic: _____ Read/Write: _____ *Your highest score suggests your dominant learning style. If you have two or more high scores, you may benefit from a multimodal approach.*		

Hemispheric Dominance: Left-Brain vs. Right-Brain Learners

Understanding hemispheric dominance can also help you tailor your learning approach. Left-brain learners often excel at logical, analytical, and sequential tasks, such as interpreting clinical protocols or memorizing detailed processes. If you find yourself naturally inclined toward structured and step-by-step methods, focusing on creating charts or detailed care plans might enhance your studies.

Right-brain learners thrive in intuitive, creative, and holistic thinking. You might enjoy visualizing patient care scenarios, engaging in empathetic storytelling, or using diagrams and color-coded notes. Recognizing whether you lean more toward left-brain or right-brain dominance can help you develop strategies that align with your natural inclinations, making the process of learning more engaging and effective.

Exercise 2.3: Left/Right Brain Coloring

Color all the left-brain activities one color and the right-brain activities another color and then give examples of all the traits you possess that pertain to each.

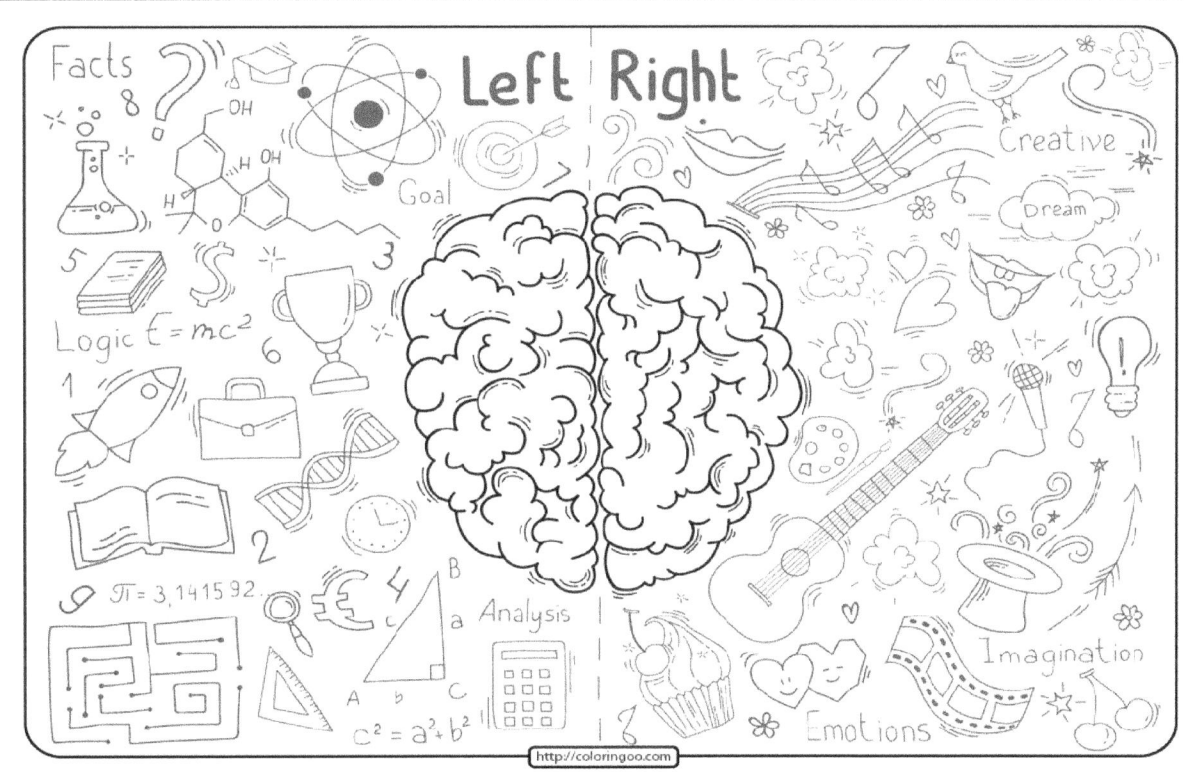

Left Brain Traits like: Analytical, Sequential, Verbal, Detail-oriented	**Right Brain Traits** like: Creative, Intuitive, Visual, Holistic

STRATEGIES FOR SUPPORTING LEARNING

As a midwifery student, you can enhance your learning by embracing strategies that cater to diverse learning styles and using tools designed to deepen your knowledge and skills:

- **Explore Varied Resources**: Make use of materials in multiple formats to match your learning preferences. If you're a visual learner, you might benefit from anatomy visualization apps, diagrams, and charts. Auditory learners can listen to recorded lectures or podcasts. Interactive tools, such as online anatomy platforms or case study simulations, are great for supporting all types of learners.
- **Engage Actively in Learning**: Hands-on practice is vital in midwifery. Participate in clinical simulations, case studies, or peer discussions whenever possible. If you're a kinesthetic learner, these activities will likely help you retain information better. Take advantage of live webinars or virtual skills labs for real-time interactions, and use self-paced tools, such as clinical skills videos or asynchronous simulations, for flexible learning.
- **Leverage Technology for Competency-Based Progress**: Utilize apps and online platforms that help you track your learning milestones and demonstrate competencies. Interactive quizzes, virtual prenatal exam simulations, and structured modules can guide your progress. For example, you could complete a self-paced clinical simulation, then review your performance with peers or instructors in a live debrief to refine your skills.
- **Embrace Reflection and Integrate Competencies**: Reflection is a powerful tool. Regularly take time to evaluate your experiences and identify areas for improvement. Consider keeping a portfolio that showcases your demonstrated competencies, or write reflective essays about specific clinical scenarios to deepen your understanding. Reflection not only supports professional growth but also helps you align your knowledge with real-world midwifery practice.

Exercise 2.4: Your Strategies for Supported Learning

List your personal strategies to address learning in these areas:

1. Explore Varied Resources:

2. Engage Actively in Learning:

3. Leverage Technology:

4. Embrace Reflection:

Asynchronous and Competency-Based Learning

Asynchronous learning environments allow students to study on their own schedules, offering flexibility to accommodate personal and professional responsibilities. Competency-based education further supports this model by focusing on mastery rather than time spent in class. These formats align well with the needs of adult learners by enabling them to:

- **Control Their Pace:** Students can spend more time on challenging areas while progressing quickly through material they grasp easily.
- **Focus on Mastery:** Competency-based programs ensure students demonstrate proficiency before advancing.
- **Integrate Learning with Life:** By fitting education into their existing routines, students maintain a balance between study and other responsibilities.

LEARNING DOMAINS AND TYPES

Midwifery education requires students to master a diverse set of competencies that span intellectual, emotional and physical domains, each of which plays a crucial role in shaping well rounded and effective practitioners. These competencies are often categorized using **Bloom's Taxonomy**, which divides learning into three primary domains: **cognitive**, **affective** and **psychomotor**. For midwifery students, developing all three domains is critical to their ability to provide safe care that is both compassionate and evidence-based, while also navigating the complex nature of childbirth, and the interpersonal relationships with the families they serve.

The interplay of these three domains reflects the multifaceted nature of midwifery. A skilled midwife must possess the intellectual *acumen* to interpret clinical evidence (cognitive), the emotional intelligence to build trust and provide information to clients in a meaningful, non-biased manner (affective) and the clinical proficiency to perform the interventions necessary to *keep birth in the community setting safe*. One domain's growth can enhance the other two domains because these domains are not compartmentalized learning experiences.

Achieving balance across all three domains in midwifery education ensures that students become competent clinicians as well as empathetic caregivers who honor the individual needs and cultural contexts of the families they serve. Recognizing the importance of all three learning domains also promotes reflective practice, a cornerstone of midwifery education, where students continually engage in assessment of their strengths and challenges, with a growth mindset which will help the midwife better meet the demands of this dynamic profession. Let's engage with each learning domain individually, in order to better understand learning goals for midwifery education.

Cognitive Domain: Understanding the Science of Clinical Midwifery Practice

The cognitive domain encompasses knowledge acquisition, critical thinking and problem-solving. These are fundamental aspects of midwifery education. IT focuses on developing the intellectual skills necessary to understand complex concepts and apply them in real-world situations. Important components include:

- **Theoretical foundations:** Midwifery students must master subjects such as anatomy, physiology, pharmacology and obstetric care. This foundational knowledge forms the basis for assessing client health and managing care competently.
- **Critical Thinking:** Students learn to analyze information, evaluate risks, engage in evidenced based decision making in all kinds of care settings.
- **Clinical Application:** The cognitive domain also includes interpreting data from diagnostic tools such as ultrasounds, lab results and antepartum/fetal monitoring.

> **Why It Matters**
> Strong cognitive skills enable midwives to engage in shared decision making from an evidence-based perspective, ensuring safety and optimal outcomes for clients and their families.

Affective Domain: Building Emotional Intelligence

Affective Domain: Developing the affective domain is not an abstract exercise—it has direct consequences for client outcomes. When midwives approach care with self-awareness and emotional intelligence, they can better recognize subtle cues from clients, de-escalate stressful situations, and create space for informed decision-making. This work also requires students to reflect on their own values, biases, and cultural frameworks, acknowledging how these shape the care they provide. Growth in the affective domain is a lifelong process, supporting midwives in building resilience and compassion throughout their careers. This domain centers on attitudes, values, and interpersonal skills essential to building trust and offering compassionate, culturally appropriate care, like:

- **Empathy and Emotional Intelligence**: Midwifery students must develop the ability to recognize and respond to clients' emotional needs while managing their own emotional growth and responses.
- **Communication and Rapport:** Effective midwifery care relies on the ability to build trust, listen actively and provide clear, supportive guidance during the birthing process.
- **Cultural Competence**: Understanding and respecting diverse cultural values around pregnancy, birth, and family is essential to creating a safe, inclusive care environment.

Psychomotor Domain: Clinical Competency and Technical Skills Development

The **psychomotor domain** focuses on the development of physical skills and technical competency, which are critical for performing hands-on skills safely and effectively. A key component of mastering these skills is muscle memory, the brain's ability to map and automate hands-on skills through repeated practice. Skill acquisition in the psychomotor domain goes beyond simply "checking off" competencies. Clinical training must balance precision with adaptability, recognizing that every birth unfolds differently. By pairing hands-on skill with critical thinking, students learn not just how to perform a technique, but when and why to use it. This integration of technical expertise with situational awareness ensures midwives can respond effectively, even under unpredictable conditions. Mastery of psychomotor skills also strengthens client trust, demonstrating professionalism and competence.

- **Technical Skills:** Midwifery students must learn procedures such as vaginal exams, suturing, administering medications and managing equipment. Muscle memory ensures these tasks can be performed with precision and confidence, even in high pressure situations.

> **Why It Matters**
> Proficiency in these skills ensures midwives can respond to both routine and emergency situations with precision and confidence.

- **Life Saving Techniques:** Emergency skills such as neonatal resuscitation or managing postpartum hemorrhage rely on well-developed clinical teaching strategies as well as repetition in practice to develop muscle memory so that you may execute them swiftly and accurately.
- **Dexterity and Confidence:** Repeated practice strengthens neural pathways, allowing actions to become automatic and freeing cognitive resources for decision making during critical moments. T Proficiency in these skills ensures midwives can respond to both routine and emergency situations with precision and confidence.

The three learning domains work together to create a learning experience that prepares students for the multifaceted demands of the profession. By weaving these domains together into a comprehensive learning program, provides students a mechanism for meeting the comprehensive and diverse needs of clients and their families. It reflects the professional commitment to combining clinical expertise with compassion, fostering better relationships, which leads to better outcomes and deeper connections.

Exercise 2.5: Integrating the Three Domains

Choose a recent learning experience from your midwifery training (a class, a clinical skill, or a client interaction). In the chart below, reflect on how each learning domain applied to that experience.

Learning Domain	How did this domain show up in your experience?
Cognitive What knowledge or critical thinking skills did you use?	
Affective How did you connect emotionally or build trust?	
Psychomotor What hands-on skills or physical techniques did you practice?	

Further Reflection:

1. Which domain do you feel strongest in right now?

2. Which one would you like to focus on improving?

Practical Application of Study Skills

Connecting Theory to Practice

A central goal of midwifery education is to integrate theoretical knowledge with clinical application. Being able to apply what one learns in textbooks, lectures, and discussions to real-world scenarios is essential for building confidence, competence, and the ability to offer safe, effective, and client-focused care. Theoretical knowledge is essential, but only clinical experience transforms it into practical skill. By applying what they learn to unpredictable situations, students develop critical thinking and learn to recognize labor progress, complications, and maternal coping in real time.

In the clinical setting, midwifery students must:

- **Navigate Unusual or Unpredictable Situations:** Birth and maternal care often involve unexpected variables that challenge theoretical models. Applying knowledge in real-time allows students to adapt and respond effectively.
- **Enhance Critical Thinking:** Clinical scenarios require midwives to synthesize information from multiple sources, assess risks, and make informed decisions under pressure.
- **Improve Patient Outcomes:** Translating theory into practice ensures that care is evidence-based and tailored to the unique needs of each client, ultimately improving health outcomes for mothers and babies.

> **Why It Matters**
> Learning happens most deeply when knowledge is applied and reflected upon. Experience without reflection risks repetition; theory without practice risks irrelevance.

Techniques for Bridging the Gap Between Study Materials and Real-World Midwifery Situations

- **Case Study Analysis:** Case studies are invaluable for connecting theory to practice. They provide a controlled environment in which students can explore complex clinical situations without real-world consequences. Students should approach them systematically by identifying key issues, applying relevant concepts, and proposing evidence-based solutions. Reflecting on case studies fosters problem-solving skills and prepares students for clinical practice.
- **Simulation-Based Learning:** Clinical scenarios replicated in a safe environment allow students to practice skills and decision-making without risking patient safety. Using manikins, role-playing, or virtual simulations, they can refine technical abilities and manage emergencies. Post-simulation debriefings provide an opportunity to analyze actions and identify areas for improvement.
- **Integrative Assignments:** Whenever students connect theoretical knowledge to hypothetical or observed clinical situations, understanding deepens. Writing care plans based on detailed scenarios encourages the application of textbook knowledge to practical decision-making.
- **Mentorship and Observation:** Observing experienced midwives bridges the gap between classroom learning and practice. Students gain insight into how seasoned practitioners apply theoretical principles, while mentors guide them in connecting concepts to patient care.
- **Reflection and Debriefing:** Reflection is critical for integrating learning. After each clinical experience, students should analyze their actions, consider alternatives, and identify areas for growth. Structured debriefings with instructors or peers offer a collaborative way to process experiences and connect them back to theory. This integration builds confidence and competence for a successful career.

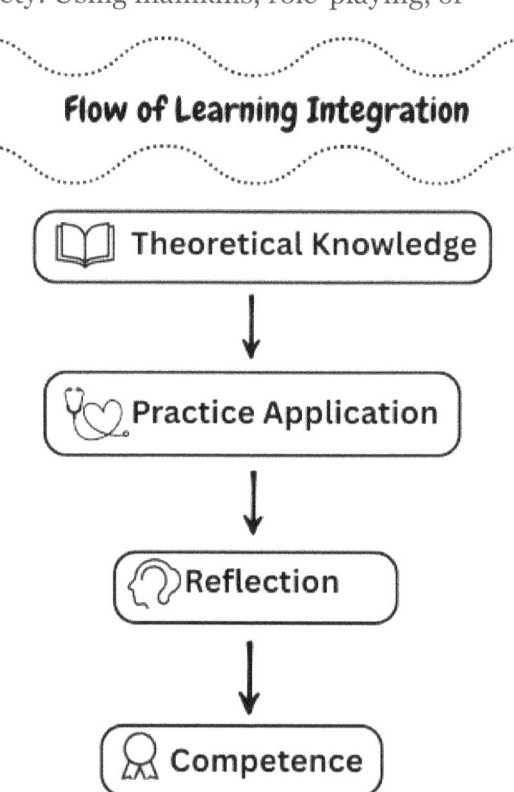

Flow of Learning Integration

Theoretical Knowledge → Practice Application → Reflection → Competence

Exercise 2.6: Clinical Scenario: Applying the Three Learning Domains

You are attending a laboring client at a birth center. They are 7 cm dilated, having regular contractions, and reporting intense lower back pain. On palpation, you note the fetal head is not well applied to the cervix, and the abdomen feels firm along the maternal flank. You recall from your studies this could indicate an occiput posterior (OP) position. Reflect on the scenario using the three learning domains below.

Cognitive Domain	Affective Domain	Psychomotor Domain
1. What do you know about fetal positioning that informs your assessment?	1. How do you support the client emotionally while assessing and managing the situation?	1. What hands-on comfort measures or position changes could you offer to encourage rotation?
2. What are the potential clinical implications of an OP position at this stage of labor?	2. How can you communicate clearly and respectfully about fetal position without increasing anxiety?	2. What hands-on comfort measures would you offer for pain?

Memory Enhancement Techniques

Midwifery students can benefit from employing memory enhancement techniques to retain critical information efficiently and effectively. These methods help organize complex material, making it easier to recall and apply in clinical settings:

- **Loci Method**: This technique involves associating information with specific physical locations. For instance, students might mentally link the stages of labor to different rooms in a birth center, creating a visual map to aid memory. This method is useful for retaining sequences or processes.
- **Chunking**: Breaking large volumes of information into smaller, manageable units improves retention. Pharmacology concepts, for example, can be categorized into groups such as analgesics, antibiotics, and uterotonic agents, allowing students to focus on one category at a time.
- **Mnemonics**: Simple phrases, acronyms, or rhymes can simplify complex information. An example in midwifery might be "**VEAL CHOP**," used to remember fetal heart rate patterns and their interpretations: **V**ariable = Cord compression, **E**arly = Head compression, **A**cceleration = Okay, **L**ate = Placental insufficiency.
- **Directed Visualization**: Visualization techniques involve creating mental images of procedures or anatomical structures. Students might visualize the steps of a prenatal exam or the process of fetal descent during labor, enhancing both understanding and confidence in clinical scenarios.

By integrating these techniques into their study routines, midwifery students can enhance their ability to retain and recall essential information, laying a solid foundation for their clinical practice. Here are some other systems of study and memory aids that may come in handy as you navigate your academic journey to midwifery excellence.

The 5-P Reading System and SQ4R Method for Active Reading and Comprehension

Both the 5-P Reading System and the SQ4R Method provide structured approaches to engaging with complex texts, making them highly effective for midwifery students navigating dense material. The 5-P Reading System emphasizes preparation and summary, guiding students to preview content, set learning goals, predict questions, process actively, and paraphrase in their own words to ensure comprehension. Similarly, the SQ4R Method builds on this by encouraging students to survey material, develop focused questions, read critically, recite key concepts, review their learning, and reflect on practical applications.

When combined, these methods offer a comprehensive strategy for mastering both theoretical and clinical content. For example, students could use the 5-P System to prepare for understanding a new protocol, then apply the SQ4R Method to analyze a case study, ensuring both retention and contextual understanding of the material.

The 5-P Reading System This system helps students approach reading assignments with a structured framework:

1. **PREVIEW** Skim headings, summaries, and keywords to get an overview.
2. **PREPARE** Set specific learning goals for the reading session.
3. **PREDICT** Formulate questions about the material to guide focused reading.
4. **PROCESS** Read actively, take notes, and highlight key points.
5. **PARAPHRASE** Summarize the material in your own words to solidify understanding.

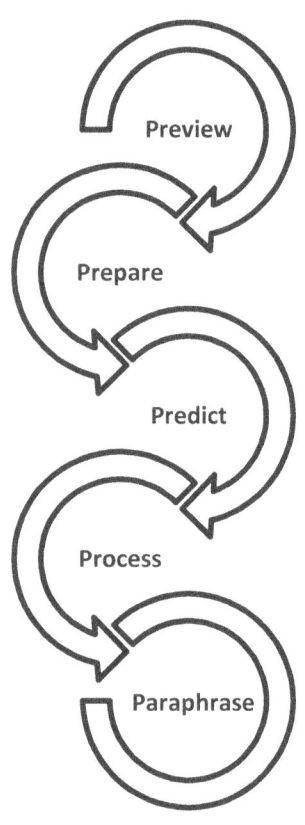

The SQ4R Method for Active Reading and Comprehension
This method encourages active engagement with texts:

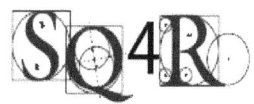

SURVEY Scan the material for an overall sense of content.

QUESTION Develop questions to focus on key concepts.

READ Dive into the text, seeking answers to your questions.

RECITE Repeat key ideas aloud or in written form to reinforce memory.

REPHRASE Write a brief summary or put in your own words.

REVIEW Revisit the material to deepen understanding and retention.

Survey - *Overview of chapter*
1. Read learning objectives.
2. Read introductory paragraph.
3. Read chapter title, headings, and subheadings.
4. Look at charts, pictures, graphs.
5. Read chapter summary, "words to remember," other help at end of chapter.
6. Read chapter questions.

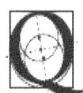

Question - *Purpose for reading*
1. Turn a heading or a subheading into a question by asking "who, what, when, where, why, or how."
2. If no headings, turn a topic sentence into a question.

Read - *For Comprehension*
1. Read one section actively to answer the question asked.
2. Compare or contrast with earlier materials studied.
3. Answer to the question should be the main idea of paragraph or section–highlight it.
4. Locate details and underline in pencil.
5. Study tables, graphs, and charts for that section, relating them to text reading.
6. Make 3x5 note cards for vocabulary.
7. Make annotations in text margins.

Recite - *For Understanding*
1. Read aloud highlighted answer to question asked.
2. State answer aloud from memory.
3. To understand – talk aloud to yourself about what is highlighted and underlined.
4. Do all of SQ4R process on one section at a time.

Rephrase - *Brief notes of chapter*
1. Write brief chapter outline; or
2. Write a brief summary on one notebook page.

Review - *For Retention*
1. Answer text questions.
2. Study highlighted and annotated information in text.
3. Use helpful memory cues.
4. Review vocabulary notecards.
5. Compare text notes to lecture notes.
6. Repeat this review weekly.

Integrating Didactic Material with Clinical Experience

Integrating didactic material with clinical practice is essential for building confidence and competence in midwifery students. This process allows theoretical concepts to take on practical meaning through direct application in real-world scenarios. Clinical rotations, placements, and long-term apprenticeship experiences immerse students in environments where they can engage with the material hands-on, connecting classroom knowledge with patient care.

By documenting clinical encounters and reflecting on their experiences, students deepen their understanding of core principles and recognize areas for growth. Practical assignments like creating shared decision-making tools or writing informed consent documents give students an opportunity to blend clinical evidence with communication strategies, preparing them to meet the needs of diverse clients. This dynamic integration ensures that students approach midwifery with both technical expertise and a nuanced understanding of patient-centered care. Assignments such as developing shared decision-making tools or informed consent documents further reinforce this learning, helping students translate evidence-based knowledge into client-centered care. These activities ensure that students not only understand theoretical material but also see its relevance in day-to-day midwifery practice.

Practical Application of Study Skills

This book supports students with exercises, quizzes, puzzles, and links to multimedia that deepen understanding of midwifery-specific material and offer interactive ways to engage with complex concepts. Midwifery education spans a wide range of topics, from anatomy and physiology to pharmacology and clinical care protocols. To manage this diverse content effectively, focus on strategies that meet your individual learning needs.

Tips for Studying Midwifery-Specific Materials
- **Prioritize key topics:** Begin with foundational areas such as fetal development, stages of labor, and common interventions. Mastery of these concepts provides a strong base for more advanced study.
- **Break it down:** Divide large subjects into manageable sections. For instance, study the anatomy of the pelvis one day and progress to fetal positioning the next.
- **Apply context:** Relating theory to real-world scenarios makes knowledge more meaningful and easier to recall.
- **Review regularly:** Frequent review reinforces learning and reduces the need for last-minute cramming. Spaced repetition—revisiting topics every few days—is especially effective.

Study Groups for Collaborative Learning

To get the most out of group study sessions:
- **Set clear goals:** Decide on a focus, such as prenatal care guidelines or postpartum assessments.
- **Assign roles:** Choose a discussion leader, note-taker, or timekeeper to keep the group on track.
- **Share perspectives:** Explore multiple approaches to clinical challenges, such as managing labor complications.
- **Teach each other:** Explaining a concept—like fetal monitoring or neonatal resuscitation—strengthens your own understanding.

Reflection and Debriefing

After each clinical experience, analyze your actions, consider alternatives, and identify areas for growth. Structured debriefing with instructors or peers offers a collaborative way to process experiences and connect them back to theory. This integration builds confidence and competence for professional practice.

Visual and Tactile Aids

Incorporate the following tools into your study routine:
- **Flashcards**: Create or use pre-made flashcards to memorize key terms and processes. For example, use cards to learn the stages of the menstrual cycle or the functions of specific medications (create some flash cards for this chapter to include).
- **Diagrams**: Study and label diagrams of anatomical structures like the pelvis, uterus, and fetal skull. Drawing or annotating these diagrams yourself can deepen your comprehension (create some diagrams to use).
- **Models**: Utilize anatomical models, such as those of the pelvis or fetal skull, to understand spatial relationships and practice skills like estimating fetal position. Midwifery programs often provide these tools, but you can also buy or borrow them for independent practice (these are already in the book).

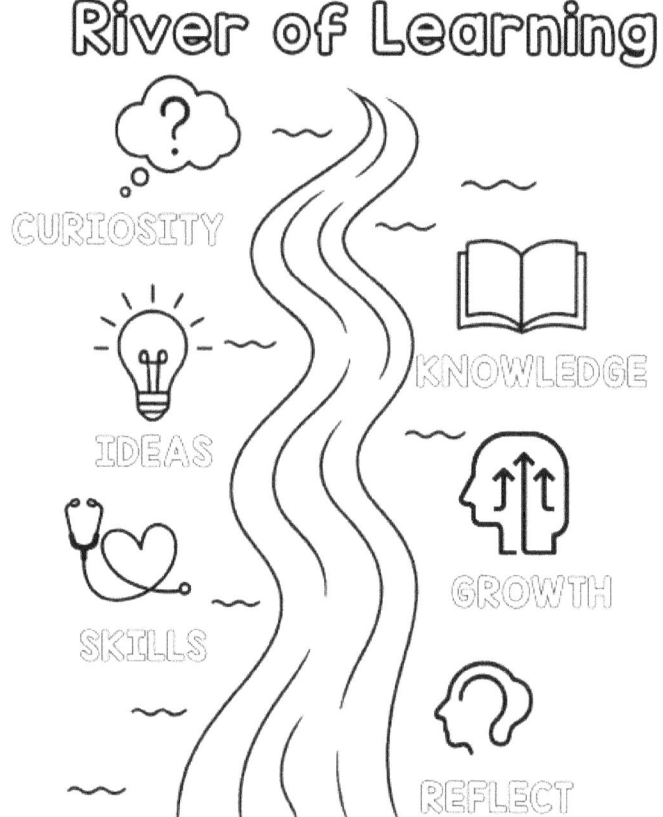

Using Grading Rubrics as a Learning Tool

Grading rubrics are not just tools for earning grades—they are guides to help you understand expectations and improve. Each educational program provides you with grading rubrics, and they all differ. Rubrics break down assignments and skills into clear, specific criteria so you can focus on what matters most. Whether you are writing SOAP notes, practicing clinical skills, or creating a client education tool, rubrics show you exactly how to succeed.

Examples of Two Types of Rubrics Scores

Analytic: Communication

4 = Consistently uses active listening and respectful language.

3 = Usually listens well, occasional lapses.

2 = Attempts active listening but misses key cues.

1 = Rarely demonstrates empathy or active listening.

Holistic: Communication

4 (Excellent): Clear, compassionate communication demonstrated consistently.

3 (Proficient): Generally effective communication; minor lapses in clarity or tone.

2 (Developing): Communication sometimes unclear; rapport inconsistently maintained.

1 (Needs Improvement): Frequent communication barriers; rapport not established.

Analytic: Technical Skill

4 = Performs procedures smoothly and accurately with confidence.

3 = Performs procedures with minor hesitation or errors.

2 = Inconsistent skills, requires frequent correction.

1 = Unable to complete procedures safely.

Holistic: Technical Skill

4 (Excellent): Skills performed accurately and confidently, inspiring client trust.

3 (Proficient): Skills generally safe and accurate, with occasional errors.

2 (Developing): Skills inconsistently safe; needs close supervision.

1 (Needs Improvement): Skills unsafe or incomplete; unable to perform independently.

How Grading Rubrics Help You Learn

- **Understanding expectations:** Rubrics outline the exact components of an assignment or skill evaluation. *Example:* A rubric for SOAP notes might include sections on documenting subjective and objective data, making an accurate assessment, and planning appropriate care.
- **Checking your work:** Use rubrics to review your own work before submitting it, and identify areas for improvement. *Example:* Before presenting a client education tool, check whether the content is accurate, easy to understand, and visually engaging.
- **Clear feedback:** A graded rubric highlights both your strengths and areas for growth. *Example:* A skills rubric might note that your sterile-glove technique was excellent but that your timing needs practice.

Structured Practice and Reflection

- **Skill practice:** Use rubrics during simulations to guide your performance. *Example:* A neonatal resuscitation rubric might include steps for preparing equipment, following the correct sequence, and communicating effectively.
- **Peer support:** Pair with a classmate to evaluate each other's practice using rubrics. This helps you learn from feedback and see different approaches.
- **Reflection and debriefing:** After each clinical experience, analyze your actions, consider alternatives, and identify areas for growth. Structured debriefings with instructors or peers provide a collaborative way to connect practice back to theory.

By applying theory through case studies, simulations, mentorship, and reflection, midwifery students build the confidence and competence necessary for a successful and meaningful career.

Exercise 2.7: Self-Assessment with a Rubric	
Choose a recent assignment or skill check. Using the rubric:	
1. Highlight the criteria where you met expectations.	1. Write down one area where you can improve.
2. Write down one concrete action you will take next time (e.g., "review fetal heart rate categories before clinical").	2. Write down one area where you need further study.

TIME MANAGEMENT FOR BUSY STUDENTS

Identifying and Mitigating Distractions

Many midwifery programs are asynchronous, meaning that much of the studying takes place in the home environment. While this flexibility allows you to tailor your study schedule, it also presents challenges such as managing distractions and integrating the demands of clinical placements into your academic routine. To achieve the best outcomes, it's crucial to approach both your study space and time with intention and structure. Start by identifying the sources of your distractions and understanding how they impact your ability to concentrate. Awareness is the first step toward implementing effective solutions.

Distractions can disrupt your focus and productivity, particularly in a home study setting. These may include:
- **Digital Distractions**: notifications, social media, and emails that pull attention away from important tasks.
- **Environmental Factors**: noise, clutter, or interruptions from family members or roommates.
- **Mental Distractions**: stress from clinical responsibilities, overthinking, or difficulty staying motivated.

Creating an Intentional Study Space

A dedicated, distraction-free study space is vital for focus. Choose an area that is separate from places used for relaxation or family activities, keeping it clean, organized, and equipped with the tools you need, such as textbooks, a computer, and a notebook. Good lighting, comfortable seating, and calming elements like plants or soft music can make your space more inviting.

If household noise is a challenge, noise-canceling headphones or a white noise machine can help. Communicate with family or housemates about your study schedule and use visual cues like a "do not disturb" sign to set boundaries and minimize interruptions.

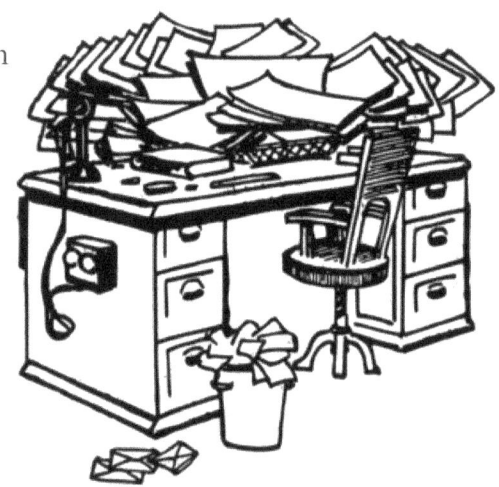

Cluttered spaces invite cluttered thinking

Integrating Clinical Placements into the Study Process

The rigors of clinical placements can make it challenging to balance study time, but integrating your clinical experiences into your learning can deepen your understanding and improve your outcomes. Here's how:

- **Reflect on Clinical Experiences**: use your study time to review and connect clinical scenarios with your academic material. For instance, after observing a specific procedure, study the associated anatomy, physiology, and best practices.
- **Link Clinical Practice with Study Goals**: if you encounter a topic in clinical placement that feels challenging, prioritize it during your next study session. This makes your learning more relevant and targeted.
- **Collaborate with Preceptors**: seek feedback from your clinical preceptors about areas for improvement and incorporate their guidance into your study routine.
- **Use Clinical Cases to Solidify Knowledge**: write brief case studies or reflections from your clinical experience to reinforce your understanding of key concepts.
- **Discuss Clinical Cases in Study Groups**: be sure to respect client privacy and not use names or personal details.
- **Keeping a birth journal** can help connect clinical practice with study goals. Remember to protect client privacy by never using full names or identifying details—use initials or general descriptions instead.

Example 1:
   Date: 4/15/26
   Birth #: 3 (observed)
   Role: Assisted with vitals and charting
   Reflections: Noted how the midwife explained informed consent before starting IV therapy—clear communication reduced the client's anxiety. I want to review pharmacology for IV fluids and practice phrasing explanations in simple, supportive language.

Example 2:
   Date: 5/20/26
   Birth #: 5 (assisted)
   Role: Practiced Leopold's maneuvers with supervision
   Reflections: Identified fetal position correctly with guidance, but found it difficult to distinguish the back from small parts. Plan to review fetal positions in anatomy text and practice more under supervision to build confidence.

Exercise 2.8: Integrating Clinical Knowledge

Write about a recent clinical experience (birth you observed, skill you practiced, or situation you discussed with your preceptor).

1. What happened? (Keep it general, protect client privacy.)

2. What did you learn from the experience?

3. What topic or skill will you study or practice next to strengthen your understanding?

Building Flexibility and Balance

Life and clinical work can be unpredictable, so build flexibility into your schedule to account for unexpected tasks or moments of rest. By adapting to changes while staying committed to your goals, you can prevent small disruptions from derailing your progress.

By recognizing distractions, creating an intentional study space, integrating clinical experiences into your learning, and structuring your time effectively, you'll set yourself up for success in both your academic and clinical responsibilities. This integrated approach ensures you're not just meeting the demands of your program but excelling in it.

Managing Your Study Time Intentionally

Effective time management helps you balance coursework, clinical responsibilities, and personal needs. Develop a weekly plan that outlines clear objectives, such as reviewing a chapter or practicing a skill.

Use tools like:

- **SMART Goal Setting**: helps keep you on track to accomplish your goals.
- **Time Blocking**: allocate specific hours for coursework, clinical review, and rest, ensuring that no area is neglected.
- **Task Prioritization**: tackle the most critical tasks during your peak focus times to maximize efficiency.
- **The Pomodoro Method**: alternate focused 25-minute study sessions with 5-minute breaks, taking a longer break after four cycles.

Be realistic about what you can accomplish and avoid overloading your schedule and inducing overwhelm. Short, intentional breaks can help recharge your energy and maintain concentration. Activities like stretching, a quick walk, or mindfulness exercises can provide a much-needed mental reset.

SMART Goal-Setting

Effective time management starts with setting clear and achievable goals. Using the **SMART** framework (Specific, Measurable, Achievable, Relevant, Time-bound) helps you stay focused and organized.

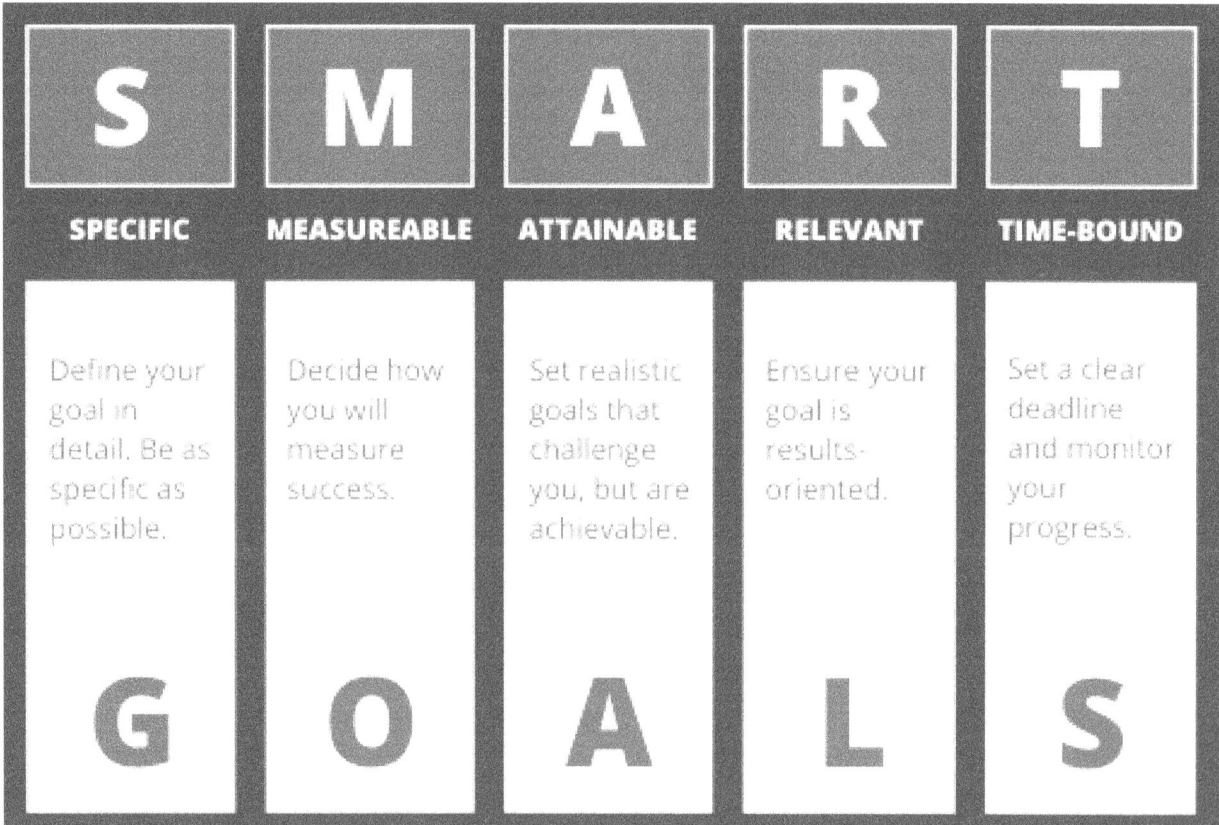

Examples of SMART goal setting:
Improving Prenatal Care Knowledge
- **Specific:** I will increase my knowledge of prenatal care by studying the most common complications of pregnancy, including preeclampsia, gestational diabetes, and placenta previa.
- **Measurable:** I will complete one chapter of a relevant textbook and one online research article weekly, summarizing key points in a study guide.
- **Achievable:** I will dedicate two hours every Wednesday to focused reading and summarizing, ensuring steady progress.
- **Relevant:** Understanding common complications is crucial for providing evidence-based care.
- **Time-bound:** I will complete my study guide and review by the end of the current semester.

Enhancing Clinical Skills
- **Specific:** I will improve my skill in performing venipunctures by practicing under supervision during clinic days.
- **Measurable:** I will successfully perform fifteen venipunctures on clients by the end of the next clinical rotation.
- **Achievable:** I will request opportunities to perform venipunctures at least twice during each clinic shift.
- **Relevant:** Developing proficiency in venipuncture is essential for a midwife.
- **Time-bound:** I will achieve this goal within the next six weeks of clinical practice.

Strengthening Communication Skills
- **Specific:** I will enhance my communication skills by learning and applying active listening techniques during client interactions.
- **Measurable:** I will incorporate active listening in at least five client visits per week, reflecting on what worked and what didn't in my journal.
- **Achievable:** I will dedicate 15 minutes at the end of each clinic day to journaling and reviewing my communication approach.
- **Relevant:** Effective communication builds trust and ensures clients feel heard and supported during their care.
- **Time-bound:** I will evaluate my progress and adjust techniques after three weeks.

Creating a Balanced Schedule

Balancing coursework, clinical rotations, and personal responsibilities can feel overwhelming, but a well-structured schedule can ease the load. Start by identifying your priorities and allotting time blocks for study, rest, and family. Use tools like digital planners or apps to track deadlines and appointments. Structured schedules with SMART goals creates a balance to responsibilities while supporting personal well-being.

Example 1: **Weekday Clinical and Study Schedule**
  Goal: Balance clinical rotation, coursework, and self-care on weekdays.
  Schedule:
  - 6:30 AM - 7:30 AM: Morning routine (breakfast, light exercise, or prayer/meditation).
  - 8:00 AM - 3:00 PM: Clinical rotation.
  - 3:30 PM - 5:00 PM: Study session (review clinical notes or assigned coursework).
  - 5:30 PM - 6:30 PM: Dinner and personal time.
  - 7:00 PM - 8:30 PM: Family time or light coursework (like reading).
  - 9:00 PM: Wind down and bedtime routine.

SMART Goal Example:
- **Specific:** I will dedicate 90 minutes to studying after clinical rotations three times per week.
- **Measurable:** I will complete one chapter or review two client cases during each session.
- **Achievable:** By keeping study sessions short and focused, I can balance learning with rest.
- **Relevant:** Consistent review will reinforce my clinical knowledge.
- **Time-bound:** I will maintain this schedule for the next four weeks and assess its effectiveness.

Example 2: **Weekend Focused Catch-Up Schedule**
　Goal: Use weekends for catching up on assignments and preparing for the week ahead.
　Schedule:
- 8:00 AM - 9:00 AM: Morning routine and review of the day's goals.
- 9:30 AM - 12:00 PM: Focused study session (assignments or exam prep).
- 12:30 PM - 1:30 PM: Lunch and relaxation.
- 2:00 PM - 4:00 PM: Skill-building (practice suturing or review procedures).
- 4:30 PM - 6:30 PM: Personal time (hobbies, family, or relaxation).
- 7:00 PM - 8:30 PM: Light reading or preparation for Monday.

SMART Goal Example:
- **Specific:** I'll complete two study sessions and one practical skill-building session every Saturday.
- **Measurable:** I'll track my progress by finishing two assignments and practicing one clinical skill.
- **Achievable:** By focusing on high-priority tasks during two sessions, I can manage my workload.
- **Relevant:** Staying on top of coursework and clinical skills ensures I meet my program requirements.
- **Time-bound:** I will follow this schedule every Saturday for the next month.

Example 3: Midweek Recharge Plan
　Goal: Include intentional rest and flexibility to recharge during busy weeks.
　Schedule:
- **7:00 AM - 8:00 AM**: Morning walk and breakfast.
- **8:30 AM - 3:00 PM**: Clinical rotation or coursework.
- **3:30 PM - 5:00 PM**: Nap, light yoga, or another restful activity.
- **5:30 PM - 7:00 PM**: Study session (summarizing key topics from the week).
- **7:30 PM - 9:00 PM**: Dinner and screen-free personal time.

SMART Goal Example:
- **Specific:** I will take a 30-minute rest break after clinical rotations twice per week.
- **Measurable:** I will log my rest activities to ensure they last 30 minutes and leave me refreshed.
- **Achievable:** A short, intentional break fits easily into my day.
- **Relevant:** Rest will help me maintain focus and avoid burnout.
- **Time-bound:** I will evaluate this habit after three weeks and adjust as needed.

Exercise 2.9: SMART Goal Setting	
Use SMART goals to create clear objectives for your own learning	
1. Specific	
2. Measurable	
3. Achievable	
4. Relevant	
5. Time Bound	

THE EISENHOWER MATRIX

The Eisenhower Matrix is a powerful tool to help midwifery students organize their task lists and manage priorities effectively. By categorizing tasks into four quadrants—**urgent and important**, **important but not urgent**, **urgent but not important**, and **neither urgent nor important**—you can focus your time and energy on what truly matters while staying organized and on track. A well-structured task list ensures that critical responsibilities, including personal and professional planning for long-term goals, are addressed in a manageable and productive way.

1. **Urgent and Important**

    Tasks in this quadrant require immediate attention and are vital for academic or clinical success. **Action**: Focus on these tasks first to avoid last-minute stress.

    Examples:
    - Completing clinical documentation due within the next 24 hours.
    - Preparing for an upcoming exam.
    - Submitting assignments by the deadline.
    - Paying the overdue electric bill.

2. **Important but Not Urgent**

    Tasks that are essential for long-term success but don't need to be completed immediately. Proactively managing these ensures steady progress toward your goals. **Action**: Plan and schedule these tasks into your calendar, breaking them into manageable steps and allotting specific time blocks for each.

    Examples:
    - Reviewing syllabi at the start of the semester to map out deadlines and assignments.
    - Creating a study schedule aligned with clinical rotations and coursework.
    - Practicing clinical skills, like fetal positioning or neonatal resuscitation.
    - Reading textbook chapters ahead of class discussions.
    - Drafting outlines for long-term projects or assignments.

3. **Urgent but Not Important**

    These tasks demand attention but do not significantly impact your learning achievements. They can often be delegated or scheduled during less productive times. **Action**: Delegate these tasks if possible, or batch them to complete efficiently without consuming valuable focus time.

Examples:
- Organizing study materials or cleaning your workspace.
- Responding to routine emails or non-urgent peer messages.
- Printing materials or preparing non-critical supplies for class.
- Addressing minor logistical issues related to your schedule or assignments.

4. Neither Urgent nor Important

Tasks in this category are distractions that do not contribute to your academic or clinical goals. Reducing or eliminating them allows you to focus more effectively. **Action**: Minimize these tasks to maintain focus on higher-priority responsibilities.

Examples:
- Scrolling through social media during study sessions.
- Watching unrelated videos or shows while procrastinating.
- Reorganizing your workspace unnecessarily instead of tackling tasks.
- Spending excessive time personalizing notes or presentations.

Integrating the Eisenhower Matrix into Task Management

By systematically categorizing and addressing tasks, this tool helps maintain organization, minimize stress, and focus on achieving learning goals and academic success. When organizing your overall task list, include all responsibilities—both immediate and long-term—such as:

Reviewing syllabi early in the semester to identify important deadlines and map out priorities.
Creating weekly outlines to plan and adjust tasks based on clinical rotations and study goals.
Scheduling time for skill practice and proactive preparation for exams or assignments.
Regularly reassess your task list to ensure alignment with your academic and clinical objectives.

Exercise 2.10: Your Personal Matrix
Place examples of your personal tasks under each category

Urgent & Important	Important Not Urgent
Do now	Do Later
Urgent but Not Important	**Neither Urgent nor Important**
Delegate	Delete

THE POMODORO TECHNIQUE

A time management method that breaks work into focused 25-minute intervals, called "pomodoros," separated by short breaks. After four pomodoros, a longer break is taken. This technique aims to improve focus and productivity by breaking down large tasks into smaller, manageable chunks.

Breakdown of the Pomodoro Technique:
1. **Choose a task:** Select the specific task you want to focus on.
- **Set a timer for 25 minutes:** This is one "pomodoro".
- **Work on the task:** Focus solely on the chosen task without distractions for the entire 25 minutes.
- **Take a short break:** After the timer rings, take a 5-minute break to rest and recharge.
- **Repeat:** Complete steps 2-4 four times.
- **Take a longer break:** After four pomodoros, take a longer break, typically 15-30 minutes.

Exercise 2.11 Pomodoro Planner		
Create a schedule for yourself using "pomodoros"		
Time Block	**Task/Goal**	**Notes/Reflection**
Block One (25 minutes)		
Five Minute Break		
Block Two (25 minutes)		
Five Minute Break		
Block Three (25 minutes)		
Five Minute Break		
Block Four (25 minutes)		
Active Break (15-30 minutes)		

IMPORTANCE OF SELF-CARE IN STUDY ROUTINES

Maintaining your physical and mental well-being is essential for effective learning and thriving in midwifery training. Balancing coursework, clinical placements, and personal responsibilities can be demanding, but incorporating self-care into your routine helps reduce stress and fosters resilience. Scheduling regular breaks, engaging in physical activity, and prioritizing healthy eating and sleep are foundational practices that enhance your ability to absorb and retain information. Midwifery requires compassion and endurance—qualities that are best nurtured by taking care of yourself first.

Why Self-Care Matters:
- **Enhanced Focus and Retention:** taking care of your body and mind allows you to concentrate better and retain information more effectively.
- **Emotional Stability:** self-care supports your ability to navigate the emotional highs and lows of clinical training.
- **Prevention of Burnout:** by managing stress proactively, you create a sustainable and less overwhelming learning experience.

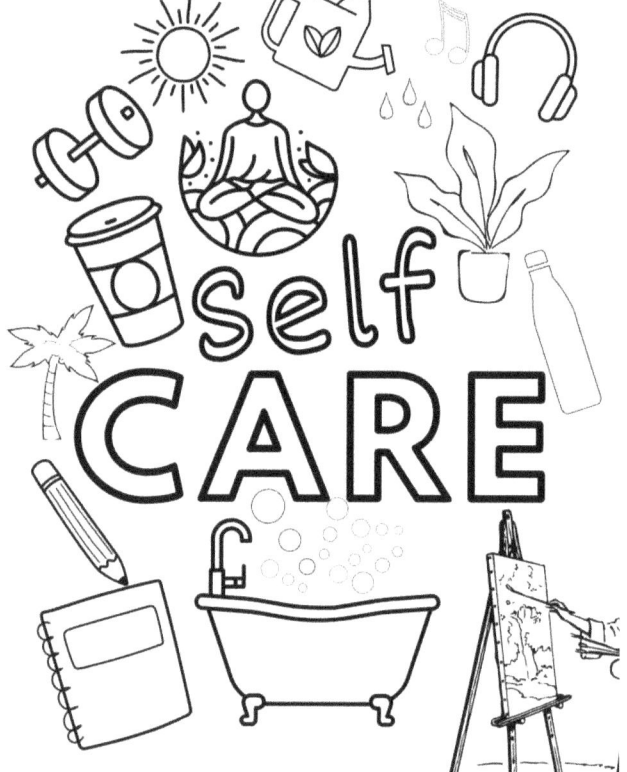

Examples of Self-Care in Action
- **Structuring Study Sessions** with Breaks.
- Use the **Pomodoro Technique** to alternate 25-minute focused study sessions with 5-minute breaks. This method prevents mental fatigue and reinforces retention.
    - *Example:* A student reviewing neonatal resuscitation could dedicate one Pomodoro session to memorizing algorithms and another to practicing steps with a study buddy.
- **Prioritizing Rest and Activity:** Incorporate light physical activities like yoga or walking into your routine to manage stress and boost energy. Pair this with consistent sleep schedules to ensure recovery.
    - *Example:* After a long clinical shift, a student might take a 10-minute walk to decompress and clear their mind before reviewing the day's notes.
- **Using a Master Calendar for Balance:** Plan your week with a calendar that includes study blocks, clinical responsibilities, self-care activities, and relaxation time.
    - *Example*: A student could schedule an hour after clinical shifts to review notes, followed by 30 minutes of unwinding with a book or favorite show.
- **Building Accountability with a Study Buddy:** Partnering with a study buddy is an excellent way to reinforce key concepts and stay motivated. Discussing material together not only deepens understanding but also creates accountability for study habits.
    - *Example:* Two students might schedule weekly sessions to review clinical scenarios or quiz each other on pharmacology, ensuring both stay on track and feel supported.
- **Mindfulness and Spiritual Practices:** Dedicate a few minutes each day to mindfulness activities like meditation, reflection, prayer, journaling, or deep breathing exercises. These practices help process emotions and maintain focus. If you have a spiritual practice, tend it like a garden, with daily attention. Attending church or cultural events can be part of your self-care. Sharing with others who have the same beliefs can strengthen your faith.
    - *Example:* A student could reflect on a particular client, perhaps one who is struggling, giving prayers or positive thoughts.

INTEGRATING EDUCATIONAL TOOLS

Leveraging technology and diverse educational resources can significantly enhance your learning experience. The following tools—ranging from apps to online platforms—provide opportunities for skill development, deeper understanding of medical concepts, and practical application of midwifery knowledge.

Apps for Medical Terminology
1. **Medical Terminology Quiz & Dictionary** *(Free)*
   Provides quick reference guides and quizzes to test your understanding of medical terms commonly used in midwifery and obstetrics.
2. **Medscape** *(Free)*
   Offers a comprehensive resource for medical terminology, drug interactions, and clinical guidelines, tailored to health care professionals.
3. **Complete Anatomy** *(Paid, Free Trial Available)*
   A 3D anatomy platform with detailed visuals and interactive features, perfect for visual learners.

Online Simulations and Case Studies
1. **Virtual Obstetric Patient Simulator** (VOPSim) *(Paid)*
   Simulates real-life scenarios in obstetrics and gynecology, allowing students to practice decision-making skills in a safe environment.
2. **Global Library of Women's Medicine** (GLOWM) *(Free)*
   Offers free access to case studies, clinical guidelines, and videos on maternal health topics.
3. **Oxford Medical Simulation** *(Paid)*
   Provides immersive clinical scenarios in midwifery and other healthcare specialties to build confidence in managing complex situations.
4. **Kahn Academy Health & Medicine** *(Free)*
   Includes videos and quizzes on human anatomy, physiology, and other foundational topics.

Using Textbooks and Supplementary Resources Effectively
1. **Open Textbook Library** *(Free)*
   A collection of openly licensed textbooks, including options for anatomy, physiology, and maternal health.
2. **Elsevier's Midwifery Resources** *(Paid)*
   Access comprehensive textbooks like *Myles Textbook for Midwives* and supplementary tools like study guides and test banks.
3. **E-Book Platforms** (e.g., Kindle, Apple Books) *(Paid)*
   Digital versions of core textbooks are often more affordable and portable than print editions.

Utilizing Charts, Graphs, and Videos
1. **The WHO Reproductive Health Library** (RHL) (Free)
   A repository of charts, infographics, and tools on evidence-based reproductive health care practices.
2. **YouTube Educational Channels** (Free). Search midwifery or the topic you are studying.
3. **MamaDoctorJones:** Videos on maternal and reproductive health.
4. **Canva for Education** (Free and Paid Plans)
   Create custom charts, infographics, and visual aids to simplify complex topics or prepare presentations.

Medical Education Lectures: Anatomy and midwifery-related tutorials.
1. **UpToDate** (Paid, Free for Some Institutions)
   A trusted resource for evidence-based charts, algorithms, and guidelines for midwifery practice.
2. **Stanford Medicine Clinical Anatomy Lectures** (Free)
   Stanford University offers free, detailed anatomy dissection videos with a clinical focus. While not midwifery-specific, they offer a deep dive into structures relevant to obstetrics and gynecology.

Tips for Integrating Educational Tools
- **Create a Study Schedule:** allocate specific times for using each resource, ensuring a balance between apps, textbooks, and simulations.
- **Combine Resources:** use multiple tools to reinforce learning. For example, review a topic in a textbook, watch a related video, and practice with a case study.
- **Use Tools Actively:** engage with the content by taking notes, answering quizzes, and applying knowledge through simulations.
- **Share and Collaborate:** discuss what you learn with peers or study buddies, leveraging tools like shared video tutorials or interactive quizzes.
- **Evaluate Effectiveness:** regularly assess whether a tool aligns with your learning style and goals, replacing less effective tools with more suitable ones.

ASSESSMENT AND FEEDBACK

Assessment and feedback are critical for mastering midwifery content and building confidence in both academic and clinical settings. This book provides not only up-to-date, applicable information but also an array of learning tools from across the educational spectrum. These tools reinforce key concepts, foster critical thinking, and prepare students for test-taking and exams. Self-assessment strategies, peer and instructor feedback, and diverse learning methodologies empower students to take ownership of their education and achieve success.

The Role of Self-Assessment in Mastering Content

Self-assessment allows students to reflect on their knowledge and skills, actively identifying strengths and areas for improvement. This reflective practice builds self-awareness and encourages a proactive approach to learning, helping students address gaps before they become barriers to success.

Strategies for Self-Assessment:
- **Knowledge Checklists:** after studying a topic, list concepts you feel confident about and those requiring further review.
- **Practice Questions:** use mock exams, online quizzes, or textbook exercises to test retention and identify weak points.
- **Tracking Progress:** keep a journal or study log to document achievements, challenges, and improvements.

The Importance of Peer and Instructor Feedback

Feedback from peers and instructors provides essential external perspectives that complement self-assessment. Constructive feedback highlights blind spots and reinforces learning through collaboration and mentorship.

How to Maximize Feedback:
- **Peer Discussions:** study groups or partnerships encourage shared learning, allowing students to explain concepts to one another and address misunderstandings collaboratively.
- **Instructor Guidance:** seek clarification on challenging topics during office hours or clinical debriefs. Instructors can provide targeted advice to improve understanding and performance.
- **Simulated Scenarios:** practice clinical skills in simulations, followed by debriefs that offer detailed feedback on technique and decision-making.

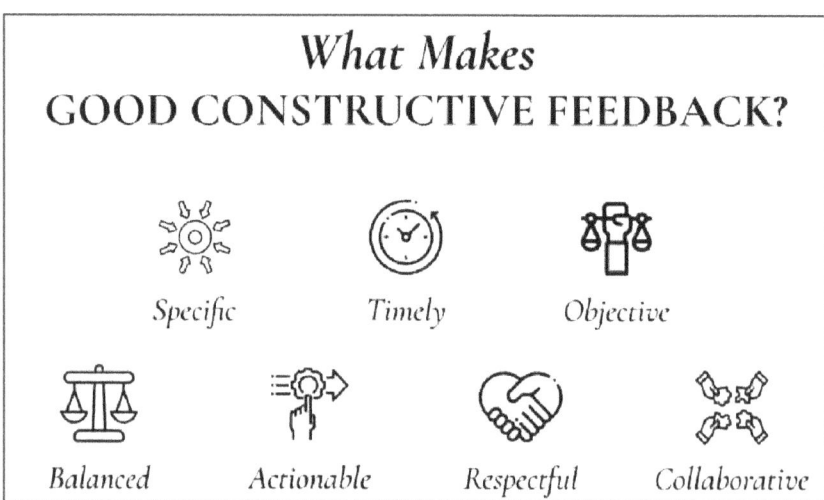

Strategies for Preparing for Exams and Certifications

Midwifery exams and certifications require not only content mastery but also effective test-taking strategies. This book integrates diverse tools and methods to help students feel confident and ready.

Exam Preparation Tips:
- **Structured Study Plans:** use calendars or planners to break down material into manageable sections and set specific goals for each session.
- **Active Recall:** practice retrieving information without looking at notes, such as answering questions or summarizing topics aloud.
- **Mock Exams:** simulate test conditions by timing yourself on practice exams and reviewing incorrect answers to target weak areas.
- **Rest and Self-Care:** prioritize sleep, nutrition, and stress management in the days leading up to the exam to ensure optimal performance.

A Holistic Approach to Learning

By leveraging self-assessment, feedback, and diverse educational tools, students can build a strong foundation of knowledge and skills while feeling well-prepared for exams and certifications. This integrated approach ensures that learning is not only effective but also adaptable to the unique challenges of midwifery education. Through reflection, collaboration, and strategic preparation, students can confidently progress toward their academic and professional goals.

The Value of Mentorship

School-based mentorship programs, such as Hivemind, Houses, Student Mentors, or Guidance Counselors offer invaluable support for midwifery students. These programs are designed to keep you on task, maintain accountability, and provide resources when challenges arise. Mentors or guidance teams can help you set achievable goals, navigate complex coursework, and advocate for you if you struggle. Regularly engaging with these programs fosters a sense of connection and support, ensuring you stay focused on your academic and professional objectives while building resilience for the journey ahead.

Exercise 2.12: Preparing for Exams
Fill out the following:
1. Choose one new strategy from this section that you will try. Write how you will apply it in your study routine.
2. List one study strategy (e.g., structured plan, active recall, mock exams, or self-care) you already use. How does it help you?
3. Who could you turn to for mentorship or support during your studies? List at least one person or program.

Printable Tips for Students Beginning their Midwifery Journey

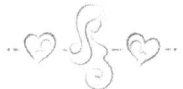

Clinical Tips to Keep You Grounded

- **Assess before acting.** Slow down, observe, and gather information. The best decisions come from a steady mind and a full picture.
- **Keep your hands warm and your voice soft**. Your presence is an intervention; let it be a calming one.
- **Chart in real time whenever possible.** Clear, contemporaneous documentation protects you and supports continuity of care.
- **When something feels "off," investigate.** Pattern changes often speak louder than numbers. Trust your training and your instincts.
- **Support physiologic processes first.** Movement, hydration, rest, privacy, and encouragement often restore progress more effectively than intervention.

Must-Know Definitions

- **Physiologic Birth:** Birth driven by the body's own hormonal and mechanical processes without unnecessary interference.
- **Uterine Tone**: The firmness of the uterus postpartum, crucial for identifying early signs of hemorrhage.
- **Station:** The measurement of fetal descent in relation to the ischial spines, ranging from −5 to +5.
- **Effacement:** The thinning and shortening of the cervix during labor, expressed as a percentage.
- **Neonatal Transition:** The newborn's shift from placental to independent breathing and circulation in the first minutes after birth.

Common Pitfalls (and How to Avoid Them)

- **Getting lost in monitoring vitals.** Always correlate numbers with the person in front of you.
- **Skipping the social history.** Emotional support systems, stress, and lived experience shape pregnancy as much as physiology.
- **Over-reassurance.** If a concern arises, explore it honestly and offer options rather than dismissing it.
- **Neglecting your own needs.** Hungry, tired midwives make mistakes. Keep snacks, water, and boundaries.
- **Forgetting the power of small things**. A sip of water, a changed position, a reassuring touch—these details often shift the course of a challenging moment.

Checklist: Essentials for Your First Clinical Bag

☐ Pen, small notebook, and backup pen

☐ Gloves, hand sanitizer, and compact first-aid kit

☐ Watch with a second hand

☐ Measuring tape and BP cuff, stethoscope, fetoscope

☐ Snacks, water bottle, spare hair tie, phone charger

☐ Compassion, patience, and curiosity (yes, pack those)

Exercise 2.14: Stepping Stone Path of Midwifery

Write the steps you take in each area:

1. Student

2. Balanced Study

3. Technology Tools

4. Compassionate Care

5. Collaboration

6. Adaptability

7. Confident Midwife

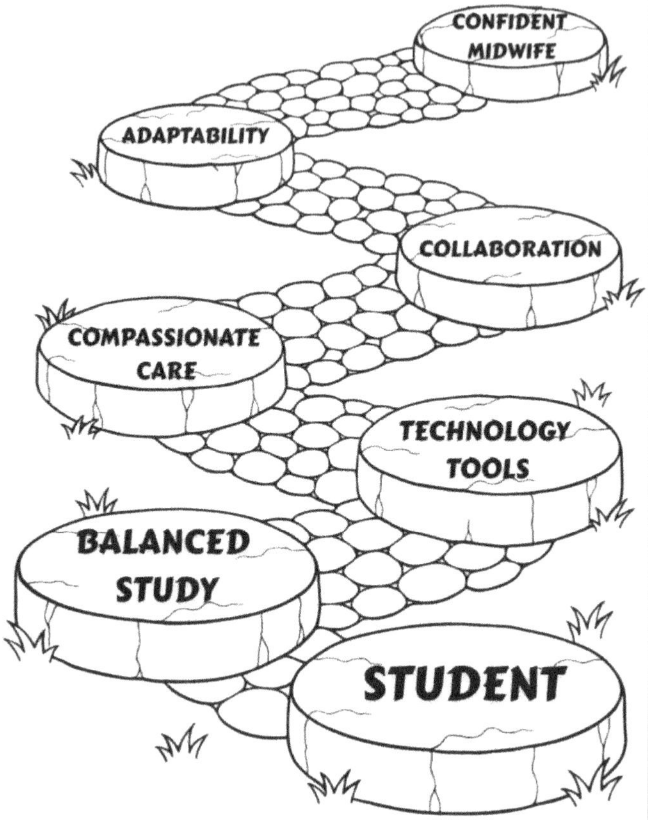

Learning to Learn Essential Takeaways

A balanced and supportive learning experience helps midwifery students thrive. Combining structured planning, effective study strategies, self-care, and collaboration enhances focus, retention, and confidence. Integrating technology and educational resources offers diverse perspectives, practical applications, and flexible access to information, deepening knowledge and preparing students for clinical excellence. Midwifery blends the rigor of science with the empathy of art, fostering evidence-based, compassionate care that honors the individuality of every client. Adaptability, both in learning styles and clinical application builds a strong foundation for lifelong growth and success in a dynamic profession.

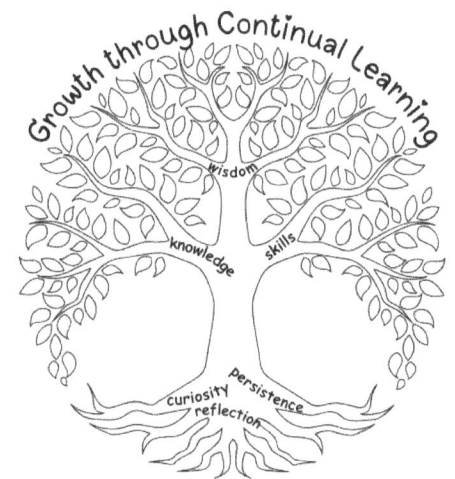

Chapter Two Self-Assessment

Multiple Choice

1. What is the primary role of the affective domain in midwifery education?
    a) Developing technical skills for clinical procedures.
    b) Enhancing emotional intelligence and cultural competence to build client trust.
    c) Strengthening interpersonal relationships through effective communication.
    d) Providing emotional support during clinical emergencies

2. Which learning style is best supported by anatomical models and clinical simulations?
    a) Auditory learners who rely on listening to lectures for understanding.
    b) Visual learners who prefer diagrams and models for studying anatomy.
    c) Kinesthetic learners who benefit from hands-on interaction.
    d) Multimodal learners who incorporate tactile tools into their broader study approach.

3. How can mentorship programs benefit midwifery students?
    a) By helping students develop professional networks and resources.
    b) By offering accountability, advocacy, and guidance during challenges.
    c) By ensuring students have fewer responsibilities during clinical rotations.
    d) By providing support for balancing academic and clinical responsibilities.

4. Which strategy best integrates clinical placements into study routines?
    a) Reflecting on clinical experiences and linking them to academic goals.
    b) Writing personal reflections on observed clinical techniques to deepen understanding.
    c) Collaborating with preceptors to improve specific skills encountered during placement.
    d) Relying solely on clinical experiences without supplemental study.

5. What is the primary purpose of using the Eisenhower Matrix in time management?
    a) To focus on completing urgent tasks before addressing other responsibilities.
    b) To categorize tasks by urgency and importance for effective prioritization.
    c) To create a balance between immediate and long-term responsibilities.
    d) To eliminate distractions without prioritizing workload.

6. How does the Pomodoro Technique improve productivity?
    a) Alternating focused study blocks with regular breaks.
    b) Requiring long, uninterrupted work sessions for better focus.
    c) Promoting balance between study and rest through structured intervals.
    d) Helping manage study time effectively across different topics.

7. Which method combines active reading with practical application in midwifery studies?
    a) Skimming material for key points without deeper engagement.
    b) Using directed visualization techniques for clinical scenarios.
    c) The SQ4R method for active reading and comprehension.
    d) The 5-P Reading System for structured engagement with texts.

8. Why is self-assessment an essential part of midwifery education?
    a) It eliminates the need for external feedback from instructors.
    b) It helps students maintain awareness of their strengths and weaknesses.
    c) It promotes proactive problem-solving for knowledge gaps.
    d) It allows students to reflect on progress and identify areas for improvement.

9. What is an example of a task in the "Important but Not Urgent" category of the Eisenhower Matrix?
    a) Reading textbook chapters ahead of class discussions.
    b) Practicing clinical skills, like neonatal resuscitation.
    c) Reorganizing study materials repeatedly instead of starting tasks.
    d) Reviewing syllabi to plan deadlines and assignments.

10. Which tool is most suitable for multimodal learning?
    a) Using charts, diagrams, and videos for comprehensive understanding.
    b) Incorporating flashcards and practice scenarios into study routines.
    c) Combining simulations, textbooks, and group discussions.
    d) Listening to audio lectures without additional engagement.

Fill in the Blank:

11. Midwifery education is a balance of _____ and _____, combining clinical precision with compassionate care.

12. The _____ Matrix is a time management tool that helps prioritize tasks based on their urgency and importance.

13. _____ learners benefit most from hands-on activities like practicing clinical skills or using anatomical models.

14. The acronym SQ4R stands for _____, _____, _____, _____, _____, and _____.

15. In the 5-P Reading System, the first step, _____, involves creating a distraction-free environment to prepare for studying.

16. The term _____ describes self-directed learning for adults, while _____ refers to teacher-directed learning for children.

17. A _____ is a tool that breaks down an assignment or skill evaluation into measurable criteria, helping students focus on expectations.

18. Logical-mathematical learners excel in tasks like _____ fetal monitoring strips or creating care algorithms.

19. One strategy for active listening is to _____ what the speaker has said to confirm understanding.

20. The primary purpose of _____ skills is to evaluate clinical information, make evidence-based decisions, and improve client care.

Chapter Two Reading & References

Recommended Reading: Adult Learning
- Brookfield, S. D. (2013). ***The Skillful Teacher: On Technique, Trust, and Responsiveness in the Classroom*** (2nd ed.). Jossey-Bass. A practical text on adult learning and teaching methods that midwifery educators and students alike can apply.
- Fleming, N. D., & Mills, C. (1992). ***VARK: A Guide to Learning Styles.*** VARK-Learn Ltd. A classic framework that helps students identify visual, auditory, reading/writing, and kinesthetic learning preferences.
- Gardner, H. (2011). ***Frames of Mind: The Theory of Multiple Intelligences*** (3rd ed.). Basic Books. Introduces the influential theory of multiple intelligences, supporting diverse learning approaches in midwifery education.
- Knowles, M. S., Holton, E. F., & Swanson, R. A. (2015). ***The Adult Learner: The Definitive Classic in Adult Education and Human Resource Development*** (8th ed.). Routledge. Foundational book on adult learning theory, highly relevant for midwifery students managing self-directed education.
- Sousa, D. A. (2016). ***How the Brain Learns*** (5th ed.). Corwin. Explores neuroscience research on memory, attention, and learning strategies applicable to midwifery study.
- St. Pierre, J. (1995). ***Lessons from a Student Midwife.*** Berkley Books. A personal account that captures the learning curve and emotional journey of becoming a midwife.
- Vincent, P. (2002). ***Baby Catcher: Chronicles of a Modern Midwife.*** Scribner. Engaging memoir of a contemporary midwife, illustrating both challenges and joys of midwifery practice.

References

Carless, D., & Boud, D. (2018). The development of student feedback literacy: Enabling uptake of feedback. *Assessment & Evaluation in Higher Education, 43*(8), 1315–1325. https://doi.org/10.1080/02602938.2018.1463354

Covey, S. R. (2020). *The 7 Habits of Highly Effective People: Powerful Lessons in Personal Change* (30th anniversary ed.). Simon & Schuster.

Cutrer, W. B., Miller, B., & Pusic, M. V. (2017). Fostering the development of master adaptive learners: A conceptual model to guide skill acquisition in medical education. *Academic Medicine, 92*(1), 70–75. https://doi.org/10.1097/ACM.0000000000001323

Gardner, H. (2006). *Multiple intelligences: New horizons in theory and practice*. Basic Books.

Goer, H., & Romano, A. (2012). *Optimal care in childbirth: The case for a physiologic approach*. Classic Day Publishing.

Harden, R. M., & Laidlaw, J. M. (2020). *Essential skills for a medical teacher: An introduction to teaching and learning in medicine* (3rd ed.). Elsevier.

Knowles, M. S., Holton, E. F., & Swanson, R. A. (2015). *The adult learner: The definitive classic in adult education and human resource development* (8th ed.). Routledge.

Merriam, S. B., & Bierema, L. L. (2013). *Adult learning: Linking theory and practice*. Jossey-Bass.

Morton, C. H., & Clift, E. G. (2014). *Birth ambassadors: Reflections on midwifery and birth activism*. Praeclarus Press.

Sadler, D. R. (2010). Beyond feedback: Developing student capability in complex appraisal. *Assessment & Evaluation in Higher Education, 35*(5), 535–550. https://doi.org/10.1080/02602930903541015

Schmidt, H. G., Rotgans, J. I., & Yew, E. H. J. (2011). The process of problem-based learning: What works and why. *Medical Education, 45*(8), 792–806. https://doi.org/10.1111/j.1365-2923.2011.04035.x

Shah, S. (2019). Adult learning theory: A primer for the medical educator. University of Maryland Medical Center. https://www.umms.org/ummc/-/media/files/ummc/for-health-professionals/gme/program-directors/faculty-development-2019/faculty-development-october-2019/adult-learning-theory_shah.pdf

Taylor, D. C. M., & Hamdy, H. (2013). Adult learning theories: Implications for learning and teaching in medical education. *Medical Teacher, 35*(11), e1561–e1572. https://doi.org/10.3109/0142159X.2013.828153

Chapter Three
Terminology for Midwifery Practice

Objectives
After completing this chapter, the student should be able to:
1. **Define** medical prefixes, suffixes, and root words commonly used in midwifery and obstetrics.
2. **Explain** how breaking down medical terms enhances comprehension and clinical accuracy.
3. **Demonstrate** the ability to interpret and construct medical terms using word components.
4. **Identify** commonly used abbreviations and mnemonics in midwifery charting and clinical communication.
5. **Explain** the importance of accuracy when using abbreviations to prevent misinterpretation.
6. **Apply** abbreviations appropriately in written documentation and verbal communication.
7. **Describe** anatomical directions such as anterior, posterior, lateral, and medial and their relevance in assessments and procedures.
8. **Recognize** key movements associated with labor positions and the cardinal movements of labor.
9. **Analyze** fetal positioning using anatomical terminology.
10. **Interpret** obstetric acronyms and abbreviations related to antepartum, labor, postpartum, and fetal monitoring.
11. **Demonstrate** the ability to use obstetrical terms correctly in documentation and communication.
12. **Practice** translating a labor and delivery report filled with acronyms into full medical terms.
13. **Utilize** medical terminology effectively in case studies and clinical scenarios.
14. **Compose** mock documentation using correct medical terminology, abbreviations, and structured charting.
15. **Evaluate** the accuracy and clarity of medical terminology usage through self-assessment exercises.
16. **Apply** knowledge of medical terminology by completing interactive activities such as crossword puzzles, matching exercises, and fill-in-the-blank scenarios.

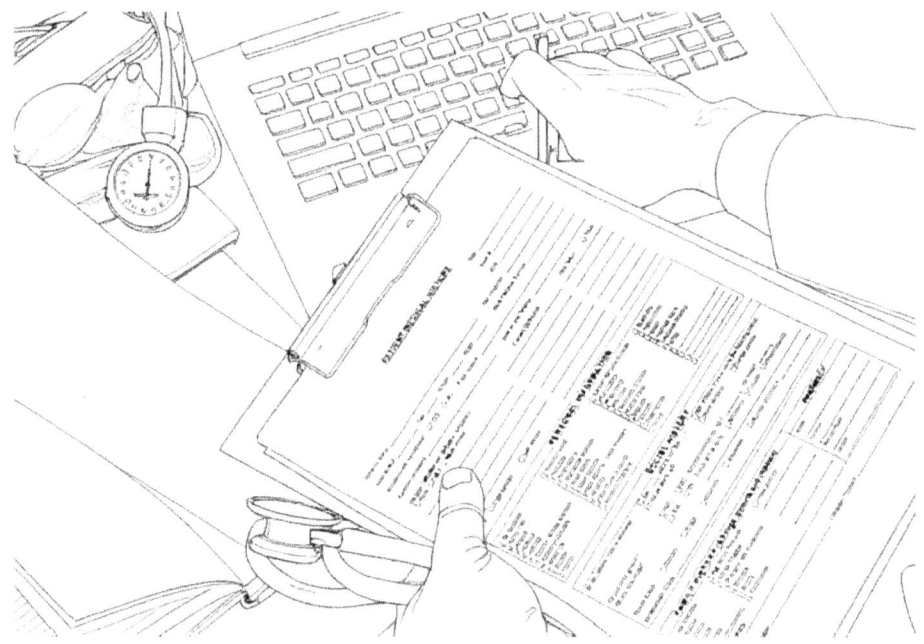

Terminology for Midwives

One of the first steps in beginning your midwifery education is to develop a strong understanding of medical terminology. Midwives are essential members of the health care team, and medical terminology facilitates clear, professional, and effective communication with other health care practitioners. Like any language, fluency in medical terminology allows student midwives to communicate efficiently and accurately within the field of medicine.

Midwives must be able to read and comprehend medical textbooks, journals, prescriptions, and medical charts. Charting is a critical component of high-quality midwifery care. Using standardized medical language ensures that documentation is clear, precise, and universally understood by other health care providers. Avoid the use of informal or midwife-exclusive terms, such as "yoni" instead of "vagina." Although a more woman-centered vocabulary might seem appealing, it could cause confusion and seem unprofessional in a clinical setting.

To retain medical terminology effectively, focus on understanding word components rather than rote memorization. By learning root words, prefixes, and suffixes, you can build a foundation upon which unfamiliar words can be understood. Breaking down complex medical terms into their parts simplifies comprehension and enhances recall.

A firm grasp of anatomical structures is also necessary for understanding medical terminology. If needed, review your anatomy and physiology knowledge to reinforce your understanding. Root words often reference specific areas of the body, which can help in interpreting terms. Consider investing in a reliable medical dictionary and referring to it whenever you encounter unfamiliar terminology.

Medical terms fall into two major categories:
1. **Descriptive terms:** These describe a characteristic such as shape, color, size, or function.
2. **Eponyms:** These are named after individuals who discovered or described an anatomical structure, diagnosed a disease, or developed a medical instrument or procedure. However, modern medical practice is moving away from eponyms, as they do not provide information on location or function. For example, the term "Fallopian tubes," named after Gabriele Falloppio, is now more commonly referred to as "uterine tubes."

Word Parts

Medical terms are composed of three basic components:

1. **Prefix** — Appears at the beginning of a word and typically specifies a subdivision, location, quantity, or time.
2. **Root word** — The central meaning of the word, to which a prefix or suffix is added.
3. **Suffix** — Appears at the end of a word and modifies the central meaning by indicating a condition, procedure, or state.

Additional word structures include:

- **Compound word** — A term containing two root words.
- **Combining form** — A root word with a vowel added to facilitate pronunciation.

Examples of word construction:

Word with a prefix and root word: **hyper/active**

Word with a suffix and root word: **tonsil/ectomy**

Word with two root words: **chole/cyst/ectomy**

Word with combining forms: **cardi/o/vascular**

Word with a prefix and a suffix only: **neo/plasm**

Word with a prefix, root word, and suffix: **peri/card/itis**

Understanding Prefix and Suffix Changes

By altering the prefix and suffix, a term's meaning can change while maintaining the same root word.

Example: Myocarditis

Prefix: **myo-** (muscle)

Root: **cardi-** (heart)

Suffix: **-itis** (inflammation)

Definition: inflammation of the heart muscle tissue

Prefix change:

Pericarditis = inflammation of the outer layer of the heart

Endocarditis = inflammation of the inner layer of the heart

Suffix change:

Cardiologist = a physician specializing in the heart

Cardiomyopathy = disease of the heart muscle

Exercise 3.1: Building Words with Prefixes and Suffixes
Use the following parts to construct new medical terms.

Examples of Word Parts to Use:

Prefixes: *brady-* (slow), *tachy-* (fast), *peri-* (around)

Roots: *gastr-* (stomach), *oste-* (bone), *derm-* (skin)

Suffixes: *-itis* (inflammation), *-ectomy* (surgical removal), *-pathy* (disease)

Start with the **root** (the main body part).

Add a **prefix** to modify speed, location, or amount.

Add a **suffix** to show a condition, disease, or procedure.

1. _____ = inflammation of the stomach
2. _____ = disease of the skin
3. _____ = surgical removal of bone
4. _____ = slow heartbeat
5. _____ = disease of bone
6. _____ = inflammation around the stomach
7. _____ = painful urination
8. _____ = inflammation of many joints
9. _____ = study of the kidney
10. _____ = excessive sugar in the blood

Common Root Words in Medical Terminology

abdomin/o	abdomen	my/o	muscle
aden/o	gland	myel/o	bone marrow; spinal cord
an/o	anus	nas/o	nose
andr/o	man	nephr/o	kidney
append/o	appendix	neur/o	nerve
angi/o	vessel	ocul/o	eye
arteri/o	artery	orchi/o, orchid/o	testicle
arthr/o	joint	oophor/o	ovary
bronch/o	bronchus	oste/o	bone
cardi/o	heart	ot/o	ear
cephal/o	head	pancreat/o	pancreas
cerebr/o	brain	pharyng/o	pharynx, throat
cheil/o	lip	phleb/o	vein
chol/e	bile, gall	pneum/o	lung
chondr/o	cartilage	proct/o	rectum
col/o	large intestine	pub/o	pubis
colp/o	vagina	pulmon/o	lung
cost/o	rib	pyel/o	renal pelvis
crani/o	skull	rect/o	rectum
cyan/o	blue	ren/o	kidney
cyst/o	bladder or sac	rhin/o	nose
dactyl/o	fingers, toes	sacr/o	sacrum
dent/o	teeth	salping/o	uterine tubes
derm/o, dermat/o	skin	splen/o	spleen
encephal/o	brain	stomat/o	mouth
enter/o	intestine	steth/o	chest
erythr/o	red	thyr/o	thyroid gland
esophag/o	esophagus	thorac/o	chest
gastr/o	stomach	trache/o	trachea
gingiv/o	gums	ureter/o	ureter
gloss/o	tongue	ur/o	urine, urinary tract
glyc/o, gluc/o	sugar	vas/o	vessel, duct
gyn/o	woman	ven/o	vein
fibr/o	fiber, connective tissue	xanth/o	yellow
hem/o, hemat/o	blood		
hepat/o	liver		
hydr/o	water		
hyster/o	uterus		
ile/o	ileum (small intestine)		
ili/o	ilium (hip bone)		
irid/o	iris		
lapar/o	abdomen		
laryng/o	larynx		
leuk/o	white		
lip/o	fat		
lymph/o	lymph		
mast/o, mamm/o	breast		
metr/o	uterus		

Exercise 3.2: Root Words

Match the root with its meaning:

1. cardi/o _____
2. gastr/o _____
3. nephr/o _____
4. oste/o _____
5. nas/o _____
6. hepat/o _____
7. colp/o _____
8. aden/o _____

A. bone
B. stomach
C. gland
D. kidney
E. vagina
F. nose
G. liver
H. heart

Common Prefixes in Medical Terminology

a-, an-	not, without	kerat/o	horn, hard
ab-, abs-	away from	kinesi/o	movement
alg/o	pain	later/o	side
amb/I	on both sides	lith/o	stone
ante-	before	macr/o	large
anti-	against	mal-	bad, poor
auto-	self	medi/o	middle
amni/o	amnion	mega-	large, great
bi-	two	men/o	menses, monthly
brachi-	arm	meta-	beyond, change
brady-	slow	micr/o	small
circum	around	mon/o	one, single
contra-	against, opposed	my/o	muscle
cyan/o	blue	myel/o	marrow, spinal cord
demi-, hemi-, semi-	half	olig/o	few, scanty
de-	from, down, away	or/o	mouth
di-	two, double	oste/o	bone
dys-	difficult, painful, abnormal	para-	alongside, abnormal
en-	in	per-	through
endo-	within	peri-	around
erythr/o	red	poly-	many
epi-	upon	post-	after
exo-	outside, outward	pre-	before
fore-	in front of (rare)	pseud/o	false
hem/o	blood	pulmon/o	lung
hemi-	half	py/o	pus
hom/o	same, similar	retro-	backward, behind
hydr/o	water	sub-	under
hyper-	above, excessive	supra-	above
hypo-	below, deficient	syn-, sym-	with, together
infra-	beneath	tachy-	fast
inter-	between	top/o	place, position
intra-	within	trans-	across, through
iso-	equal	troph/o	nutrition, growth
juxta-	near	xanth/o	yellow

Exercise 3.3: Prefixes

A. Match each prefix with its meaning.

1. brady- _____
2. tachy- _____
3. pre- _____
4. sub- _____
5. poly- _____

A. many   **B.** before   **C.** fast
D. slow   **E.** under, below

B. Use the correct prefix to complete each term.

_____cardia = slow heart rate
_____dermal = beneath the skin
_____natal = before birth
_____pnea = rapid breathing
_____uria = excessive urination

Common Suffixes in Medical Terminology

-al	pertaining to	-lysis	breakdown, destruction
-algia	pain	-logy	study of, science of
-emia	blood condition	-metry	measurement
-esthesia	sensation, feeling	-oid	resembling
-algesia	pain sensitivity	-oma	tumor, mass
-ase	enzyme	-osis	abnormal condition
-cele	hernia, protrusion	-ostomy	surgical opening
-cyte	cell	-otomy	cutting into
-dynia	pain	-paresis	partial paralysis, weakness
-ectomy	surgical removal	-pathy	disease
-emesis	vomiting	-penia	deficiency
-genesis, -genic	producing, causing	-phobia	fear
-graphy	recording, writing	-plasm	formation, growth
-ia	condition	-plegia	paralysis
-ic	pertaining to	-pnea	breathing
-itis	inflammation	-rrhea	flow, discharge
-ize	to treat, make, or become	-sclerosis	hardening
-ism	condition, process, theory	-scopy	visual examination
-kinesis	movement	-trophic, -trophy	nutrition, development

Exercise 3.4: Suffixes

A. Match each suffix with its meaning.

1. -itis _____
2. -ectomy _____
3. -algia _____
4. -emia _____
5. -logy _____

A. pain **B.** study of
C. inflammation **D.** blood condition
E. surgical removal

B. Fill in the blank with the correct suffix.

1. Tonsil_____ = surgical removal of the tonsils
2. Cardi_____ = inflammation of the heart
3. Hemat_____ = condition of the blood
4. Neuro_____ = study of the nervous system

Exercise 3:5 Obstetric Terms

Draw lines where the prefix, root, and suffix divide. (Example: P o s t | p a r t u m   after birth)

1. Multipara _____
2. Tocolysis _____
3. Hyperemesis _____
4. Pelvimetry _____
5. Postpartum _____
6. Primagravida _____
7. Antepartum _____
8. Amniocentesis _____

General Medical Abbreviations

In midwifery practice, abbreviations are widely used to facilitate efficient charting and clinical communication. They provide a shorthand system that allows essential information to be documented quickly and clearly. Correct use of abbreviations is critical for patient safety. Misinterpretation or misuse can lead to serious errors, affecting maternal and fetal outcomes. Midwives, birth assistants, and other team members must be familiar with standard abbreviations to maintain consistency and avoid confusion in clinical records.

Common General Abbreviations

aa	of each
ac	before meals (ante cibos)
ad lib	as desired
aq	water
bid	twice a day
BP	blood pressure
c	with
CBC	complete blood count
cm	centimeter
dr	dram
Dx	diagnosis
ENT	ear, nose, throat
ext	extract
FUO	fever of unknown origin
G	gram (gm outdated)
h	hour
Hb or Hgb	hemoglobin
Hct	hematocrit
Hg	mercury
HR	heart rate
hs	at bedtime (hora somni)
IM	intramuscular
inf	infusion
IV	intravenous
IVF	intravenous fluids
mcg	microgram
mg	milligram
ml	milliliter (preferred over cc)
NPO	nothing by mouth (nil per os)
O2	oxygen
Oz	ounce
pc	after meals (post cibos)
per	by
PO	by mouth (per os)
PR	per rectum
pt	patient
q2h	every 2 hours
q3h	every 3 hours
q4h	every 4 hours
qh	every hour
qid	four times a day (quater in die)
qod	every other day *
qs	quantity sufficient
RR	respiratory rate
Rx	take (prescription)
s	without (sine)
SOB	shortness of breath
sp gr	specific gravity
stat	immediately (statim)
subq	subcutaneous
supp	suppository
susp	suspension
tab	tablet
tbsp	tablespoon
tid	three times a day (ter in die)
top	apply topically
TPR	temperature, pulse, respiration
tsp	teaspoon
ung	ointment
v/s	vital signs
WBC	white blood cell
WNL	within normal limits

> ***Discouraged Abbreviations**
>
> Some abbreviations are unsafe because they can be misread; use the recommended terms instead. They may still appear in older records, so recognize them but avoid in current documentation.
>
> - **cc**: cubic centimeter; can look like "oo" or "u." Use **ml**.
> - **qd**: every day; can be read as "qid." Use **daily**.
> - **qod**: every other day; can be read as "qd." Write out **every other day**.
> - **U**: unit; can be mistaken for "o" or "4." Spell out **unit**.
>
> **os**: by mouth (per os); may be confused with "OS" (left eye). Use **PO** or **oral**.

Common Midwifery Abbreviations

Antepartum (AP)–Prenatal Abbreviations

AFI	Amniotic Fluid Index
AFP	Alpha-Fetoprotein
BPP	Biophysical Profile
CVS	Chorionic Villus Sampling
EDD/EDC	Estimated Due Date / Estimated Date of Confinement
FHR/FHT	Fetal Heart Rate/ Fetal Heart Tones (older usage)
FM	Fetal Movement
G/P	Gravida/Para
GA	Gestational Age
GBS	Group B Streptococcus
GDM	Gestational Diabetes Mellitus
GTPAL	Gravida, Term, Preterm, Abortions, Living
HELLP	Hemolysis, Elevated Liver enzyme levels, and Low Platelet levels
IAB	Induced Abortion
IUGR	Intrauterine Growth Restriction
LGA	Large for Gestational Age
LMP	Last Menstrual Period
NST	Non-Stress Test
NT	Nuchal Translucency
PEC	Preeclampsia
PIH	Pregnancy-Induced Hypertension
PPROM	Preterm Premature Rupture of Membranes
PROM	Premature Rupture of Membranes
PTL	Preterm Labor
Rh	Rhesus Factor
SAB	Spontaneous Abortion (miscarriage)
SGA	Small for Gestational Age
UA	Urinalysis

Intrapartum (IP)–Labor & Birth Abbreviations

AROM	Artificial Rupture of Membranes
BOW	Bag of Waters
C/S	Cesarean Section
Ctx	Contractions
Cx	Cervix
Epi	Episiotomy (sometimes epidural, clarify context)
Fetal Positions	LOA=Left Occiput Anterior, ROA=Right Occiput Anterior, LOP=Left Occiput Posterior, ROP=Right Occiput Posterior
NST	Non Stress Test
Pit	Pitocin (oxytocin; often spelled out)
PPH	Postpartum Hemorrhage
PRN	As Needed
PROM	Premature Rupture of Membranes
ROM	Rupture of Membranes
SROM	Spontaneous Rupture of Membranes
SVD	Spontaneous Vaginal Delivery
TOLAC	Trial of Labor After Cesarean
VBAC	Vaginal Birth After Cesarean
VE	Vaginal Exam

Postpartum (PP) – After Birth Abbreviations

BF	Breastfeeding
BUBBLE-HE	Postpartum assessment: (Breasts, Uterus, Bladder, Bowel, Lochia, Episiotomy/laceration, Homan's sign, Emotional status)
EBF	Exclusive Breastfeeding
FF	Formula Feeding
LATCH	Latch Score (breastfeeding assessment)
Lochia	Postpartum vaginal discharge
PP	Postpartum
PPD	Postpartum Depression
PPH	Postpartum Hemorrhage
REEDA	Redness, Edema, Ecchymosis, Discharge, Approximation
RhoGAM	Rh immunoglobulin (if indicated for Rh-negative clients)
TDAP	Tetanus, Diphtheria, Pertussis vaccine

Newborn (NB) Abbreviations

AGA	Appropriate for Gestational Age
APGAR	Appearance, Pulse, Grimace, Activity, Respiration
Bili	Bilirubin
CPAP	Continuous Positive Airway Pressure
ELBW	Extremely Low Birth Weight
LBW	Low Birth Weight
LGA	Large for Gestational Age
MEC	Meconium
NB	Newborn
NBS	Newborn Screening
PKU	Phenylketonuria (metabolic screen)
RA	Room Air
SGA	Small for Gestational Age
TSB	Total Serum Bilirubin
TTN	Transient Tachypnea of the Newborn
VLBW	Very Low Birth Weight

Exercise 3.6: OB Abbreviations
Match the abbreviation with its meaning:

1. _____ AFI	A. Postpartum perineal healing assessment
2. _____ GDM	B. Trial of labor after cesarean
3. _____ PROM	C. Transient tachypnea of the newborn
4. _____ TOLAC	D. Amniotic fluid index
5. _____ REEDA	E. Premature rupture of membranes
6. _____ APGAR	F. Newborn assessment at 1 and 5 minutes
7. _____ TTN	G. Gestational diabetes mellitus

Exercise 3.6: Interpreting a Chart Note
Read the following chart note and write out what each abbreviation means in full sentences:

Ms. Sanchez, G3T2P0A1L2, admitted in L&D on 11/23/25 at 13:50 with SROM. FHT WNL throughout labor. SDVB at 18:36 on 11/23/25. PP stable, EBL 350cc, NB skin-to-skin, BF initiated, APGAR 8/9.

DEFINITIONS OF PREGNANCY

- **Gravida** ("to bear"): any pregnancy, including the current one.
- **Para** ("to give birth"): a woman who has given birth at ≥ 20 weeks' gestation, whether the infant was born alive or stillborn.
- **Nulligravida**: a woman who has never been pregnant.
- **Primigravida**: a woman pregnant for the first time.
- **Multigravida**: a woman who has been pregnant more than once.
- **Nullipara**: a woman who has never given birth at ≥ 20 weeks' gestation.
- **Primipara**: a woman who has given birth once at ≥ 20 weeks' gestation.
- **Multipara**: a woman who has given birth two or more times at ≥ 20 weeks' gestation.
- **Grand multipara**: a woman who has given birth to five or more infants at ≥ 20 weeks' gestation.

Gestational Age Terms
- **Term:** Birth between 37–42 weeks (some sources further divide term into early, full, and late term).
- **Preterm:** Birth after 20 weeks and before 37 completed weeks.
- **Postterm:** Birth after 42 weeks.

GTPAL System
A more detailed system, GTPAL, is now commonly used to describe a woman's obstetric history:
- **G** = Gravida (number of pregnancies)
- **T** = Term births
- **P** = Preterm births
- **A** = Abortions (spontaneous or induced < 20 weeks)
- **L** = Living children

Notes:
- *A multiple pregnancy (twins, triplets, etc.) is considered one pregnancy (gravida), but the number of **births** (para) reflects the number of birth events, not the number of infants delivered.*
- *Abortions (spontaneous or induced) before 20 weeks are counted as gravida but not para.*
- *The current pregnancy is counted as gravida until delivery.*

Exercise 3.7: Pregnancy Definition & GTPAL
Fill in the Blank

1. A woman who has been pregnant three times and has never given birth at ≥20 weeks is called a _____.

2. Maria had a stillbirth at 28 weeks. It was her only previous pregnancy; she is now pregnant again.
   Chart: G ____ T ____ P ____ A ____ L ____

3. Jane has four children: one set of twins, one child born at term, and one child born at 35 weeks. She has had one abortion, and she is pregnant again.
   Chart: G ____ T ____ P ____ A ____ L ____

4. Debbie had one miscarriage at 16 weeks and is pregnant now.
   Chart: G ____ T ____ P ____ A ____ L ____

5. Sarah delivered triplets at 32 weeks and is now pregnant again.
   Chart: G ____ T ____ P ____ A ____ L ____

Exercise 3.8: Charting Abbreviations	
Translate these terms:	
1. G3P2 at 39+4 weeks presents with SROM at 2300 hours. BP 120/80, HR 78, RR 16. FHR 140, reactive NST. Awaiting AROM.	
2. G4P3 at 38+2 weeks reports PIH symptoms. NST non-reactive, and EFW 3500g.	
3. G2P1 at 37+5 weeks presents with CTX q5 minutes, reporting LOF since midnight. Initial assessment: BP 118/76, HR 82, AFI normal, EFW 3200g.	
4. G1P0 at 40+1 weeks presents with CTX q3 minutes and reports decreased FM. FHR is 130 with moderate variability, reactive NST.	

Exercise 3.9: Interpreting Prescription Orders
Read each prescription and write out in plain language what it means.
1. Amoxicillin 250 mg 1 po qid ac
2. Pitocin 20 U IM prn for a hypotonic uterus
3. Comfrey ung ss oz apply to affected area hs
4. Vit C 1 gm po q4h × 7 days
5. Meperidine 50 mg qid prn for pain
6. Chamomile & hops 2 oz aa for inf. Use prn sleep
7. Nifedipine 10 mg po q6h for PTL

The Use of Mnemonics in Midwifery Practice

Midwifery is a dynamic field that requires quick decision-making, recall of vast amounts of clinical information, and the ability to assess and respond to both normal and emergency situations. Mnemonics serve as valuable tools in midwifery practice by helping students and providers remember key concepts, assessments, and interventions in an efficient and structured way. These simple memory aids allow for faster recall of protocols and assessments, ensuring that midwifery care remains thorough, efficient, and evidence-based.

Mnemonics can be particularly useful in:

- **Antenatal care**–Tracking pregnancy history (GTPAL) and assessing fetal well-being (VEAL CHOP for fetal heart rate patterns).
- **Labor and birth**–Evaluating the progress of labor (4 P's of Labor) and assessing amniotic fluid after rupture of membranes (COAT).
- **Postpartum care**–Performing structured postpartum assessments (BUBBLE HE) and assessing newborn health immediately after birth (APGAR).

EMERGENCY RESPONSE–MANAGING COMPLICATIONS SUCH AS POSTPARTUM HEMORRHAGE (3 T'S OF PPH) OR SEVERE PREECLAMPSIA (HELLP SYNDROME). OB MNEMONICS: QUICK REFERENCE

Antenatal

GTPAL: **G**ravida, **T**erm, **P**reterm, **A**bortions, **L**iving

HELLP: **H**emolysis, **E**levated **L**iver enzymes, **L**ow **P**latelets

Intrapartum

4 P's of Labor: **P**assenger, **P**assageway, **P**owers, **P**syche

COAT: **C**olor, **O**dor, **A**mount, **T**ime (amniotic fluid)

7 Cardinal Movements of Labor –
"*Every Darn Fool In Egypt Eats Eggs*" → **E**ngagement, **D**escent, **F**lexion, **I**nternal Rotation, **E**xtension, **E**xternal Rotation, **E**xpulsion

VEAL CHOP –
- **V** = Variable → **C** = Cord compression
- **E** = Early → **H** = Head compression
- **A** = Accelerations → **O** = Okay
- **L** = Late → **P** = Placental insufficiency

Postpartum

BUBBLE HE: **B**reasts, **U**terus, **B**ladder, **B**owel, **L**ochia, **E**pisiotomy/laceration, **H**oman's sign, **E**motional status

3 (or 4) T's of Postpartum Hemorrhage: **T**one, **T**issue, **T**rauma, (**T**hrombin)

Newborn

APGAR: **A**ppearance, **P**ulse, **G**rimace, **A**ctivity, **R**espiration

Anatomical Directions

Understanding anatomical directions is essential in midwifery for accurate assessment and communication to describe the position of the fetus, locate anatomical landmarks, and ensure precise documentation and procedures.

Anatomical Planes

1. MEDIAN PLANE or **midsagittal** plane, divides the body into equal right and left halves. It runs exactly down the midline, while a **parasagittal** plane is off-center. Movements in this plane include flexion and extension (e.g., bending and straightening the knee).

2. SAGITTAL PLANE divides the body into left and right sections.

3. TRANSVERSE PLANES or **horizontal** planes are perpendicular to the long axis of the body and divide the body into superior (upper) and inferior (lower) sections. Movements in this plane include rotational movements (e.g., twisting the torso).

4. FRONTAL PLANES or **coronal** planes divide the body into anterior (front) and posterior (back) sections. Movements in this plane include abduction and adduction (e.g., raising the arms sideways).

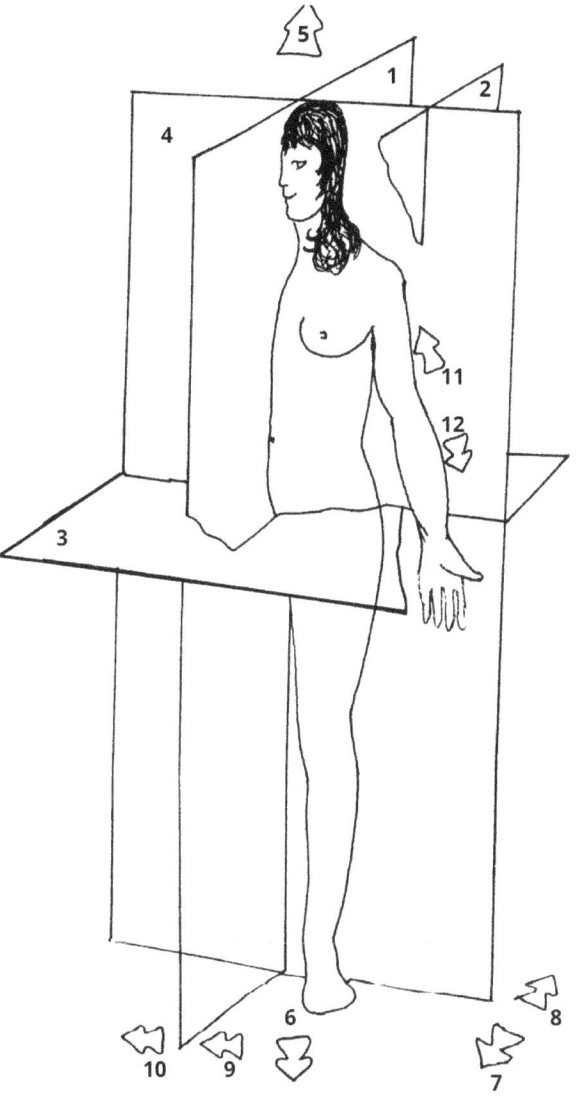

Directions

5. SUPERIOR or **cranial** is closer to the head or above another structure.

6. INFERIOR is closer to the feet, or lower than another structure.

7. ANTERIOR is towards the front of the body.

8. POSTERIOR is towards the back of the body.

9. MEDIAL is toward the midline of the body.

10. LATERAL is away from the midline of the body further away from the median plane.

11. PROXIMAL is closer to the point of origin, for example closer to the origin of the limb.

12. DISTAL is farther from the point of origin.

Application in Midwifery:

Fetal Positioning: anatomical terms are used to describe fetal positions, such as occiput anterior (OA), occiput posterior (OP), left occiput transverse (LOT), and right sacrum anterior (RSA) in breech presentations. Understanding these terms helps in labor assessment and delivery planning.

Fundal Height Measurement: determining fundal height involves recognizing anatomical references, such as the symphysis pubis (inferior landmark) and the xiphoid process (superior landmark), ensuring accurate assessment of fetal growth.

Pelvic Examinations: directional terms assist in describing findings during vaginal examinations, including cervical position (anterior/posterior) and fetal descent (station relative to ischial spines).

Procedures and Documentation: proper use of anatomical language aids in charting, interdisciplinary communication, and consistent documentation of procedures which leads to a reduction in charting errors in maternal and fetal assessments.

> **Why It Matters**
> Directional terms and anatomical planes are the "map language" of the body. Midwives use these words to describe fetal position, chart exam findings, and communicate clearly with other providers.
>
> *Example:* "laceration at the posterior fourchette" → everyone knows exactly where that is.
>
> *Example:* "fetus in left occiput anterior (LOA) position" → combines left/right, anterior/posterior, and occiput as landmarks.

HUMAN BODY CAVITIES

The human body is divided into several large body compartments, known as body cavities, which house and protect vital organs. These cavities provide structural organization and allow for functional separation of different organ systems. The two largest body cavities are the dorsal (posterior) cavity and the ventral (anterior) cavity.

Body Cavities and Membranes

Protective membranes, which provide support, lubrication, and protection from friction during movement surround many organs within these cavities. The major membranous linings include:

Cavity	Principal Contents	Membranous Lining
Dorsal Body Cavity		
Cranial Cavity	Brain	Meninges
Vertebral (Spinal) Canal	Spinal Cord	Meninges
Ventral Body Cavity		
Thoracic Cavity	Heart, Lungs	Pericardium (heart), Pleura (lungs)
Abdominal Cavity	Digestive Organs, Spleen, Kidneys	Peritoneum
Pelvic Cavity	Bladder, Reproductive Organs	Peritoneum

Human Body Cavities

1. **DORSAL BODY CAVITY** is located along the back (posterior) side of the body and is responsible for enclosing and protecting the central nervous system. *It consists of:*

   a. **Cranial Cavity**: located within the skull and contains the brain.
   b. **Spinal (Vertebral) Cavity**: a narrow, elongated space that runs along the spine, enclosing and protecting the spinal cord. The brain and spinal cord are further protected by cerebrospinal fluid (CSF), which cushions and nourishes these structures, as well as the meninges, a specialized set of protective membranes.

2. **VENTRAL BODY CAVITY** is the larger, front-facing (anterior) compartment of the body, housing many of the body's essential organs. It is divided into two main subdivisions:

   Thoracic Cavity: Located in the chest and enclosed by the ribcage, it contains:

   a. **Pleural cavities**: surround each lung.
   b. **Pericardial cavity**: surrounds the heart and is located within the mediastinum, the central space between the lungs.
   c. **The diaphragm**, a dome-shaped muscle important for breathing, separates the thoracic cavity from the abdominopelvic cavity.

3. **ABDOMINOPELVIC CAVITY** is located below the diaphragm. It is the largest cavity in the body and can be further divided into:

   a. **Abdominal cavity**: houses digestive organs such as the stomach, intestines, liver, gallbladder, pancreas, kidneys, and spleen.
   b. **Pelvic cavity**: contains the bladder, reproductive organs, and rectum. Particularly relevant in midwifery, as it houses the uterus during pregnancy and expands to accommodate fetal growth and birth.

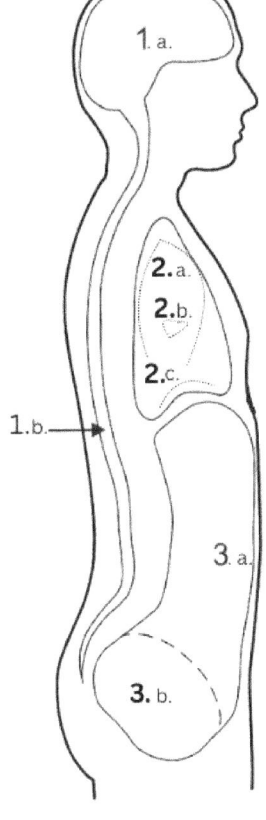

Relevance to Midwifery

Helps assess maternal comfort, understanding physiological changes during pregnancy and birth, and responding to potential complication particularly regarding:

- **Pregnancy:** the expanding uterus shifts organs within the abdominopelvic cavity, impacting digestion, circulation, and respiration.
- **Labor and Birth:** the pelvic cavity plays a crucial role in fetal descent and passage during labor.
- **Fetal Positioning**: midwives assess fetal position and engagement within the pelvic inlet and outlet, which are anatomical landmarks within the pelvic cavity.

> **Why It Matters?**
> Body cavities describe the major compartments where organs are located. Knowing them helps midwives understand where symptoms or procedures apply.
>
> *Example:* Amniotic sac is within the pelvic cavity.
>
> *Example:* Spinal anesthesia is injected near the vertebral canal (dorsal cavity).
>
> *Example:* Heartburn in pregnancy is due to pressure in the abdominal cavity.

Anatomical General Motion

Understanding anatomical motion is essential for medicine in general and midwifery practice in particular, as it relates to maternal positioning, fetal movements, and biomechanics during pregnancy, labor, and birth. Movement plays a critical role in fetal positioning, descent, and rotation through the birth canal, and midwives can use this knowledge to optimize birth outcomes and promote comfort.

Movements Along the Sagittal (Median) Plane

- **Flexion**: a movement that decreases the angle between two body parts. *Example:* Bending the elbow to bring a hand toward the face or bowing forward from the waist. .In labor, flexion of the fetal head is crucial for optimal passage through the birth canal.

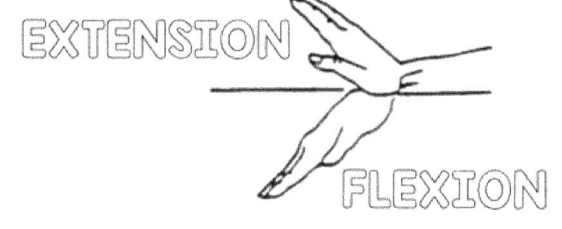

Birth Application: Encouraging maternal forward-leaning positions (e.g., hands and knees, leaning on a birth ball) may help align the baby in the optimal position for descent.

- **Extension**: a movement that increases the angle between two body parts.
  Example: Arching the back or straightening a flexed joint.

Application for Birth: As the baby moves through the birth canal, the head extends to navigate the perineum. Maternal movements that encourage this, such as an upright or hands-and-knees position, may facilitate easier birth.

Movements Along the Coronal (Frontal) Plane

- **Abduction**: moving a limb away from the midline of the body.
  Example: lifting the arms or legs outward.

> **Why It Matters**
> *The same motions that joints make are mirrored in the birth process:*
> - **Flexion**: Baby tucks chin to present the smallest head diameter.
> - **Extension**: Baby's head stretches back as it passes under the pubic bone.
> - **Internal rotation**: Baby rotates shoulders and head to fit through the pelvis.

Application for Birth: Encouraging the birthing person to open their knees wide (e.g., squatting or hands-and-knees positions) increases pelvic diameter, allowing for more space for the baby's descent.

- **Adduction**: moving a limb toward the midline of the body.
  Example: bringing the legs together after being apart.

External rotation: baby turns back to align shoulders for delivery.

Application for Birth: In some cases, positioning that involves bringing the knees inward while keeping the ankles apart (such as in asymmetrical lunges) may help disengage a baby that is stuck and facilitate rotation.

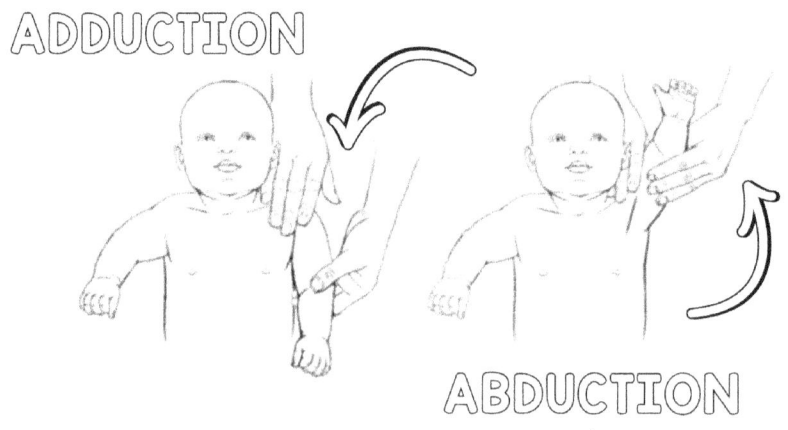

The following terms describe different types of movement:

- **Circumduction** is the movement of the limb, hand, or fingers in a circular pattern, using the sequential combination of flexion, adduction, extension, and abduction motions. *Example:* Moving the arm in a circular motion or rotating the hips.

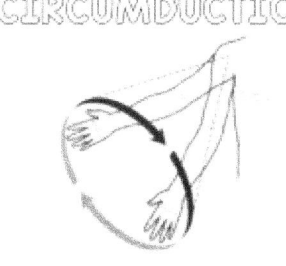

Application for Birth: Hip circles, figure-eight movements, and belly dancing motions encourage optimal fetal positioning, relieve tension, and help with fetal descent.

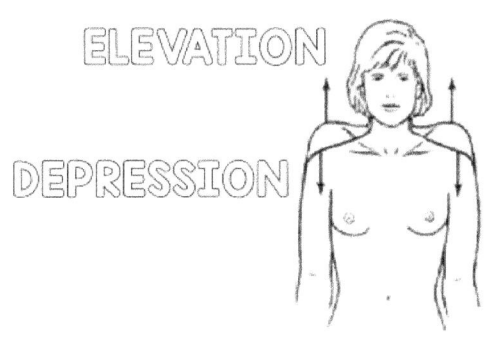

- **Elevation and Depression:** Elevation moves a structure upward (superiorly), while depression moves it downward (inferiorly). These terms are commonly applied to the scapula (shoulder blades) and mandible (jaw). For example, shrugging the shoulders involves elevation, while lowering them is depression.

- **Rotation**: turning a body part around its axis. *Example:* Turning the head side to side.

Application for Birth: Relaxing the shoulders during contractions reduces tension and allows for better oxygenation, helping to promote an effective labor pattern.

- **Medial (Internal) Rotation**: rotating a limb toward the midline.

Application for Birth: Internally rotating the thighs (e.g., knees together, feet apart) may widen the lower pelvis and help shift the baby's position.

- **Lateral (External) Rotation**: rotating a limb away from the midline.

Application for Birth: Encouraging the birthing person to externally rotate their hips (e.g., deep squatting or wide-legged kneeling) may open the pelvis for descent.

- **Hand and Forearm Movements**

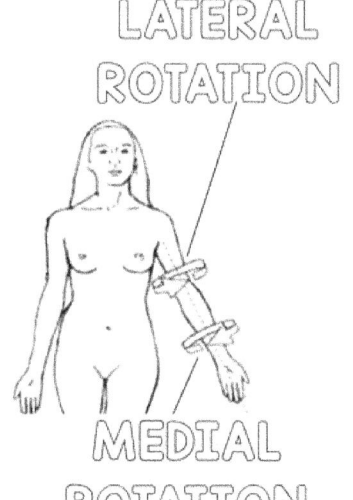

PRONATION: rotating the forearm so the palm faces downward.

SUPINATION: rotating the forearm so the palm faces upward.

Application for Birth: Hand positioning during pushing (e.g., gripping a squat bar, pressing against a surface) can affect upper body stability and engagement of core muscles.

Jaw and Shoulder Movements

- **Protrusion**: moving a structure forward (e.g., pushing the jaw outward).
- **Retrusion**: moving a structure backward (e.g., pulling the jaw inward).

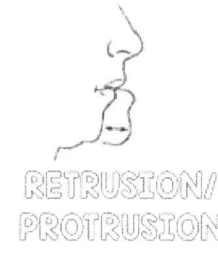

Application for Birth: Relaxing the jaw and face (a principle known as "sphincter law") helps reduce tension in the pelvis, promoting smoother labor progress. Open mouth breathing and sound-making can encourage this relaxation.

Exercise 3.10: Applying Anatomical Terms
In the following pairs of body parts, circle one pair that matches the term.

1. Circle the one that is **distal**:
   Finger / Hand   Elbow / Wrist   Foot / Knee   Elbow / Shoulder

2. Circle the one that is **superior**:
   Head / Neck   Foot / Knee   Elbow / Hand   Breast / Umbilicus
   Kidneys / Bladder   Ovaries / Uterus

3. Circle the one that is **anterior**:
   Umbilicus / Spine   Liver / Kidneys   Uterus / Bladder   Nose / Ears

4. Circle the one that is **superficial**:
   External Oblique Muscle / Internal Oblique Muscle
   Rib Cage / Lungs   Endometrium / Myometrium

5. Circle the one that is **lateral**:
   Lungs / Heart   Sternum / Breasts   Ovaries / Uterus

Exercise 3.11: Anatomical Movement
Match each anatomical movement with the best example.

1. ___ Circumduction		A. Turning the palm downward to rest on a table
2. ___ Elevation		B. Shrugging the shoulders upward toward the ears
3. ___ Depression		C. Lowering the shoulders back to a neutral position
4. ___ Lateral rotation		D. Moving the arm in a circular motion at the shoulder
5. ___ Medial rotation		E. Rotating the thigh so the toes point outward
6. ___ Pronation		F. Rotating the thigh so the toes point inward
7. ___ Supination		G. Turning the palm upward as if holding a bowl of soup
8. ___ Protrusion		H. Pushing the lower jaw forward
9. ___ Retrusion		I. Pulling the lower jaw backward

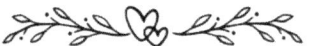

TERMINOLOGY FOR MIDWIFERY PRACTICE ESSENTIAL TAKEAWAYS

Understanding medical terminology is a foundation skill for every midwife. Mastery of roots, prefixes, and suffixes allows quick interpretation of unfamiliar terms and supports clear, accurate charting. Abbreviations save time but must be used with care, since misinterpretation can lead to errors. Midwives should know both the commonly used shorthand and which outdated abbreviations are discouraged.

Anatomical terms, planes, body cavities, and motions provide the shared language of health care. These concepts are not abstract—they are applied daily when describing fetal position, performing assessments, and communicating with the birth team. Mnemonics, quick reference charts, and consistent practice make this vocabulary easier to retain.

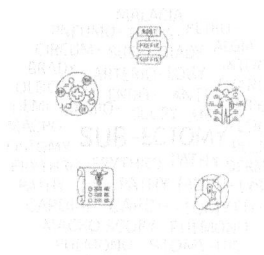

Clear and precise language does more than keep records neat—it builds trust, prevents mistakes, and helps midwives speak with authority in both community and professional settings. As midwifery continues to integrate within larger health systems, fluency in medical terminology is part of what strengthens interprofessional collaboration while preserving the midwife's distinct voice.

The more fluent you become in this language, the more confident and effective you will be as a midwife, able to advocate for safe, respectful, and culturally responsive care.

Chapter Three Self-Assessment

Multiple Choice
1. Which of the following is the correct meaning of the prefix brady-?
   a) Fast
   b) Slow
   c) Irregular
   d) Strong

2. The suffix -itis means:
   a) Tumor
   b) Surgical removal
   c) Inflammation
   d) Enlargement

3. Which plane divides the body into left and right halves?
   a) Frontal
   b) Sagittal
   c) Transverse
   d) Coronal

4. Which of the following represents the correct order of the seven cardinal movements of labor?
   a) Descent, Flexion, Engagement, Internal Rotation, Extension, External Rotation, Expulsion
   b) Engagement, Descent, Flexion, Internal Rotation, Extension, External Rotation, Expulsion
   c. Flexion, Descent, Engagement, Extension, Internal Rotation, External Rotation, Expulsion
   d. Engagement, Flexion, Descent, Internal Rotation, External Rotation, Extension, Expulsion

5. What does the abbreviation "AROM" stand for?
   a) Assisted removal of membranes
   b) Active rupture of membranes
   c) Accurate removal of membranes
   d) Artificial rupture of membranes

Fill in the Blank
6. Low blood sugar _____
7. Fast heart rate _____
8. Low blood pressure _____
9. LMP _____
10. IAB _____
11. EDD _____
12. EDC _____

13. WBC _____
14. WNL _____
15. PROM _____
16. QID _____
17. SAB _____
18. TPR _____

19. Use the GTPAL system to assess the following situation: A 32-year-old client presents with a positive pregnancy test. She tells you she has 3 children. She also says she had a stillborn baby at 28 weeks, and 3 losses before 12 weeks, as well as a loss at 16 weeks.
G_____ T_____ P_____ A_____ L_____

True/False
20. _____ EDD and EDC have the same meaning.
21. _____ All medical terms are a combination of a prefix or a suffix and a root.
22. _____ Proximal is close to the central body.
23. _____ Anterior refers to the back of the body.
24. _____ A multigravida may have never given birth to a term child.
25. _____ The transverse plane divides the body into upper and lower portions.
26. _____ The suffix -ectomy means inflammation.
27. _____ A primigravida refers to a woman who is pregnant for the first time.
28. _____ Tachycardia means a slow heart rate.
29. _____ The posterior position refers to the baby's occiput (back of the head) pointing toward the mother's sacrum.

Matching
30. Match the root with its meaning:
    1. cardi/o _____   A. bone
    2. gastr/o _____   B. stomach
    3. nephr/o _____   C. kidney
    4. oste/o _____   D. nose
    5. rhin/o _____   E. heart

31. Match each anatomical plane with its description:
    1. _____ Divides body into left and right halves   A. Sagittal
    2. _____ Divides body into front and back portions   B. Frontal (Coronal)
    3. _____ Divides body into upper and lower portions C. Transverse

32. Match the abbreviation with its full term:
    1. _____ FHR   A. Estimated fetal weight
    2. _____ NST   B. Fetal heart rate
    3. _____ PT   C. Electronic fetal monitoring
    4. _____ EFM   D. Non-stress test
    5. _____ TOLAC   E. Spontaneous rupture of membranes
    6. _____ EFW   F. Preterm Labor
    7. _____ PIH   G. Pregnancy-induced hypertension
    8. _____ SROM   H. Trial of labor after cesarean

Chapter Three Reading & References

Recommended Reading: Medical Terminology
- Bickley, L. S. (2021). ***Bates' Guide to Physical Examination and History Taking*** (13th ed.). Wolters Kluwer. Classic clinical reference that reinforces anatomical terminology in practical assessments.
- Chabner, D. A. (2021). ***The Language of Medicine*** (12th ed.). Elsevier. A standard text for mastering medical terminology through word parts, widely used in health care education.
- Ehrlich, A., & Schroeder, C. L. (2020). ***Medical Terminology for Health Professions*** (9th ed.). Cengage. Focuses on real-world application of prefixes, suffixes, and root words with review exercises.
- Fischbach, F. T., & Dunning, M. B. (2021). ***Manual of Laboratory and Diagnostic Tests*** (10th ed.). Wolters Kluwer. Helpful for understanding lab abbreviations and diagnostic terminology encountered in clinical settings.
- Kapit, W., Elson, L. M., & Latif, M. (2017). ***The Anatomy Coloring Book*** (4th ed.). Pearson. An interactive approach to learning anatomy and terminology through coloring.
- Moore, K. L., Dalley, A. F., & Agur, A. M. (2018). ***Clinically Oriented Anatomy*** (8th ed.). Wolters Kluwer. Detailed anatomy text; helpful for students who want deeper understanding of body planes, cavities, and motion.
- Mosby. (2021). ***Mosby's Dictionary of Medicine, Nursing & Health Professions*** (11th ed.). Elsevier. Comprehensive reference dictionary, widely used for accurate definitions in health care.
- Taber's Cyclopedic Medical Dictionary. (2022). ***Taber's Cyclopedic Medical Dictionary***. F.A. Davis Company. Concise, portable dictionary with clinical focus, useful for quick look-up in practice.

References

Bickley, L. S. (2021). Bates' guide to physical examination and history taking (13th ed.). Wolters Kluwer.

Chabner, D. A. (2021). The language of medicine (12th ed.). Elsevier.

Ehrlich, A., & Schroeder, C. L. (2020). Medical terminology for health professions (9th ed.). Cengage.

Fischbach, F. T., & Dunning, M. B. (2021). Manual of laboratory and diagnostic tests (10th ed.). Wolters Kluwer.

Frazier, M., & Drzymkowski, J. (2017). Essentials of human diseases and conditions (6th ed.). Elsevier.

Gylys, B. A., & Masters, R. (2017). Medical terminology simplified: A programmed learning approach by body system (6th ed.). F.A. Davis Company.

Kapit, W., Elson, L. M., & Latif, M. (2017). The anatomy coloring book (4th ed.). Pearson.

Marieb, E. N., & Hoehn, K. (2018). Human anatomy & physiology (11th ed.). Pearson.

Mosby. (2021). Mosby's dictionary of medicine, nursing & health professions (11th ed.). Elsevier.

Moore, K. L., Dalley, A. F., & Agur, A. M. (2018). Clinically oriented anatomy (8th ed.). Wolters Kluwer.

Pagana, K. D., & Pagana, T. J. (2021). Mosby's diagnostic and laboratory test reference (15th ed.). Elsevier.

Stedman's medical dictionary. (2020). Wolters Kluwer.

Taber's cyclopedic medical dictionary. (2022). F.A. Davis Company.

Tortora, G. J., & Derrickson, B. (2017). Principles of anatomy and physiology (15th ed.). Wiley.

Turley, S. (2020). Medical language: Immerse yourself (5th ed.). Pearson.

Chapter Four
Reproductive Anatomy & Physiology

Objectives
After completing this chapter, the student should be able to:
1. **Identify** all the parts of the pelvic girdle.
2. **Locate** all the ligaments of the pelvis.
3. **Describe** the four classic pelvic types.
4. **Locate** the structures and **explain** the functions of the parts of the female and male reproductive systems, including
    a. organs;
    b. musculature;
    c. ligaments;
    d. nerves; and
    e. blood supply.
5. **Define** and **explain** the functions of ovarian hormones.
6. **Describe** how ovulation and menstruation work.
7. **List** the sources of all the hormones involved in the menstrual cycle.
8. **Describe** the four phases of the menstrual cycle.
9. **Explain** the changes that occur in the uterus throughout the four phases of the menstrual cycle.
10. **Explain** how the ovum is moved down the uterine tube toward the uterus.
11. **Examine** how culture affects feelings and practices around menstruation
12. **Trace** the path of sperm from the testes to the vagina.
13. **List** each of the glands that add secretion to the semen along the way.

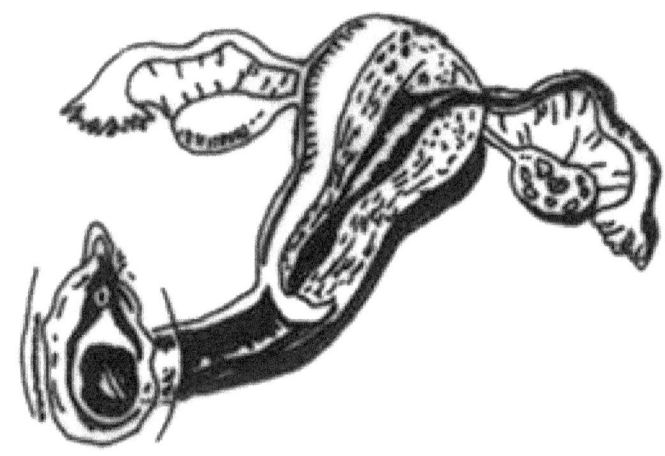

The Bony Pelvis

A thorough understanding of the pelvic anatomy is essential for student midwives, as the pelvis plays a critical role in pregnancy, labor, and birth. The shape, size, and structure of the pelvis directly influence the progress of labor and the baby's ability to navigate through the birth canal. By studying the bony landmarks such as the symphysis pubis, ischial spines, sacrum, and pelvic inlet and outlet, midwives can assess fetal descent, engagement, and rotation during childbirth. Knowledge of the ligaments, muscles, and joints, including the sacroiliac joint and the symphysis pubis, helps in understanding pelvic mobility and how hormonal changes, such as the release of relaxin, affect labor. A well-informed midwife can identify potential challenges, such as cephalopelvic disproportion or malpositioning, and take appropriate measures to support a safe and efficient birth process.

Additionally, understanding pelvic anatomy aids in postpartum recovery, pelvic floor health, and recognizing complications like pelvic pain or dysfunction. Mastering the pelvis is fundamental to providing skilled, compassionate, and evidence-based care for birthing individuals.

The **innominate bone**, also known as the coxal or hip bone, is a large, fused structure that forms one half of the pelvis. *It is comprised of three distinct parts:*

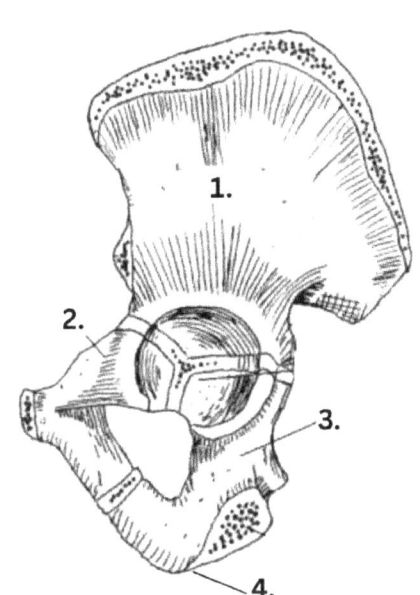

1. ILIUM this is the broad, flaring portion that forms the upper part of the hip bone. It features the iliac crest, a prominent ridge that serves as an attachment site for numerous muscles and ligaments, contributing to the overall stability of the trunk.

2. ISCHIUM located in the lower and posterior region, the ischium includes the ischial tuberosity—a robust projection that bears weight when sitting. This part plays a significant role in supporting the body during various activities.

3. PUBIS found at the anterior and inferior portion, the pubis contributes to the formation of the pubic symphysis, where the left and right pubic bones meet. This joint helps absorb shock and maintain the integrity of the pelvic ring.

Together, these three parts fuse during development to create a sturdy and integral component of the pelvic skeleton, essential for weight-bearing, movement, and the protection of pelvic organs.

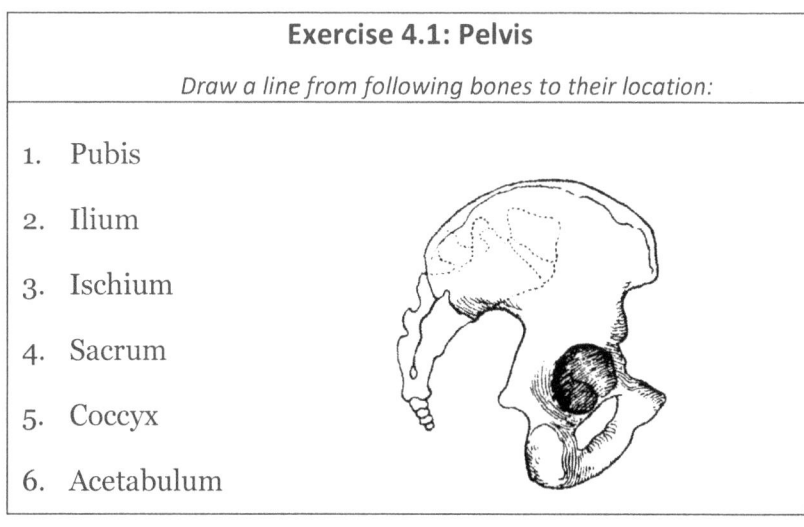

Exercise 4.1: Pelvis

Draw a line from following bones to their location:

1. Pubis
2. Ilium
3. Ischium
4. Sacrum
5. Coccyx
6. Acetabulum

The Pelvis

The pelvis consists of four bones: Two **innominate** bones (also called hip bones or coxal bone); the **sacrum**; and the **coccyx**. They are united by four joints. By adulthood, these bones are fused together.

A. ILIAC CREST the rounded, superior border of the ilium; it serves as a key attachment site for several muscles and ligaments, contributing to trunk stability.

B. SACRUM a large, triangular bone formed by the fusion of sacral vertebrae; it forms the posterior wall of the pelvic cavity and connects with the ilia at the sacroiliac joints.

C. ANTERIOR SACRAL FORAMINA small openings on the front of the sacrum that allow nerves and blood vessels to pass, facilitating communication between the pelvic organs and the spinal cord.

D. ANTERIOR INFERIOR ILIAC SPINE a bony projection on the front of the ilium that provides an attachment point for muscles such as the rectus femoris and contributes to the stability of the hip joint.

E. ISCHIAL SPINE a pointed projection on the ischium that serves as an important landmark in obstetrics and as an attachment site for ligaments that support the pelvic floor.

F. COCCYX commonly known as the tailbone, this small, triangular bone at the base of the spine consists of fused vestigial vertebrae and provides support when sitting.

G. ACETABULUM is a deep, cup-shaped cavity formed by the ilium, ischium, and pubis; it articulates with the head of the femur to form the hip joint, enabling a wide range of motion.

H. PUBIC TUBERCLE a prominent bump on the superior aspect of the pubis that serves as an attachment point for the inguinal ligament, playing a role in stabilizing the anterior pelvis.

I. PUBIC SYMPHYSIS A cartilaginous joint where the two pubic bones meet in the front of the pelvis; it absorbs shock during movement and provides stability to the pelvic ring.

J. OBTURATOR FORAMEN is a large, oval opening bordered by the pubis and ischium, largely covered by a membrane; it allows the passage of nerves and blood vessels to the lower limb.

K. BODY OF PUBIS the central portion of the pubic bone that forms part of the anterior pelvic ring, contributing to the overall stability and structure of the pelvis.

PELVIC LIGAMENTS

The pelvis is stabilized and supported by several key ligaments that connect the bones and provide structural integrity. These ligaments help maintain posture, allow movement, and play a critical role in childbirth.

The most important pelvic ligaments include:

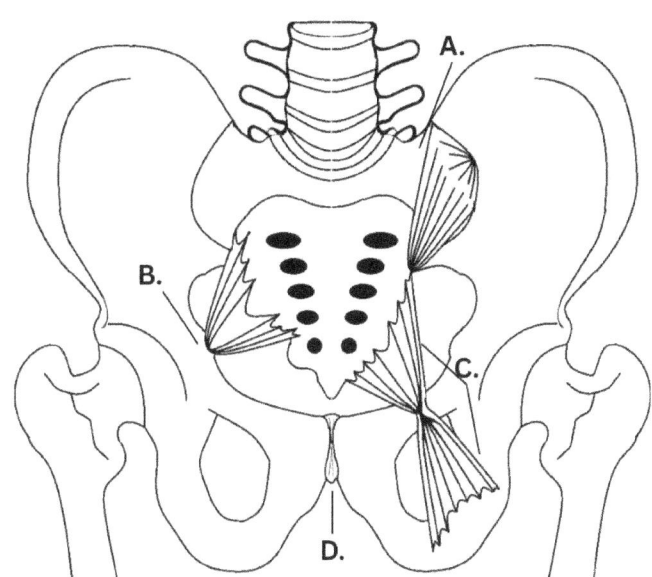

A. SACROILIAC LIGAMENTS The sacroiliac ligaments play a crucial role in maintaining pelvic stability. They securely connect the sacrum to the ilium, limiting excessive movement at the sacroiliac joints. This connection is essential for effective load transfer between the spine and the lower extremities, ensuring balance and proper function during everyday activities.

B. SACROSPINOUS LIGAMENTS Extending from the sacrum to the ischial spines, these ligaments provide stability to the lower pelvis and prevent excessive movement of the sacrum.

C. SACROTUBEROUS LIGAMENTS Running from the sacrum to the ischial tuberosities, these ligaments help create the greater and lesser sciatic foramen, which allows passage of nerves and blood vessels. They also contribute to pelvic floor support.

D. PUBIC LIGAMENTS (Anterior & Posterior) These reinforce the symphysis pubis, ensuring stability at the front of the pelvis and allowing slight flexibility during childbirth.

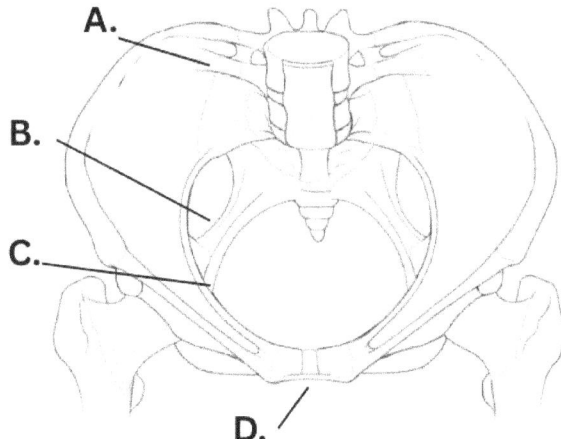

Ligament	Function / Connection
Broad Ligament	Stabilizes uterus side-to-side; contains vessels and nerves
Suspensory Ligament	Anchors ovary to pelvis; contains ovarian vessels
Round Ligament of the Uterus	Maintains anteversion; passes to labia majora
Uterosacral Ligament	Anchors cervix to sacrum; maintains uterine position
Ovarian Ligament	Connects ovary to uterus near tubal insertion

How the Pelvis Functions in Daily Life

In everyday life, the pelvis serves as the foundation for movement and weight distribution. The pelvic ligaments and joints work together to:
- Support the spine and transfer body weight to the legs
- Provide stability for walking, running, and sitting
- Allow limited movement while maintaining structural integrity
- Anchor important core and pelvic floor muscles, assisting in posture

Because of these functions, strong pelvic ligaments and muscles are essential for daily activities such as lifting, bending, and maintaining balance.

How the Pelvis Adapts During Pregnancy

During pregnancy, the pelvis undergoes significant changes to accommodate the growing baby and prepare for labor:
- The hormone **relaxin** increases ligament flexibility, allowing the pelvic joints to loosen and widen slightly.
- The **symphysis pubis** may widen, which can sometimes lead to pubic symphysis dysfunction (SPD) and cause pelvic pain and instability.
- Increased weight and postural changes place extra strain on the sacroiliac joints and lower back.

These adaptations help prepare the body for labor but may also lead to discomfort as the pelvis shifts.

Pelvic Function During Labor and Childbirth

During labor and birth, the pelvis plays a critical role in guiding the baby through the birth canal. The process involves:
1. **Pelvic widening**: relaxed ligaments and softened joints allow the pelvic bones to shift slightly, increasing the diameter of the birth canal.
2. **Fetal descent and engagement**: the baby's head moves downward into the pelvis, guided by the shape of the pelvic inlet and the ischial spines.
3. **Rotation and passage through the pelvic outlet**: the baby rotates to navigate the narrowest points of the pelvis, aided by the flexibility of the sacrum and coccyx.
4. **Delivery**: as the baby crowns, the pubic arch and perineal tissues stretch to accommodate the head.

> **Practice Tip**
> When teaching clients about pelvic changes in pregnancy, use simple analogies. Comparing the pelvis to a flexible ring or basket that widens just enough to let the baby pass can help families visualize the process.

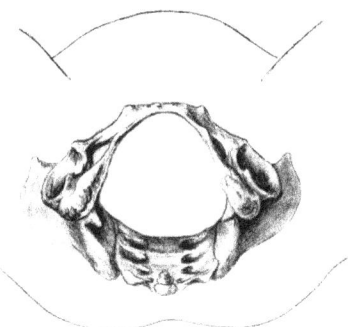

Exercise 4.2: Pelvic Function and Adaptation	
Match each situation to the correct pelvic function or adaptation:	
1. _____Standing upright without falling over	**A.** Fetal descent and engagement
2. _____A woman feels pain at her pubic bone during pregnancy	**B.** Structural support and posture
3. _____The baby's head moves down into the pelvis	**C.** Symphysis pubis widening (possible SPD)
4. _____The pelvic bones shift slightly during labor	**D.** Pelvic widening in labor

Exercise 4.3: Pelvis

Place the letter of the following bone markings on the diagram:

    a. ischial tuberosities
    b. ischial spines
    c. greater sciatic notch
    d. anterior superior iliac spine
    e. iliac crest
    f. obturator foramen
    g. acetabulum
    h. inferior rami of the pubis
    i. sacral promontory

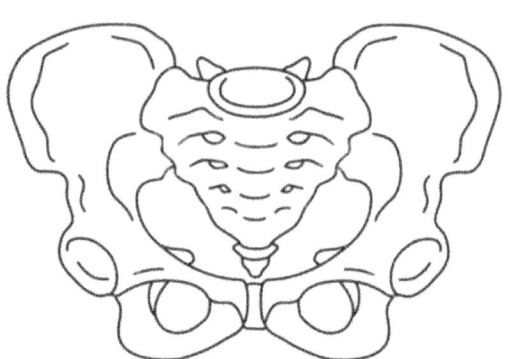

Draw a line from following to where the joints are:

1. sacro-iliac joint

2. symphysis pubis

3. sacrococcygeal joint

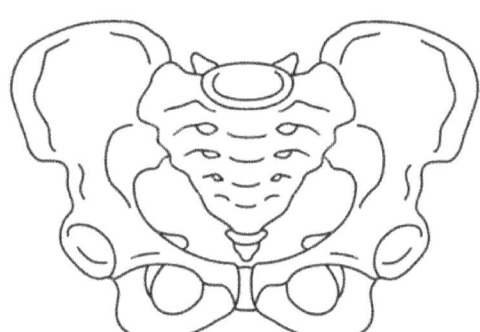

Place the letter of the following ligaments on the diagram:

  a. sacrospinous ligament

  b. sacrotuberous ligament

  c. anterior pubic ligament

  d. sacrococcygeal ligament

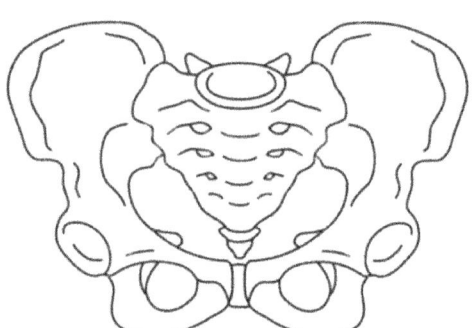

The Uterine Ligaments

The uterus is anchored in the pelvis by several supportive ligaments that help maintain its position and orientation in both pregnant and non-pregnant states. These structures are composed of connective tissue and often carry blood vessels, lymphatics, and nerves.

Key Uterine Ligaments

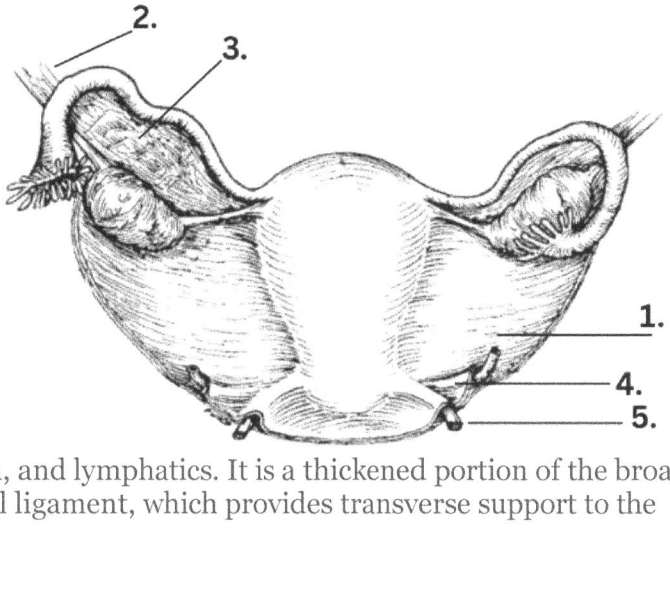

1. **BROAD LIGAMENT** The broad ligaments are wide, wing-like folds of peritoneum that extend from the lateral sides of the uterus to the pelvic sidewalls. Although they provide minimal structural support, they enclose important structures such as the uterine tubes, ovarian ligaments, blood vessels, and lymphatics. They also help maintain the uterus in a central position.

2. **SUSPENSORY LIGAMENT** of the the ovary (Infundibulopelvic Ligament). This ligament extends from the lateral pole of the ovary to the pelvic wall and contains the ovarian artery, vein, and lymphatics. It is a thickened portion of the broad ligament and should not be confused with the cardinal ligament, which provides transverse support to the cervix.

3. **OVARIAN LIGAMENT** The ovarian ligament is a short, fibrous band that connects the medial surface of the ovary to the lateral side of the uterus, just below the uterine tube. It helps stabilize the ovary's position in relation to the uterus.

4. **CARDINAL LIGAMENTS** (Transverse Cervical Ligaments): The cardinal ligaments run transversely from the cervix and lateral vagina to the pelvic sidewalls, at the level of the ischial spines. They provide the primary support for the cervix and upper vagina and contain the uterine arteries and veins.

5. **ROUND LIGAMENT** Arising near the uterine horn (cornu), the round ligaments pass anteriorly through the inguinal canals to the labia majora. They assist in maintaining the uterus in an anteverted position. During pregnancy, these ligaments stretch significantly, often causing discomfort.

6. **UTEROSACRAL LIGAMENTS** These strong fibrous bands extend from the posterior cervix and upper vagina around the rectum to insert on the sacrum. They provide posterior support and help maintain the forward tilt of the uterus by pulling the cervix backward. They also define the lateral borders of the rectouterine pouch (pouch of Douglas).

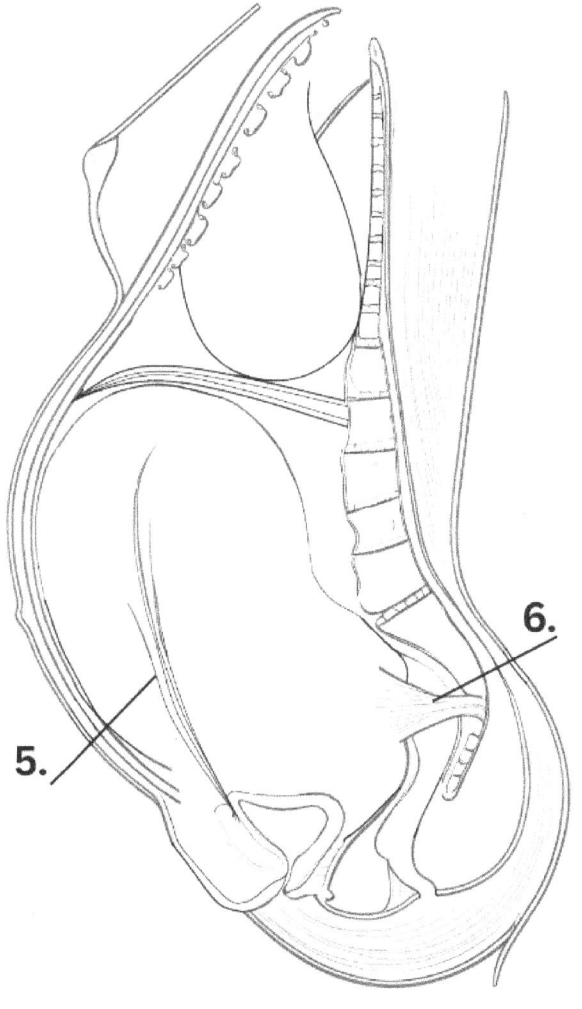

PELVIC ORGANS

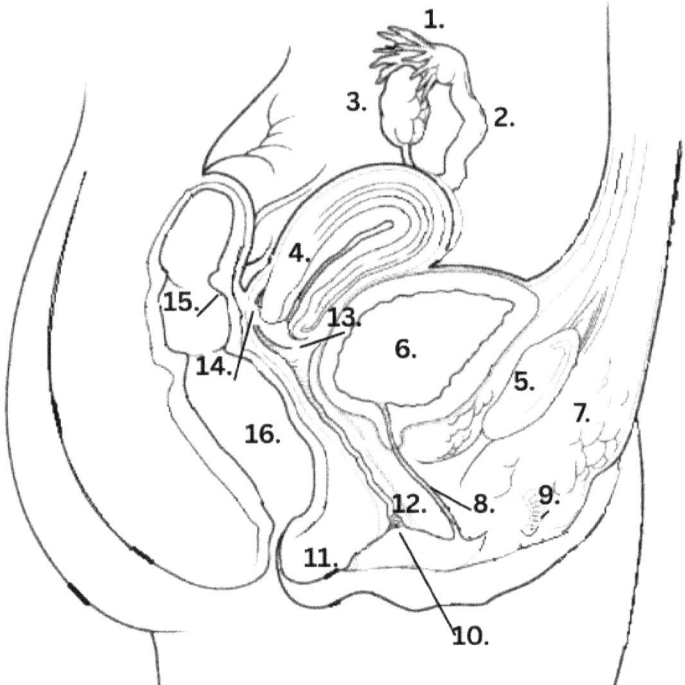

1. **FIMBRIAE** fingerlike projections at the end of the uterine tube that help guide the ovum from the ovary into the tube after ovulation.
2. **UTERINE TUBE** (*formerly* fallopian tube): a narrow, muscular tube that carries the ovum from the ovary to the uterus; primary site of fertilization.
3. **OVARY** the female reproductive organ that produces and releases eggs (ova) and secretes the hormones estrogen and progesterone.
4. **UTERUS** a pear-shaped muscular organ where the fertilized egg implants and develops into a fetus during pregnancy.
5. **PUBIS** the front part of the pelvis, forming part of the pubic bone that meets at the midline at the symphysis pubis.
6. **BLADDER** a hollow organ in front of the uterus that stores urine before it is expelled through the urethra.
7. **MONS PUBIS** a fatty, rounded pad covering the pubic bone, providing cushioning and protection; covered with hair after puberty.
8. **URETHRA** a short tube that carries urine from the bladder to the outside of the body, located above the vaginal opening (introitus).
9. **CLITORIS** a small, highly sensitive erectile organ at the top of the vulva, involved in sexual arousal; homologous to the penis.
10. **INTROITUS** the external opening of the vagina leading into the vaginal canal.
11. **PERINEUM** the tissue-covered area between the vaginal opening and the anus, supporting the pelvic floor and stretching during childbirth.
12. **VAGINA** a muscular canal connecting the external genitalia to the cervix; involved in sexual intercourse, menstrual flow, and childbirth.
13. **ANTERIOR VAGINAL FORNIX** a shallow recess between the cervix and anterior vaginal wall, allowing some movement of the cervix.
14. **POSTERIOR VAGINAL FORNIX** a deeper recess behind the cervix, adjacent to the rectouterine pouch (pouch of Douglas); sometimes used for medical procedures such as culdocentesis.
15. **RECTOUTERINE POUCH** (pouch of Douglas) the lowest part of the peritoneal cavity, between the rectum and posterior uterus, where fluid may collect.
16. **RECTUM** the final portion of the large intestine, located behind the vagina and uterus; stores and expels feces.

THE UTERUS

The uterus is a dynamic muscular organ located in the pelvis between the bladder and rectum. It plays a central role in the menstrual cycle, implantation, and the growth and birth of a baby and placenta. It is typically shaped like an inverted pear and measures approximately 7.5 cm long, 5 cm wide, and 1.75 cm thick in a non-pregnant state, though size and shape vary between individuals and across the reproductive lifespan.

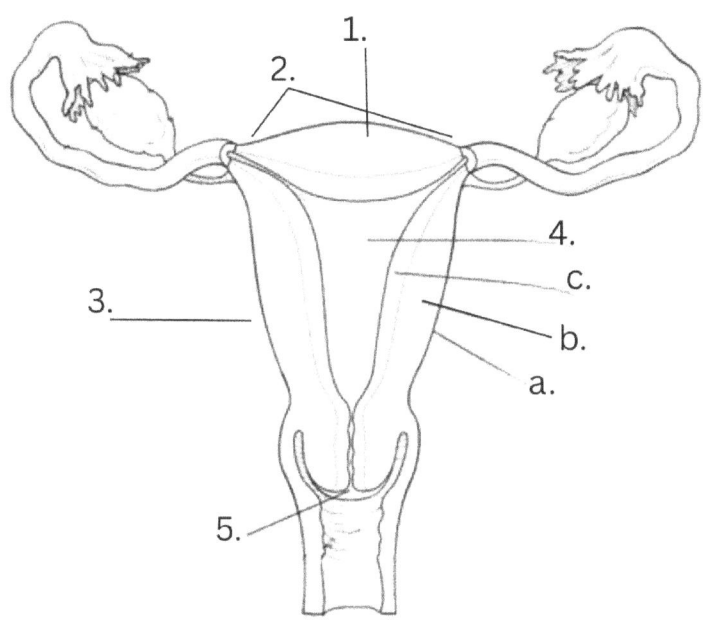

1. FUNDUS The top of the uterus, located above the openings to the uterine tubes.
2. CORNUA (Horns) The upper outer corners where the uterus meets the uterine tubes.
3. CORPUS (Body) The central, tapering portion that expands significantly during pregnancy.
4. UTERINE CAVITY The hollow space inside the uterus where implantation occurs and the fetus develops during pregnancy.
    a. PERIMETRIUM The outermost layer, also called the serous layer, is a continuation of the peritoneum. It protects the uterus and connects it laterally to the broad ligaments.
    b. MYOMETRIUM This is the thick muscular layer responsible for the strong, coordinated contractions during labor and menstruation. In the corpus, muscle fibers run in **longitudinal fibers** in the outer layer, the middle layer has **figure-eight fibers**, and the inner layer has **circular fibers**. They are interlaced with connective tissue and blood vessels. In the cervix, the muscle fibers are fewer and embedded in dense collagen, giving the cervix its firm structure.

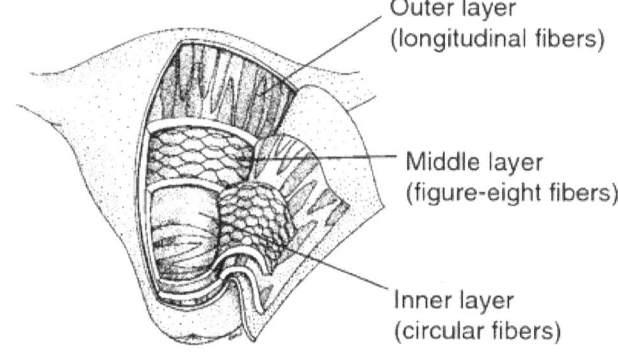

   c. ENDOMETRIUM The inner mucosal lining of the uterus, which thickens and sheds in response to hormonal cycles.

It has two functional layers:

- STRATUM FUNCTIONALIS The top layer that builds up and is shed during menstruation.
- STRATUM BASALIS The deeper layer that regenerates a new functionalis each cycle.

Uterine Blood Supply

The arterial blood flow to the uterus follows a branching pathway:

1. **UTERINE ARTERY** The main source of blood for the uterus, it originates from the internal iliac artery, which is a major vessel of the pelvis.
   A. **Radial arteries**: from the arcuate arteries, radial arteries branch inward to supply the myometrium, the muscular layer of the uterus.
   B. **Basal arteries:** supply the basal layer of the endometrium, which is the permanent tissue that regenerates after menstruation. These are not hormone-sensitive.
   C. **Spiral arteries:** supply the functional layer of the endometrium, the tissue that is shed during menstruation. These are sensitive to hormonal changes and play a critical role in the menstrual cycle and during pregnancy.
2. **OVARIAN ARTERY** Arising directly from the abdominal aorta, the ovarian artery also contributes to the uterine blood supply.
3. **VAGINAL ARTERIES** The vaginal artery branches off the internal iliac artery.

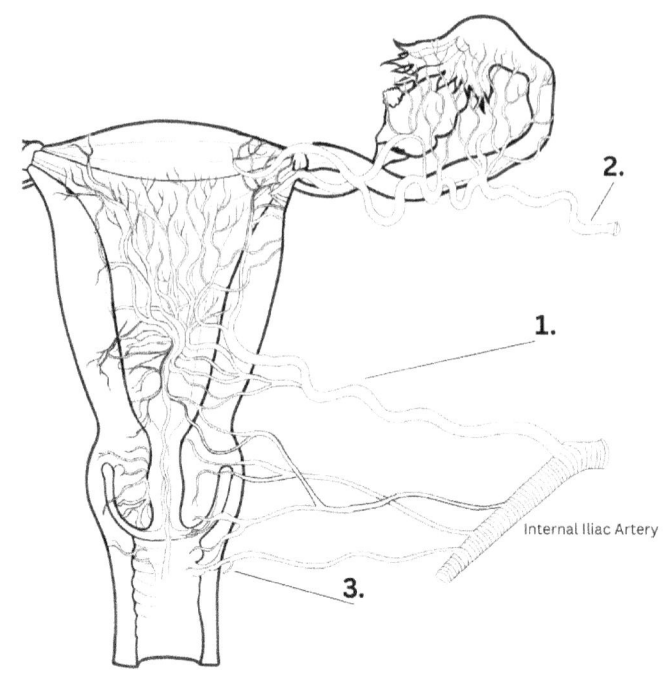

Uterine Nerve Supply

The main supply to the uterus is considered to come from the pelvic autonomic system are the sympathetic and parasympathetic nervous systems. Nerve impulses to the uterus are in response to chemical agents within the uterus or hormonal factors in the feto-placental unit. Sympathetic nerves from the pelvic plexus pass to the para-cervical ganglia, which are sheaths of sympathetic nerve fibers situated close behind and on either side of the cervix. The contact or pressure on the cervix of a well-fitting presenting part results in the transmission of a stimulus through the para-cervical ganglia from the nerve endings in the cervix. Pressure on the cervix stimulates afferent nerves via the pelvic plexus, contributing to the Ferguson reflex and increased oxytocin release.

The uterine nerves pass to the spinal cord accompanying sympathetic nerves in the:

A. **INFERIOR HYPOGASTRIC PLEXUS** and

B. **SUPERIOR HYPOGASTRIC PLEXUS** and the **hypogastric nerve**. They then pass through the lumbar and lower thoracic sympathetic chain and enter the spinal cord through the...

C. **POSTERIOR NERVE ROOTS** of spinal cord. The pudendal nerve supplies structures in the pelvis.

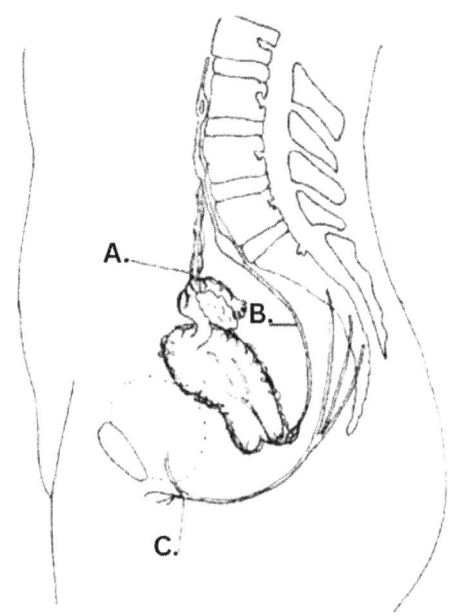

Cervix: Structure and Function

The cervix, or "neck" of the uterus, extends into the upper portion of the vagina and is formed from the lower uterine segment. *It has three key features:*

1. **INTERNAL OS** The opening at the junction between the uterus and cervical canal.
2. **CERVICAL CANAL** The narrow passageway between the internal and external os.
3. **EXTERNAL OS** The visible and palpable portion of the cervix inside the vaginal canal.

The cervix is surrounded by four **fornices** of the vagina, named by their position: These fornices accommodate the cervix and allow for flexibility and expansion, which is important for gynecologic procedures and vaginal delivery.

3. a. **ANTERIOR FORNIX**

3. b. **POSTERIOR FORNIX**

3. c. **RIGHT AND LEFT LATERAL FORNICES**

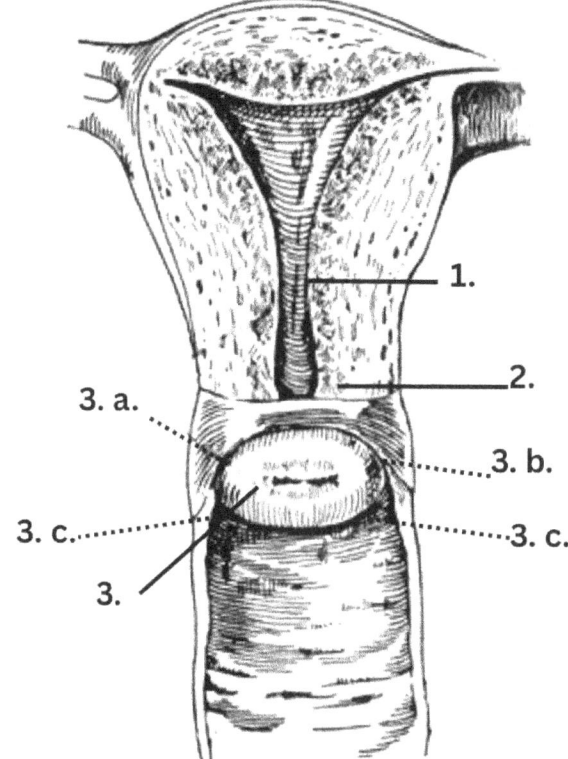

The external os changes shape after childbirth. In multiparous women, the external os is typically wider and more irregular in shape compared to a nulliparous cervix.

Cervical and Vaginal Secretions

The cervical glands secrete mucus that exits into the vaginal canal, forming part of normal vaginal discharge. This discharge plays a key role in maintaining the vaginal environment at a slightly acidic pH (~4.5), which helps protect against infections by suppressing the growth of harmful microbes. During ovulation, the pH becomes more alkaline, creating a sperm-friendly environment to facilitate fertilization. Regular douching can disrupt this balance and is not recommended especially for youth, unless medically indicated.

VAGINA STRUCTURE AND FUNCTION

The vagina is a flexible, muscular canal that extends from the vulva (external genitalia) to the uterus. The anterior wall of the vagina is positioned near the bladder and urethra, while the posterior wall lies in proximity to the rectum. The posterior wall is typically longer due to the cervix's positioning and angulation into the vaginal vault.

It plays multiple vital roles in reproductive and sexual health:
- Serves as a passage for menstrual flow and mucous discharge
- Functions as a muscular pathway for penetration during sexual intercourse
- Allows for natural lubrication and self-cleaning
- Acts as the birth passageway during vaginal delivery

Vaginal Rugae and Wall Structure

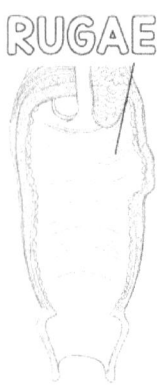

A distinctive feature of the vaginal wall is the presence of rugae—folds or ridges in the mucosal lining that allow the vaginal canal to expand significantly during sexual arousal, insertion of medical instruments, or childbirth. These rugae contribute to the elasticity and capacity of the vaginal walls, especially in individuals who have not yet given birth vaginally.

The vaginal wall is made up of four integrated layers:

1. MUCOSAL LAYER The inner layer, lined with non-keratinized stratified squamous epithelium, this layer features rugae and is lubricated by cervical secretions and transudation from underlying capillaries.

2. SUBMUCOSAL LAYER (lamina propria): Contains vascular elastic connective tissue, supporting the mucosa and accommodating changes in diameter.

3. MUSCULAR LAYER is composed of involuntary smooth muscle fibers, arranged in circular and longitudinal layers, allowing for contraction and flexibility.

4. ADVENTITIAL LAYER The outer connective tissue layer containing blood vessels, lymphatics, and nerve fibers, providing support and sensation.

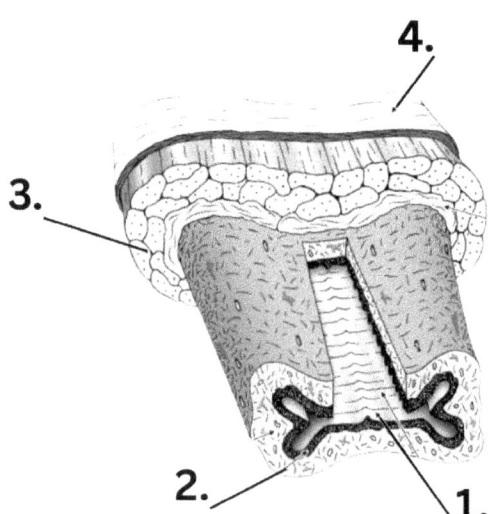

Additional Structures:

1. The HYMEN is a thin membrane that may partially cover the vaginal introitus in some individuals. It varies greatly in size, shape, and elasticity and may be absent, stretched, or disrupted due to physical activity, tampon use, or sexual activity.

2. The INTROITUS is the external opening of the vagina, situated between the urethral meatus and anus.

3. The LABIA MINORA are the inner folds of skin that protect the vaginal and urethral openings. They contain sebaceous glands, sensory nerve endings, and help direct urine flow. Superiorly, they converge to form the clitoral hood; inferiorly, they attach near the posterior commissure and contribute to the opening of the vaginal canal.

Exercise 4.4: Pelvic Organ Functions
Match each structure with its correct description. Write the letter of the description next to the number.

1. _____Ovary	A. Rounded top portion of the uterus, used to measure growth in pregnancy
2. _____Uterine tube	B. Female reproductive organ that produces eggs and hormones
3. _____Fundus	C. Narrow lower portion of the uterus, connecting to the vagina
4. _____Cervix	D. Muscular canal transporting ovum from ovary to uterus; site of fertilization
5. _____Perineum	E. Tissue between vaginal opening and anus that stretches during childbirth

The Vulva

The vulva refers to the external genital structures of individuals assigned female at birth. It includes multiple components that serve protective, sensory, and reproductive functions.

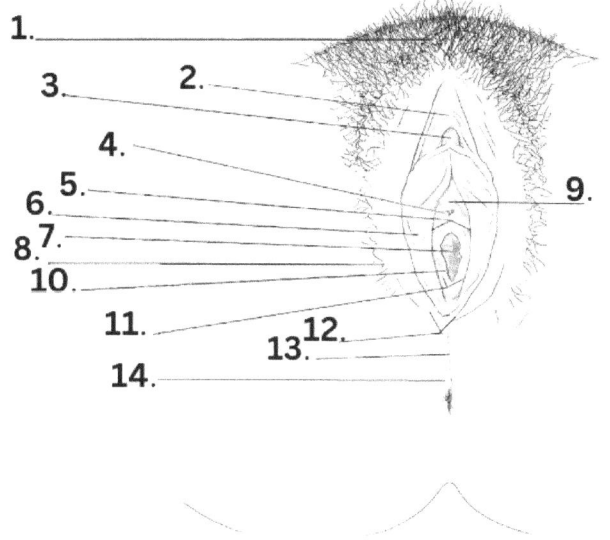

1. **MONS PUBIS** A fatty cushion located over the pubic bone (symphysis pubis). It provides protection and cushioning and becomes covered with pubic hair after puberty.
2. **PREPUCE OR CLITORAL HOOD** is located over the clitoris.
3. **CLITORIS** A highly vascular and sensitive erectile organ involved in sexual pleasure. The frenulum is a small band of tissue that connects the clitoral shaft to the labia minora.
4. **URETHRAL MEATUS** A small opening located just below the clitoris, through which urine is expelled from the bladder.
5. **PARAURETHRAL GLANDS** (Skene's Glands) Small glands located on either side of the urethral opening that produce secretions and may contribute to sexual response.
6. **LABIA MINORA** Two inner folds of mucosal tissue that extend from the clitoral hood (prepuce) downward toward the fourchette. They help protect the vestibule and contain numerous nerve endings and blood vessels for sensation.
7. **INTROITUS** (Vaginal Opening) The entrance to the vaginal canal. It varies in size and shape and may be partially covered by the hymenal tissue in some individuals.
8. **LABIA MAJORA** Two outer folds of skin extending from the mons pubis to the perineum. The outer surface is typically covered with pubic hair, while the inner surface contains sweat and sebaceous glands that help maintain moisture and protection.
9. **VESTIBULE** The area between the labia minora that houses the urethral opening, vaginal opening (introitus), and glands that contribute to lubrication.
10. **HYMENAL RING** A thin, elastic membrane that partially covers the vaginal opening in some individuals. It may stretch or tear due to various activities, including sexual activity, tampon use, or physical exercise.
11. **VESTIBULAR GLANDS** (Bartholin's Glands) : Glands located near the introitus that secrete lubricating fluid to enhance comfort during sexual activity.
12. **FOURCHETTE** A fold of skin at the posterior end of the labia minora, located near the perineum. It can stretch during childbirth.
13. **PERINEAL BODY** The area between the vaginal opening and the anus. It supports pelvic floor structures and stretches significantly during childbirth.
14. **ANUS** The external opening of the rectum, located at the posterior end of the perineum. It allows for the excretion of feces and is surrounded by muscles that control bowel movements.

BLOOD SUPPLY OF THE EXTERNAL GENITALIA

The external genitalia, collectively referred to as the vulva, receives a rich vascular supply that supports sensory function, tissue health, and sexual arousal. The internal pudendal artery, a terminal branch of the internal iliac artery, is the primary vessel responsible for delivering oxygenated blood to this region. It travels through the pudendal canal (Alcock's canal) and courses along the ischial spine, then forward along the pubic arch to supply multiple branches:

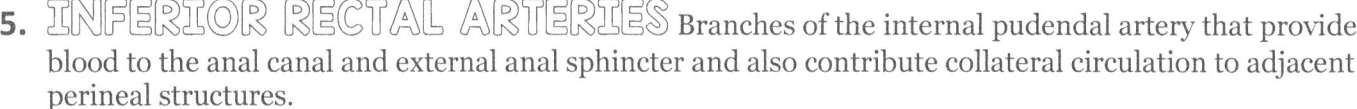

1. **DORSAL ARTERY OF THE CLITORIS** Travels along the dorsal surface of the clitoral shaft, supplying the glans clitoris and prepuce. It also contributes to the blood supply of the vestibule and anterior vaginal wall.

2. **DEEP ARTERY OF THE CLITORIS** (Artery of the Corpus Cavernosum) Penetrates the clitoral body, supplying the erectile tissue of the corpora cavernosa, which are responsible for clitoral tumescence.

3. **PERINEAL ARTERIES** Arise from the internal pudendal artery and supply the skin and superficial muscles of the perineum, including the posterior labial region and external anal sphincter.

4. **POSTERIOR LABIAL ARTERIES** Branch from the perineal artery to supply the labia majora and minora, contributing to the vascular network that supports tactile sensation and engorgement during sexual arousal.

5. **INFERIOR RECTAL ARTERIES** Branches of the internal pudendal artery that provide blood to the anal canal and external anal sphincter and also contribute collateral circulation to adjacent perineal structures.

These arteries **anastomose** (interconnect) with branches from the external **pudendal arteries** (derived from the femoral artery) and contribute to a highly vascularized and responsive network. Venous drainage follows a similar pattern, largely via the pudendal veins, and is important for maintaining vascular homeostasis and thermoregulation in the genital area.

The Clitoris

The clitoris is a highly sensitive, erectile organ that plays a central role in sexual pleasure. Though often thought of as a small external nub, the clitoris is far more extensive than it appears on the surface.

> **Key Fact**
> The clitoris has over 8,000 sensory nerve fibers in the glans alone, which is more than twice the number in the glans penis. This makes it the most sensitive organ in the human body.

Location of the Clitoris in the Vulva and Pelvic Floor

The clitoris sits at the anterior junction of the labia minora, tucked just under the mons pubis and above the urethra. Its internal structures run deep into the pelvis, anchoring around the pubic arch. It shares close anatomical relationships with the urethra, anterior vaginal wall, and pelvic floor muscles, particularly the bulbospongiosus and ischiocavernosus muscles, which support clitoral erection and rhythmic contraction during orgasm.

ANATOMY OF THE CLITORIS

The clitoris is composed of several parts:

1. **CLITORAL HOOD** (Prepuce) A fold of skin that protects the glans, formed by the upper portion of the labia minora.
2. **CLITORAL SHAFT** (Body) The internal continuation of the glans, made of erectile tissue that becomes engorged with blood during arousal.
3. **GLANS** The visible portion located just beneath the clitoral hood (prepuce), above the urethral opening. It contains a dense concentration of nerve endings.
4. **CRURA** Two legs of erectile tissue that extend downward and backward along the pubic bones, anchoring the clitoris to the pelvis.
5. **BULBS OF THE VESTIBULE** Paired masses of erectile tissue located beneath the labia majora on either side of the vaginal opening. Though not technically part of the clitoris, they functionally contribute to sexual arousal and are sometimes grouped with clitoral structures.

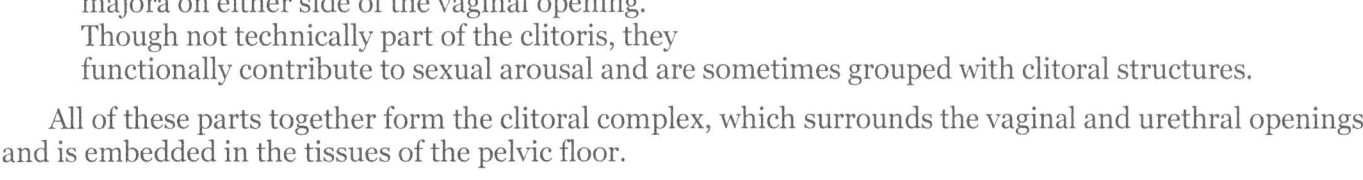

All of these parts together form the clitoral complex, which surrounds the vaginal and urethral openings and is embedded in the tissues of the pelvic floor.

How Birth May Affect the Clitoris

While the clitoris itself is not directly involved in childbirth, it may be affected in several ways:

- **Swelling and Trauma:** Pressure from crowning or the use of instruments (like forceps) during birth can cause swelling or bruising to the vulva, including the clitoral glans and hood
- **Perineal Tearing or Episiotomy:** Tearing that extends toward the anterior perineum can involve or affect the clitoral hood or labia minora, impacting sensitivity or tissue integrity.
- **Neurological Changes:** Stretching or compression of pelvic nerves may temporarily reduce sensation or cause heightened sensitivity.
- **Pelvic Floor Dysfunction:** Changes in the tone or coordination of the pelvic floor muscles can affect the blood flow and neuromuscular support of the clitoral complex, which may influence arousal and orgasm postpartum.

> **Clinical Tip**
> Swelling or bruising of the clitoris and vulva after birth is common. Applying cold packs in the immediate postpartum period can help reduce swelling and discomfort.
>
> Always assess tissue integrity carefully and reassure clients that sensation often returns as healing progresses.

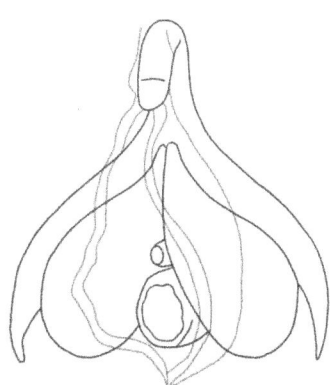

MUSCLES OF THE PERINEUM

The muscles of the perineum form a supportive and dynamic part of the pelvic floor, contributing to continence, sexual function, and core stability. They are arranged in both deep and superficial layers and may be stretched or injured during childbirth.

Levator Ani Complex (Deep Layer)

The levator ani is a sling-like group of muscles that forms most of the pelvic diaphragm. It supports pelvic organs and helps maintain continence. It consists of three paired muscles:

1. ILIOCOCCYGEUS
2. PUBOCOCCYGEUS
3. PUBORECTALIS (often included in newer classifications)

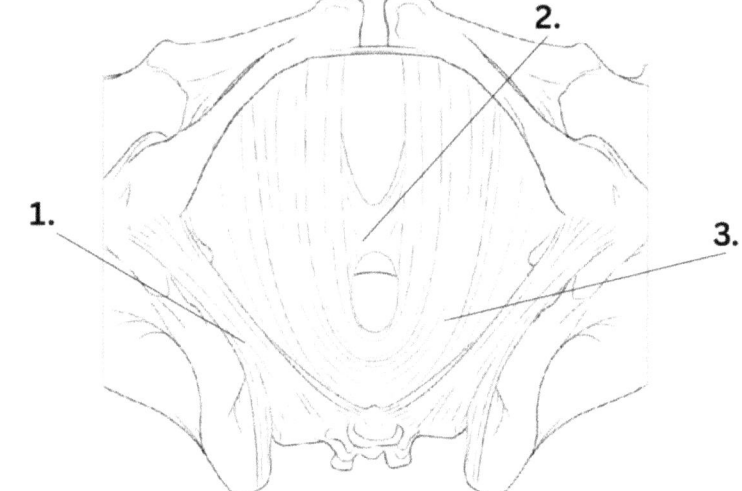

Together, these muscles surround and support the urethra, vagina, and rectum. They are critical for pelvic floor tone and function. *Note:* The ischiococcygeus (or coccygeus) is sometimes grouped with the levator ani, but it is technically a separate muscle that stabilizes the sacrum and coccyx.

Perineal Body and Converging Muscles (Superficial Layer)

The perineal body is a fibromuscular node between the vaginal opening and the anus. It serves as the central point of attachment for several important superficial muscles:

1. ISCHIOCAVERNOSUS Runs from the ischial tuberosity along the sides of the clitoral crura. It helps maintain clitoral erection and is involved in orgasmic function.
2. BULBOCAVERNOSUS (Bulbospongiosus): Surrounds the vaginal opening and clitoral bulbs, contributing to clitoral engorgement and vaginal tightness during arousal.
3. SUPERFICIAL TRANSVERSE Perineal Muscle: Extends from the perineal body to the ischial tuberosities, providing lateral support to the perineum.
4. EXTERNAL ANAL SPHINCTER: Encircles the anus and is essential for fecal continence. It may be injured or torn during childbirth, especially with deep perineal lacerations.

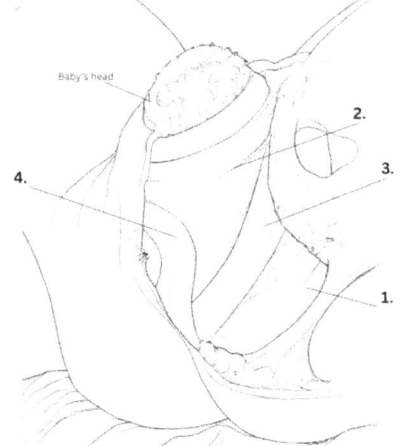

Pelvic muscles during crowning

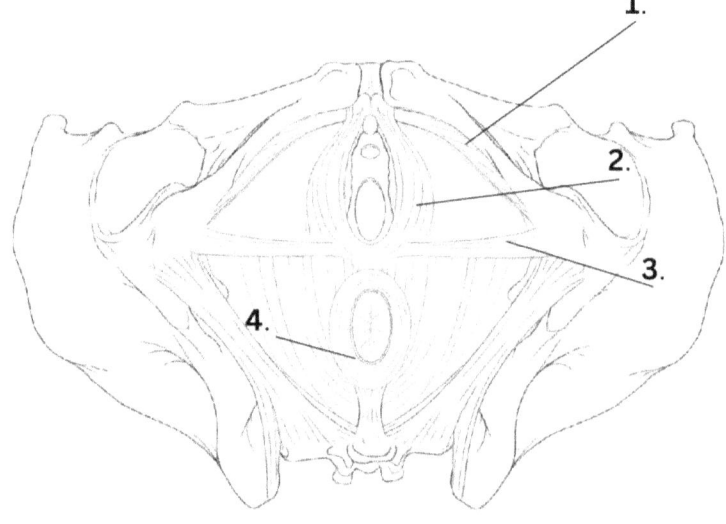

These muscles work together to support the pelvic floor, aid in sexual function, and maintain continence. During birth, they undergo intense stretching and pressure, which can lead to temporary dysfunction, laceration, or long-term changes. Postpartum recovery of the perineum often benefits from pelvic floor therapy, gentle movement, and body awareness practices.

THE PELVIC FLOOR AS A DYNAMIC SYSTEM

The pelvic floor is a group of muscles, ligaments, and connective tissue that stretches like a hammock from the pubic bone to the tailbone and side to side between the sitting bones. It supports the pelvic organs—bladder, uterus, and rectum—while also playing crucial roles in:

- Continence (controlling urination and defecation)
- Sexual function
- Core stability
- Support for breathing and posture
- Labor and delivery mechanics

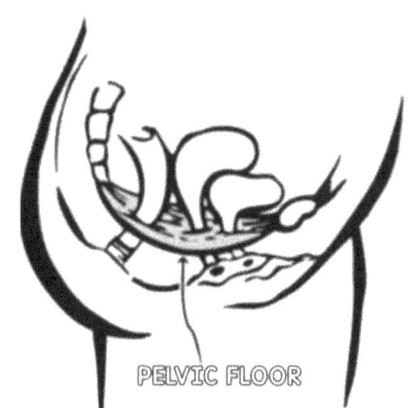

During Pregnancy

As the body transforms to support new life, the pelvic floor muscles respond with remarkable adaptability. These muscles carry the increasing weight of the uterus while adjusting to hormonal shifts that soften and relax the pelvic tissues. This natural softening, combined with changes in posture and alignment, affects how the pelvic floor functions, requiring a careful balance of tone and flexibility. Increased blood flow and fluid retention can lead to swelling of the vulva and perineum, while the perineal body becomes more elastic in preparation for labor. Supporting pelvic floor health during pregnancy involves cultivating both strength and release, ensuring the body is responsive and resilient for birth and postpartum recovery. *During pregnancy, the pelvic floor undergoes major adaptations to support the growing uterus and baby:*

Increased Load
- The uterus steadily increases in weight, pressing down on the pelvic floor.
- The muscles must remain strong enough to support the organs, yet flexible enough to allow for birth.

Hormonal Changes
- Relaxin and progesterone soften ligaments and connective tissue, preparing the body for birth.
- These hormones also reduce pelvic floor tone, which can lead to sensations of pressure or heaviness.

Postural Shifts
- As posture changes with the growing belly, the alignment of the pelvis can shift, influencing how the pelvic floor functions.
- Poor alignment may overwork or weaken certain areas of the pelvic floor.

Increased Circulation and Swelling
- Increased blood and fluid flow can cause visible swelling of the vulva and perineum.
- The perineal body becomes more elastic in preparation for stretching during birth.

Exercise 4.5: Muscle Changes in Pregnancy

Match letter to its correct description.

1. _____ Hormones that soften ligaments and connective tissue
2. _____ Becomes more elastic in preparation for birth_____
3. _____ May swell due to increased circulation during pregnancy
4. _____ Affects how pelvic muscles are used during pregnancy
5. _____ Group of muscles that support bladder, uterus, and rectum

A. Relaxin & Progesterone
B. Perineal body
C. Vulva & Perineum
D. Postural shifts
E. Pelvic floor

During Labor and Birth

As labor begins, the pelvic floor shifts from supporting to yielding. These deep and superficial muscles, especially the **levator ani** group, must stretch dramatically to allow the baby to pass through the birth canal. Far from being passive, the pelvic floor actively guides the baby's descent and rotation with each contraction and push. During the second stage of labor, the perineum thins and expands as the baby crowns, sometimes stretching up to three times its normal length. This intense transformation can result in tearing, particularly if the tissues are tense or under strain. A responsive pelvic floor, capable of both engagement and release, can support a more efficient, intuitive birth and may reduce trauma. Awareness, breath, and body alignment all play key roles in how these muscles function during the birthing process.

1. **Engagement and Descent**
   - The baby's head navigates through the pelvis—rotating and descending through the birth canal.
   - The pelvic floor muscles stretch and yield to guide the baby downward. The **levator ani**, especially the **pubococcygeus** and **puborectalis**, must lengthen significantly—up to three times their resting length.

2. **Pushing Phase**
   - During the second stage of labor, the pelvic floor muscles soften and thin out to make space for the baby.
   - A coordinated release of muscle tension is just as important as strength. If the muscles are too tight, they may slow descent or contribute to tearing.

3. **Perineal Stretching**
   - The **bulbospongiosus** and **superficial transverse perineal muscles** stretch around the baby's head.
   - The perineal body is under immense pressure and may tear, especially in first-time births or with precipitous deliveries.

4. **Anal Sphincter and Trauma**
   - In some cases, the external anal sphincter may also be injured during childbirth (third- or fourth-degree tears), affecting continence and requiring careful repair.

Exercise 4.6: Pelvic Floor in Labor & Birth
Match letter to its correct description.

1. _____ Muscles that stretch to guide the baby through the pelvis	**A.** Levator ani
2. _____ Muscles thin and soften to allow the baby through	**B.** Pushing phase
3. _____ Important during crowning; may stretch up to 3x	**C.** Perineal stretching
4. _____ May tear in severe births; affects continence	**D.** External anal sphincter
5. _____ Prevents tearing and supports smoother birth	**E.** Pelvic floor release

UTERINE (FALLOPIAN) TUBES

The uterine tubes (also called fallopian tubes) are two narrow, flexible structures that transport the ovum (egg cell) from the ovaries to the uterus. Each tube is approximately 10 centimeters (4 inches) long and lies within the broad ligament, connecting the ovary to the uterus. Fertilization typically occurs within these tubes.

Four Main Parts of the Uterine Tube

1. **INTERSTITIAL PORTION**: The narrowest section (about 1 millimeter wide), which passes through the uterine wall.
2. **ISTHMUS**: A short, narrow segment adjacent to the uterus.
3. **AMPULLA**: The widest and longest section, where fertilization most often occurs.
4. **INFUNDIBULUM**: The funnel-shaped, distal end of the tube near the ovary. It contains **fimbriae**, fingerlike projections that help guide the ovum into the tube after ovulation.

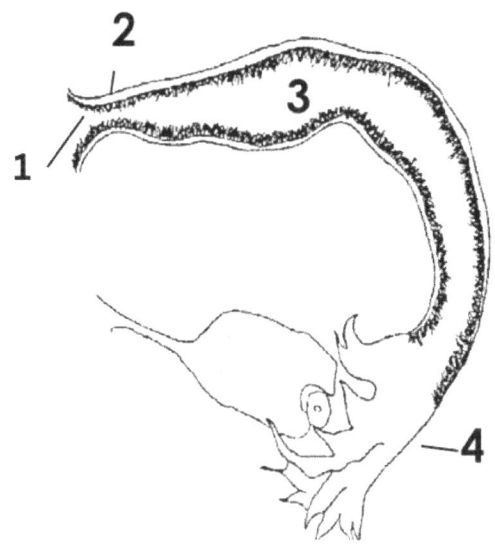

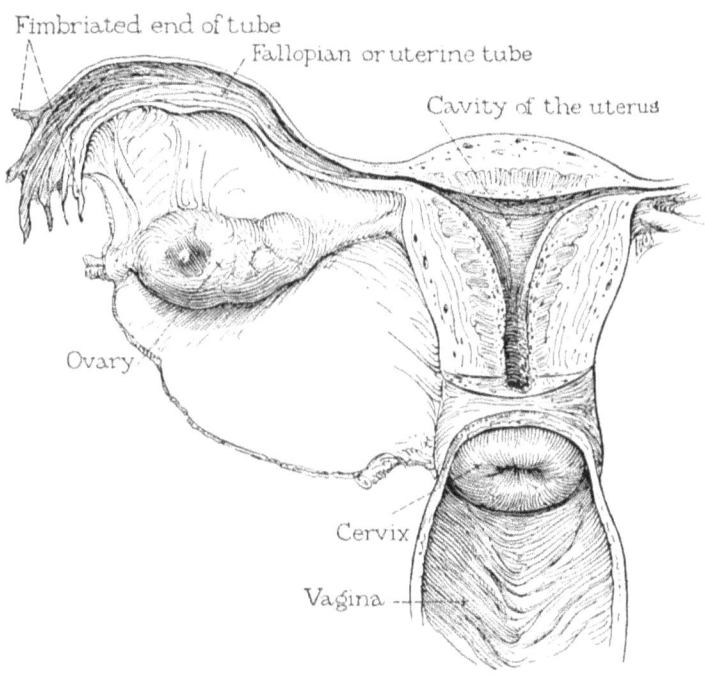

Three Layers of the Uterine Tube

1. **SEROUS MEMBRANE**: The outer protective covering.
2. **MUSCULARIS**: The middle muscular layer that produces **peristalsis** (wave-like contractions) to move the ovum toward the uterus.
3. **MUCOSA**: The inner lining, made of **ciliated** cells that help propel the ovum and secretory cells that nourish it.

Exercise 4.7: Uterine Tube
Match letter to its correct description.

1. ____ Funnel-shaped end near the ovary with fingerlike projections	**A.** Interstitial portion
2. ____ Widest and longest section where fertilization usually happens	**B.** Isthmus
3. ____ Short, narrow section closest to the uterus	**C.** Ampulla
4. ____ Narrowest part that passes through the uterine wall	**D.** Infundibulum

The Ovary

The ovaries are two almond-shaped reproductive organs located in the upper pelvic cavity, one on each side of the uterus. They are held in place by the ovarian ligaments (which connect the ovaries to the uterus) and the suspensory ligaments (which connect them to the pelvic wall). Each ovary measures approximately 4 centimeters long, 2 centimeters wide, and 1.25 centimeters thick, though size and shape can vary with age, cycle phase, and hormonal status.. While the ovaries are the main producers of reproductive hormones during the menstrual years, sex hormones are also produced by other body systems, including the placenta during pregnancy and the adrenal glands throughout life, in both females and males. These hormones play important roles even outside of the ovulatory cycle

Primary Functions of the Ovaries
- Maturation of ova (egg cells) for fertilization
- Release of an ovum (ovulation) during the menstrual cycle
- Hormone production, including estrogen, progesterone, and small amounts of androgens

Structural Layers of the Ovary

1. GERMINAL EPITHELIUM A thin outer layer of cuboidal epithelial cells covering the ovary
2. TUNICA ALBUGINEA A dense connective tissue layer beneath the epithelium
3. STROMA The internal framework, divided into:
   - A. CORTEX The outer region containing follicles at various stages of development
   - B. MEDULLA The inner region containing blood vessels, lymphatics, and nerves

Ovarian Follicle Development

A. OVARIAN FOLLICLES Located in the cortex; these house the developing oocytes (immature ova), which are surrounded by hormone-secreting support cells

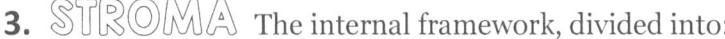

B. GRAAFIAN FOLLICLE A mature follicle that enlarges and eventually ruptures during ovulation; it also secretes estrogens

C. CORPUS LUTEUM After ovulation, the follicle becomes a temporary endocrine structure that secretes progesterone and small amounts of estrogen
- If pregnancy occurs, the corpus luteum supports early pregnancy until the placenta takes over hormone production
- If no pregnancy occurs, it degenerates into the **corpus albicans**

> **Why It Matters?**
> - The ovaries are small but powerful organs that do more than just release eggs.
> - They produce the hormones that shape the menstrual cycle, mood, energy, and bone health.
> - Their follicles are like little ecosystems, supporting early life before anyone even knows they're pregnant.
> - Whether you're supporting a birth, learning your own cycle, or helping someone navigate menopause, knowing the ovaries matters.

Comparative Reproductive Cell Development:

At birth, baby girls are born with all the oocytes (immature egg cells) they will ever have—approximately 1 to 2 million. This number declines significantly over time, with only about 400–500 ovulated across the entire reproductive lifespan.

In contrast, males are not born with mature sperm. Instead, they begin producing sperm at puberty and continue throughout their life. Spermatogenesis is a continuous process in the testes, taking roughly 90 days for each new batch of sperm to mature.

OVARIAN AND RELATED HORMONES

Hormones produced by the ovaries, pituitary gland, placenta, and adrenal glands work together to regulate the menstrual cycle, ovulation, pregnancy, and the development of secondary sex characteristics.

Estrogens

Sources: Primarily produced by the Graafian follicles during the follicular phase and by the placenta during pregnancy. Smaller amounts are synthesized in the adrenal glands and adipose tissue.

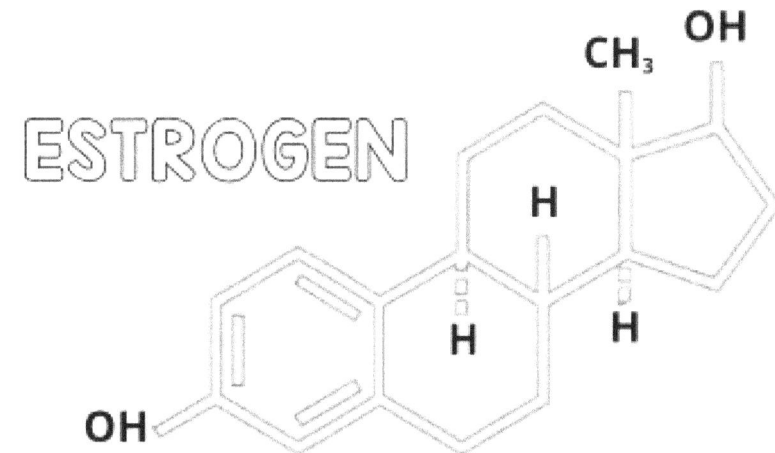

Types:
- Estradiol (E2): Dominant during reproductive years
- Estrone (E1): More prevalent post-menopause
- Estriol (E3): Prominent in pregnancy

Key Roles:
- Stimulates breast development and secondary sexual traits
- Promotes endometrial proliferation
- Regulates cervical mucus and maintains vaginal epithelium
- Supports bone density and cardiovascular health
- Increases uterine contractility and fallopian tube motility

Progesterone

Sources: Secreted mainly by the corpus luteum after ovulation and by the placenta during pregnancy; also produced in small amounts by the adrenal glands.

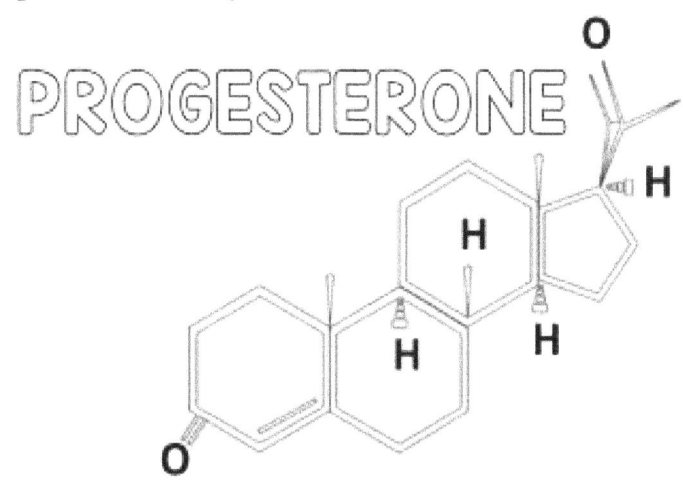

Key Roles:
- Prepares the endometrium for implantation
- Maintains the uterine lining during early pregnancy
- Suppresses uterine contractility to protect implantation
- Supports breast tissue development
- Inhibits lactation until after delivery

Luteinizing Hormone (LH)
Source: Anterior pituitary gland

Key Roles:
- Triggers ovulation (release of the mature ovum)
- Stimulates development and maintenance of the corpus luteum
- Works in concert with FSH during the menstrual cycle

Follicle-Stimulating Hormone (FSH)
Source: Anterior pituitary gland

Key Roles:
- Stimulates follicular growth in the ovaries
- Encourages estrogen secretion from developing follicles
- Critical in the early phase of the menstrual cycle

Androgens
Includes testosterone and dehydroepiandrosterone (DHEA). Produced mostly by the adrenal glands, with a minor contribution from the ovaries.

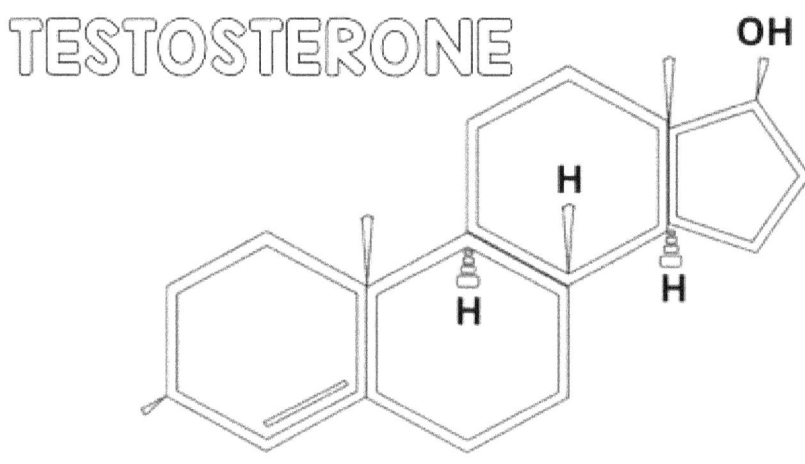

Key Roles:
- Support libido and sexual response
- Influence fat and hair distribution
- Serve as precursors for estrogen synthesis, using peripheral conversion by aromatase enzyme
- Play a role in skin changes during pregnancy

Relaxin
Sources: Secreted by the corpus luteum and later the placenta during pregnancy.

Key Roles:
- Softens the cervix in preparation for labor
- Relaxes pelvic ligaments
- Increases flexibility of the birth canal

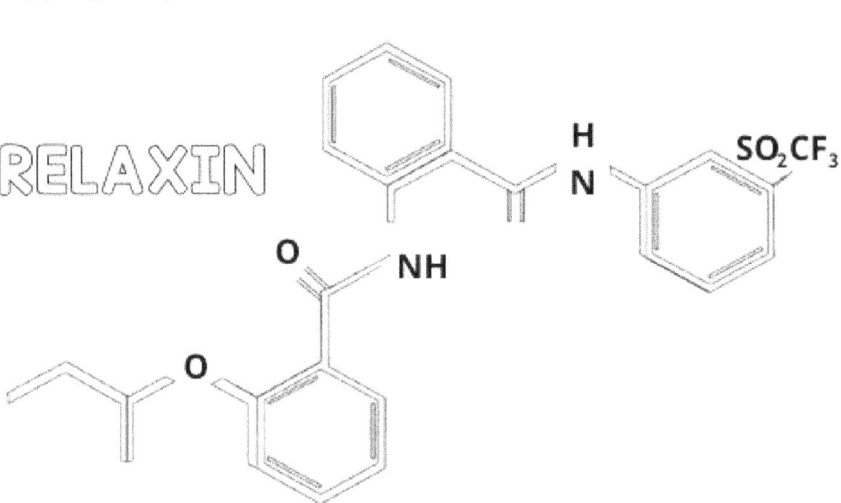

Hormones produced by the ovaries, pituitary gland, placenta, and adrenal glands work together to regulate the menstrual cycle, ovulation, pregnancy, and secondary sex characteristics.

Hormonal Regulation of the Menstrual and Ovulation Cycle

Understanding the menstrual cycle is not just foundational—it is indispensable to midwifery. This cyclical process governs ovulation, endometrial changes, menstruation, and hormonal feedback. It underlies fertility, influences mood and energy, and prepares the body for pregnancy month after month. For midwives, mastery of this process is essential for cycle tracking, fertility counseling, hormonal assessments, and the management of reproductive transitions from menarche to menopause. *The menstrual cycle is composed of two parallel but intimately connected processes:*

1. The **ovarian (hormonal) cycle**—describing changes in the ovary related to egg development and hormone production.
2. The **endometrial (uterine) cycle**—describing changes in the uterine lining in preparation for implantation.

These two cycles unfold simultaneously across approximately 21–35 days, most commonly 28, and are regulated by hormones produced by the hypothalamus, pituitary gland, ovaries, and eventually, in pregnancy, the placenta.

THE OVARIAN (HORMONAL) CYCLE

The ovarian cycle describes the development, maturation, and release of an ovum (egg), along with the hormonal changes that regulate this process. It includes three phases:

1. Follicular Phase (Days 1–13)
1. Initiated by the **hypothalamus**, which secretes gonadotropin-releasing hormone (GnRH)
2. GnRH signals the **anterior pituitary** to release follicle-stimulating hormone (FSH)
3. FSH stimulates several ovarian follicles to grow. As they mature, they begin producing estradiol, the dominant form of estrogen
4. Rising estrogen exerts negative feedback on FSH (limiting excess follicle development) and initiates proliferation of the endometrial lining in the uterus

Hormones involved:
- **GnRH** – From the hypothalamus; triggers pituitary hormone release
- **FSH** – Stimulates follicular growth and estrogen secretion
- **Estrogen** – Promotes follicle maturation, prepares cervical mucus, supports endometrial proliferation

> **Why It Matters?**
> A clear, detailed understanding of the menstrual and ovulation cycle allows midwives to:
>
> - **Evaluate** menstrual patterns as a vital sign of reproductive health
> - **Educate** clients on natural fertility awareness and contraceptive methods
> - **Identify** cycle-related disorders, such as luteal phase defects, anovulation, or endometrial insufficiency
> - **Interpret** hormonal labs and time diagnostic procedures appropriately
> - **Support** early pregnancy recognition and management, including hCG monitoring

2. Ovulation (~Day 14)
1. When estrogen peaks, it briefly switches to positive feedback, causing a surge in luteinizing hormone (LH)
2. The LH surge induces rupture of the dominant follicle, releasing the mature ovum into the fallopian tube
3. Estrogen supports tubal motility and cervical mucus changes to facilitate fertilization

Hormones involved:
- **LH** – Triggers ovulation and final follicle maturation
- **Estrogen (peak)**: Signals the LH surge and supports sperm transport

3. Luteal Phase (Days 15–28)
1. The ruptured follicle becomes the corpus luteum, which secretes progesterone and some estrogen
2. Progesterone stabilizes the endometrial lining, reduces uterine contractility, and prepares the uterus for implantation
3. If no pregnancy occurs, the corpus luteum degenerates after approximately 14 days, causing a hormonal decline and the onset of menstruation

Hormones involved:
- **Progesterone**: Secreted by the corpus luteum; prepares and maintains the endometrium
- **Estrogen**: Supports the effects of progesterone
- **Relaxin**: Secreted in small amounts; begins softening the uterus and pelvic tissues
- **Inhibin**: Inhibin from corpus luteum helps suppress FSH, contributing to inhibition of new follicular recruitment in luteal phase. However, estrogen and progesterone also play important roles — inhibin alone may not guarantee absolute suppression.

The Endometrial (Uterine) Cycle

While the ovaries prepare and release an ovum, the uterus prepares to receive a potential embryo. The endometrial cycle describes the growth, differentiation, and breakdown of the functional layer of the uterine lining. *It includes three phases:*

1. Menstrual Phase (Days 1–5)
1. Marked by the shedding of the functional layer of the endometrium due to falling estrogen and progesterone levels
2. Spiral arteries constrict, leading to ischemia and necrosis of endometrial tissue
3. The basal layer remains intact and regenerates regenerates the functionalis layer in the next cycle.

Hormonal context:
- Low progesterone and estrogen due to corpus luteum degeneration

2. Proliferative Phase (Days 6–14)
1. Rising estrogen from growing follicles stimulates endometrial regrowth
2. Endometrial glands elongate and blood vessels regenerate
3. Cervical mucus becomes clear, elastic, and sperm-friendly

Hormonal context:
- Estrogen-dominant phase; prepares for ovulation and supports sperm transport

3. Secretory Phase (Days 15–28)
1. Triggered by progesterone from the corpus luteum after ovulation
2. Endometrial glands become coiled and secretory, releasing glycogen-rich fluids to nourish a potential embryo
3. Spiral arteries grow deeper and increase blood flow

If implantation occurs, human chorionic gonadotropin (hCG) is released by the embryo to preserve the corpus luteum. If not, hormonal support ends, and the ischemic phase begins.

Hormonal context:
- Progesterone-dominant phase; supports implantation and early pregnancy

2. Ischemic Phase (Final 1–2 Days of Secretory Phase)
1. Occurs only if implantation does not occur
2. Withdrawal of progesterone causes spiral arteries to constrict, leading to hypoxia and cell death in the functional layer
3. Inflammatory mediators break down tissue in preparation for menstruation
   This phase initiates the next menstrual cycle.

Coordination of Ovarian and Endometrial Phases

Ovarian Cycle	Endometrial Cycle	Hormonal Profile
Follicular (Days 1–13)	Menstrual + Proliferative	Rising FSH and estrogen
Ovulation (~Day 14)	Late Proliferative	LH surge, estrogen peak
Luteal (Days 15–28)	Secretory	Progesterone dominant, moderate estrogen
Corpus luteum dies	Ischemic + Menstrual begins	Sharp fall in progesterone and estrogen

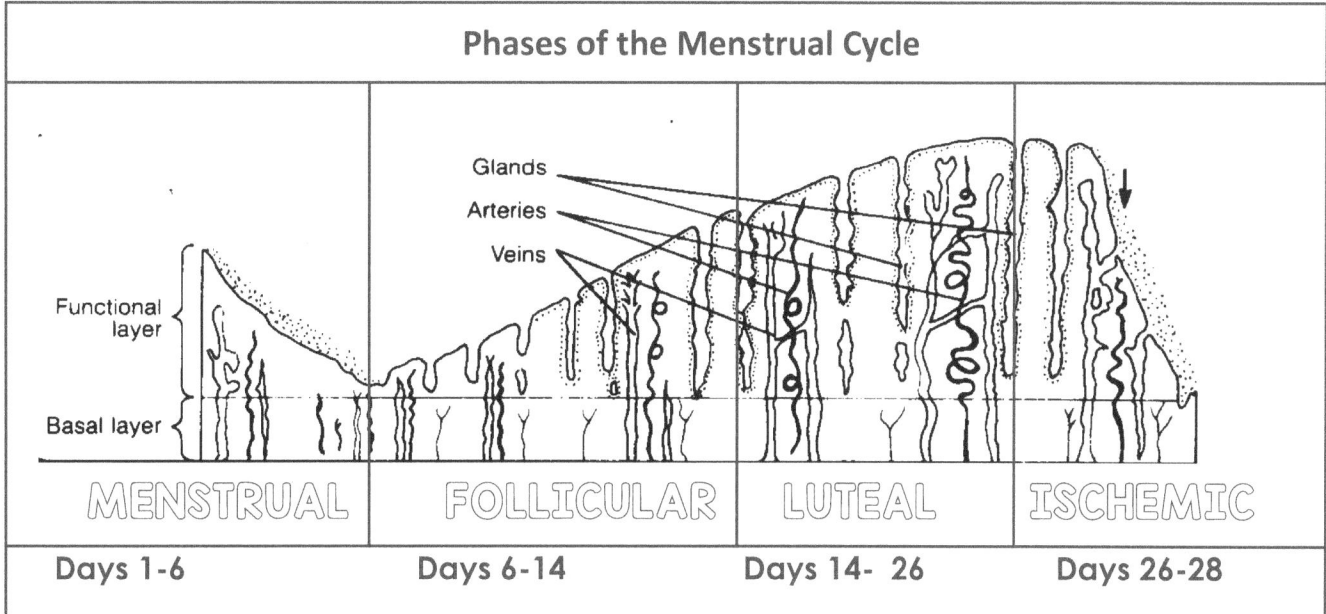

Clinical Tip
Irregular cycles are most often due to changes in the follicular phase. If the luteal phase is shorter than 10 days, it may indicate luteal phase defect, which can affect fertility.

Key Fact
The average menstrual cycle is 28 days, but normal cycles can range from 21–35 days in adults. Variations in timing often come from differences in the length of the follicular phase, while the luteal phase is typically a consistent 14 days.

Exercise 4.8: Menstrual Cycle Phase Matching Activity
Below are four key phases of the menstrual cycle (excluding menstruation) and their typical timing in a 28-day cycle. Match each phase to the correct time frame.

1. _____ Ischemic
2. _____ Follicular
3. _____ Luteal
4. _____ Ovulation

A. Days 1-13
B. Day 14
C. Days 15-28
D. Days 27-28

Additional Hormones in the Cycle

Androgens
- *Sources:* Ovaries and adrenal glands
- *Functions:* Support libido, serve as precursors for estrogen, influence hair and skin during the cycle

Relaxin
- *Sources:* Corpus luteum (later placenta)
- *Functions:* In early cycles, begins softening uterine tissues; later facilitates cervical ripening and ligament relaxation in pregnancy

Inhibin
- *Sources:* Granulosa cells of the follicle and corpus luteum
- *Functions:* Suppresses FSH production to ensure only one dominant follicle develops per cycle

Human Chorionic Gonadotropin (hCG)
- *Source:* Trophoblast cells of the embryo (if fertilization occurs)
- *Function:* Preserves the corpus luteum and its progesterone output to sustain the early pregnancy
- Hormones from the hypothalamus, pituitary, ovaries, placenta, and adrenal glands coordinate the menstrual cycle, ovulation, and pregnancy.

Hormone	Source	Primary Roles
GnRH	Hypothalamus	Stimulates pituitary release of FSH & LH
FSH	Anterior pituitary	Stimulates follicle growth, estrogen production
LH	Anterior pituitary	Triggers ovulation, supports corpus luteum
Estrogen	Ovaries (follicles), placenta	Thickens endometrium, cervical mucus, secondary sex traits
Progesterone	Corpus luteum, placenta	Maintains uterine lining, suppresses contractions
Androgens	Adrenal glands, ovaries	Libido, estrogen precursor, skin/hair influence
Relaxin	Corpus luteum, placenta	Softens cervix, relaxes pelvic ligaments
Inhibin	Follicles, corpus luteum	Inhibits further FSH release
hCG	Embryo (trophoblast)	Sustains corpus luteum in early pregnancy

Exercise 4.10: Hormone Functions			
Match each hormone listed in the left column with its correct source and its main function			
Hormone	Source	Function	Peaks (on/around day __)
Estrogen			
Progesterone			
Testosterone			
Relaxin			
Follicle Stimulating Hormone			
Luteinizing Hormone			

Ovulation

Ovulation is the process by which an ovum (egg) matures and is released from the ovary. At birth, the total ovarian reserve is usually around 1 to 2 million **primordial follicles**, with around 200,000 per ovary present during puberty. With the onset of puberty and under the influence of estrogen, a primordial follicle matures into a **Graafian follicle**. Each month, one of these follicles develops and begins to protrude from the surface of the ovary. As it enlarges, the surrounding capsule thins and stretches. Eventually, the follicle ruptures, releasing the ovum and its surrounding follicular fluid—this is ovulation.

Some individuals can feel ovulation as it occurs. A sharp, cramping sensation known as **mittelschmerz** (German for "middle pain") may be experienced on one side of the lower abdomen. The **fimbrial end** of the uterine (fallopian) tube lies close to the ovary and catches the ovum as it is released. **Ciliated epithelial cells** and the **muscularis layer** of the tube help propel the ovum toward the uterus.

Ovulation is regulated by a complex hormonal cascade during the menstrual cycle. The **hypothalamus** releases **gonadotropin-releasing hormone (GnRH)**, which stimulates the **anterior pituitary gland** to secrete **follicle-stimulating hormone (FSH)**. FSH promotes the development of the Graafian follicle, which secretes increasing amounts of estrogen. When estrogen levels peak, a brief **positive feedback loop** causes a surge in **luteinizing hormone (LH)**, which triggers ovulation.

After ovulation, the site on the ovary where the ovum was released becomes the **corpus luteum** (Latin for "yellow body"), which secretes **progesterone**. This hormone prepares the endometrium for implantation and supports early pregnancy. If pregnancy occurs, the corpus luteum enlarges and continues to produce progesterone until the placenta takes over hormone production around the fourth or fifth month. If pregnancy does not occur, the corpus luteum degenerates after approximately fourteen days and becomes the **corpus albicans** ("white body"), marking the end of the luteal phase.

Hormonal Effects of Ovulation

1. HYPOTHALAMUS
2. GONADOTROPHIC HORMONES
3. ANTERIOR PITUITARY
4. OVARY
5. OVARIAN HORMONES
6. GRAAFIAN FOLLICLE
7. OVULATION
8. CORPUS LUTEUM
9. CORPUS ALBICANS

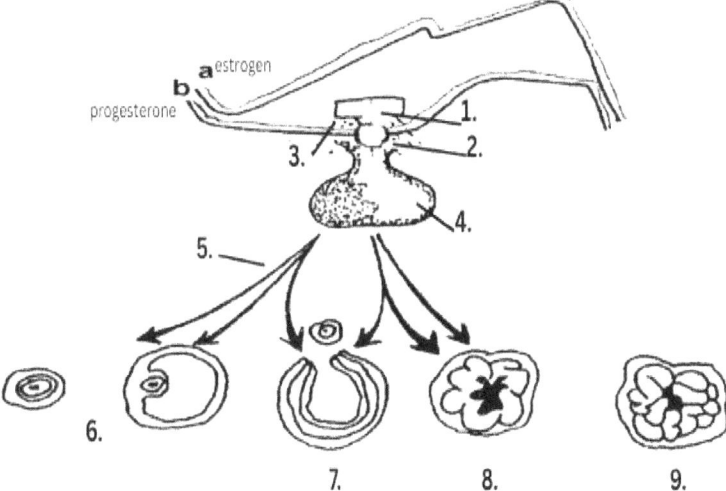

Exercise 4.11: Steps of Ovulation
Write the correct number when it occurs next to each step

_____Anterior pituitary releases FSH

_____Corpus luteum releases progesterone and estrogen

_____Hypothalamus releases LHRF

_____LH triggers ovulation

_____Graafian follicles produce estrogens

_____Anterior pituitary releases LH

_____FSH stimulates the Graafian follicle to develop

_____Hypothalamus releases FSHRF

Exercise 4.12: Menstrual Feelings & Menarche Reflection
Culture, family, and personal experience shape how menstruation is understood.
This reflection encourages midwifery students to explore their own story and its impact on their care for others.

Reflective Questions:
1. What, if anything, did you know about menstruation before your first period?
2. Where did you learn it?
3. Were there any misconceptions?
4. What do you wish you had known?
5. How did you feel about your first period before it happened?
6. How did the experience match or not match your expectations?
7. Did it have symbolic meaning for you?
8. Have you ever felt shame or embarrassment about menstruation?
9. Have you ever concealed your period? Why?
10. How do you feel about your period now?
11. How could you help a young person have a positive relationship with their changing body?
12. For my daughter's first period I will…

The Male Reproductive System

The male reproductive system is designed to produce, mature, and deliver sperm. It includes both primary reproductive organs (the testes) and accessory glands and ducts that contribute to the formation and transport of semen. The penis, scrotum, and associated structures also play roles in sexual function and fertility.

Midwifery and Male Reproductive Health

While midwifery primarily focuses on the reproductive health of women and birthing people, an understanding of the male reproductive system is essential for comprehensive care. Midwives often counsel couples, assess fertility challenges, and support reproductive decision-making across partnerships. They also examine newborn male infants as part of routine assessment—checking for the presence of testes, urethral placement, and signs of congenital anomalies. Knowing the structures and functions of the male system—including sperm production, hormonal influences, and common dysfunctions—enables midwives to educate, refer, and advocate effectively for all aspects of reproductive wellness.

Although midwives do not directly manage male reproductive conditions, they play a vital role in supporting the reproductive health of men and sperm-producing partners. Recognizing that fertility is a dyadic process, midwives help improve outcomes for the entire family unit.

Ways midwives support male reproductive health:
- Educating clients and partners about sperm health and timing of intercourse
- Encouraging sperm-safe practices (e.g., avoiding heat, tobacco, alcohol, and endocrine disruptors)
- Counseling on fertility evaluations and semen analysis when conception is delayed
- Referring individuals for evaluation of erectile dysfunction, testicular pain, or infertility
- Discussing permanent contraception options like vasectomy in shared family planning conversations

Primary Organs

1. TESTES The testes are the paired male gonads located in the scrotum. Each testis is approximately 5 cm in length and 2.5 cm in width. It is divided into lobules that contain seminiferous tubules—the site of spermatogenesis (sperm production), and Leydig cells, located between tubules, which produce the hormone testosterone.

Functions: Production of spermatozoa secretion of testosterone, which regulates male secondary sex characteristics, libido, and and spermatogenesis.

2. SCROTUM is a loose pouch of skin that houses and protects the testes. It acts as a thermoregulatory organ, maintaining the testes at a temperature approximately 2–4°F below core body temperature—a critical requirement for healthy sperm production.
Clinical Relevance: Excess heat (e.g., tight clothing, frequent hot tubs) may impair sperm quality. Scrotal abnormalities, such as varicoceles or testicular torsion, can contribute to infertility

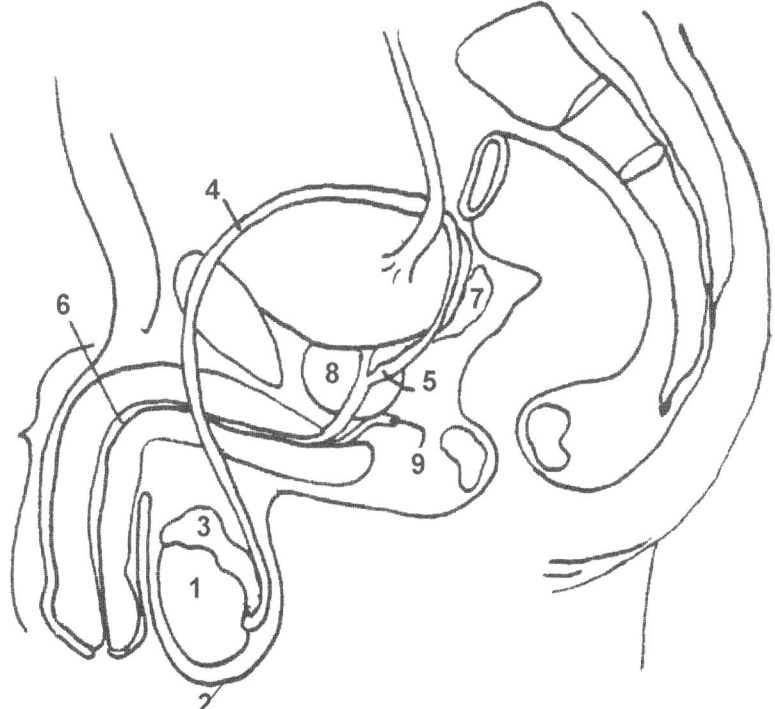

Duct System

3. EPIDIDYMIS is a tightly coiled tube (about 6 meters in length) lying along the posterior surface of each testis. It functions as the site for sperm maturation and storage. During ejaculation, the epididymis propels sperm toward the urethra via peristaltic contractions.

4. VAS DEFERENS (Ductus Deferens) is a muscular tube approximately 45 cm long. It transports sperm from the epididymis into the ejaculatory ducts. This duct also contributes to the formation of semen through the addition of fluid from the seminal vesicles and prostate. *Clinical Note:* Vasectomy is a form of permanent contraception performed by severing the vas deferens.

5. EJACULATORY DUCTS These short ducts (~2 cm) are continuations of the vas deferens that pass through the prostate and empty into the urethra. They transport semen during ejaculation.

6. URETHRA The urethra in males serves a dual purpose—transporting both urine and semen. It extends from the bladder, passes through the prostate, urogenital diaphragm, and penis, and opens at the external urethral meatus.

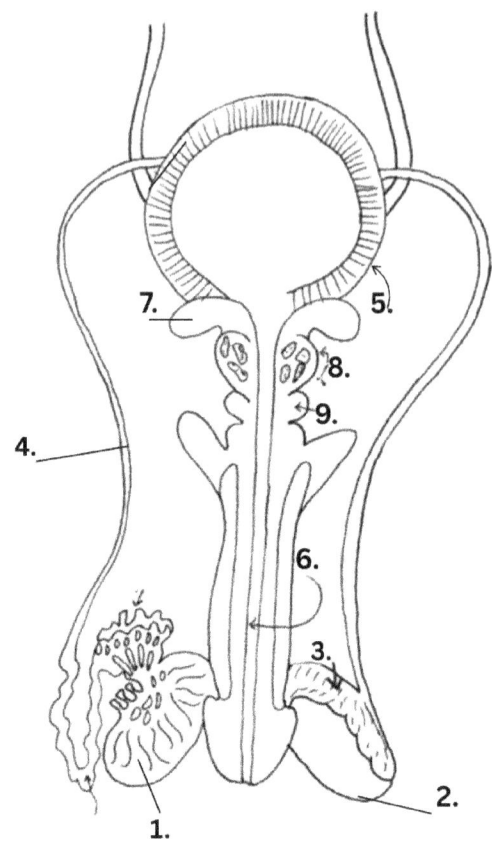

Accessory Glands

7. SEMINAL VESICLES These paired glands are located at the base of the bladder and secrete a fructose-rich, alkaline fluid that nourishes sperm and contributes to semen volume. Their secretions help neutralize vaginal acidity, enhancing sperm survival.

8. PROSTATE GLAND Located just below the bladder and encircling the urethra, the prostate produces a milky alkaline secretion that makes up about 25% of the semen. This fluid aids in sperm motility and longevity. *Clinical Relevance:* Prostatic hypertrophy can interfere with urination or ejaculation. Prostate inflammation (prostatitis) can impact fertility and comfort

9. BULBOURETHRAL (COWPER'S) GLANDS These small pea-sized glands lie beneath the prostate and secrete a clear mucous fluid during sexual arousal. This pre-ejaculatory fluid lubricates the urethra and neutralizes acidic urine residue.

EXTERNAL GENITALIA

PENIS

The penis is composed of three columns of erectile tissue and functions in both urination and sexual intercourse. The shaft contains the **corpora cavernosa** and **corpus spongiosum**, which engorge with blood during erection. The **glans** is the sensitive tip, and the **prepuce** (foreskin) may be present unless removed via circumcision.

Uncircumcised Penis   Circumcised Penis

Spermatogenesis: The Sperm Life Cycle

Sperm production occurs within the seminiferous tubules of the testes and takes approximately 64–90 days from start to finish. Full sperm maturation (including epididymal transit) brings the total to ~90 days before sperm are ejaculated. The process involves several stages:

1. **Spermatogonia** (stem cells) undergo mitosis and meiosis to form **spermatocytes**, then spermatids, and finally mature spermatozoa
2. Developing sperm are nourished and supported by **Sertoli cells**
3. Mature sperm migrate to the **epididymis,** where they complete maturation and gain motility

Each day, a healthy adult male produces millions of sperm. However, only a fraction are viable, motile, and morphologically normal, which is critical when assessing fertility.

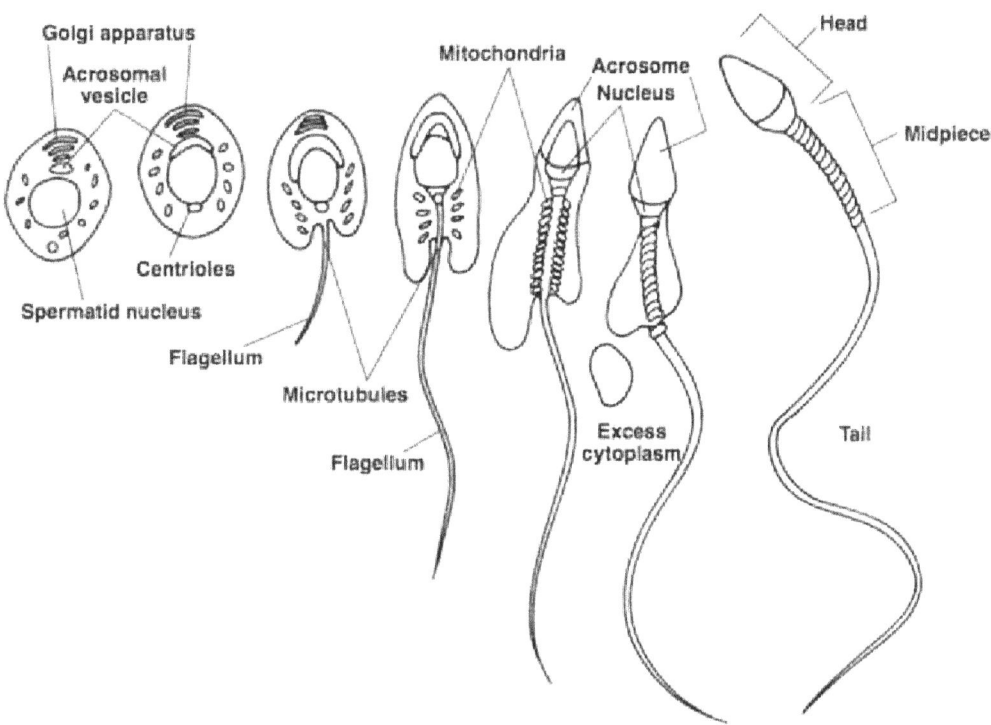

Exercise 4.12: Matching Male Reproduction
Match each structure to its function:

1. _____Stores and matures sperm
2. _____Produces sperm and testosterone
3. _____Transports sperm to the urethra
4. _____Contributes fluid to semen that nourishes sperm
5. _____Produces fluid that helps sperm motility

A. Testes
B. Epididymis
C. Vas deferens
D. Prostate gland
E. Seminal vesicles

Exercise 4.13: Sperm Journey Review
Describe the pathway sperm follows from creation to ejaculation:

1.

2.

3.

Case Study: Delayed Conception

A couple has been trying to conceive for over a year. The female partner's menstrual cycles are regular, and ovulation has been confirmed. The male partner reports he has no known health problems but mentions he takes hot baths daily, smokes occasionally, and recently started testosterone supplements purchased online.

Discussion Questions:
1. What lifestyle factors might be affecting this individual's fertility?
2. What role can a midwife play in helping this couple?
3. When should a referral for semen analysis be considered?

> **Why It Matters?**
> Although midwifery care centers on women, fertility is a shared process. Midwives are uniquely positioned to educate both partners about sperm health, hormone balance, and anatomy. Understanding the male reproductive system supports holistic counseling, improves fertility outcomes, and strengthens the midwife's role as a family-centered provider.

Exercise 4.14: Reproductive A&P Review
Fill in the Blank

1. Which structure houses developing follicles and produces sex hormones? _____
2. Name two hormones essential for ovulation and where they originate.
    a. _____
    b. _____
3. What is the role of the levator ani muscle group in reproductive health? _____
4. List one function of the epididymis and one of the uterine tubes.

    → Epididymis: _____

    → Uterine tube: _____

REPRODUCTIVE ANATOMY AND PHYSIOLOGY ESSENTIAL TAKEAWAYS

Understanding reproductive anatomy and physiology is foundational to midwifery care. This chapter explores the bony pelvis, uterine ligaments, internal and external reproductive structures, and the hormonal orchestration of ovulation, menstruation, and pregnancy. Students learn how the pelvis functions in pregnancy and labor, how uterine layers and ligaments adapt, and how organs like the uterus, ovaries, and vagina work together to support fertility and birth. Special attention is given to the dynamic pelvic floor—its structure, role in labor, and postpartum recovery—as well as variations in pelvic types and their clinical implications.

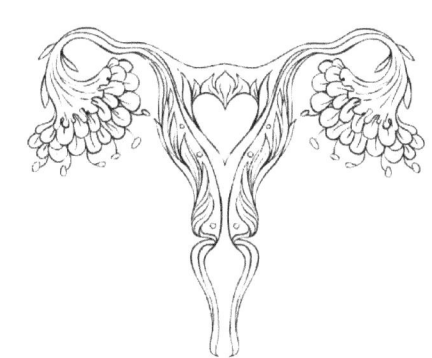

The chapter also includes thorough explanations of male reproductive anatomy and function, reinforcing midwives' role in assessing fertility holistically and supporting reproductive decision-making for all individuals. By tracing hormone production, gamete development, and the coordination of the menstrual and ovarian cycles, students gain a framework to interpret signs of health and imbalance, provide education, and guide clients through reproductive transitions from puberty to menopause and beyond.

Chapter Four Self-Assessment

Multiple Choice
1. The cardinal ligament:
   a) Suspends the ovary to the pelvic side walls
   b) Attaches to the uterus just below the fallopian tubes and inserts in the labia majora
   c) Drapes over the uterus and ovaries
   d) Connects to the uterus at the junction between the cervix and the body of the uterus

2. The round ligament:
   a) Suspends the ovary to the pelvic side walls
   b) Attaches to the uterus just below the fallopian tubes and inserts in the labia majora
   c) Drapes over the uterus and ovaries
   d) Connects to the uterus at the junction between the cervix and the body of the uterus

3. The broad ligament:
   a) Suspends the ovary to the pelvic side walls
   b) Attaches to the uterus just below the fallopian tubes and inserts in the labia majora
   c) Drapes over the uterus and ovaries
   d) Connects to the uterus at the junction between the cervix and the body of the uterus

4. The soft mucosal lining of the uterus is the:
   a) Perimetrium
   b) Myometrium
   c) Peritoneum
   d) Endometrium

5. The levator ani consists of three muscle pairs:
   a) Iliococcygeus, bulbocavernosus, and pubococcygeus
   b) Pubococcygeus, superficial transverse muscle, bulbocavernosus
   c) Iliococcygeus, bulbocavernosus, ischiocavernosus
   d) Iliococcygeus, pubococcygeus, ischiococcygeus

6. The function of the uterine tubes is to:
   a) Store ova until fertilization occurs
   b) Transport the ovum from the ovary to the uterus
   c) Support the uterus during pregnancy
   d) Produce progesterone and estrogen

7. Which structure is located between the bladder and the rectum?
   a) Vagina
   b) Uterus
   c) Cervix
   d) Perineum

8. The ovarian cycle is primarily regulated by which two pituitary hormones?
   a) Estrogen and progesterone
   b) FSH and LH
   c) Prolactin and oxytocin
   d) Cortisol and insulin

9. Which phase of the menstrual cycle immediately follows ovulation?
   a) Follicular phase
   b) Ischemic phase
   c) Luteal phase
   d) Menstrual phase

10. The function of cervical mucus during ovulation is to:
    a) Block sperm entry into the uterus
    b) Increase lubrication for comfort
    c) Facilitate sperm movement and survival
    d) Thicken to prevent infection

11. The structure that produces estrogen during the follicular phase is the:
    a) Corpus luteum
    b) Developing follicle
    c) Anterior pituitary gland
    d) Hypothalamus

12. The average volume of blood lost during a normal menstrual period is approximately:
    a) 10–20 mL
    b) 30–50 mL
    c) 60–100 mL
    d) 150–200 mL

13. The hormone primarily responsible for stimulating milk ejection (let-down reflex) is:
    a) Estrogen
    b) Prolactin
    c) Oxytocin
    d) Progesterone

14. The term *retroverted uterus* refers to a uterus that:
    a) Tilts forward toward the bladder
    b) Tilts backward toward the spine
    c) Rotates to the left side of the pelvis
    d) Lies transversely in the abdominal cavity

Number in Order
15. Number each part of the vulva in the order it occurs from anterior to posterior:

    ____ Mons pubis
    ____ Clitoris
    ____ Urethra
    ____ Introitus (vaginal opening)
    ____ Fourchette
    ____ Perineum
    ____ Anus

Matching
16. Match the menstrual cycle phase to its timeline (based on a 28-day cycle):

    1. ____ Luteal phase   A. Days 26–28
    2. ____ Follicular phase   B. Day 14
    3. ____ Menstrual phase   C. Days 1–13
    4. ____ Ovulation   D. Days 15–28
    5. ____ Ischemic phase   E. Days 1–5

Fill in the Blank
17. The hormone that stimulates follicle growth is _____
18. The hormone responsible for triggering ovulation is _____
19. The hormone that maintains the endometrial lining is _____
20. The structure that produces progesterone after ovulation is the _____
21. The _____ is the rounded upper portion of the uterus, used to measure growth during pregnancy.
22. The _____ are fingerlike projections that help guide the ovum into the uterine tube.
23. The _____ is the hollow muscular organ where a fertilized egg implants and develops.
24. The _____ is the tissue between the vaginal opening and the anus that stretches during birth.
25. The _____ is the most common site of fertilization in the uterine tube.
26. The _____ pelvis type is considered most favorable for vaginal birth due to its rounded shape.

True or False
27. _____ The thick muscular middle layer of the uterus is called the myometrium.
28. _____ The paraurethral glands are another name for Bartholin's glands.
29. _____ Mittelschmerz is the stretchy, transparent cervical mucus that occurs around ovulation.
30. _____ The fimbriae are at the proximal end of the uterine tube.
31. _____ Perianal means inside the anus.
32. _____ The broad ligament extends from the peritoneum.
33. _____ Semen is slightly acid.
34. _____ The corpus luteum secretes FSH.
35. _____ Estrogen is produced by the anterior pituitary gland.
36. _____ The ovarian follicles contain immature ova that develop under hormonal influence.
37. _____ The hymen is a thick muscular layer separating the vagina from the cervix.
38. _____ The corpus luteum forms from the ruptured follicle after ovulation.
39. _____ Prolactin levels increase significantly during pregnancy and peak after birth.
40. _____ The pelvic floor muscles provide essential support for the uterus, bladder, and bowel
41. _____ The broad ligament originates at the base of the uterine tube and inserts into the labia majora.

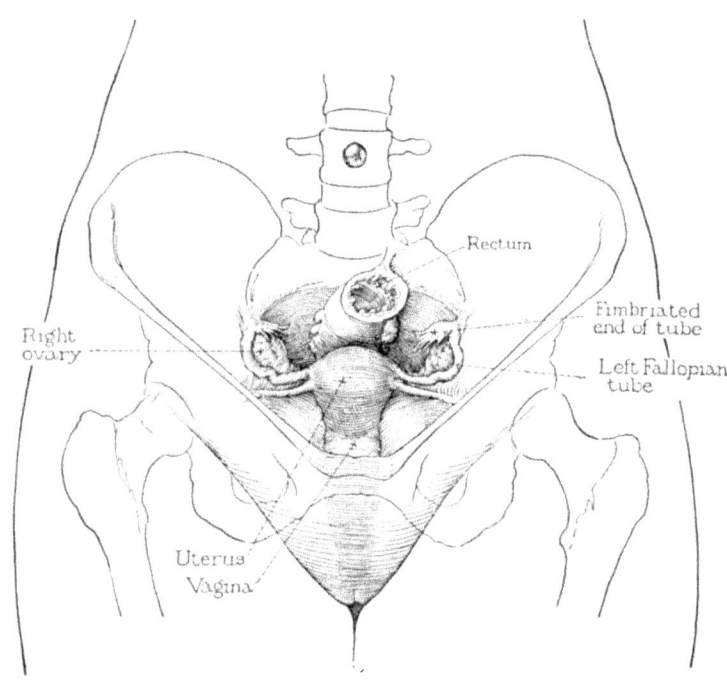

Chapter Four Reading & References

Recommended Reading: Reproductive Anatomy and Physiology
- Drake, R. L., Vogl, W., & Mitchell, A. W. M. (2019). ***Gray's Anatomy for Students*** (4th ed.). Elsevier. Student-friendly adaptation of the classic Gray's Anatomy with clear reproductive system coverage.
- Kapit, W., Elson, L. M., & Latif, M. (2017). ***The Anatomy Coloring Book*** (4th ed.). Pearson. Interactive tool reinforcing reproductive anatomy through visual learning and labeling.
- Marieb, E. N., & Hoehn, K. (2018). ***Human Anatomy & Physiology*** (11th ed.). Pearson. Provides accessible explanations of the reproductive system, ideal for students beginning anatomy studies.
- Miles, S. H. (1997). ***The Nurse–Midwifery Handbook*** (2nd ed.). Springer. Offers concise anatomical and physiological reference points useful for student midwives.
- Miles, D. ***A Midwife's Guide to Anatomy and Physiology in Pregnancy and Childbirth*** (3rd ed.). An accessible and beautifully illustrated overview of reproductive anatomy, fetal development, and physiologic adaptation during pregnancy.
- Moore, K. L., Dalley, A. F., & Agur, A. M. (2018). ***Clinically Oriented Anatomy*** (8th ed.). Wolters Kluwer. Standard anatomy reference with strong coverage of reproductive structures and clinical correlations.
- Netter, F. H. (2018). ***Atlas of Human Anatomy*** (7th ed.). Elsevier. Classic anatomical atlas with detailed illustrations of male and female reproductive systems.
- Snell, R. S. (2018). ***Clinical Anatomy by Systems*** (9th ed.). Wolters Kluwer. Organ-system approach that contextualizes reproductive anatomy with clinical applications.
- Tortora, G. J., & Derrickson, B. (2017). ***Principles of Anatomy and Physiology*** (15th ed.). Wiley. Comprehensive yet approachable text linking structure and function of reproductive anatomy.
- Varney, H., Kriebs, J. M., & Gegor, C. L. (2018). ***Varney's Midwifery*** (6th ed.). Jones & Bartlett Learning. Midwifery text with detailed sections on reproductive anatomy and physiology in clinical context.

References

Drake, R. L., Vogl, W., & Mitchell, A. W. M. (2019). *Gray's anatomy for students* (4th ed.). Elsevier.

Grant, J. C. B. (1972). *Grant's method of anatomy: A clinical problem-solving approach* (7th ed.). Williams & Wilkins.

Gray, H. (1973). *Gray's anatomy of the human body* (35th ed.). Longman. (Revised by Warwick & Williams)

Kapit, W., Elson, L. M., & Latif, M. (2017). *The anatomy coloring book* (4th ed.). Pearson.

Marieb, E. N., & Hoehn, K. (2018). *Human anatomy and physiology* (11th ed.). Pearson.

Miles, S. H. (1997). *The nurse–midwifery handbook* (2nd ed.). Springer.

Moore, K. L., Dalley, A. F., & Agur, A. M. (2018). *Clinically oriented anatomy* (8th ed.). Wolters Kluwer.

Netter, F. H. (2018). *Atlas of human anatomy* (7th ed.). Elsevier.

Snell, R. S. (1981). *Clinical anatomy for medical students* (2nd ed.). Little, Brown.

Tortora, G. J., & Derrickson, B. (2017). *Principles of anatomy and physiology* (15th ed.). Wiley.

Varney, H., Kriebs, J. M., & Gegor, C. L. (2018). *Varney's midwifery* (6th ed.). Jones & Bartlett Learning.

Chapter Five
Biology for Midwives

Objectives
After completing this chapter, the student should be able to:
1. **Describe** the structure and function of a human cell and its major organelles.

2. **Explain** how substances move across cell membranes and why this matters in midwifery.

3. **Differentiate** between mitosis and meiosis, including their roles in growth, repair, and gamete formation.

4. **Summarize** the role of stem cells in early development.

5. **Define** key genetic terms (chromosomes, genes, alleles, dominant/recessive, genotype, phenotype, X-linked).

6. **Interpret** simple inheritance patterns using Punnett squares and carrier diagrams.

7. **Recognize** the difference between Mendelian traits and polygenic/complex traits.

8. **Explain** the importance of the human microbiome for newborn health and midwifery practice.

9. **Describe** how epigenetics shows the interaction between genes and environment.

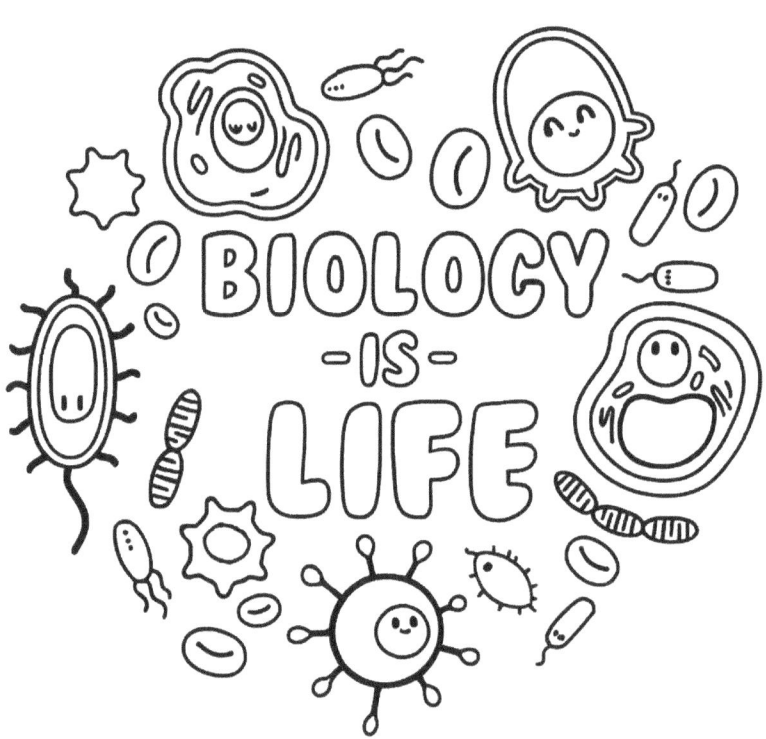

Foundations of Biology for Student Midwives

Understanding the building blocks of life—cells, cell division, and genetic inheritance—is essential for safe, informed midwifery care. A strong foundation in biology and microbiology equips student midwives to explain early development, assess reproductive health, and communicate complex processes like conception, implantation, and genetic screening in clear, compassionate ways.

Midwives draw on this knowledge when helping clients interpret early pregnancy tests, discuss miscarriage risk, navigate prenatal genetic screenings, or recover from pregnancy loss. The ability to translate biology into accessible language strengthens trust, promotes body literacy, and affirms the midwife's role as a bridge between science and care.

This chapter invites students to root their midwifery practice in biology while honoring the sacred complexity of life. From microscopic cell structures to the transformation of embryogenesis, each topic explored here reinforces the midwife's role in making life's invisible processes visible, meaningful, and empowering.

Understanding the building blocks of life—cells, division, and transport—is essential for safe, informed midwifery care. From interpreting lab results to explaining embryonic development, a strong biology foundation helps midwives translate science into compassionate guidance.

> **Key Vocabulary: Cell Energy and Transport**
>
> - **Diffusion:** Passive movement of molecules from an area of high concentration to low concentration.
> - **Osmosis:** Diffusion of water across a semi-permeable membrane.
> - **Facilitated diffusion:** Passive transport using a protein carrier to move larger or charged particles.
> - **Active transport:** Movement of substances against their concentration gradient using cellular energy (ATP).
> - **Sodium-potassium pump:** Active transport system that pumps Na^+ out and K^+ into the cell to maintain electrical balance.
> - **Endocytosis:** Process where the cell engulfs material (includes phagocytosis and pinocytosis).
> - **Exocytosis:** Release of substances from the cell via vesicles.
> - **ATP (Adenosine Triphosphate):** Main energy currency of the cell, required for active processes.

CELLS: STRUCTURE AND FUNCTION

Cells are the smallest living units, forming the foundation of every tissue, organ, and system. The human journey begins with a single fertilized cell. In midwifery, understanding cell biology supports everything from fetal development to wound healing.

Key Features of a Cell:

1. **PLASMA MEMBRANE:** A flexible, semi-permeable boundary that controls what enters or exits the cell, maintaining internal balance.
2. **NUCLEUS:** The command center, containing DNA and directing cell behavior, growth, and replication. It houses the nucleolus, which helps build ribosomes.
3. **CYTOPLASM:** A gel-like interior that supports and cushions the organelles while hosting metabolic reactions.

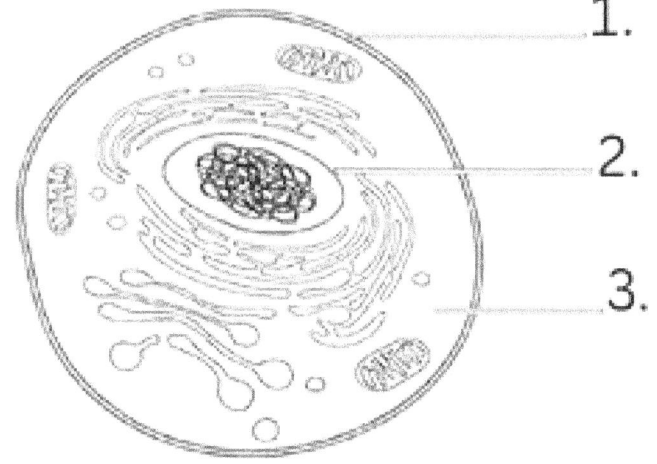

Cellular Transport and Energy

Cells must move water, nutrients, gases, and waste across their membranes to stay alive. These transport processes keep the body in balance, support fetal development, regulate hydration, and maintain healthy tissues during pregnancy. The two major categories of membrane transport are passive transport and active transport.

Passive transport requires no energy. Diffusion and osmosis are the most common forms. Diffusion occurs when molecules move from an area of higher concentration to an area of lower concentration. This natural spreading process explains how oxygen crosses from the mother's bloodstream into the placenta, how carbon dioxide leaves fetal tissues to be exhaled, and how topical herbs or medications enter cells.

Osmosis is a type of diffusion in which water moves across a semi-permeable membrane. Water shifts toward the side with more dissolved particles until the concentrations are balanced. The osmosis diagram shows water moving into the saltier compartment because the membrane allows water to pass but not the solute. Osmosis is central to hydration, swelling, IV fluid balance, electrolyte changes, and placental exchange. Midwives use these principles when guiding hydration, interpreting electrolyte panels, managing swelling in pregnancy, and explaining how excess water can dilute sodium levels.

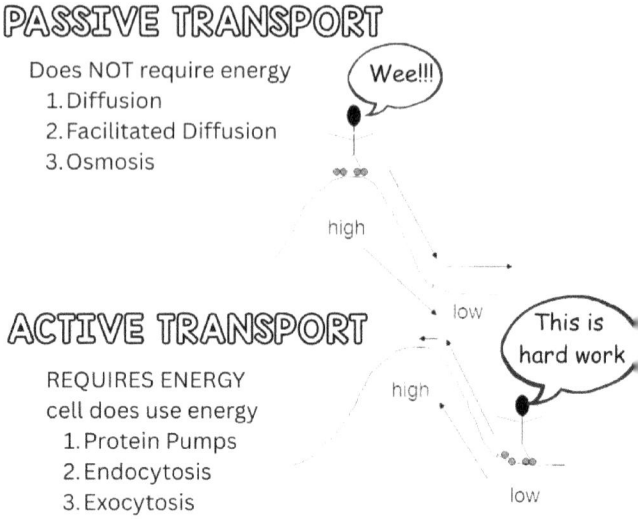

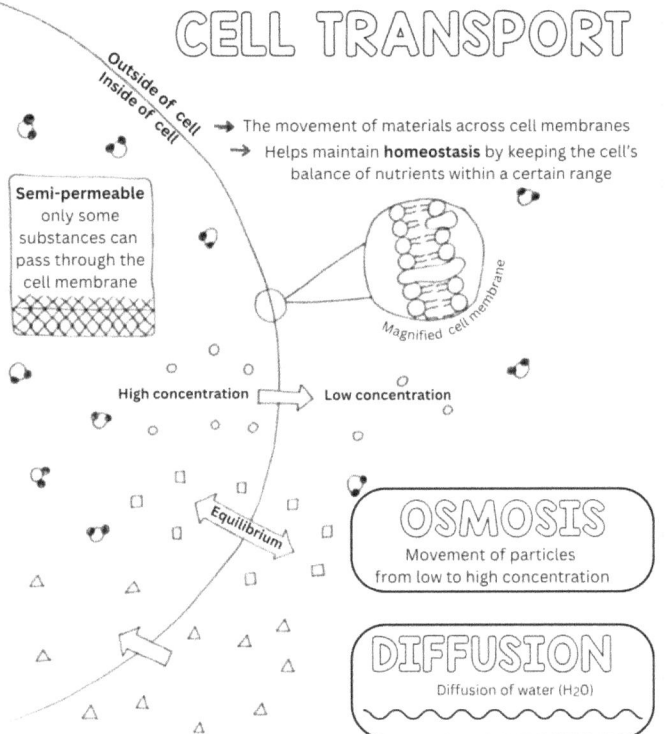

Active transport requires energy in the form of ATP. Cells use active transport to move substances from low concentration to high concentration. The sodium–potassium pump is a well-known example and is essential for nerve signals, muscle contractions, and normal heart rhythm. Endocytosis (taking substances in) and exocytosis (sending substances out) are additional forms of active transport that allow cells to take in nutrients, release hormones, remove waste, and communicate with other cells.

Together, diffusion, osmosis, and active transport explain how the placenta exchanges nutrients and gases, how hydration affects labor, how swelling forms, how medications move into cells, and how the newborn maintains fluid balance after birth. A clear understanding of membrane transport helps midwives interpret laboratory findings, manage IV fluids, support physiologic birth, and teach families how the body maintains balance throughout pregnancy and the postpartum period.

Exercise 5.1: Passive or Active?
Match the correct term next to each example below.

1. _____ Oxygen moving from maternal blood into the placenta
2. _____ Water shifting toward the saltier side of a solution
3. _____ A cell using ATP to pump sodium out and potassium
4. _____ A hormone packaged and released from a cell
5. _____ A medication diffusing through a cell membrane

A. Diffusion
B. Osmosis
C. Active transport
D. Exocytosis
E. Diffusion

Organelle Functions

Each organelle has a specialized task that keeps the cell — and the body — running smoothly.

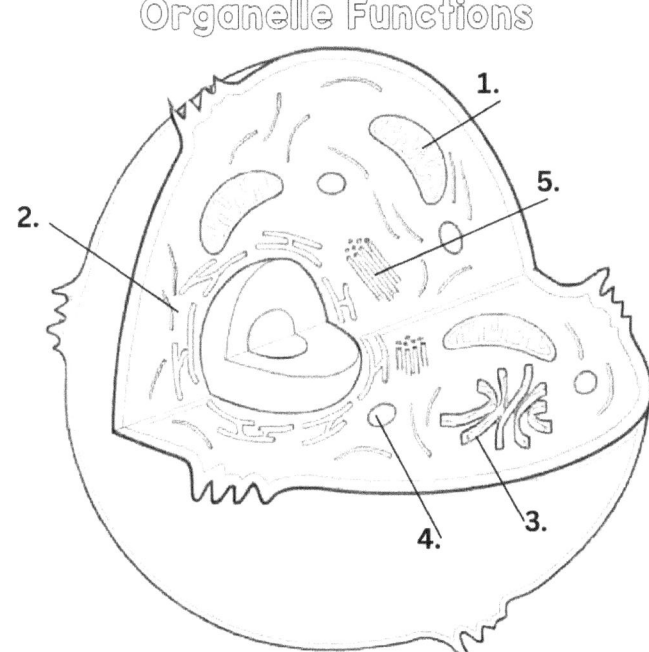

1. **MITOCHONDRIA**: Powerhouses of the cell. They produce ATP, essential for energy-intensive functions like placental development, brain activity, and uterine contraction.
2. **RIBOSOMES**: Are protein builders and are critical for fetal growth and tissue repair.
3. **ENDOPLASMIC RETICULUM (ER)**:
   • **Rough ER** Builds proteins, especially those bound for membranes or export (think: hormones).
   • **Smooth ER** Synthesizes lipids and detoxifies substances — especially important in placental hormone production.
4. **GOLGI APPARATUS**: Packages and ships proteins, helping cells communicate and grow.
5. **LYSOSOMES**: Break down debris and bacteria. Crucial in inflammation and recovery after birth.
6. **CENTRIOLES**: Organize microtubules to ensure accurate cell division — essential for embryonic development and healing.

Organelle	Function	Why It Matters in Midwifery
Nucleus	Stores DNA; controls cell activity	Supports understanding of genetic inheritance
Mitochondria	Produces cellular energy (ATP)	Explains maternal fatigue, placental function, metabolic health
Ribosomes	Synthesizes proteins	Key to tissue development and healing
Endoplasmic Reticulum	Processes proteins and lipids	Impacts hormone production and fetal development
Plasma Membrane	Regulates entry/exit of substances	Relevant in implantation, immune response

| Lysosomes | Breaks down waste and cellular debris | Helps explain cell turnover, and tissue degeneration in miscarriage |

Exercise 5.2: Cells
Match the descriptions in Column I with the names in Column II

1. _____ Holds nucleus together.
2. _____ Surface for chemical activity.
3. _____ Units of heredity.
4. _____ Digestion center.
5. _____ Where proteins are made.
6. _____ Structures involved in mitosis.
7. _____ Hollow cylinder that supports
8. _____ Spherical body within nucleus.
9. _____ Controls entry into and out of cell.
10. _____ Chromosomes are found here.
11. _____ Jellylike substance within cell.
12. _____ Contains code which guides all cell activities.
13. _____ Minute hole in nuclear membrane.
14. _____ "Powerhouse" of cell.
15. _____ Contains water and dissolved minerals.
16. _____ Stores food or contains pigment.

A. Golgi bodies
B. nucleus
C. chromosomes
D. vacuole
E. ribosomes
F. endoplasmic reticulum
G. nuclear membrane shapes cell
H. centrioles
I. cytoplasm
J. cell (plasma) membrane
K. mitochondria
L. lysosome
M. genes
N. nuclear pore
O. nucleolus
P. microtubule

Exercise 5.3: Types of Organisms
Color each type and discuss the midwifery application.

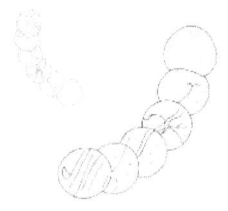

Group B Strep
BACTERIA

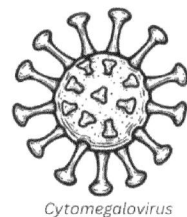

Cytomegalovirus
VIRUS

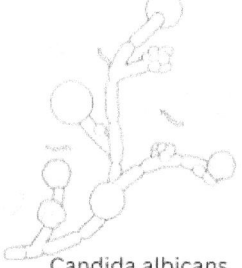

Candida albicans
FUNGI

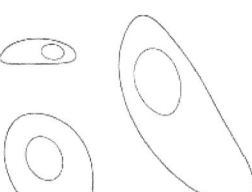

Toxoplasma gondii
PROTOZOA

CELL DIVISION AND REPAIR

Cells divide in two main ways: **mitosis** and **meiosis**.

Mitosis produces two identical daughter cells. This process supports tissue growth, regeneration, and repair—crucial for uterine lining renewal, placental development, and postpartum healing. Mitosis preserves the full set of chromosomes, ensuring genetic stability.

Meiosis, by contrast, occurs only in the ovaries and testes. It creates gametes (eggs and sperm), each with **half** the normal number of chromosomes. This reduction ensures that fertilization results in the correct number of chromosomes in the embryo.

When cell division is disrupted, it can lead to problems such as chromosomal abnormalities, cancer, molar pregnancy, or poor tissue healing. Midwives apply this knowledge when counseling clients on ovulation, interpreting genetic screening, and explaining tissue repair or pregnancy loss. A working understanding of mitosis and meiosis strengthens both clinical care and communication.

Quick Comparison: Mitosis vs. Meiosis

Mitosis	Meiosis
Occurs in all body cells	Occurs only in ovaries and testes
Produces 2 identical cells	Produces 4 genetically unique gametes
Maintains full chromosome count	Halves the chromosome count
Supports growth and repair	Enables sexual reproduction

Phases of the Cell Cycle and Mitosis:

1. **INTERPHASE** The cell performs normal functions and replicates its DNA in preparation for division. Though not part of mitosis itself, it is the longest phase of the cycle.
2. **PROPHASE** Chromatin condenses into visible chromosomes. The nuclear envelope breaks down, and spindle fibers form from centrosomes.
3. **METAPHASE** Chromosomes align along the metaphase plate at the center of the cell, connected to spindle fibers at their centromeres.
4. **ANAPHASE** Spindle fibers shorten, pulling sister chromatids apart toward opposite poles.
5. **TELOPHASE** Chromatids reach the poles and de-condense. Nuclear envelopes re-form around each set of chromosomes.
6. **CYTOKINESIS** Often overlaps with telophase. The cell membrane pinches inward, dividing the cytoplasm and completing the formation of two genetically identical daughter cells.

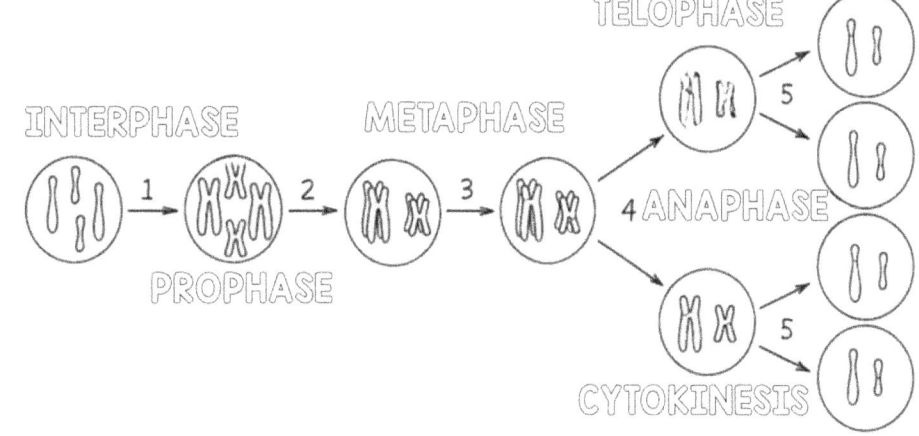

Each daughter cell produced by mitosis is diploid and genetically identical to the original parent cell. This process ensures genomic stability across cell generations and supports the constant renewal needed for reproductive and general health.

Meiosis

Meiosis is a specialized type of cell division that produces gametes, sperm in males and ova (eggs) in females. Unlike mitosis, which results in two genetically identical diploid cells, meiosis produces four genetically diverse haploid cells, each with half the original chromosome number. This reduction is essential for maintaining chromosome balance across generations and enabling sexual reproduction.

Functions of meiosis:
- Production of gametes (sperm and eggs)
- Reduction of chromosome number from diploid (2n) to haploid (n)
- Introduction of genetic diversity through recombination and independent assortment

Phases of meiosis: Meiosis occurs in two sequential stages: Meiosis I and Meiosis II, each with distinct phases.

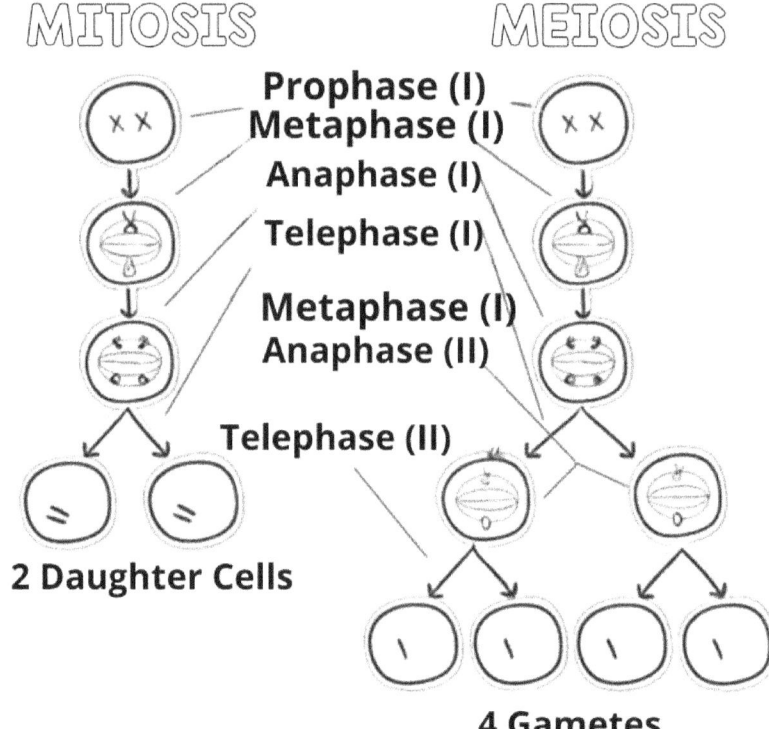

Meiosis I (Reduction Division)

1. **PROPHASE I** Homologous chromosomes pair up in a process called synapsis and exchange genetic material via crossing over. This promotes genetic diversity.
2. **METAPHASE I** Paired homologous chromosomes align along the metaphase plate.
3. **ANAPHASE I** Homologous chromosomes (not sister chromatids) are pulled to opposite poles of the cell.
4. **TELOPHASE I AND CYTOKINESIS** Two haploid daughter cells are formed, each containing half the original number of chromosomes, but still in the form of sister chromatids.

Meiosis II (Equational Division)

1. **PROPHASE II** Chromosomes re-condense in both haploid cells; spindle fibers reform.
2. **METAPHASE II** Chromosomes align individually along the metaphase plate.
3. **ANAPHASE II** Sister chromatids are finally separated and drawn to opposite poles.
4. **TELOPHASE II AND CYTOKINESIS** Four non-identical haploid cells are formed, each with a unique combination of genetic material.

Unlike mitosis, which preserves genetic identity, meiosis enhances genetic variation, which is critical for evolution and adaptation in sexually reproducing populations.

Trigger for Meiosis II

Meiosis II begins without another round of DNA replication. In most cells, it proceeds shortly after Meiosis I. However, in human egg cells, Meiosis II arrests at metaphase II and only completes if fertilization occurs. When a sperm enters the egg, the oocyte completes division to form a mature ovum and releases a small, non-functional cell called the second polar body.

Exercise 5.4: Mitosis/Meiosis
Color and label the stages

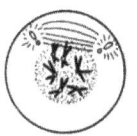 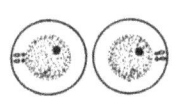 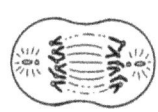 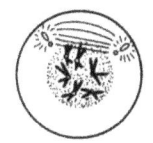 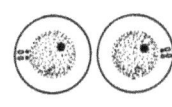 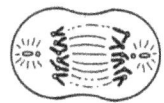

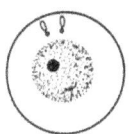 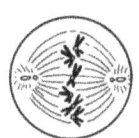 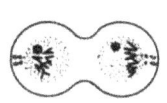 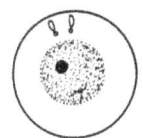 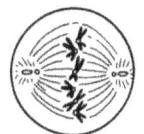 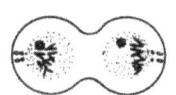

Exercise 5.5: Cells
Mark where each occurs

	Meiosis	Mitosis
No pairing of homologs occurs		
Two divisions		
Four daughter cells produced		
Used in growth and maintenance, asexual reproduction		
Associated with sexual reproduction		
One division		
Two daughter cells produced		
Involves duplication of chromosomes		
Chromosome number is maintained		
Chromosome number is halved		
Crossing over between homologous chromosomes may occur		
Daughter cells are identical to parent cells		
Produce gametes		
Synapses occurs in prophase		

Stem Cells in Early Development

Stem cells are the foundational cells of life. They are unspecialized cells with the unique ability to develop into different types of cells, tissues, and organs. Stem cells are particularly important in the earliest stages of pregnancy, when the embryo is rapidly dividing and forming the structures needed for development.

There are several types of stem cells, each with different levels of potential:

1. **TOTIPOTENT** These are the most versatile stem cells. They can become any cell type in the body or placenta. The fertilized egg and the first few divisions are totipotent.
2. **PLURIPOTENT** These cells can become any cell type in the body (but not placenta). Pluripotent stem cells arise shortly after implantation and give rise to the three germ layers: ectoderm, mesoderm, and endoderm.
3. **MULTIPOTENT** These are more specialized. They can form cells within a related group (e.g., blood cells, muscle cells, nerve cells). Hematopoietic stem cells in the bone marrow are a good example.

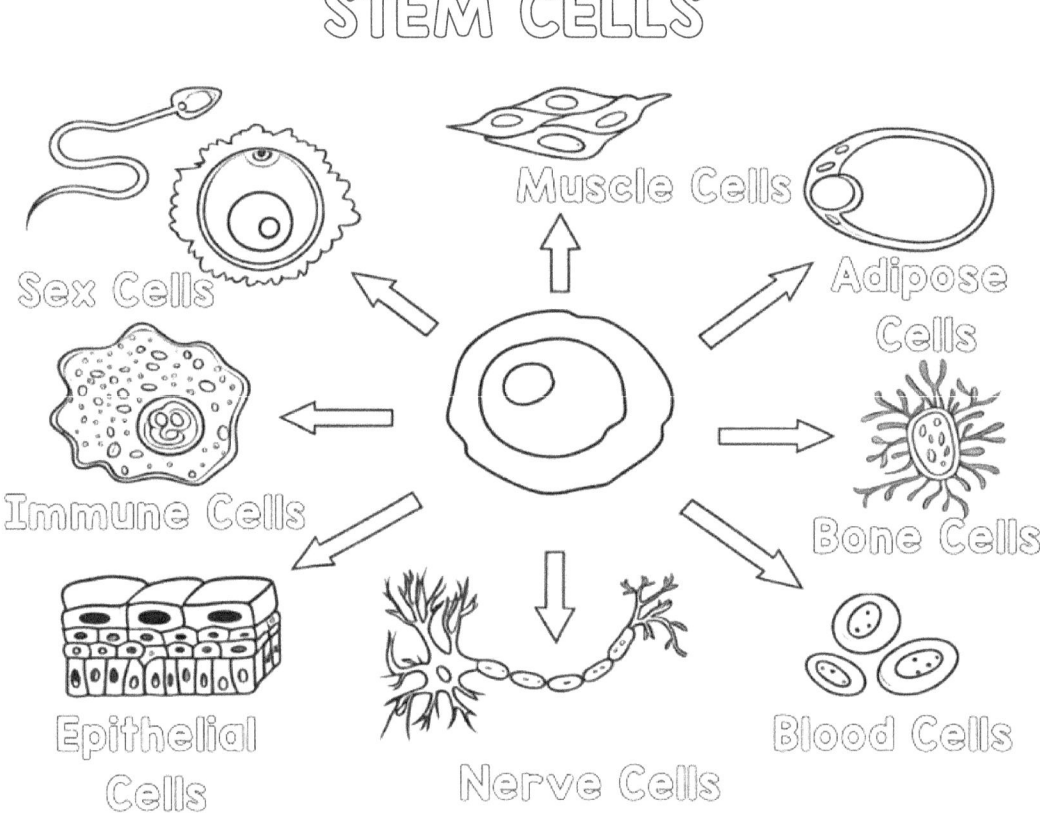

As the embryo grows, these stem cells begin to specialize, guiding the formation of tissues and organs. Midwives may encounter the topic of stem cells when discussing fetal development, umbilical cord blood banking, or emerging therapies. While midwives do not manipulate stem cells in practice, understanding their role helps in educating clients about early development and potential research applications in the future.

Scenario for Practice

During a prenatal visit, a client asks about cord blood banking and wonders why it might be important.

How would you briefly explain what stem cells are and how they could be useful in the future, in a way that is accessible and empowering?

The Human Microbiome

Maternal Microbiome in Pregnancy
The maternal microbiome is now recognized as a functional "organ" of pregnancy, contributing to nutrition, metabolism, and fetal development. These microbial communities shift during pregnancy to support both mother and baby:
- **Gut microbiome:** Diversity decreases, while certain bacteria become more abundant to increase energy extraction from food. These changes help transfer nutrients to the fetus but can also be linked to conditions such as gestational diabetes or preeclampsia.
- **Oral microbiome:** Hormonal changes may increase gum inflammation and bleeding. Poor oral health has been associated with preterm birth and low birth weight, making dental care an important part of midwifery care.
- **Vaginal microbiome:** Becomes dominated by *Lactobacillus* species, which produce lactic acid to lower vaginal pH and protect against infection. This balance is also essential for seeding the infant microbiome during vaginal birth.
- **Placental microbiome:** Research suggests the placenta hosts its own microbial community, potentially influencing fetal development and priming the immune system.

How Babies Acquire Their First Microbes
- **During birth:** As the baby passes through the birth canal, they are coated in the mother's vaginal and intestinal bacteria. These microbes are swallowed and seeded on the skin, mouth, and gut.
- **After birth:** Skin-to-skin contact, breastfeeding, and exposure to the home environment continue to build the baby's microbiome. Breast milk contains prebiotics (food for good bacteria) and probiotics (beneficial bacteria) that help the infant gut thrive.
- **Skin-to-skin** and breastfeeding immediately after birth are two of the most effective ways to establish a healthy infant microbiome.
- **Cesarean birth:** Babies born by cesarean may have a different early microbiome, often more influenced by skin and hospital bacteria. Skin-to-skin and early breastfeeding are especially important for these babies.

Why Delaying the First Bath Matters
For many years, it was common practice to wash newborns right after birth. We now know that early bathing can remove the vernix caseosa (the white, creamy coating on a newborn's skin). Vernix is more than just a temporary covering, it:
- Contains antimicrobial peptides that help prevent infections.
- Helps regulate body temperature.
- Acts as a natural moisturizer and protective barrier.
- Transfers beneficial bacteria that seed the baby's microbiome.
- Helps vernix do its job and supports the baby's early microbial colonization.

The World Health Organization (WHO) and many professional midwifery bodies recommend delaying the first bath for at least 24 hours, or if not possible, for at least 6 hours after birth. Delayed bathing allows the baby's skin to absorb protective properties from vernix and supports the establishment of healthy bacteria on their skin.

The Microbiome and Long-Term Health
Research shows that the microbiome influences more than digestion — it plays a role in immune system development, metabolism, and even risks for conditions like allergies, asthma, and obesity later in life. The early hours and days after birth are a "window of opportunity" when microbial communities are seeded and begin to flourish.

MICROBIOME CHANGES

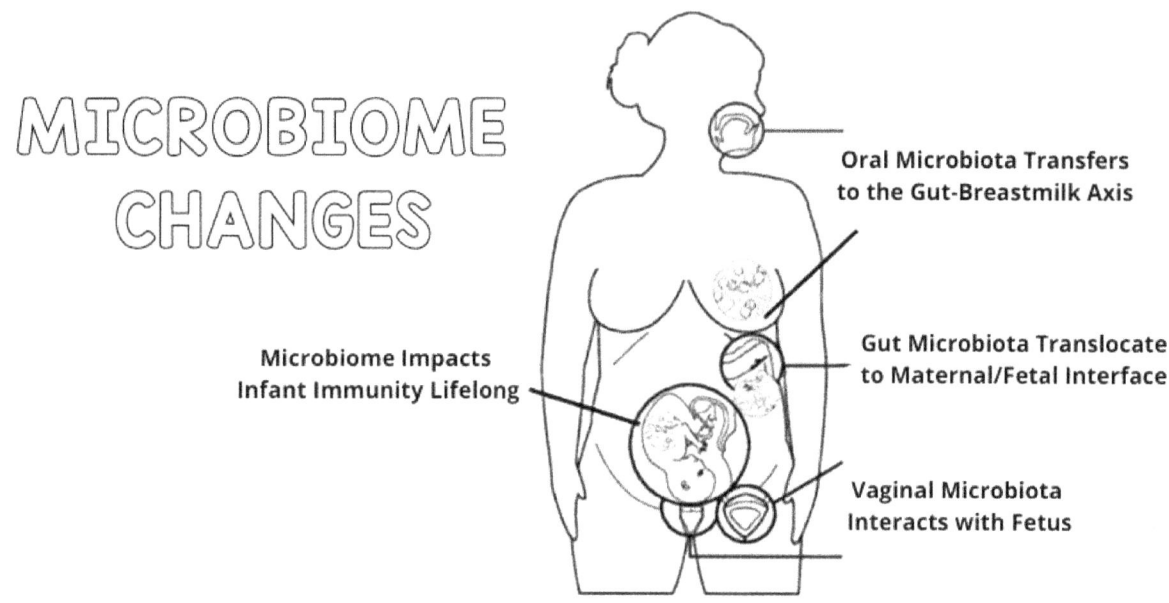

Exercise 5.3: Applications of Biology

Answer the following:

1. **Cellular Transport**
   How does understanding osmosis and diffusion help you make decisions about IV fluids for mothers in labor or postpartum?

2. **Cell Organelles**
   Mitochondria are the "powerhouses" of the cell. Why might mitochondrial health be important during pregnancy, birth, and recovery?

3. **Cell Division and Repair**
   Healing after birth involves rapid cell division. How does knowledge of mitosis help explain the body's ability to recover from birth-related tissue changes?

4. **Meiosis and Genetics**
   Meiosis ensures genetic diversity and accurate chromosome number. Why is this process especially important for understanding fertility, conception, and birth defects?

5. **Stem Cells**
   Stem cells can differentiate into many types of cells. How could this concept be important when thinking about fetal development or future medical treatments like cord blood banking?

6. **Microbiome**
   The microbiome begins forming during and after birth. How can midwives support healthy microbial colonization for newborns?

Genetics for Midwives

What Is Genetics?
Genetics is the study of how biological traits are passed from one generation to the next. These traits are carried on genes, which are located on chromosomes within each cell's nucleus. Every person inherits a unique combination of genetic material from their biological parents, making each individual both distinct and connected to their ancestry.

Every cell in the human body carries a complete set of instructions stored on chromosomes. These instructions, written in genes, influence everything from hair color and blood type to hormone production and disease risk.

For midwives, genetics is not about predicting the future with certainty, but about understanding **patterns of inheritance**. Some traits follow simple rules; a single gene can determine whether a condition appears, is hidden as a carrier state, or does not show up at all. Other traits are influenced by many genes and by environment, making outcomes more complex. While midwives do not diagnose or manage genetic disorders, we play a vital role in educating, supporting, and referring clients with informed, compassionate care.

Tools like the **Punnett square** (which shows possible combinations of parental alleles) and diagrams of **carrier inheritance** (such as when both parents carry a recessive gene) help us visualize risk. These tools are especially useful in midwifery when explaining why a baby may inherit a condition, why some conditions "skip" generations, or how a parent can carry a gene without showing the trait.

> **Key Vocabulary**
> - **Allele:** One of two or more versions of a gene; inherited from each parent.
> - **Carrier:** An individual who has one recessive allele and one dominant allele but does not express the trait.
> - **Chromosome:** A structure made of tightly coiled DNA and proteins; humans have 23 pairs.
> - **DNA (Deoxyribonucleic Acid):** The molecule that contains the genetic code used to build and operate the body.

DNA and Chromosomes
DNA (deoxyribonucleic acid) is the instruction manual for life. It contains all the information needed to build and operate every cell in the body. DNA is composed of two twisting strands that form a double helix, made up of repeating units called nucleotides. These nucleotides use four chemical bases—**adenine** (A), **thymine** (T), **cytosine** (C), and **guanine** (G)—to carry genetic information.

This DNA is tightly coiled into chromosomes, which are housed in the nucleus of nearly every human cell. Humans have 46 chromosomes, organized into 23 pairs:

- 22 pairs of autosomes: These carry the majority of our genetic information.
- 1 pair of sex chromosomes: These determine biological sex (XX or XY).

Each chromosome contains hundreds to thousands of genes—segments of DNA that influence everything from hair color and blood type to enzyme function and metabolism. The different versions of each gene are called alleles, and the specific combination inherited from each parent is what makes each person genetically unique.

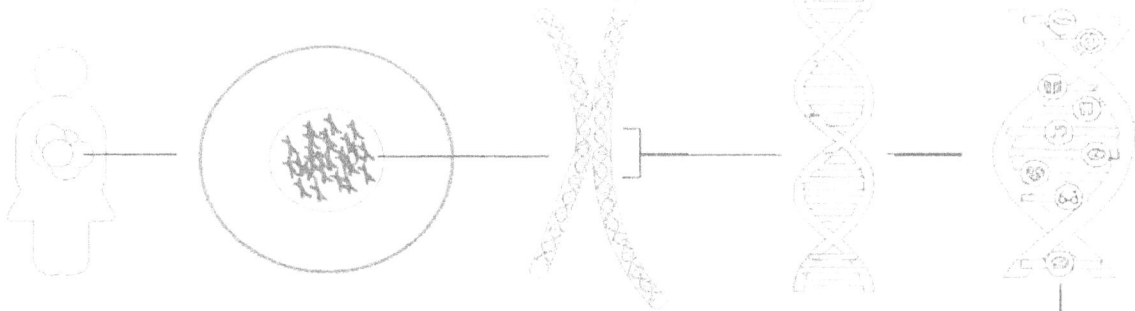

| Your body is made of cells | Each cell has your chromosomes | Every chromosome contains our DNA | In your DNA are your genes | Your genes carry your traits |

DNA, RNA, and Protein Synthesis

DNA (deoxyribonucleic acid) is the cell's master instruction manual. DNA is like a recipe book. But the cell doesn't cook directly from that book. Instead, it makes a copy of the recipe (RNA), carries it to the kitchen (cytoplasm), and then builds the meal (protein). Proteins are the body's workers: they form tissues, carry signals, and regulate growth.

Step 1: REPLICATION

Before a cell divides, it makes a complete copy of its DNA so that each new cell gets the full instruction book.

Step 2: TRANSCRIPTION

Inside the nucleus, a single recipe (gene) is copied from DNA into messenger RNA (mRNA).
The mRNA leaves the nucleus through a nuclear pore and carries the instructions to the cytoplasm.

Step 3: TRANSLATION

Ribosomes (the cell's "chefs") read the mRNA instructions in groups of three letters called **codons**. Transfer RNAs (tRNA) bring in the matching **amino acids** (the ingredients). The amino acids are linked together into a chain, which folds into a protein.

Key Vocabulary

- **Dominant Trait:** A trait that is expressed when at least one dominant allele is present.
- **Gene:** A segment of DNA that carries instructions for a specific trait.
- **Genotype:** The genetic makeup or combination of alleles (e.g., AA, Aa, or aa).
- **Heterozygous:** Having two different alleles for a specific gene (e.g., Aa).
- **Homozygous:** Having two identical alleles for a specific gene (e.g., AA or aa).
- **Phenotype:** The observable characteristics or traits expressed from the genotype.
- **Recessive Trait:** A trait that is expressed only when two recessive alleles are present.
- **X-linked Trait:** A trait associated with a gene carried on the X chromosome; often more likely to affect individuals with XY chromosomes.

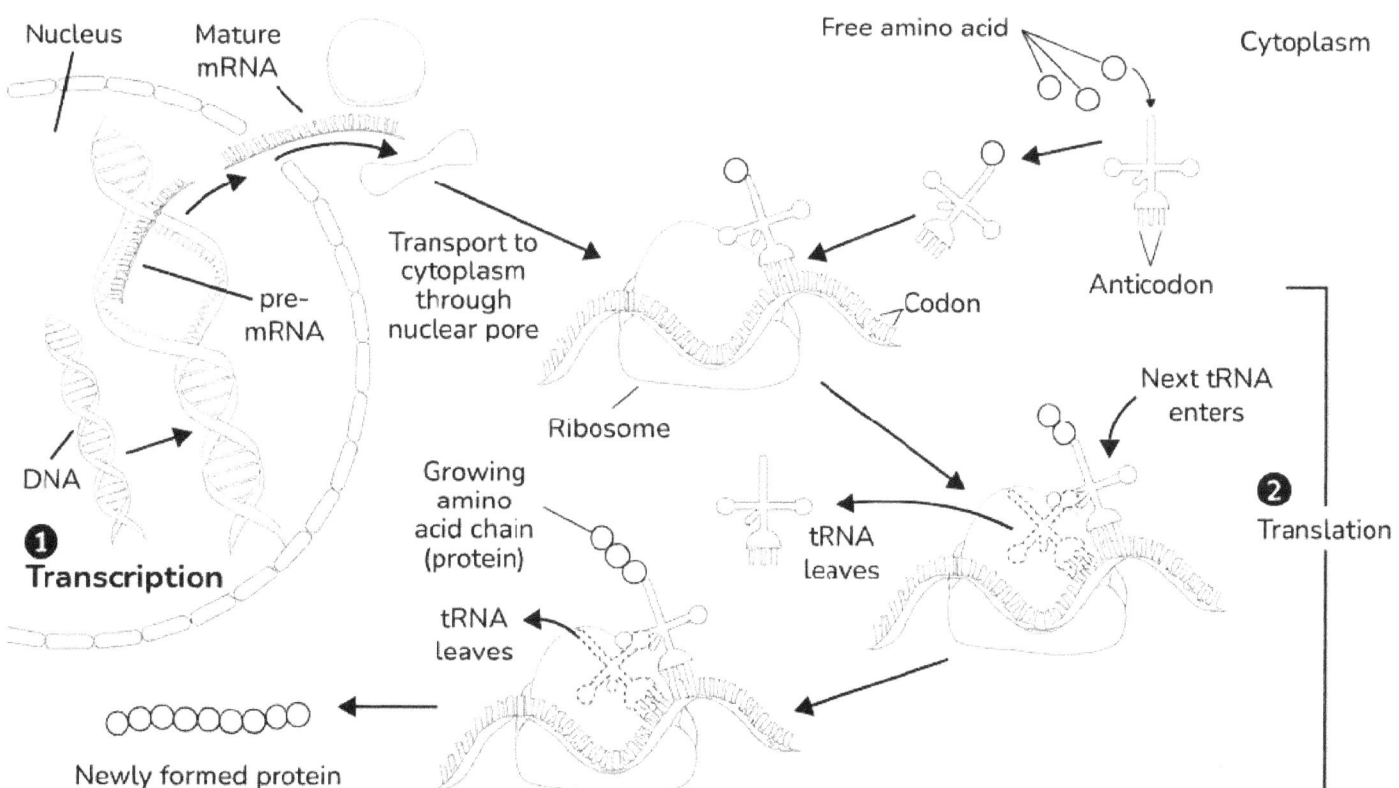

Punnett Square

The Punnett square is a simple tool that helps visualize how traits are inherited from parents to offspring. It shows the possible combinations of alleles that a child might receive, based on the genetic makeup of the parents. This chart is especially useful when explaining dominant and recessive inheritance patterns.

For example, if both parents carry one dominant allele for brown eyes (B) and one recessive allele for blue eyes (b), the following outcomes are possible:

	Genotype	
	Parent 1	
	b	b
Parent 2 B	Bb	Bb
Parent 2 b	bb	bb

bb	50%
Bb	50%
BB	0%

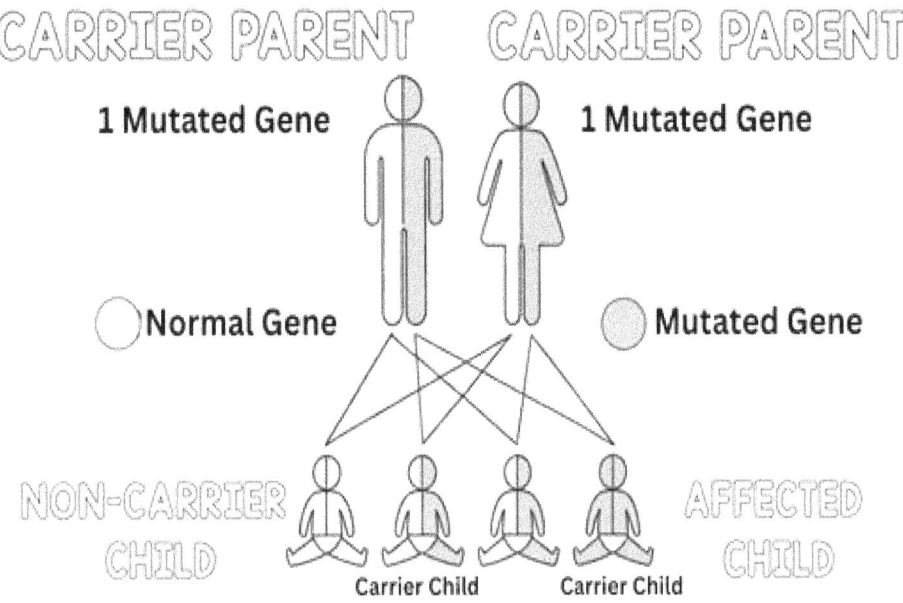

Exercise 5.7: Genetics
Match numbers with the correct letter

1. _____ What's the difference between genotype and phenotype?
2. _____ If two parents carry a recessive gene for blue eyes, what are the chances their baby will have blue eyes?
3. _____ Why are X-linked traits more likely to affect people with XY chromosomes?
4. _____ Can a baby inherit a trait that neither parent visibly expresses? Why or why not?

A. Yes—if both parents carry the gene without expressing it (they are carriers)
B. 25% chance, if both are carriers.
C. People with XY chromosomes have no second X to mask recessive traits.
D. Genotype is the internal genetic code; phenotype is what we see.

Chromosomal Abnormalities

Most pregnancies progress with normal chromosomal division, but sometimes errors occur. These errors can lead to conditions such as Down syndrome (Trisomy 21), Turner syndrome (Monosomy X), or Edwards syndrome (Trisomy 18). While midwives do not diagnose these conditions, understanding their existence is important when supporting families through prenatal screening, early pregnancy loss, or discussions of genetic results.

Epigenetics: Genes and Environment Working Together

Not all traits are determined strictly by DNA. **Epigenetics** refers to chemical "tags" on DNA that turn genes on or off without changing the genetic code. Epigenetics helps explain why two people with the same genetic risk may experience different health outcomes. These tags can be influenced by factors such as environment, nutrition, stress, or exposure to toxins.

Examples:
- Adequate folate in pregnancy can prevent neural tube defects.
- Chronic stress may influence birth outcomes through hormonal pathways.

Why Epigenetics Matters in Midwifery

Epigenetics helps midwives explain why genes are not destiny. Health outcomes depend not only on DNA, but also on how genes are expressed in response to environment and care. Nutrition, toxins, and stress can all influence these changes. Midwives can use epigenetics to encourage healthy behaviors in pregnancy while honoring the complexity of how life and environment interact with DNA.

Studies show that **generational trauma** can affect gene expression and immune function, shaping how the body responds to stress across generations. These effects do not alter the genetic code but can influence hormone levels, immune balance, and emotional regulation. Supportive care, healing environments, and nurturing relationships can help restore balance and promote healthier outcomes for both mother and baby — and for future generations.

Examples in Midwifery Practice
- **Nutrition:** Adequate folate during pregnancy can "switch on" protective genes that prevent neural tube defects.
- **Stress:** Chronic stress may alter gene expression, associated with an increased risk of preterm birth.
- **Breastfeeding:** Human milk provides compounds that shape infant gene expression and immune development.
- **Environmental exposures:** Smoking, alcohol, and toxins can silence or activate genes in ways that affect fetal growth.
- **Intergenerational impact:** Some epigenetic changes can be passed to future generations, shaping health beyond one pregnancy.

Exercise 5.8: Applying Genetic Knowledge
Answer the following real-world examples of how genetic knowledge impacts midwifery practice:
1. A client asks why a chromosomal abnormality might lead to miscarriage.
2. A pregnant woman with fatigue wants to understand what mitochondria have to do with energy levels.
3. You're reviewing a lab result that mentions white blood cell count, and the client wants to know what it means.
4. Everyone in my family has dimples. My partner doesn't. Do you think our baby will?"

Selected Hereditary Traits in Humans

Genetics is often taught using simple "dominant vs. recessive" examples, but modern science emphasizes most human traits are influenced by many genes working together (polygenic) as well as environmental factors such as nutrition, lifestyle, and exposures. Only a few traits follow a clear single-gene (Mendelian) inheritance pattern. The chart below separates some **true Mendelian traits** from **polygenic or complex traits** to help you recognize the difference.

Mendelian (Single-Gene) Traits	Polygenic or Complex Traits
Widow's peak hairline: often taught as dominant (though inheritance may be more complex)	**Hair texture (straight, wavy, curly)**: multiple genes involved
Attached earlobes: traditionally described as recessive, though not purely single-gene	**Hair color (black, brown, blond, red)**: many genes + environment
Polydactyly (extra fingers/toes): usually autosomal dominant, variable expression	**Eye color (brown, blue, green, hazel, gray)**: polygenic
Cystic fibrosis: autosomal recessive disorder	**Skin pigmentation**: polygenic and influenced by environment
Sickle-cell disease: autosomal recessive; carriers have some malaria resistance	**Height and body build**: strongly polygenic and environment-influenced
Huntington's disease (chorea): autosomal dominant, late onset	**Male-pattern baldness**: polygenic, influenced by hormones
Albinism: usually autosomal recessive	**Vision (near- or farsightedness)**: polygenic + environmental
Tay–Sachs disease: autosomal recessive	**Most hearing loss**: many genetic and environmental causes
Hemophilia A & B: X-linked recessive disorders	**Susceptibility/resistance to common diseases**: multifactorial
	Mental health conditions (e.g., schizophrenia, bipolar disorder): complex, multifactorial
	Congenital anomalies (e.g., cleft lip/palate, Hirschsprung disease): usually multifactorial

Exercise 5.9 Hereditary Traits
Match each trait with the correct letter, either A or B

1. ____Cystic fibrosis	**A.** Mendelian Trait
2. ____Eye color	**B.** Polygenic/Complex Trait.
3. ____Huntington's disease	
4. ____Skin pigmentation	
5. ____Sickle-cell disease	
6. ____Height	
7. ____Hemophilia A &	
8. ____Mental health conditions (e.g., schizophrenia, bipolar disorder)	

FOUNDATIONS OF BIOLOGY FOR MIDWIVES ESSENTIAL TAKEAWAYS

Biology provides the foundation for understanding how pregnancy and birth unfold, and for midwives it is the bridge between science and care. Every pregnancy begins with a single cell, nourished through cellular transport and guided by DNA. From that beginning, mitosis explains how tissues grow, heal, and regenerate after birth, while meiosis accounts for the genetic balance and uniqueness of each new life. Stem cells remind us of the body's remarkable capacity for growth and repair, and genetics and inheritance show how family traits, strengths, and vulnerabilities may appear across generations. Epigenetics extends this knowledge by revealing how nutrition, stress, and environment can influence outcomes, teaching us that biology is not fixed but responds dynamically to lived experience.

The microbiome further demonstrates that health is shaped not only by human cells but also by trillions of microbial partners. Vernix, skin-to-skin contact, and breastfeeding are not simply cultural practices but biologically grounded strategies that protect newborns and strengthen long-term health. These insights help midwives explain why delayed bathing matters, why nutrition and rest during pregnancy affect both mother and baby, and why screening tests provide valuable information for family decision-making. They also inform counseling about fertility, conception, age-related risks, and the prevention of infection.

By weaving biological knowledge into everyday care, midwives can translate complex science into clear, compassionate guidance. This integration allows families to understand that pregnancy is at once universal in its patterns and unique in each expression. Grounding midwifery in biology strengthens our ability to educate, advocate, and walk beside families through pregnancy, birth, and the beginnings of life.

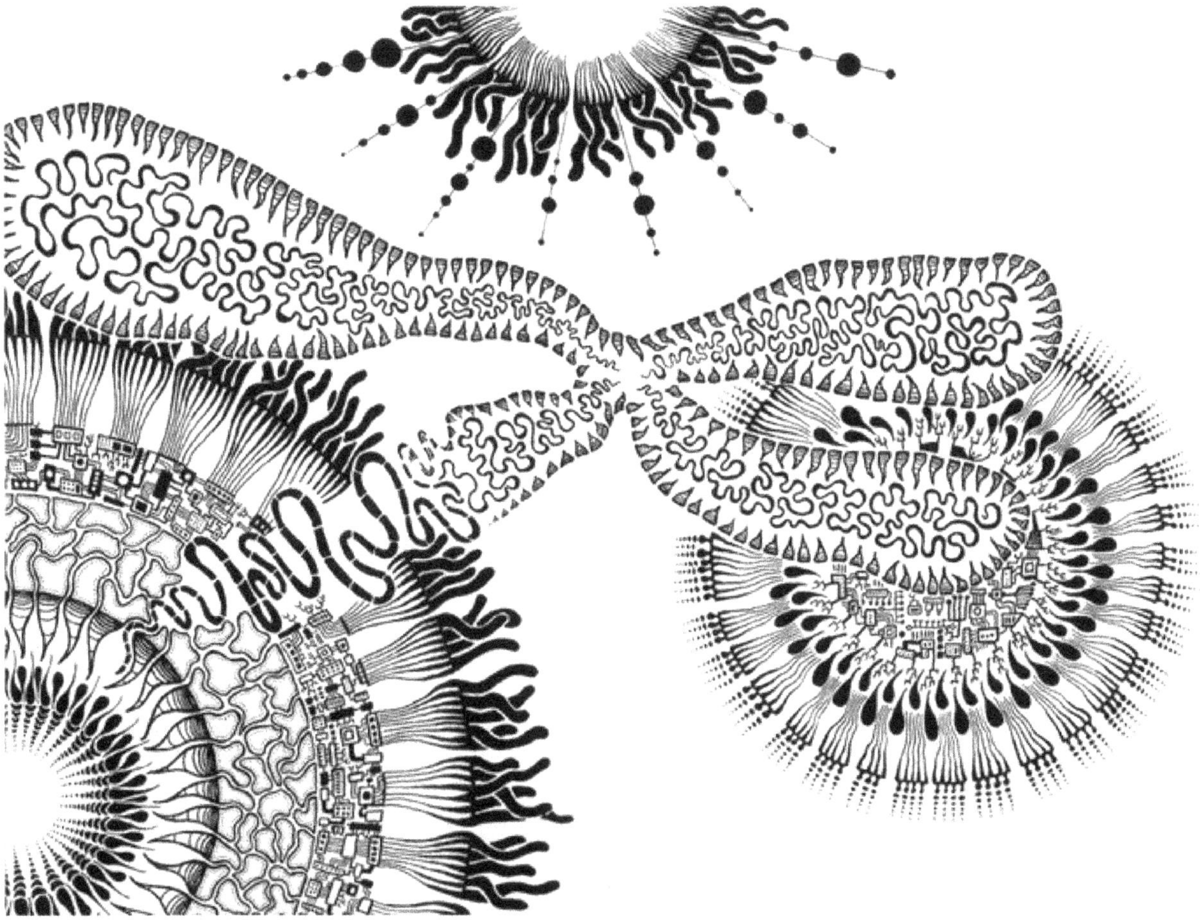

Chapter Five Self-Assessment

Multiple Choice

1. The "powerhouse" of the cell, responsible for producing ATP, is:
   a) Nucleus
   b) Mitochondria
   c) Ribosome
   d) Golgi apparatus

2. Which process requires energy (ATP)?
   a) Diffusion
   b) Osmosis
   c) Active transport
   d) Facilitated diffusion

3. Ribosomes are responsible for:
   a) Breaking down waste
   b) Producing proteins
   c) Storing genetic material
   d) Transporting oxygen

4. The plasma (cell) membrane is best described as:
   a) A rigid wall that never changes
   b) A semi-permeable barrier that regulates entry and exit
   c) The site of photosynthesis
   d) The location of DNA storage

5. Which type of stem cell can become any cell in the body or placenta?
   a) Pluripotent
   b) Totipotent
   c) Multipotent
   d) Unipotent

6. Mitosis results in:
   a) Two identical diploid cells
   b) Four genetically diverse haploid cells
   c) Growth of bacteria
   d) DNA transcription

7. Which of the following occurs only in meiosis (not mitosis)?
   a) DNA replication
   b) Formation of spindle fibers
   c) Crossing over between homologous chromosomes
   d) Cytokinesis

8. The microbiome of a newborn is most strongly influenced by:
   a) Genetics only
   b) Bathing immediately after birth
   c) Mode of birth, skin-to-skin, and breastfeeding
   d) Placental circulation

9. Epigenetics refers to:
   a) Changes in the DNA code itself
   b) Chemical tags that turn genes on or off
   c) Extra chromosomes
   d) Gene mutations

10. Which of the following is a Mendelian (single-gene) trait?
    a) Eye color
    b) Skin pigmentation
    c) Huntington's disease
    d) Height

Fill in the Blank

11. The command center of the cell, which stores DNA, is the _____.

12. The process where a section of DNA is copied into mRNA is called _____.

13. During _____, a cell divides to form four unique gametes, each with half the number of chromosomes.

14. The creamy substance covering newborns that protects the skin and seeds the microbiome is called _____.

15. Traits influenced by multiple genes and environment are called _____ traits.

True/False

_____16. Diffusion requires energy (ATP).
_____17. Lysosomes help break down waste and bacteria inside the cell.
_____18. In mitosis, the chromosome number is cut in half.
_____19. A Punnett square shows the possible combinations of parental alleles in offspring.
_____20. Delaying newborn bathing helps protect the baby's microbiome.
_____21. Epigenetics changes the DNA code permanently.
_____22. Ribosomes are where proteins are made in the cell.
_____23. Sickle-cell disease is a polygenic trait.
_____24. The microbiome only affects digestion and not other systems.
_____25. In meiosis, crossing over between homologous chromosomes promotes genetic diversity.

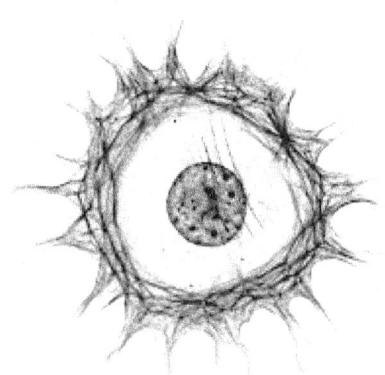

Chapter Five Reading & References

Recommended Reading: Biology

- Kaplan, E. S., & Ehrenstein, D. (2023). ***The Biology Coloring Book*** (2nd ed.).
  A classic interactive book that reinforces cell biology, genetics, and physiology through coloring.
- Knight, R. (2015). ***Follow Your Gut: The Enormous Impact of Tiny Microbes on Our Health and Well-Being.*** A short, engaging book on the microbiome and its role in health and development.
- Krogh, D. (2016). ***Biology: A Guide to the Natural World*** (6th ed.).
  A clear, visual introduction to biology, widely used in nursing and allied health programs.
- Mader, S. S., & Windelspecht, M. (2018). ***Essentials of Biology*** (6th ed.).
  A concise text designed for pre-nursing and pre-health students. Covers cell structure, genetics, and microbiology in accessible language.
- Moalem, S. (2014). ***Inheritance: How Our Genes Change Our Lives—and Our Lives Change Our Genes.*** A narrative, easy-to-read book exploring genetics and epigenetics.
- Sadava, D., Hillis, D., Heller, H., & Berenbaum, M. (2017). ***Life: The Science of Biology*** (11th ed.) A more comprehensive text for students who want deeper exploration.
- Wright, R., & Boore, J. (2019). ***Biology for Nurses*** (3rd ed.).
  Connects biological principles directly to nursing and midwifery practice.

References

American Academy of Pediatrics. (2016). Delayed bathing of the newborn: Infant care practices to support health and bonding. *Pediatrics, 138*(3), e20161889. https://doi.org/10.1542/peds.2016-1889

Centers for Disease Control and Prevention. (2020). *Genetics basics*. U.S. Department of Health and Human Services. https://www.cdc.gov/genomics/disease/genetics.htm

Kaplan, E. S., & Ehrenstein, D. (2023). *The biology coloring book* (2nd ed.). Harper Perennial.

Knight, R. (2015). *Follow your gut: The enormous impact of tiny microbes on our health and well-being*. Simon & Schuster.

Krogh, D. (2016). *Biology: A guide to the natural world* (6th ed.). Pearson.

Mader, S. S., & Windelspecht, M. (2018). *Essentials of biology* (6th ed.). McGraw-Hill Education.

Midwifery Today. (n.d.). Selected articles on microbiome, delayed bathing, and birth practices. https://www.midwiferytoday.com

Moalem, S. (2014). *Inheritance: How our genes change our lives—and our lives change our genes*. Grand Central Publishing. National Human Genome Research Institute. (2022). *Epigenetics fact sheet*. https://www.genome.gov/about-genomics/fact-sheets/Epigenomics-Fact-Sheet

National Institutes of Health. (2018). *The human microbiome*. https://commonfund.nih.gov/hmp

Sadava, D., Hillis, D. M., Heller, H. C., & Berenbaum, M. R. (2017). *Life: The science of biology* (11th ed.). W. H. Freeman.

Wright, R., & Boore, J. (2019). *Biology for nurses* (3rd ed.). Routledge.

World Health Organization. (2017). *Protecting, promoting and supporting breastfeeding in facilities providing maternity and newborn services: Guideline*. https://apps.who.int/iris/handle/10665/259386

Chapter Six
How Life Begins

Objectives
After completing this chapter, the student should be able to:
1. **Explain** the process of conception, including ovulation, fertilization, zygote formation, and the sequence of early embryonic development up to implantation.
2. **Differentiate** between types of twins (monozygotic and dizygotic), including how and when they form and the clinical implications of chorionicity and amnionicity.
3. **Describe** the stages of pre-embryonic, embryonic, and fetal development, from the formation of the blastocyst through the third trimester.
4. **Identify** and explain the functions of the decidua, including its regions and its role in implantation, placental development, and immune tolerance.
5. **Explain** the role and formation of the placenta, chorionic villi, and umbilical cord, and describe how these structures support fetal nutrition, waste elimination, and hormone production.
6. **Describe** the formation, structure, and function of the amniotic membranes and amniotic fluid, including their role in fetal protection and development.
7. **Summarize** the principles of fetal circulation, including key shunts and the transition to neonatal circulation at birth.
8. **Explain** the timeline and significance of fetal sensory development (touch, taste, hearing, and vision) and its implications for bonding and newborn behavior.
9. **Describe** the timing and mechanism of sexual differentiation, including genetic, gonadal, and hormonal influences, and the clinical relevance of differences in sexual development (DSDs).
10. **Identify** critical periods of susceptibility during embryonic and fetal development, and list common teratogens and their associated risks.
11. **Explain** the significance of embryonic folding and germ layer differentiation, and list the major tissues derived from the ectoderm, mesoderm, and endoderm.
12. **Apply** microbiological and developmental knowledge to support fertility counseling, prenatal education, and early pregnancy assessment in clinical practice.

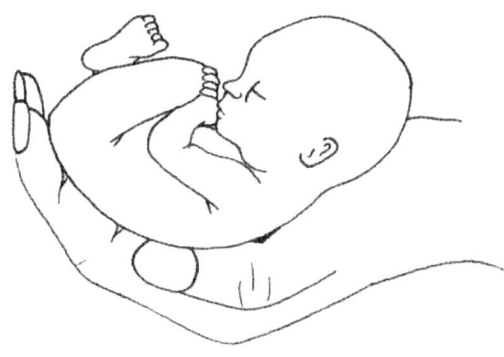

How Life Begins

Conception: The Beginning of Pregnancy

When **ovulation** occurs, the ovarian follicle releases a mature egg into the fallopian tube. At the same time, the cervical glands produce mucus that becomes less acidic and more fluid, with a slippery, stretchy quality called **spinnbarkeit**. This change helps sperm survive longer and move more easily through the cervical canal.

During sexual intercourse, millions of sperm are released, but only a small fraction survive the acidic environment of the vagina and the long passage through the cervix and uterus to reach the fallopian tube. Fertilization usually takes place in the **ampulla**, the widest section of the tube.

The egg is surrounded by the **zona pellucida** and the **corona radiata**. Hundreds of sperm release enzymes to help break down these protective layers, but ultimately only **one sperm** succeeds in penetrating the egg. Immediately afterward, the egg forms a **fertilization membrane** that prevents additional sperm from entering.

Once inside, the sperm sheds its tail, leaving only the head, which contains the male genetic material. This nucleus, with 23 chromosomes, unites with the egg's nucleus, which also contains 23 chromosomes. When these pronuclei fuse, fertilization is complete. The resulting **zygote** now has a full set of 46 chromosomes — half from each parent.

Key Vocabulary

- **Gamete**: A reproductive cell — sperm in males and egg (ovum) in females — each containing half the number of chromosomes (haploid).
- **Ovulation**: The release of a mature egg from the ovary.
- **Fertilization**: The union of a sperm and an egg to form a zygote.
- **Zona Pellucida**: A protective glycoprotein layer surrounding the egg.
- **Corona Radiata**: The outer layer of cells surrounding the egg that helps protect it and provides nutrients.
- **Spinnbarkeit**: The slippery, stretchy quality of cervical mucus at ovulation that helps sperm survive and move more easily.
- **Fertilization Membrane**: A barrier formed after one sperm penetrates the egg, preventing additional sperm from entering.
- **Aneuploidy**: The presence of an abnormal number of chromosomes in a cell.

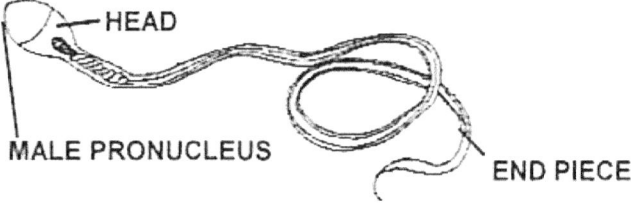

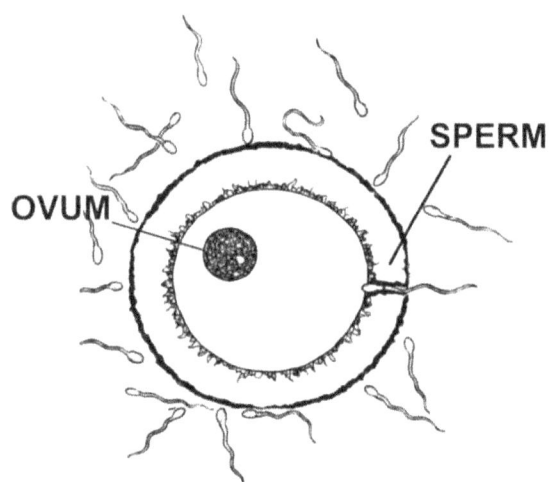

Midwifery Applications

Midwives use knowledge of conception to explain fertilization and early development, counsel clients on fertility and pregnancy, and identify potential complications. Understanding ovulation, fertile windows, and implantation supports accurate dating, early loss care, and informed reproductive choices.

Key Facts

- Sperm can survive in the female reproductive tract for up to five days.
- An egg is usually viable for twelve to twenty-four hours after ovulation.
- Fertilization triggers a reaction that blocks additional sperm from entering the egg.

Rarely, a fertilized egg implants outside the uterus, causing an ectopic pregnancy.

Exercise 6.1: Conception Review
Answer the questions below:

1. What change occurs in cervical mucus at ovulation that helps sperm survive and move?

2. Where in the uterine tube does fertilization usually occur?

3. What prevents more than one sperm from entering the egg?

4. How many chromosomes does a zygote contain, and where do they come from?

GAMETE AGING AND REPRODUCTIVE HEALTH

As people age, the quality of their gametes changes in ways that influence fertility and pregnancy outcomes. These changes affect both conception and the health of future pregnancies.

In individuals with ovaries:
- The number of eggs is set at birth and declines steadily with age.
- After about age thirty-five, egg quality decreases more rapidly, leading to higher rates of chromosomal abnormalities such as trisomy 21 (Down syndrome), trisomy 18, and trisomy 13.
- The risk of miscarriage increases, often due to these chromosomal errors.
- Older oocytes are also more likely to fail to implant or to result in very early pregnancy loss.

> **Key Fact**
> The average age at first birth has risen in many countries, making knowledge of gamete aging increasingly relevant for midwives.

In individuals with testes:
- Sperm production continues throughout life, but aging can reduce sperm motility and lower semen volume.
- DNA fragmentation in sperm increases with age, which can impair embryo development.
- These changes are linked to higher rates of miscarriage and have also been associated with certain neurodevelopmental conditions, including autism spectrum disorder and schizophrenia.

Application in Midwifery

Midwives must understand how age-related changes in egg and sperm quality affect conception, pregnancy risks, and prenatal screening. Recognizing when gamete aging may contribute to miscarriage, chromosomal abnormalities, or developmental concerns supports timely referrals for fertility evaluation and genetic counseling. It also allows midwives to provide compassionate, inclusive guidance to families exploring pregnancy later in life.

> **Clinical Tip**
> Offer early discussion about fertility planning and prenatal testing options for clients who are thirty-five or older, or whose partners are older fathers.

CONCEPTION OF TWINS

Twins can form in two main ways:

1. **MONOZYGOTIC (identical) twins** result from a single fertilized egg that splits into two embryos. The timing of this split determines the number of placentas and amniotic sacs:
    * **Days 1–3:** Each twin develops its own placenta and sac (**dichorionic, diamniotic**).
    * **Days 4–8:** Twins share a placenta but have separate sacs (**monochorionic, diamniotic**).
    * **Days 8–13:** Twins share both a placenta and a sac (**monochorionic, monoamniotic**).
    * **After day 13:** Incomplete separation may result in **conjoined twins**.

2. **DIZYGOTIC (fraternal) twins** occur when two eggs are released during ovulation and fertilized by two separate sperm. These twins always have their own placentas and sacs (**dichorionic, diamniotic**), though the placentas may fuse.

Clinical Note: Determining **chorionicity** (number of placentas) and **amnionicity** (number of amniotic sacs) is essential in assessing risk. Monochorionic twins share a placenta, which can lead to complications such as **twin-to-twin transfusion syndrome (TTTS)**. Ultrasound between ten and fourteen weeks is used to identify chorionicity and guide care.

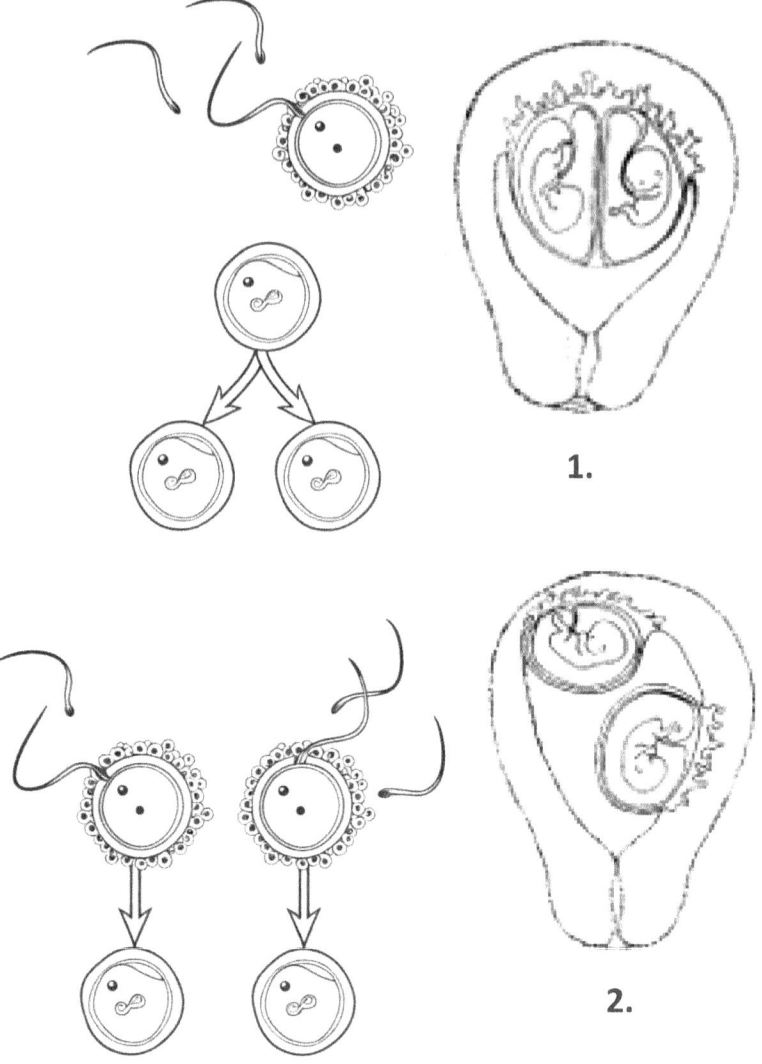

1.

2.

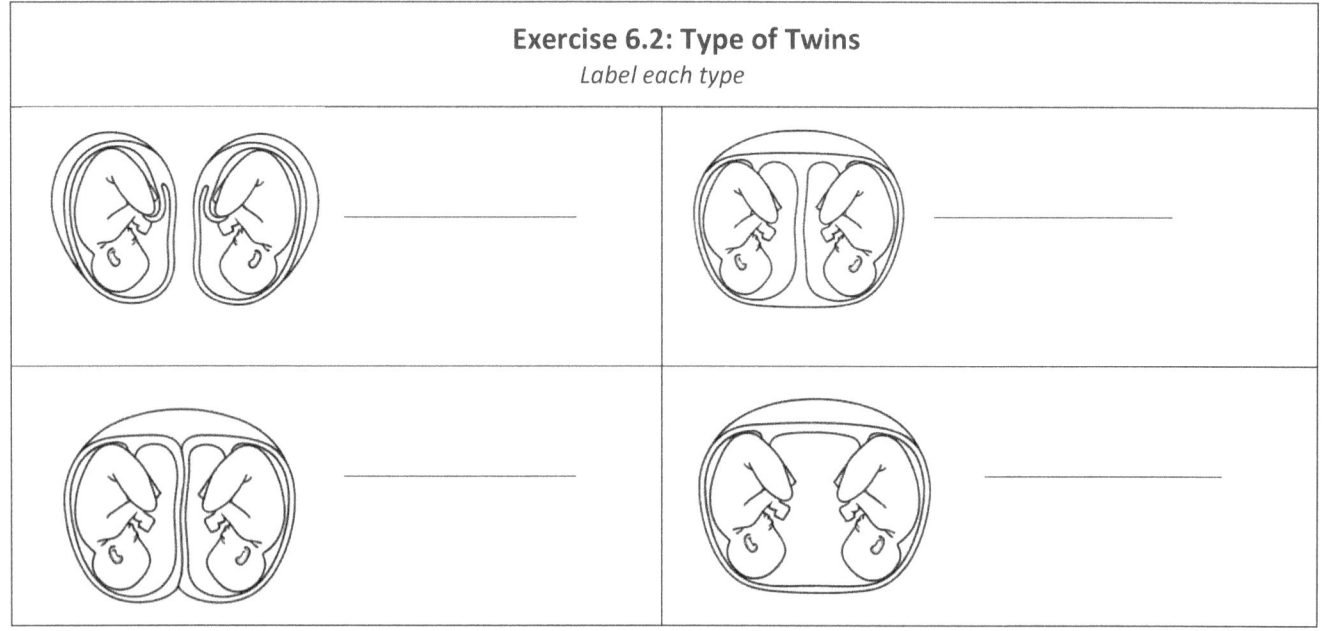

Exercise 6.2: Type of Twins
Label each type

The Process of Early Development

This sequence of stages — from the zygote through cleavage, morula, blastocyst, gastrula, and membrane formation — is essential for establishing a viable pregnancy and supporting the developing embryo.

By about the **fourth day** after fertilization, the dividing cells form a solid mass called the **morula**, meaning "mulberry" because of its clustered appearance. Around the **fifth day**, the morula enters the uterine cavity and develops into a **blastocyst**, a hollow ball of cells surrounded by a fluid-filled cavity called the **blastocele**. This stage is also known as the **blastula phase**.

On the **seventh or eighth day** after conception, the blastocyst begins **implantation** into the **endometrium**, which transforms into the **decidua** during pregnancy. Sometimes a small amount of **implantation bleeding** occurs. The endometrium, rich in blood vessels and glandular secretions during the post-ovulatory (secretory) phase, nourishes and supports the blastocyst until it can develop its own circulatory system.

> ### Key Vocabulary
>
> - **Zygote:** A single cell formed from the union of an egg and sperm, containing a complete set of 46 chromosomes (23 from each parent).
>
> - **Cleavage:** A series of rapid mitotic divisions that increase the number of cells without increasing overall size.
>
> - **Morula:** A solid ball of cells (16–32) formed by the third day after fertilization.
>
> - **Blastocyst:** A fluid-filled hollow structure formed about the fifth or sixth day after fertilization that will implant in the uterus.
>
> - **Embryoblast** (inner cell mass): The group of cells inside the blastocyst that will develop into the embryo.

By about **day fourteen**, cells of the blastocyst continue to grow and divide. At one point, cells move inward, creating a pocket that pushes into the hollow center. This marks the:

1. **GASTRULA** stage. Within the double-walled gastrula, the inner cell mass separates into three **primary germ layers**:

    A. **ECTODERM**: Develops into the skin, nervous system, hair, nails, and tooth enamel.

    B. **MESODERM**: Forms muscles, bones, connective tissue, the cardiovascular system, and reproductive organs.

    C. **ENDODERM**: Becomes the lining of the gastrointestinal tract, respiratory system, and several internal organs.

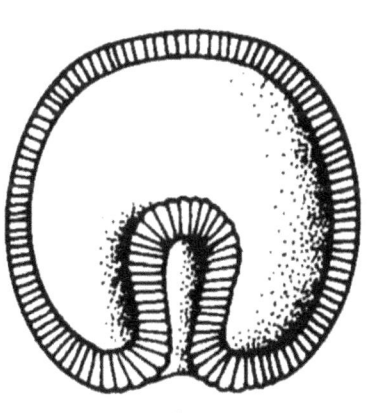

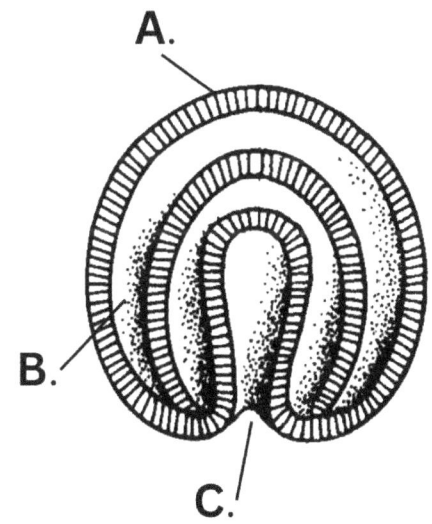

The outer cells of the blastocyst, the **trophoblast** (or **trophectoderm**), develop into the **chorion**, which surrounds the embryo. From this layer, **chorionic villi** form as fingerlike projections that extend into the decidua. These will later develop into the placenta.

Another important layer, the **extraembryonic mesoderm**, does not form part of the embryo itself. Instead, it develops into the **chorion, amnion, allantois,** and **yolk sac**. These extraembryonic membranes lie outside the embryonic disc and provide protection and nourishment for the embryo and, later, the fetus.

1. The AMNION surrounds the embryo, creating the **amniotic cavity** (where the blastocele once was). It eventually produces amniotic fluid, which cushions and protects the fetus.
2. The YOLK SAC provides early nutrition and plays a role in the initial formation of blood cells.
3. The ALLANTOIS is a vascular membrane whose blood vessels contribute to the **umbilical cord** and help establish maternal–fetal circulation.
4. The CHORION surrounds the blastocyst. Part forms the placenta, while another portion fuses with the amnion to create the double-layered **fetal membranes**.

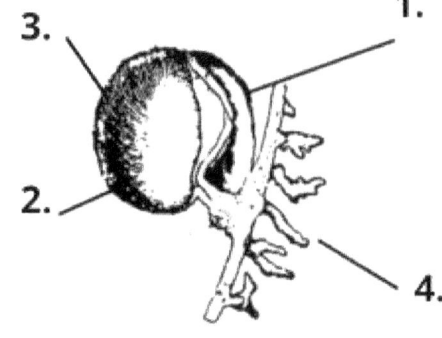

After fertilization, the zygote begins a tightly orchestrated series of developmental events as it moves toward the uterine cavity:

1. ZYGOTE: The single-cell stage immediately after fertilization, containing a diploid set of 46 chromosomes (23 from each parent).
2. CLEAVAGE: Rapid mitotic divisions increase the number of cells without increasing overall size.
3. MORULA: by around day 3, the zygote has divided into a solid ball of 16–32 cells.
4. BLASTOCYST: by days 5–6, the morula develops into a hollow, fluid-filled structure called the blastocyst.
    - **Trophoblast**: The outer layer of cells, which will form the placenta and membranes.
    - **Embryoblast (inner cell mass)**: The cluster of cells inside the blastocyst that will become the embryo.
    - **Cytotrophoblast**: The inner trophoblast layer, maintaining cellular boundaries.
    - **Syncytiotrophoblast**: The outer trophoblast layer, which invades the uterine lining and initiates placental development.
5. IMPLANTATION: between days 6–10, the blastocyst embeds into the thickened endometrium, securing nutrients and establishing the foundation for pregnancy.

This period, known as the **pre-embryonic stage**, is critical for establishing a viable pregnancy. Proper cellular organization, signaling, and implantation lay the groundwork for embryogenesis and the development of all future tissues and organ systems.

Midwifery Applications

Understanding early embryonic development helps midwives provide accurate explanations of fertilization and implantation, assess early pregnancy progress, and support clients with counseling, fertility awareness, or early loss. This knowledge also underpins the ability to interpret early ultrasounds, anticipate developmental milestones, and guide clients with clarity and compassion.

First 23 Days of Development

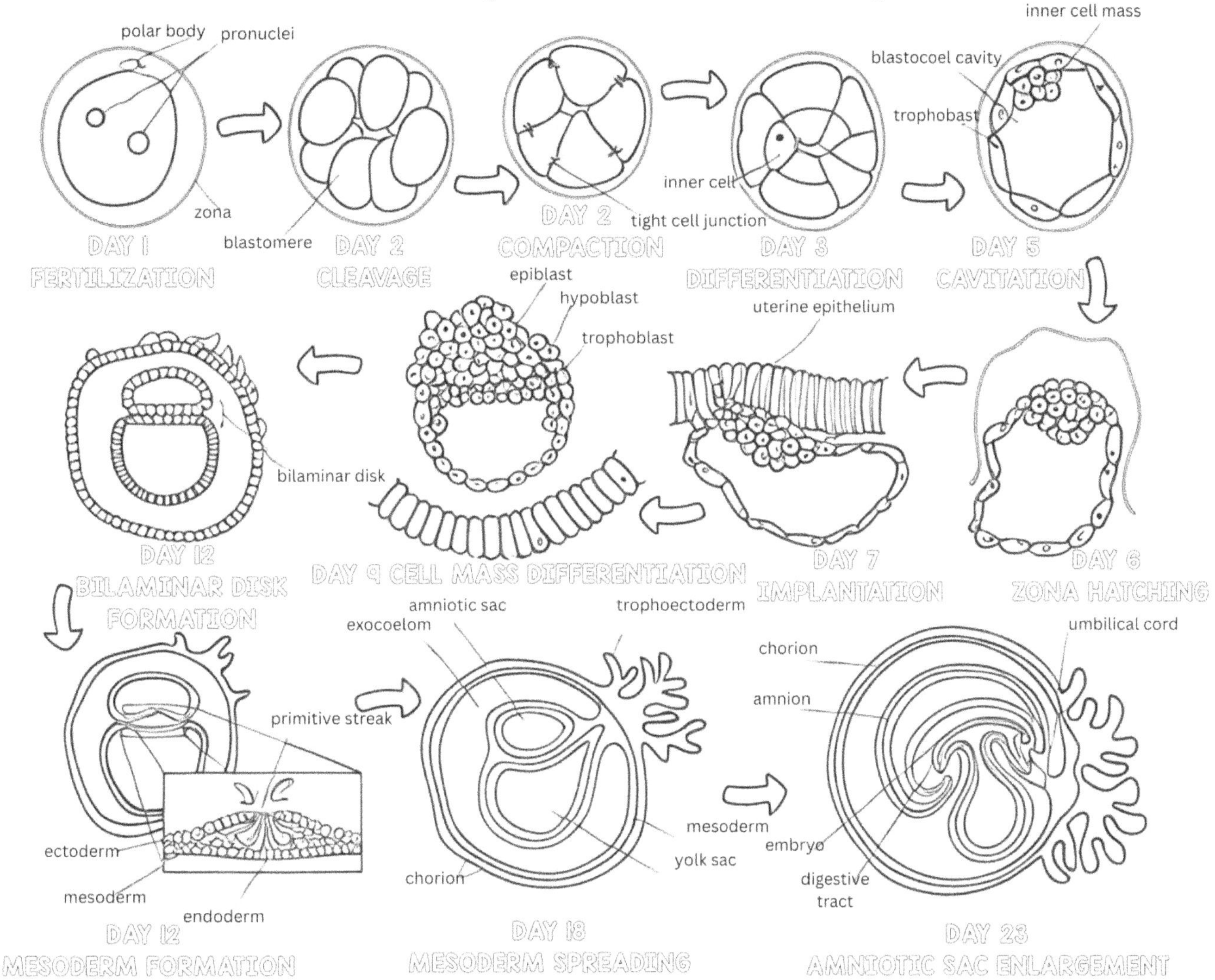

polar body
pronuclei
zona
DAY 1
FERTILIZATION
blastomere
DAY 2
CLEAVAGE
DAY 2
COMPACTION
tight cell junction
inner cell
DAY 3
DIFFERENTIATION
inner cell mass
blastocoel cavity
trophobast
DAY 5
CAVITATION
epiblast
hypoblast
trophoblast
uterine epithelium
bilaminar disk
DAY 12
BILAMINAR DISK FORMATION
DAY 9 CELL MASS DIFFERENTIATION
DAY 7
IMPLANTATION
DAY 6
ZONA HATCHING
amniotic sac
exocoelom
trophoectoderm
primitive streak
ectoderm
mesoderm
endoderm
DAY 12
MESODERM FORMATION
chorion
mesoderm
yolk sac
DAY 18
MESODERM SPREADING
umbilical cord
chorion
amnion
embryo
digestive tract
DAY 23
AMNIOTIC SAC ENLARGEMENT

EMBRYONIC FOLDING AND GERM LAYER DERIVATIVES

By the fourth week, the flat embryonic disc folds in two directions to create a three-dimensional body:

- **Longitudinal folding** (head to tail): Defines the head and tail regions.
- **Lateral folding** (side to side): Brings the body walls together to form the body cavity and primitive gut.

As folding continues, the germ layers specialize:

- **Ectoderm** → skin, brain, spinal cord, sensory organs.
- **Mesoderm** → muscles, bones, blood, heart, and reproductive organs.
- **Endoderm** → lining of the digestive tract, lungs, pancreas, liver, and other internal organs.

LONGITUDINAL FOLDING
NEURAL TUBE
ECTODERM
MESODERM
ENDODERM
NEURALTUBE

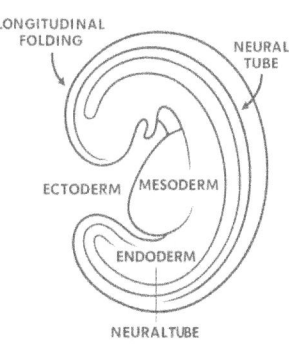

Disruptions in folding can lead to midline defects such as omphalocele or gastroschisis (where abdominal organs push outside the body through a hole in the abdominal wall).

Exercise 6.3: Folding Check	
Match the fold with the outcome.	
1. _____Longitudinal folding 2. _____Lateral folding	A. Brings body walls together to close the ventral body wall B. Establishes head-to-tail axis and primitive gut tube

SEXUAL DIFFERENTIATION

Developmental Process: At fertilization, the **genetic sex** of the embryo is established — typically XX for female or XY for male. Beginning around **week 7**, the **SRY gene** (if present on the Y chromosome) directs the undifferentiated gonads to become **testes**. These begin producing **testosterone** and **anti-Müllerian hormone** (AMH), which promote the development of male internal and external genitalia.

In the absence of the SRY gene and these hormones, the gonads develop into ovaries, and the reproductive tract follows the typical female pathway.

By **weeks 11–13**, external genitalia begin to differentiate visibly, although sex assignment by ultrasound is usually not reliable until the second trimester.

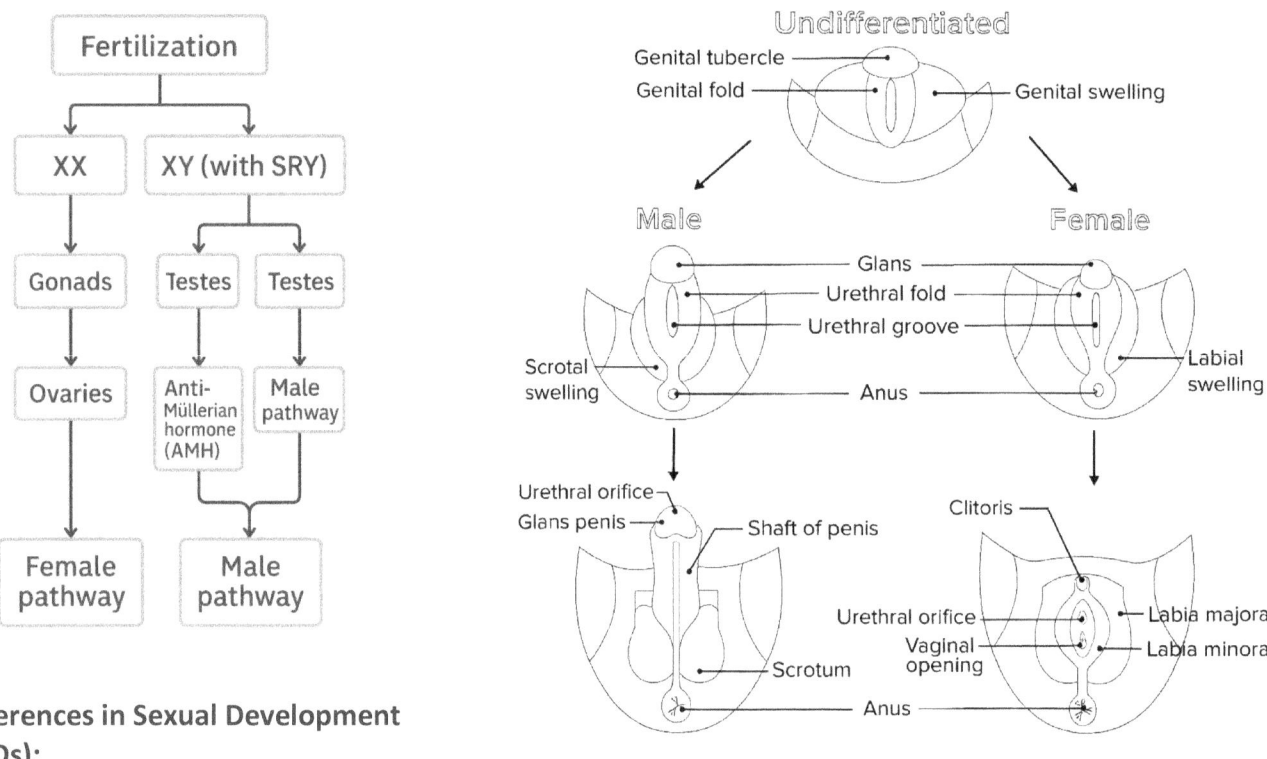

Differences in Sexual Development (DSDs):

Variations in chromosomal, gonadal, or anatomic sex that may not align in a typical binary pattern. These variations require sensitive, inclusive, and well-informed midwifery care.

Midwifery Applications
- Midwives may be asked about fetal sex early in pregnancy or during anatomy scans.
- Provide accurate answers and set realistic expectations.
- Use inclusive language and avoid assumptions.
- Support clients facing unexpected findings with compassion and appropriate referral.

Decidua

Structure and Function

After fertilization, the endometrial lining of the uterus transforms into a specialized tissue called the **decidua**. This transformation is essential for implantation, early nourishment, and the development of the placenta. The decidua provides a thick vascular bed, immunological tolerance, and structural support, while also regulating how deeply the trophoblast invades the uterine wall.

The decidua can be described in two ways:

1. By tissue layers of the endometrium:

    A. COMPACT LAYER: The thin surface layer next to the uterine cavity, made up of tightly packed cells.

    B. SPONGY LAYER: The middle layer containing large decidual (stromal) cells; helps prevent the placenta from embedding too deeply.

    C. BASAL LAYER: The layer closest to the myometrium; it regenerates the new endometrium after birth.

> **Key Vocabulary**
> - **Decidua:** The hormonally primed and structurally altered endometrium during pregnancy.
> - **Decidua basalis:** The part of the decidua beneath the implanted embryo; forms the maternal portion of the placenta.
> - **Decidua capsularis:** The part of the decidua that surrounds the embryo and separates it from the uterine cavity.
> - **Decidua parietalis** (decidua vera): The remaining endometrium not directly involved in implantation.
> - **Trophoblast:** The outer cell layer of the blastocyst that becomes the placenta and membranes.
> - **Cytotrophoblast:** The inner layer of trophoblast cells.
> - **Syncytiotrophoblast:** The outer layer of trophoblast cells that invades the endometrium and initiates placental development.

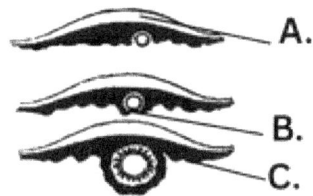

2. By relationship to the implanted embryo:

    A. DECIDUA BASALIS: The portion of the decidua directly beneath the implanted embryo; forms the maternal side of the placenta.

    B. DECIDUA CAPSULARIS: The portion that surrounds the embryo and separates it from the uterine cavity.

    C. DECIDUA PARIETALIS (vera): The remainder of the uterine lining not directly involved in implantation.

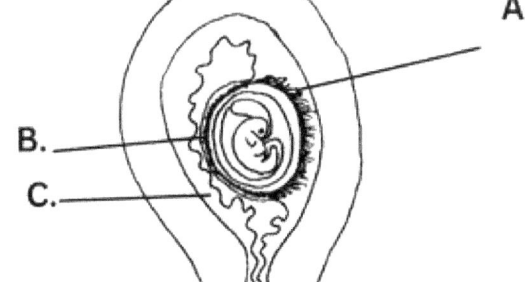

As pregnancy progresses, the decidua capsularis thins and eventually merges with the decidua parietalis around the twelfth week, closing the uterine cavity. The transformation of the endometrium into the decidua creates the foundation for implantation. From this point, the developing embryo establishes its vital connection with maternal blood supply through the formation of the placenta.

Midwifery Applications

The decidua supports implantation, immune tolerance, and placental development. Abnormal decidualization can lead to miscarriage, ectopic pregnancy, preeclampsia, or placenta accreta spectrum. Midwives use this knowledge to interpret early ultrasounds, counsel clients about concerning symptoms, monitor those with uterine risk factors, and provide timely referrals with compassionate care.

PLACENTAL EARLY DEVELOPMENT

Early Formation
The placenta begins to form soon after **implantation**, when the trophoblast cells of the blastocyst invade the **decidua basalis**.

These cells differentiate into:
- **Cytotrophoblast**: the cellular inner layer.
- **Syncytiotrophoblast**: the outer layer that invades maternal tissue and establishes blood flow.

Finger-like **chorionic villi** develop, extending into maternal blood spaces and creating the first exchange pathways. By the end of the first trimester, the placenta is fully functional as the lifeline between parent and fetus.

In early pregnancy, the placenta:
- Produces **hCG**, which supports the corpus luteum and maintains progesterone.
- Facilitates **nutrient and gas exchange** through the developing villous circulation.
- Acts as an **immune buffer**, preventing maternal rejection of the embryo.

Key Vocabulary

- **Placenta**: A temporary organ formed from fetal tissue that supports the pregnancy.
- **Chorionic villi**: Finger-like projections that extend into the maternal lining, establishing circulation.
- **Spiral arteries**: Maternal blood vessels that supply oxygen and nutrients to the intervillous space.
- **hCG (human chorionic gonadotropin)**: A hormone produced by the placenta in early pregnancy that maintains progesterone production.

Early Placental Development

1. PLACENTA
2. UTERUS WALL
3. AMNIOTIC SAC (amnion)
4. AMNIOTIC FLUID
5. EMBRYO
6. UMBILICAL CORD
7. NETWORK OF CAPILLARIES IN PLACENTA
8. OXYGENATED MATERNAL BLOOD (to embryo)
9. DEOXYGENATED BLOOD (from embryo to mother)

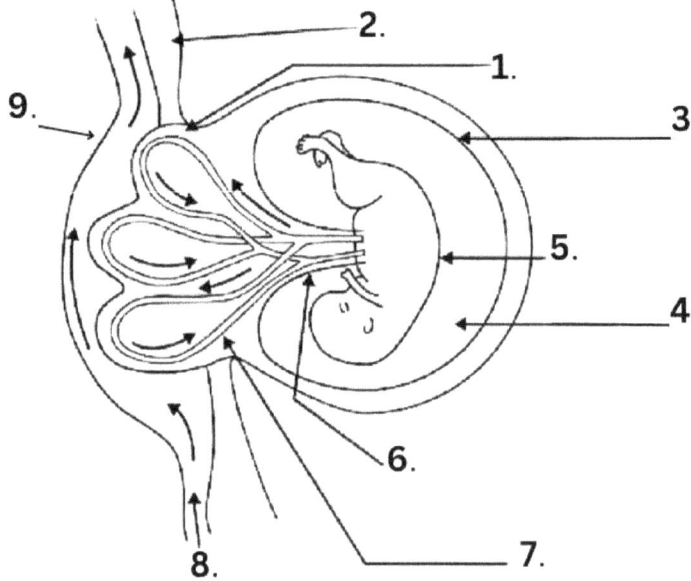

Color oxygenated blood red
Deoxygenated blood blue

Midwifery Applications
- Explain the role of **hCG** in sustaining pregnancy and the basis of early pregnancy tests.
- Recognize the importance of placental attachment (decidua basalis) in establishing a healthy pregnancy.
- Identify early warning signs, such as abnormal bleeding, which may indicate implantation or placental development concerns.

Amniotic Membranes

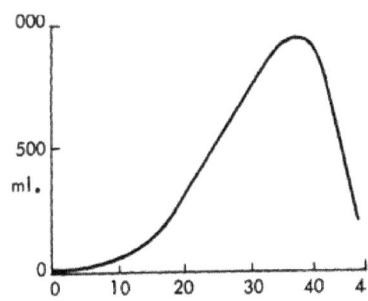

Formation and Composition
Amniotic fluid begins forming soon after conception, initially derived from maternal plasma. Amniotic fluid is later composed of fetal urine, respiratory tract secretions, and cellular debris. It contains water, electrolytes, proteins, carbohydrates, lipids, hormones, and fetal cells.

Volume increases steadily during the first and second trimesters, peaking around 34–36 weeks at approximately 800–1000 mL. After 37 weeks, fluid volume may gradually decrease.

Anatomy
The amniotic membranes consist of two layers:

1. **Amnion** (inner layer): thin, transparent, and avascular. It lines the amniotic cavity and directly encloses the fetus.
2. **Chorion** (outer layer): thicker and fibrous. It connects to the decidua (uterine lining) and contributes to placental formation.

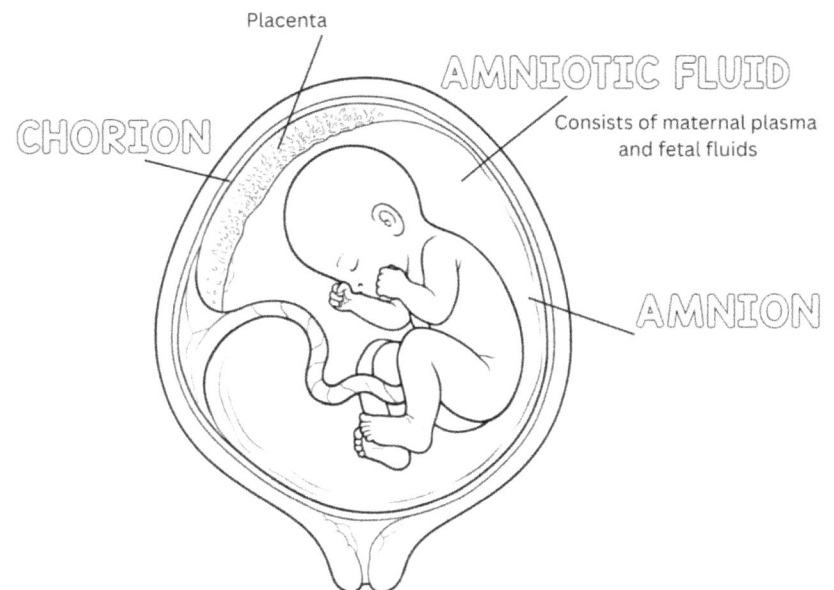

Together, they form the **amniotic sac**, which:

- Provides a **barrier** against infection.
- Maintains the shape and integrity of the gestational sac.
- Helps regulate and contain **amniotic fluid,** cushioning and protecting the fetus.

Functions of Amniotic Fluid
- **Protection**: cushions the fetus from external pressure and trauma.
- **Temperature regulation**: maintains a stable environment for growth.
- **Movement and growth**: provides a buoyant space for symmetrical musculoskeletal development.
- **Lung development**: enables fetal breathing-like movements that help the lungs mature.
- **Infection barrier**: creates a shield against pathogens by forming a physical seal around the fetus.
- **Structural support**: maintain the shape and integrity of the gestational sac.
- **Fluid regulation**: contain and manage amniotic fluid volume and composition.
- **Biochemical signaling**: produce cytokines and prostaglandins that may help initiate labor and respond to inflammation.
- Prevents **fetal parts from adhering** to the amnion and allows the fetus to expand and grow symmetrically in all directions.

Midwifery Applications
- Recognize the importance of intact membranes in sustaining pregnancy.
- Identify signs of rupture, which may require prompt evaluation.
- Explain the role of amniotic fluid in protecting and supporting the fetus.
- Teach clients that amniotic fluid volume changes across pregnancy but is normally replenished regularly.
- Recognize that ultrasound is used to monitor fluid levels and fetal well-being.

UMBILICAL CORD AND VESSELS

Anatomy

1. The UMBILICAL CORD is the fetus's lifeline, ensures continuous circulation between fetus and placenta, providing nutrients and oxygen while removing waste. The cord provides enough flexibility for fetal movement.
2. It contains: two ARTERIES carrying deoxygenated blood from fetus to the placenta.
3. One VEIN returning oxygenated blood back to the fetus.
4. WHARTON'S JELLY is a gelatinous tissue that cushions and protects the vessels.
5. An outer covering of AMNION Membrane layer that surrounds the cord, continuous with the amniotic sac.

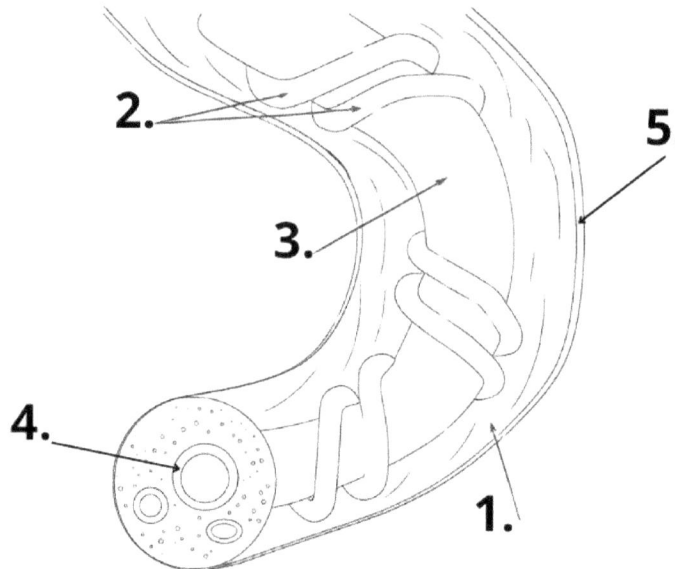

Color oxygenated venous blood red
Deoxygenated arterial blood blue

Umbilical Cord Circulation

In fetal circulation, the usual pattern of blood flow is reversed:
1. **Umbilical arteries** carry deoxygenated blood away from the fetus to the placenta
2. **Umbilical vein** carries oxygenated, nutrient-rich blood from the placenta back to the fetus

Midwifery Applications
- Explain basic cord function during prenatal visits.
- Recognize and document cord details at birth (e.g., number of vessels, insertion site).
- Monitor fetal movement and know when to assess for possible cord involvement.
- Understand when referral or additional monitoring may be needed (e.g., single artery, abnormal insertion, cord prolapse).
- Counting the vessels of the cord when examining the placenta after birth.

Cultural Tradition
Preserving the Umbilical Cord
Across the world, families have honored the umbilical cord as more than a biological remnant, a symbol of life's beginning and a child's connection to family, land, and spirit.

- **Indigenous North America:** The cord may be sewn into a beaded pouch and carried through life for protection and identity.
- **West Africa:** Families often dry and preserve the cord or bury it at the home, linking the child to land and lineage.
- **Asia & Europe:** Parents may save the dried stump as a charm for health and good fortune, placing it in a keepsake box or prayer book.

Lakota beaded umbilical turtle pouch

Fetal Circulation

In the womb, the fetus does not breathe air. Oxygen and nutrients are provided through the **placenta**, which functions as the lungs, kidneys, and digestive system during pregnancy. The **fetal circulation** is specially designed to deliver the most oxygen-rich blood to vital organs, particularly the brain and heart, while bypassing the non-functioning lungs. Because the placenta performs the work of gas exchange and waste removal, several unique vessels and shunts temporarily alter the normal postnatal pattern of blood flow.

1. SUPERIOR VENA CAVA Returns deoxygenated blood from the head and upper body to the right atrium.

2. FORAMEN OVALE A small opening between the right and left atria that allows blood to bypass the fetal lungs.

3. INFERIOR VENA CAVA Receives mixed blood from the lower body and the ductus venosus; carries it to the right atrium.

4. DUCTUS VENOSUS A temporary vessel that carries oxygen-rich blood from the umbilical vein past the liver into the inferior vena cava.

5. HEPATIC PORTAL VEIN Channels blood through the liver; in the fetus, part of the flow is shunted by the ductus venosus.

6. UMBILICAL VEIN Brings oxygenated blood from the placenta to the fetus. It is the only fetal vein that carries oxygen-rich blood.

7. PLACENTA Acts as the lungs, kidneys, and digestive system of the fetus, exchanging gases, nutrients, and wastes with the mother's blood.

8. UMBILICAL ARTERIES Two arteries that return deoxygenated blood and waste from the fetus to the placenta.

9. UMBILICAL VEIN (SECOND VIEW) Shown again in the lower diagram entering the fetal abdomen and connecting to the ductus venosus.

10. ABDOMINAL AORTA Main artery carrying blood from the heart to the lower body and umbilical arteries.

11. LIVER Partially bypassed in fetal life; receives a small portion of umbilical venous blood for growth and metabolism.

12. DUCTUS ARTERIOSUS Connects the pulmonary artery to the aorta so most blood can bypass the non-functioning lungs.

13. PULMONARY ARTERY Carries blood from the right ventricle toward the lungs; most passes through the ductus arteriosus.

14. PULMONARY VEINS Return oxygenated blood from the lungs after birth; minimal flow before breathing begins.

Color oxygenated venous blood red
Deoxygenated arterial blood blue

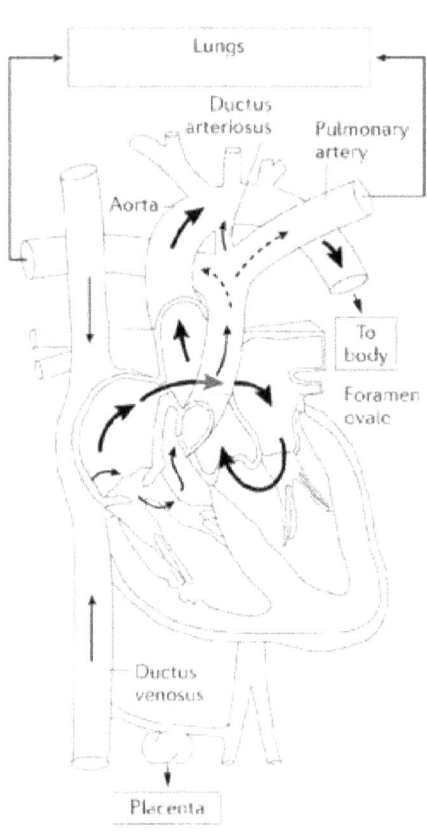

Transition at Birth

At birth, the umbilical cord circulation stops, and the baby's lungs expand with the first breaths. Blood flow increases to the lungs, closing the **foramen ovale**, while rising oxygen levels cause the **ductus arteriosus** to constrict. The **ductus venosus** stops functioning as placental flow ceases. These rapid changes shift the newborn's circulation from placental dependence to full lung function. Midwives observe this transformation in the newborn's breathing, color, and tone—key indicators of a smooth transition to independent life.

Midwifery Applications

Understanding fetal circulation helps midwives interpret how oxygen and nutrients reach the fetus, recognize signs of compromised placental exchange, and appreciate the dramatic transition that occurs at birth. This knowledge also supports informed choices such as **delayed cord clamping**, which allows additional placental blood to enter the newborn's circulation, improving oxygenation, iron stores, and overall stability in the first minutes of life.

Exercise 6.4: Fetal Circulation

List the four layers which separate fetal blood from maternal blood:

1. _____
2. _____
3. _____
4. _____

List the four temporary structures of fetal circulation:

1. _____
2. _____
3. _____
4. _____

Label the parts:

1. _____
2. _____
3. _____
4. _____
5. _____

Fetal Development

Embryonic Period (Weeks 2 to 8):

The first trimester is the architecture phase of pregnancy. Though invisible to the outside world, it marks a time of intense internal transformation. Most clients may not yet feel pregnant, yet their bodies are engaged in continuous, intricate work. For midwives, this trimester calls for both attentiveness and respect. We are charged with safeguarding what cannot yet be seen, relying on the deep intelligence of the body as it begins to shape new life.

During the **embryonic period** (conception to 8 weeks), the developing conceptus is called an **embryo**. This is a time of rapid morphogenesis, organogenesis, and cell differentiation. By the end of week 8, all major organ systems are present in rudimentary form, though highly vulnerable to teratogens.

> **Key Vocabulary**
> - **Fetal period:** The stage from week 9 until birth, when tissues and organs grow and mature.
> - **Quickening:** The first sensation of fetal movement felt by the pregnant woman, usually between 16 and 20 weeks.
> - **Surfactant:** A substance made in the fetal lungs in the third trimester that reduces surface tension in the alveoli and enables breathing after birth.
> - **Viability:** The stage when the fetus can survive outside the uterus, generally around 22–25 weeks with intensive medical support.
> - **Brown fat:** A special type of fat that produces heat to help newborns regulate body temperature after birth.

Weeks 1–4: Fertilization to Implantation
- Fertilization occurs in the uterine tube, forming a zygote.
- Rapid mitotic division leads to a morula, then a blastocyst.
- Implantation begins around day 6 to 10 in the uterine lining.
- The three germ layers (ectoderm, mesoderm, endoderm) begin forming, setting the foundation for every organ and structure.

Weeks 5–6: Early Organogenesis
- The **neural tube begins closing**; brain and spinal cord formation begins.
- The **primitive heart tube** begins beating by day 22 to 24.
- Limb buds, primitive facial features, and early internal organs begin forming.
- **Placental circulation** begins contributing to nutrient and waste exchange.

Weeks 7–8: Defining Human Form
- **Facial features** become more defined; arm and leg buds grow and shape.
- **Major organs** continue forming: lungs, liver, kidneys, intestines.
- **Brain regions** differentiate, and cranial nerves appear.
- Crown to Rump Length (**CRL**): ~1.5 to 2 cm.

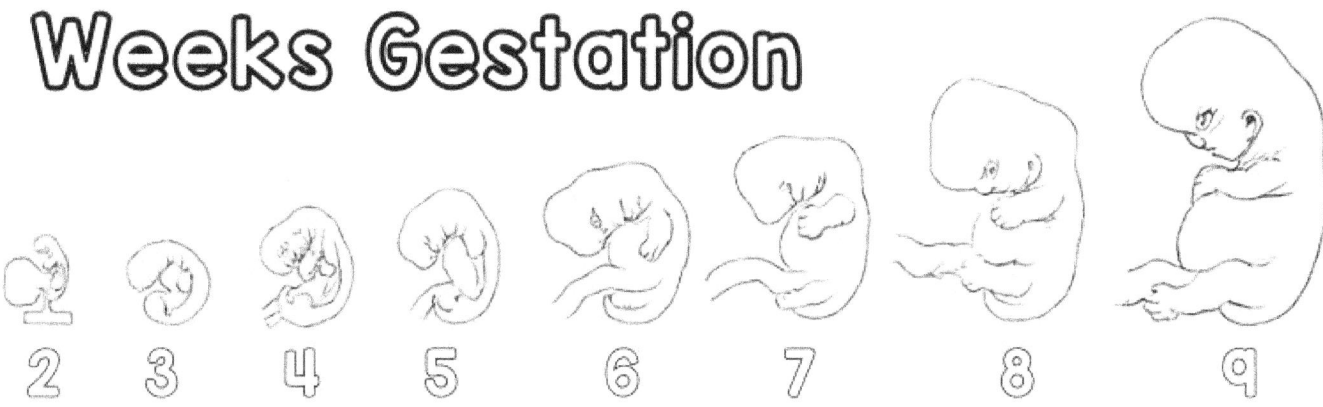

First Trimester (Weeks 1–12)
(Some medical sources define the first trimester as 13 weeks and 6 days)

From **week 9 onward**, the developing human is called a **fetus**. The first trimester establishes the foundations of growth, with organs continuing to mature in structure and function. The head is proportionally large, making up nearly half the fetal length, and the face becomes more human in appearance. Reflex movements begin, though they are not yet felt. The **placenta** is now fully formed, supporting nutrient and waste exchange and producing hormones that sustain pregnancy.

Weeks 9–12: *Now termed a fetus rather than an embryo.*
- Fingernails, toenails, and early hair begin to form.
- External genitalia begin to differentiate, though still difficult to identify.
- Intestines return to the abdominal cavity from the cord.
- External genitalia begin to differentiate.
- Fingers and toes form; nails begin to develop.
- Fetal movements begin but are not yet felt by the pregnant woman.
- The heart is fully formed and visible on ultrasound.
- Heartbeat can typically be detected via Doppler by 10–12 weeks.
- The fetus makes spontaneous movements.

Clinical Note: First Trimester
- Most **miscarriages** (spontaneous abortions) occur in the first trimester, often due to chromosomal abnormalities.
- **Rising hCG** levels may cause nausea and fatigue.
- **Ultrasound** can confirm viability, number of fetuses, and gestational dating.

Milestones
- **Maternal**: Hormonal changes lead to early pregnancy symptoms.
- **Fetal**: Organs take shape, and the heartbeat becomes detectable by ultrasound.
    - By the end of the first trimester, the fetus has distinct fingerprints that will remain unique for life.

The Fetal Period (Week 9 to Birth)

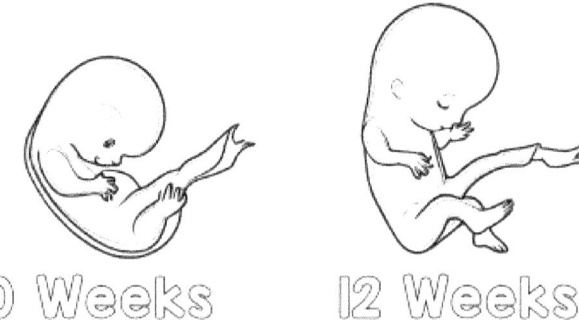

10 Weeks   12 Weeks

Exercise 6.5: First Trimester Check-In

Fill in the Blank:

1. By week ___, the embryo is now called a fetus.
2. The fetal heart is fully formed and can usually be detected by Doppler at – weeks.
3. The first felt fetal movements are called _____.
4. During the first trimester, the fetus develops ___, ___, and early hair.

SECOND TRIMESTER (WEEKS 13–27)

(Some medical sources define the second trimester as 14 weeks to 27 weeks and 6 days)

In the second trimester, pregnancy becomes visible. The fetus grows steadily, and its presence becomes more real to the parents. The mystery of development unfolds into a rhythm of kicks, images, and sound. This is a time of increasing connection, and for midwives, a chance to offer grounded guidance. Anatomy scans, fetal movement, and growth all take center stage. The risk of early loss lessens, and excitement often rises.

Weeks 13–16: Growth and Refinement

- Facial features are clearly defined; eyes and ears shift into position.
- Bones begin to ossify and are visible on ultrasound.
- External genitalia become more distinct and may be seen on ultrasound.
- The fetus begins moving limbs and may suck its thumb.
- Lanugo (fine hair) starts to form.
- CRL: ~9 to 12 cm.

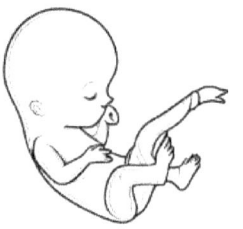
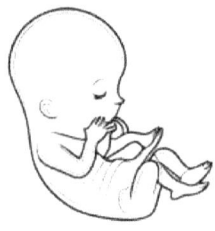

Weeks 17–20: Sensory Awareness and Movement

- Clients often report **quickening**—feeling the fetus move. Earlier in those who have been pregnant before.
- **Brown fat** begins to form, supporting future thermal regulation.
- Vernix caseosa (a white, waxy coating) starts covering the skin.
- Ears are structurally complete; the fetus begins responding to sound.
- Heart sounds audible via fetoscope by 18 to 20 weeks.
- Fundus typically at the level of the umbilicus by 20 weeks.

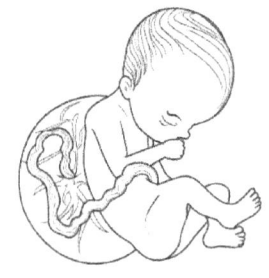

Weeks 21–24: Threshold of Viability

- Surfactant production begins in the alveolar cells.
- Skin is translucent, and fine hair covers the body.
- Fetal reflexes such as startle and grasp appear.
- Eyelids begin to separate, and REM sleep is observed.
- **Weight**: ~600 to 800 grams by 24 weeks.
- Infants born at **22 weeks** now have about a 25% chance of survival with intensive medical support. Survival increases with each week: roughly 40–60% at 24 weeks and up to 70–75% at 25 weeks.

Weeks 25–27: Neural and Respiratory Maturity

- Brain growth accelerates; gyri and sulci begin forming.
- Eyes open and begin tracking light.
- Lungs continue branching and producing surfactant.
- Fetus begins forming patterns of alertness and rest.
- Weight: ~1 to 2 pounds by end of the second trimester.

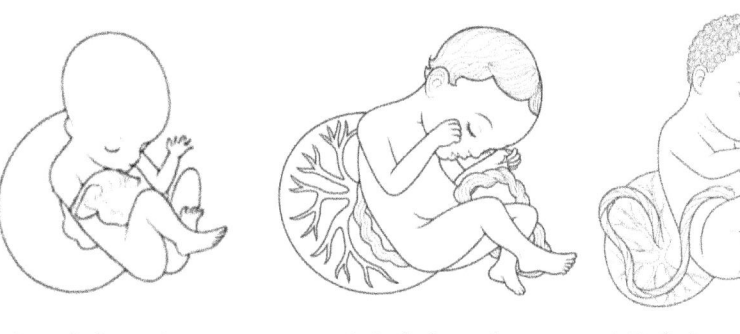

24 Weeks 26 Weeks 27 Weeks

Third Trimester (Weeks 28 to 40+)

The third trimester is a season of refinement and readiness. The fetus is preparing for life outside the womb, and the pregnant woman is navigating physical, emotional, and relational transitions. For midwives, this time calls for grounded presence. We monitor fetal position, growth, and well-being while preparing clients for labor, birth, and postpartum. There is a growing sense of mystery and anticipation, as each day brings the baby closer to meeting the world.

Weeks 28–31: Functional Maturation

- Central nervous system can now regulate temperature and basic breathing.
- Lungs continue maturing; alveoli multiply.
- Eyelids open; blinking reflex appears.
- Sleep-wake cycles emerge and may align with maternal rhythms.
- Skin is still thin, but fat layers begin to form.
- Fetus often moves into a head-down position during this period.

Weeks 32–36: Fat Storage and Reflex Readiness

- Lanugo starts to disappear; skin appears less wrinkled.
- More brown fat is deposited, especially over the back and shoulders.
- Sucking reflex becomes stronger; coordination improves.
- Practice breathing movements increase.
- Fetal position stabilizes; engaged head may be palpable by 36 weeks.
- Weight gain is rapid; up to ½ pound per week.
- The **lungs mature between 34 and 37 weeks**, producing enough **pulmonary surfactant**, a mixture of phospholipids (including **lecithin** and **sphingomyelin**). Surfactant coats the air sacs (**alveoli**) and keeps them from collapsing after exhalation.

Weeks 37–40+: Full Term

- Full term is defined as 39 to 40+6 weeks gestation.
- Lungs are typically mature, and surfactant is adequate.
- Skin is smooth; vernix begins to decrease.
- Reflexes are well developed; the baby practices breathing, sucking, and blinking.
- Placenta reaches functional maturity and begins aging.
- Estimated average weight: 6 to 9 pounds; length: ~19 to 21 inches.

> **Key Vocabulary:**
> - **Surfactant:** A substance produced by fetal lungs that reduces surface tension and helps keep the alveoli open for breathing after birth.
> - **Cortisol Surge:** A rise in fetal cortisol levels during late pregnancy that promotes maturation of the lungs, liver, and digestive system, and contributes to the initiation of labor.
> - **Thermoregulation:** The fetus's ability to regulate body temperature, supported by brown fat accumulation and neurologic development.
> - **Neurobehavioral Regulation:** Maturation of fetal neurologic systems that support reflexes, sensory processing, sleep-wake cycling, and adaptation to extrauterine life.
> - **Transition:** The process by which a newborn shifts from placental to independent respiration and circulation following birth.

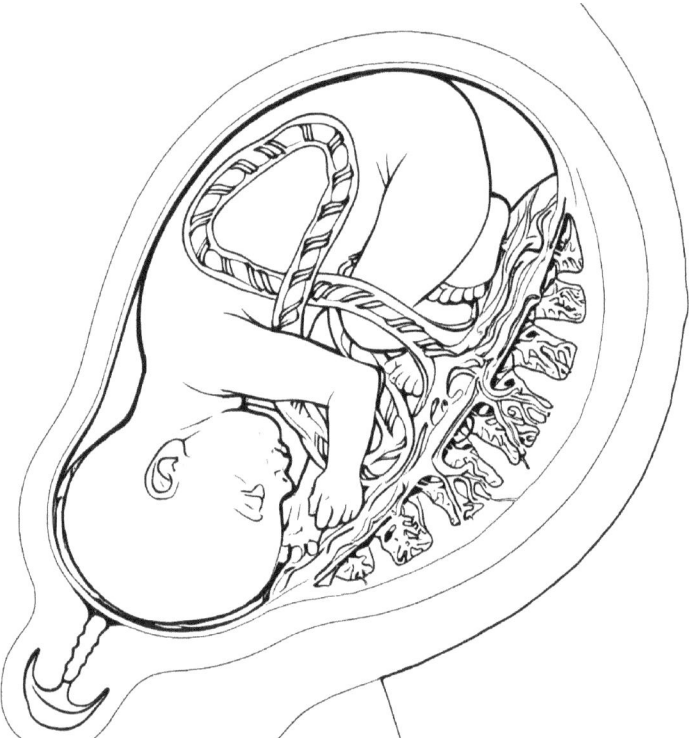

During the Third Trimester
- **Surfactant** production is critical for independent breathing at birth.
- **Brown fat** and subcutaneous fat help the newborn regulate temperature.
- Rapid brain growth supports reflexes and sensory development.
- Full-term birth offers the best outcomes, even though survival before term is now possible.

Midwifery Applications:
- Estimate gestational age and compare growth with expected milestones.
- Recognize complications such as intrauterine growth restriction (IUGR), early pregnancy loss, preeclampsia, and abnormal placental attachment.
- Counsel clients about prenatal screening.
- Provide reassurance and support bonding by helping families understand their baby's development.
- Explain key milestones such as heartbeat detection, quickening, and lung maturity.
- Counsel clients on maternal nutrition, which is vital for fetal growth and health.
- Provide anticipatory guidance and reassurance to support bonding and informed decision-making.

Fetal Readiness for Labor

In the final weeks of pregnancy, the fetus reaches a stage of integrated readiness for labor and birth. Maturation of the lungs, brain, and digestive system enables the transition to extrauterine life. Surfactant production peaks, the fetal brain integrates behavioral reflexes like suck-swallow-breathe, and endocrine changes such as the fetal cortisol surge help prime multiple organ systems. The skin thickens, fat accumulates for thermoregulation, and the sleep-wake cycle aligns more clearly with the maternal rhythm.

These changes are not isolated—they occur in a synchronized and interdependent way. The placenta, fetal brain, and maternal body engage in hormonal cross-talk that helps initiate spontaneous labor. This readiness allows the fetus to survive and thrive after birth—not only physiologically, but relationally, with the capacity to engage, connect, and bond.

> **Key Landmarks**
> - **Heartbeat audible** by Doppler: 10–12 weeks
> - **Heartbeat audible** by fetoscope: 18–20 weeks
> - **Quickening** reported by pregnant mother: 16–20 weeks
> - **Viability** threshold begins: 23–24 weeks
> - Head-down (**vertex**) position common by: 32–36 weeks
> - **Full term** defined: 39–40+6 weeks
> - **Post-dates** monitoring begins: 41 weeks

Midwifery Applications
- **Clinical Assessment:** Monitoring for signs of physiologic maturity, such as fetal position, movement patterns, and growth.
- **Labor Counseling:** Supporting clients in understanding the value of spontaneous labor timing when medically appropriate.
- **Education:** Explaining the relationship between gestational age and system readiness to support informed decision-making.
- **Risk Identification:** Recognizing when fetal readiness may be delayed or incomplete (e.g., in late preterm birth, IUGR, or gestational diabetes).
- **Newborn Transition Support:** Observing breathing, tone, and reflexes to ensure the newborn is adapting well after birth.

Post-Term

Beyond **42 weeks**, the fetus is considered **post-term**. The decidua capsularis has already disappeared, and the fetus may show signs of post-maturity such as dry or peeling skin, reduced vernix, and decreased fat stores, and potential placental insufficiency.

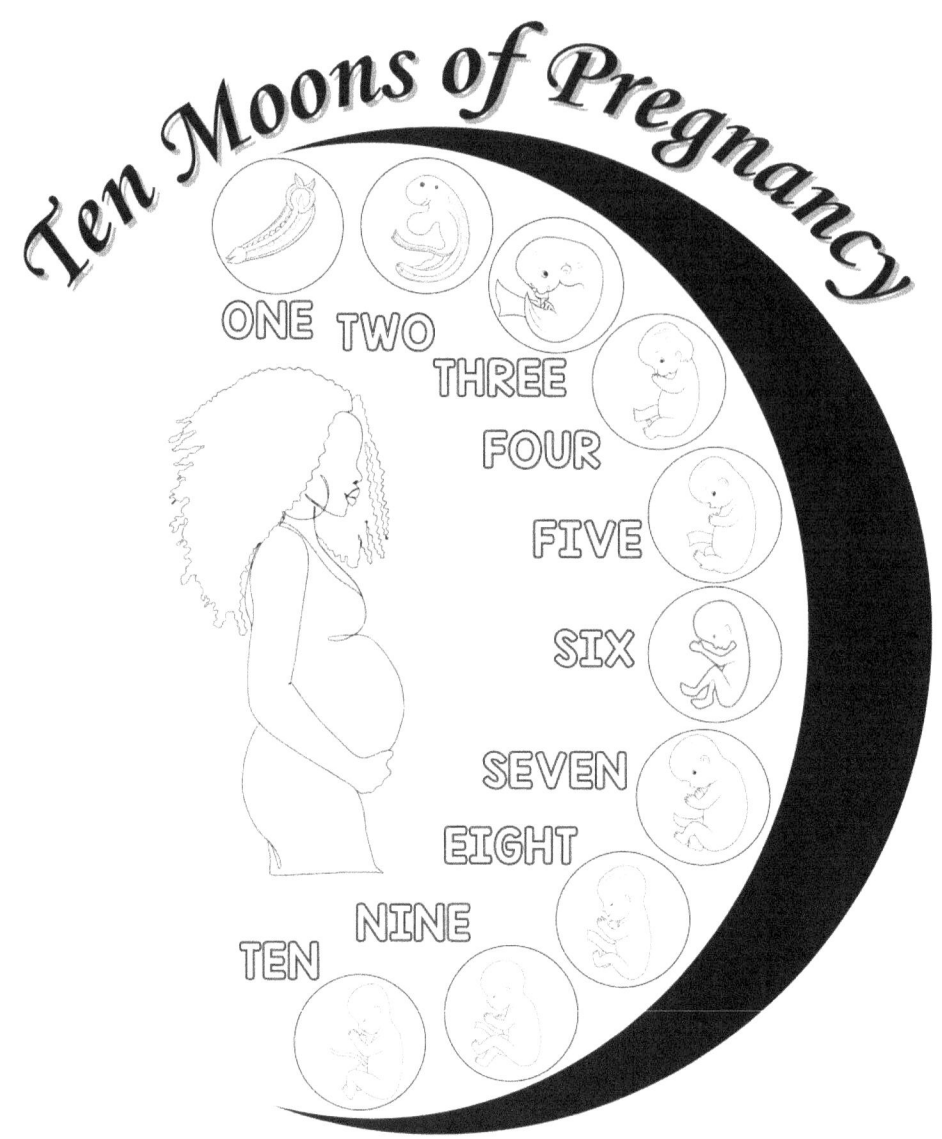

FETAL DEVELOPMENT CHART

Weeks	Length (approx.)	Weight (approx.)	Developmental Characteristics
8	2.5–3 cm	~2 g	Organs and blood vessels forming; embryo becomes a fetus
12	7–9 cm (crown–rump)	20–30 g	Face more humanlike; nails, hair buds, reflex movements; placenta fully formed
20	25 cm	~300 g	Quickening felt; lanugo and vernix present; eyelashes and eyebrows visible
28	35 cm	~1,000 g	Rapid brain growth; fat storage; improved chance of survival with intensive care
34–37	45 cm	2,000–2,500 g	Lungs maturing; surfactant (lecithin and sphingomyelin) sufficient for breathing
40	48–52 cm	3,000–3,600 g	Full term; adequate fat stores; ready for birth

Exercise 6.6: Fetal Development Milestones by Trimester

Match each milestone to the trimester A, B, or C, when it typically occurs:

1. _____ Heart is fully formed and visible on ultrasound
2. _____ External genitalia begin to differentiate
3. _____ Quickening (first fetal movements felt by the pregnant woman)
4. _____ Facial features become more distinct
5. _____ Formation of lanugo and vernix caseosa
6. _____ Brown fat begins to develop
7. _____ Lungs mature and produce surfactant
8. _____ Rapid brain growth and nervous system maturation
9. _____ Full-term birth (39–40 weeks)

A. **First trimester** (weeks 9–13)
B. **Second trimester** (weeks 14–27)
C. **Third trimester** (weeks 28–birth)

Teratogens and Critical Windows of Susceptibility

A **teratogen** is any substance, infection, or environmental factor that disrupts normal growth and development. The effect depends on the **type of exposure, dose, duration,** and — most importantly — the **timing** during pregnancy.

Key Timeframes

- **Pre-implantation (0–2 weeks):** "All-or-nothing" period — severe damage usually results in loss of the conceptus.
- **Embryonic period (3–8 weeks):** Highest risk for major structural abnormalities during active organogenesis.
- **Fetal period (9 weeks–birth):** Risks shift toward growth restriction and functional problems, especially in the brain, eyes, ears, and genitalia.

Common Teratogens

- **Infections:** Rubella, cytomegalovirus (CMV), toxoplasmosis, varicella.
- **Medications:** Isotretinoin, ACE inhibitors, warfarin, certain anticonvulsants.
- **Substances:** Alcohol, tobacco, cannabis, cocaine, methamphetamines. *Alcohol exposure may cause fetal alcohol spectrum disorders (FASD), leading to growth restriction and neurodevelopmental challenges.*
- **Environmental exposures:** Lead, mercury, radiation, certain pesticides.

Midwifery Applications

A clear understanding of teratogenic risks enables midwives to support preconception planning, protect fetal development, and empower clients with accurate, non-judgmental information. Midwives play an essential role in prevention and counseling by:

- Taking thorough medical, occupational, and substance-use histories.
- Advising on safe medication use before and during pregnancy.
- Teaching infection prevention strategies such as handwashing, safe food handling, and vaccinations.
- Supporting individuals with substance-use disorders through trauma-informed care and referral.
- Providing reassurance and accurate information if accidental exposure occurs.

Exercise 6.7: Match the Teratogen to Its Effect

Match the number of each teratogen with the letter of its potential effect:

1. _____ Alcohol
2. _____ Rubella (German measles)
3. _____ Isotretinoin (Accutane)
4. _____ Cigarette smoke
5. _____ Mercury

A. Hearing loss and cataracts in the newborn
B. Fetal alcohol spectrum disorders (growth restriction, neurodevelopmental delays)
C. Neural tube defects and heart malformations
D. Low birth weight, impaired lung development
E. Neurologic damage

FETAL SENSORY DEVELOPMENT

Sensory Development

As the fetus matures, sensory systems become active in preparation for life outside the womb. These early experiences influence brain development and support bonding after birth.

- **Touch** develops first, beginning around **8 weeks**, with widespread skin sensitivity by 20 weeks.
- **Taste and smell** receptors form early; flavors from the maternal diet enter the **amniotic fluid**, allowing the fetus to taste and smell what the mother eats.
- **Hearing** develops around **18–20 weeks**. By 25 weeks, the fetus responds to sound and may recognize voices and rhythms. Studies show that babies can remember stories or songs heard repeatedly in the womb and show preference for their mother's voice soon after birth.
- **Vision** develops last. By the third trimester, the fetus can sense light and shadow, though sight remains limited until after birth.

> **Key Vocabulary**
> - **Touch:** The first sense to develop, beginning around 8 weeks.
> - **Quickening**: The first felt fetal movements, often interpreted as an early sensory connection.
> - **Amniotic fluid:** Fluid in the amniotic sac that carries flavors and scents from the maternal diet.
> - **Surfactant**: A lung secretion necessary for breathing after birth; indirectly tied to sensory readiness.
> - **Fetal learning:** The ability of the fetus to perceive, process, and remember sensory experiences before birth.

Fetal Awareness and Learning

Research demonstrates that fetuses are capable of **learning and memory**. By about **32 weeks**, fetuses show signs of **short-term memory** (about 10 minutes) and even **long-term memory** (at least 24 hours). Exposure to repeated sounds, such as music or a parent's voice, can calm the fetus and shape recognition after birth. Music in particular has been shown to influence fetal heart rate and movement, suggesting that late-term fetuses can process complex sounds and sustain attention longer as they mature.

Maternal environment also plays a role. Stress, anxiety, or trauma during pregnancy may affect fetal brain development and later emotional regulation. Conversely, positive sensory input — such as a calm environment, spoken words, or songs — can support bonding and may enhance newborn recognition and comfort.

Midwifery Applications
- Encourage parents to talk, sing, or read to their baby to promote bonding.
- Explain how maternal nutrition, stress, and environmental exposures influence fetal sensory experiences.
- Reassure families that many newborn responses, such as recognizing a parent's voice, begin in utero.
- Advocate for quiet, supportive birth environments that respect the newborn's sensory readiness.

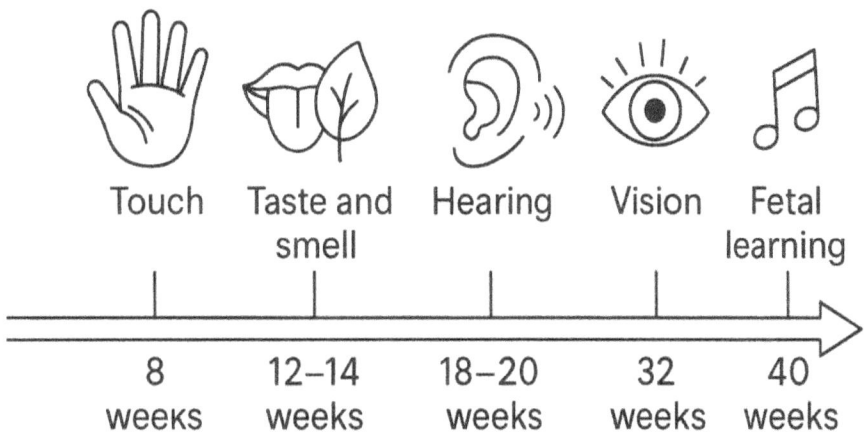

Exercise 6.8: Fetal Senses	
Match each fetal sensory milestone with the trimester A, B, or C when it usually occurs	
1. _____Touch begins (~8 weeks; widespread by 20 weeks)	A. First trimester (weeks 9–13)
2. _____Flavors and scents from the maternal diet reach the amniotic fluid	B. Second trimester (weeks 14–27)
3. _____Responds to sound by about 25 weeks; may recognize familiar voices and music	C. Third trimester (weeks 28–birth)
4. _____Vision develops; fetus perceives light and shadow in the third trimester	

How Life Begins Essential Takeaways

Conception begins when a sperm fertilizes an ovum in the uterine tube, creating a zygote with 46 chromosomes. This cell divides into a morula and then a blastocyst, which implants into the uterine lining. Germ layers form and develop into all the body's tissues and organs. Midwives use this knowledge to explain early pregnancy and reassure families about implantation and development.

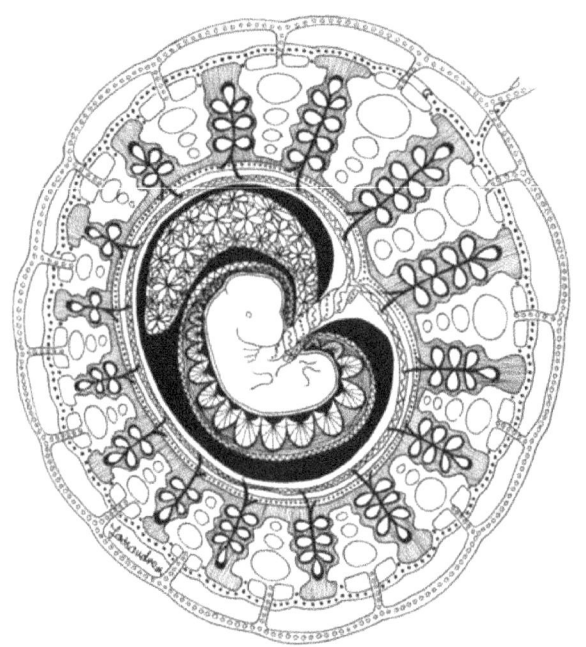

Pregnancy may involve twins, either identical (from one fertilized egg) or fraternal (from two eggs). Chorionicity and amnionicity influence outcomes, making ultrasound interpretation and timely referral an important midwifery skill.

The quality of gametes changes with age. For those with ovaries, egg quality declines after about age thirty-five, increasing the risks of infertility, miscarriage, and chromosomal abnormalities such as trisomy 21. For those with testes, aging can reduce sperm motility and increase DNA fragmentation, raising miscarriage risk and developmental concerns. Midwives support families by offering education, counseling, and referrals for screening when age may affect pregnancy outcomes.

Healthy pregnancy depends on the transformation of the decidua and the development of the placenta, membranes, and amniotic fluid. These structures nourish, protect, and regulate the embryo and fetus. The umbilical cord, with its two arteries and one vein cushioned by Wharton's jelly, acts as the lifeline between mother and child. Understanding these processes equips midwives to explain diagnostic findings and identify when further evaluation is needed.

Fetal circulation relies on placental oxygen and specialized shunts that bypass the liver and lungs until birth. Development progresses from organ formation in the first trimester to growth, sensory development, and preparation for birth in later stages. The senses emerge in sequence, with touch first and vision last, and fetuses begin responding to sound before birth, knowledge that helps midwives encourage bonding through voice and touch.

Teratogens pose the greatest risk during weeks three to eight, but exposures at any stage can affect growth and function. Midwives play a central role in education and prevention, guiding families on safe choices and offering compassionate counseling if concerns arise.

Chapter Six Self-Assessment

Multiple Choice
1. Fertilization most often takes place in the:
    a) Cervix
    b) Uterine tube (ampulla)
    c) Uterus
    d) Vagina

2. Quickening (the first felt fetal movements) usually occurs:
    a) 8–10 weeks
    b) 12–14 weeks
    c) 16–20 weeks
    d) 24–28 weeks

3. Surfactant production begins around:
    a) 12 weeks
    b) 20 weeks
    c) 24 weeks (functional by 34–36 weeks)
    d) 40 weeks

4. By which week is the placenta considered fully mature and ready to sustain the pregnancy until birth?
    a) 20 weeks
    b) 28 weeks
    c) 34 weeks
    d) 39–40 weeks

5. Which structure forms the maternal side of the placenta?
    a) Chorionic villi
    b) Decidua basalis
    c) Amnion
    d) Umbilical vein

7. Which sense develops *first* in the fetus?
    a) Vision
    b) Taste
    c) Hearing
    d) Touch

8. Which germ layer gives rise to the reproductive organs?
    a) Ectoderm
    b) Mesoderm
    c) Endoderm
    d) Trophoblast

9. Implantation usually occurs:
    a) Immediately after fertilization
    b) Between days 6–10 after fertilization
    c) Around 3 weeks after fertilization
    d) At 12 weeks of gestation

10. The umbilical vein carries:
    a) Deoxygenated blood from the fetus to the placenta
    b) Oxygenated blood from the placenta to the fetus
    c) Blood between the fetal lungs and heart

    d) Blood from the fetal liver to the kidneys

11. The structure that first produces progesterone before the placenta takes over is the:
    a) Corpus luteum
    b) Chorionic villi
    c) Amniotic sac
    d) Decidua basalis

12. The outer membrane that contributes to forming the placenta is the:
    a) Chorion
    b) Amnion
    c) Decidua capsularis
    d) Zona pellucida

13. The fetal heartbeat begins around which gestational age?
    a) 2 weeks
    b) 4 weeks
    c) 6 weeks
    d) 10 weeks

True/False

14. _____ Fraternal twins come from one fertilized egg that splits.
15. _____ Conjoined twins occur when the split happens after day 13.
16. _____ Monochorionic twins are always monoamniotic.
17. _____ Ultrasound between 10–14 weeks can help determine chorionicity.
18. _____ Surfactant is a protein that helps the fetus digest amniotic fluid.
19. _____ Identical twins always share a placenta.
20. _____ The placenta acts as the lungs, kidneys, and digestive system for the fetus before birth.
21. _____ The yolk sac provides early nutrition and forms the first red blood cells for the embryo.
22. _____ The amniotic fluid volume is entirely fetal urine by the end of the first trimester.
23. _____ The umbilical cord normally contains two arteries and one vein.
24. _____ The placenta produces both estrogen and progesterone after about 10–12 weeks of gestation.
25. _____ Fetal breathing movements before birth help develop the lungs and strengthen respiratory muscles.

Fill in the Blank

26. Fertilization most often occurs in the _____ of the uterine tube.
27. Sperm can survive up to _____ days in the female reproductive tract.
28. The egg is usually viable for _____ to _____ hours after ovulation.
29. The fetal circulation includes three major shunts: _____, _____, and _____.
30. The _____ is a gelatinous material in the umbilical cord that cushions and protects blood vessels.

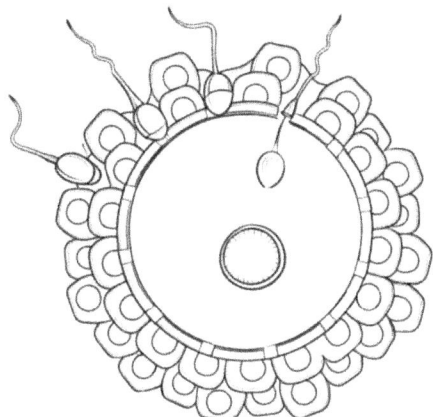

Chapter Six Reading & References

Recommended Reading: How Life Begins
- Carlson, B. M. (2014). ***Human Embryology and Developmental Biology*** (5th ed.). Elsevier. Bridges embryology with developmental biology, providing molecular and genetic insights into early human development.
- Gilbert, S. F., & Barresi, M. J. F. (2020). ***Developmental Biology*** (12th ed.). Sinauer/Oxford University Press. A broad classic in developmental biology, helping students understand the cellular and molecular mechanisms that underlie embryonic growth and differentiation.
- Larsen, W. J., Sherman, L. S., Potter, S. S., & Scott, W. J. (2017). ***Larsen's Human Embryology*** (5th ed.). Elsevier. Comprehensive reference integrating molecular biology, genetics, and developmental anatomy to explain human growth from conception through birth.
- Moore, K. L., & Persaud, T. V. N. (2015). ***Before We Are Born: Essentials of Embryology and Birth Defects*** (9th ed.). Elsevier. Companion to *The Developing Human*, offering a concise overview of embryology with emphasis on clinical implications and congenital anomalies.
- Moore, K. L., Persaud, T. V. N., & Torchia, M. G. (2020). ***The Developing Human: Clinically Oriented Embryology*** (11th ed.). Elsevier. A widely used textbook offering detailed descriptions and illustrations of embryonic and fetal development, with strong clinical correlations.
- Nayak, B. S., & Somayaji, S. N. (2014). ***Human Embryology: An Educational Coloring Book***. Jaypee Brothers Medical Publishers. A visual learning tool that reinforces key concepts of embryonic and fetal development through interactive diagrams.
- Netter, F. H., & Machado, C. A. (2019). ***Netter's Atlas of Human Embryology*** (1st ed.). Elsevier. Richly illustrated atlas linking early embryologic structures with clinical practice.
- Sadler, T. W. (2019). ***Langman's Medical Embryology*** (14th ed.). Wolters Kluwer. Concise and accessible embryology text emphasizing key developmental processes and their relevance to congenital anomalies.

References

Carlson, B. M. (2014). *Human embryology and developmental biology* (5th ed.). Elsevier.

Cathelijne, F., van Heteren, P., Boekkooi, F., Henk, W., Jongsma, J., & Nijhuis, G. (2000). Fetal learning and memory. *The Lancet, 356*(9236), 1169–1170.

Chism, O. (1999, January 12). Classical: The thinking child's music; Studies suggest link between exposure and improved brain functioning. *The Dallas Morning News*, 5C.

Gilbert, S. F., & Barresi, M. J. F. (2020). *Developmental biology* (12th ed.). Oxford University Press.

Hopson, J. (1998). Fetal psychology. *Psychology Today*. http://www.leaderu.com/orgs/tul/psychtoday9809.html

James, D. K., Spencer, C. J., & Stepsis, B. W. (2002). Fetal learning: A prospective randomized controlled study. *Ultrasound in Obstetrics & Gynecology, 20*(5), 431–438.

Kisilevsky, B. S., Hains, S. M. J., Jacquet, A.-Y., Granier-Deferre, C., & Lecanuet, J. P. (2004). Maturation of fetal responses to music. *Developmental Science, 7*(5), 550–559.

Larsen, W. J., Sherman, L. S., Potter, S. S., & Scott, W. J. (2017). *Larsen's human embryology* (5th ed.). Elsevier.

Levy, Y. (n.d.). *The effects of background music on learning: A review of recent literature*. San Diego State University. http://edweb.sdsu.edu/Courses/Ed690DR/Examples/LitRev/Levy.htm

Moore, K. L., & Persaud, T. V. N. (2015). *Before we are born: Essentials of embryology and birth defects* (9th ed.). Elsevier.

Moore, K. L., Persaud, T. V. N., & Torchia, M. G. (2020). *The developing human: Clinically oriented embryology* (11th ed.). Elsevier.

Nayak, B. S., & Somayaji, S. N. (2014). *Human embryology: An educational coloring book*. Jaypee Brothers Medical Publishers.

Sadler, T. W. (2019). *Langman's medical embryology* (14th ed.). Wolters Kluwer.

Chapter Seven
Physiology of Pregnancy

Objectives
After completing this chapter, the student should be able to:
1. **Define** pregnancy and describe its stages.
2. **Explain** how to determine the length of gestation and calculate an estimated due date.
3. **Identify** the signs and symptoms of pregnancy.
4. **Differentiate** between presumptive, probable, and positive signs of pregnancy.
5. **Describe** the physiological changes of pregnancy across the following systems:
    a. Circulatory
    b. Respiratory
    c. Urinary
    d. Gastrointestinal
    e. Musculoskeletal
    f. Neurological
    g. Integumentary
    h. Reproductive
6. **State** the usual timing of common signs and symptoms of pregnancy.
7. **Explain** the causes and describe treatments for common discomforts of pregnancy.
8. **Identify** when these discomforts typically occur.
9. **Describe** the physical changes that predispose pregnant individuals to these discomforts.
10. **Distinguish** between normal discomforts of pregnancy and possible complications.
11. **Recommend** strategies for preventing, alleviating, or minimizing common discomforts.
12. **Describe** the four psychological tasks of pregnancy, recognizing diverse family structures, identities, and cultural contexts. List possible feelings, concerns, and needs associated with each.
13. **Discuss** physiologic, emotional, and relational aspects of sexuality during pregnancy.

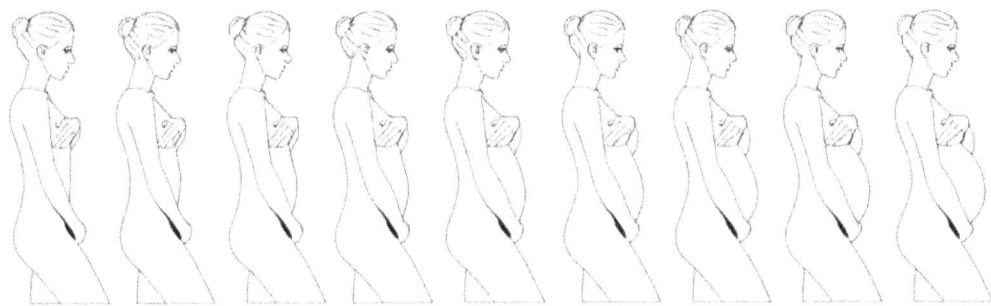

Physiology of Normal Pregnancy

The Midwife's Role in Normal Pregnancy

Pregnancy is most often a healthy, normal process. The role of the midwife is to safeguard this normalcy while remaining prepared to recognize when deviations arise. Unlike a model of care that frames pregnancy primarily as a medical condition, midwifery views pregnancy and birth as profound, physiologic life events.

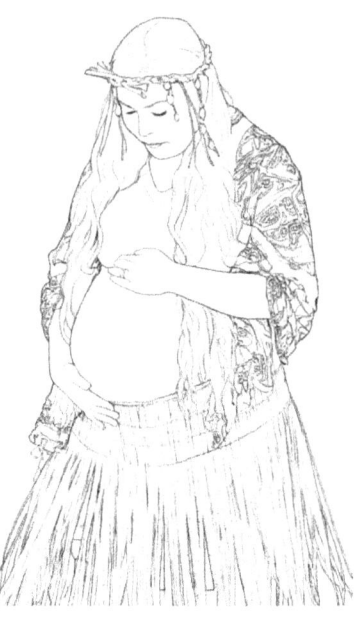

Midwives encourage women to trust their bodies and to view pregnancy as natural and healthy, even in cultures where it is often medicalized. By helping clients understand the body's adaptations and systemic changes, midwives empower them to optimize their own health and their baby's well-being, while also minimizing common discomforts. During pregnancy, every system in the body changes to support fetal growth and prepare for birth. With a thorough knowledge of these normal processes, midwives can reassure families, identify early signs of deviation, and strengthen trust in both the birth process and their own abilities.

Midwives also draw upon the wisdom carried through generations. Across cultures, pregnancy has been recognized as a time of heightened awareness and sensitivity. By encouraging women to listen closely to their own instincts and inner knowledge, midwives validate the idea that the body carries ancestral memory of how to give birth. Integrating this embodied wisdom with modern evidence-based practice allows midwives to honor both tradition and science in their care.

Pregnancy brings emotional and psychological changes as well, as the pregnant woman, her partner, and her family adapt to new roles and responsibilities. Whether partnered or single, every woman needs care and support to prepare for parenting. This often means reframing concerns as part of normal adaptation. A client who worries that her early fatigue signals a problem can be reassured that increased metabolic demands and hormonal shifts commonly cause tiredness. Mood changes or fluctuations in libido, likewise, can be explained as natural responses to pregnancy's physiologic and emotional transitions.

This perspective, which centers the client's lived experience while maintaining clinical vigilance, reflects a core difference between midwifery and conventional obstetric care. By normalizing rather than pathologizing these changes, midwives preserve trust, reduce unnecessary fear, and provide safe, evidence-based care.

> **Clinical Tip**
> When explaining normal pregnancy changes, use simple, body-positive language. This helps clients reframe discomforts as meaningful adaptations rather than problems, reducing anxiety and increasing trust in the process.

Holistic Midwifery Care

- Pregnancy reflects the *wisdom of nature* and the body's remarkable capacity for adaptation.
- Listening to one's body and to ancestral knowledge helps women approach pregnancy with awareness and trust.
- Understanding normal physiology allows midwives to recognize early deviations while affirming the natural strength of the process.

- Holistic care addresses body, mind, emotions, and spirit, honoring pregnancy as both a biological and a transformative life experience.

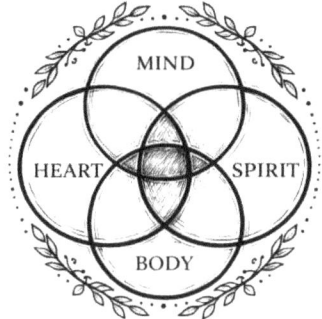

Exercise 7.1: Midwifery Role in Normal Pregnancy

Fill out the following:

1. Why is it important for midwives to frame pregnancy as a normal process?

2. How does understanding physiology help reassure clients?

3. A client has read about every possible pregnancy complication online and arrives fearful. How can a midwife respond in a way that both validates her concern and restores confidence?

4. How can emphasizing normalcy in pregnancy influence the experience of labor and birth for the client and midwife?

Length of Gestation and Estimated Due Date (EDD)

Midwives often use multiple methods together to determine dating. The length of gestation is traditionally counted from the first day of the last menstrual period (LMP). A typical pregnancy lasts about 40 weeks (280 days), nine months and seven days, or ten moons. When counted from the time of conception, pregnancy is about 38 weeks (267 days), eight months and three weeks, or nine and one-half lunar cycles.

Gestation length varies between individuals. A pregnancy lasting 37 to 42 weeks is considered within the normal range, and fewer than five percent of women deliver on their exact due date.

- **Preterm pregnancy:** A pregnancy that ends before 37 completed weeks.
- **Late preterm:** 34 weeks 0 days through 36 weeks 6 days.
- **Early term:** 37 weeks 0 days through 38 weeks 6 days.
- **Full term:** 39 weeks 0 days through 40 weeks 6 days.
- **Late term:** 41 weeks 0 days through 41 weeks 6 days.
- **Postterm pregnancy:** A pregnancy that continues beyond 42 weeks.

Estimating Due Dates

Accurate estimation of the Estimated Date of Delivery (EDD) — also called the Estimated Date of Birth (EDB) or in older texts Estimated Date of Confinement (EDC) — is important, since both prematurity and postmaturity carry risks. For calculation purposes, dates are usually counted from the LMP (sometimes written LNMP, Last Normal Menstrual Period).

> **Key Vocabulary:**
> - **Gestational age:** The age of the pregnancy measured from the first day of the last menstrual period (LMP).
> - **Estimated Due Date (EDD):** The predicted date of birth, calculated from the LMP or confirmed by other clinical methods.
> - **Conceptional age:** The actual age of the embryo or fetus from the time of fertilization, usually about two weeks less than gestational age.
> - **Quickening:** The first felt movements of the fetus, usually between 16 and 20 weeks, which can help confirm dating.
> - **Fundal height:** A measurement of the uterus from the pubic bone to the top of the uterus, used to estimate gestational age after 20 weeks.

> **Key Fact**
> Fewer than **5 percent** of women deliver on their exact due date. Most births occur between 37 and 42 weeks

Naegele's Rule is the most common method for calculating the EDD although useful has limitations with irregular cycles or uncertain recall.

1. Subtract three months from the first day of the LMP.
2. Add seven days.

Example: If the first day of the LMP is April 10, subtract three months = January 10. Add seven days = January 17. The EDD is January 17.

This method is reliable only if:

- The client is sure of her LMP.
- Cycles are regular (28–30 days).
- Oral contraceptives were not used in the three months prior to conception.
- The client was not breastfeeding at the time.

> **Exercise 7.2: Estimating EDD**
> *Fill in the Blank using Naegele's Rule.*
>
> 1. If a woman's LMP is 3/11/24, her EDD is _____
> 2. If a woman's LMP is 1/26/25, her EDD is _____
> 3. If a woman's LMP is 12/3/25, her EDD is _____
> 4. If a woman's LMP is 7/12/25, her EDD is _____

Other Methods of Estimating Gestational Age

Early ultrasound dating is usually accurate using crown–rump length is accurate to approximately ±5–7 days, while accuracy decreases in the second trimester to approximately ±10–14 days and in the third trimester to ±21 days due to:

- **Early growth is very consistent.** In the first trimester, embryos and early fetuses develop at nearly the same rate across all pregnancies. Measuring the crown–rump length (CRL) provides a highly accurate estimate of gestational age.
- **Later growth varies more.** In the second and third trimesters, genetic factors, nutrition, and placental function cause babies to grow at different rates. A measurement at 30 weeks might reflect a naturally small or large baby rather than an incorrect due date.

Other approaches include:

- Early bimanual **pelvic exam** by an experienced practitioner, although it is subjective.
- **Quickening** (first fetal movement, usually around 18–20 weeks in nulliparous women and earlier, around 16–18 weeks, in multiparas).
- **Fetal heart rate** heard with Doppler at 10–12 weeks, or with a fetoscope at 18–20 weeks.
- **Fundal height measurement**: fundal height in centimeters usually correlates with weeks of gestation; at 20 weeks, the fundus is at the umbilicus (about 20 cm).
- **Coital history** (if dates are limited and known).
- **Birth control history** (when contraception stopped or if a failure occurred).

Application in Midwifery

Midwives combine menstrual history, clinical findings, and ultrasound when needed to establish gestational age. Rather than treating the EDD as a fixed point, they frame it as a **window of expected arrival**—typically from 37 to 42 weeks. This perspective helps clients understand natural variation while still monitoring carefully for signs of postterm pregnancy or other concerns. By presenting the due date as a flexible guide rather than a hard deadline, midwives promote informed choice, reduce pressure for unnecessary interventions, and uphold maternal autonomy and fetal well-being.

Exercise 7.3: Due Dates
Fill in the Blank

1. Why is first trimester ultrasound more reliable than later ultrasounds for dating?

2. A client with irregular cycles does not recall her LMP. Which dating tools would you rely on and why?

3. A client is "late" at 40 weeks and feels pressured to consider induction. How might a midwife reframe this using updated definitions of term?

SIGNS AND SYMPTOMS OF PREGNANCY

Before the widespread use of home pregnancy tests and diagnostic ultrasound, midwives and physicians relied primarily on signs and symptoms to determine whether conception had occurred. Today, modern diagnostics are widely available, but learning to identify and interpret clinical signs remains a vital midwifery skill, especially in low-resource settings.

Signs of pregnancy are traditionally grouped into three categories: **presumptive, probable, and positive**. Because many symptoms can have causes other than pregnancy, no single sign is conclusive on its own. Midwives consider the whole clinical picture, combining history, physical findings, and, when available, laboratory or ultrasound confirmation. This holistic approach emphasizes careful observation and client-centered care.

Presumptive Signs (Subjective) Reported by the pregnant woman, but not conclusive on their own.
- **Amenorrhea:** absence of menstruation, most common sign. Can also result from breastfeeding, stress, malnutrition, hormonal disorders, or chronic illness.
- **Frequent urination** may result from pressure on the bladder but can also be caused by infection.
- **Breast changes:** soreness, tingling, fullness, or darkened areolae may occur in pregnancy, PMS, or ovulation.
- **Nausea and vomiting:** common in pregnancy, but may also be due to illness.
- **Quickening:** first perception of fetal movement, usually around 16 weeks. Can be overlooked or mistaken. Fatigue.
- **Mood changes** (emotional lability, irritability)
- **Food cravings or aversions**

Probable Signs (Objective) *Also called Predictive Signs.* Observed by the examiner, suggesting but not confirming pregnancy.
- **Skin changes:** striae gravidarum (stretch marks), linea nigra, chloasma (mask of pregnancy).
- **Abdominal enlargement:** may be due to pregnancy, but also fat, edema, or tumors.
- **Palpation of fetal parts:** may be mistaken for tumors.
- **Pregnancy tests:** detect hCG in urine or blood. Highly accurate, though hCG can appear in other conditions.

Pelvic exam findings:
- **Hegar's sign:** softening of the uterine isthmus (7–12 weeks).
- **Chadwick's sign:** bluish discoloration of cervix and vagina (early pregnancy).
- **Goodell's sign:** softening of the cervix.
- **McDonald's sign:** ease in flexing the body of the uterus against the cervix.
- **Internal ballottement:** fetus rebounds against examining finger when tapped.

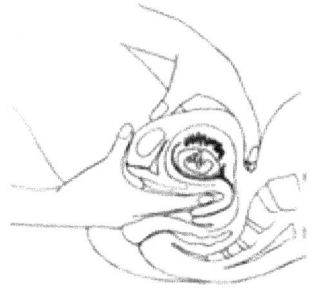
HEGAR'S SIGN

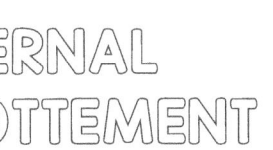
INTERNAL BALLOTTEMENT

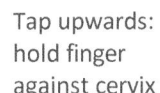 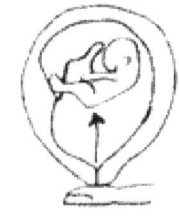 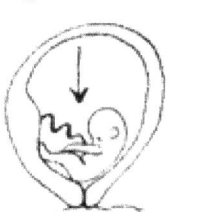

Tap upwards: hold finger against cervix

The fetus floats upwards in the amniotic fluid

As the fetus sinks a gentle tap is felt on the examining finger

Positive Signs (Diagnostic)
Reported by the pregnant woman, but not sufficient on their own to confirm pregnancy.

- Visualization of the fetus on ultrasound (gestational sac visible at ~5 weeks, heartbeat by 6 weeks)
- Auscultation of fetal heart tones (Doppler at 9–12 weeks, fetoscope at 18–20 weeks)
- Palpation of fetal movement by an experienced examiner (18–20 weeks)

Application in Midwifery

- **Early care:** Clients may seek care before confirmation. Midwives can combine reported symptoms with clinical findings to establish provisional care and plan follow-up.
- **Pattern recognition:** A cluster of signs (e.g., amenorrhea, nausea, and uterine enlargement) increases likelihood, but inconsistencies may signal ectopic pregnancy, miscarriage, or inaccurate dating.
- **Client education:** Clear explanations reduce fear and build trust. For example: "Your test is positive and I can feel the uterus growing. These are strong indicators of early pregnancy."
- **Low-resource practice:** In settings without lab or imaging tools, observing uterine size, cervical changes, and fetal heart tones becomes essential.

> **Clinical Tip**
> When reviewing early symptoms, emphasize that signs like nausea, breast tenderness, or fatigue can have many causes. Combining multiple findings gives a clearer picture than relying on one symptom alone.

Exercise 7.4: Pregnancy Signs
Fill in the Blank

1. Why are presumptive signs not considered diagnostic?

2. How does a positive pregnancy test fit into the classification of signs?

3. At what gestational age are fetal heart tones usually detectable with Doppler and with a fetoscope?

4. A client presents with breast tenderness and a missed period but a negative pregnancy test. How would you approach this situation as a midwife?

Changes in System Physiology During Pregnancy

Pregnancy is a time of profound transformation. Nearly every organ system in the body adapts to sustain the growing fetus and prepare for birth. These changes are not signs of illness, but examples of the body's remarkable capacity for adaptation. Blood volume expands to support increased circulation, respiration adjusts to meet higher oxygen demands, digestion slows to optimize nutrient absorption, and hormones coordinate the growth and development of both parent and baby.

For midwives, learning these changes is more than memorizing a list of symptoms and lab values. It is about seeing pregnancy as a normal physiologic state rather than a pathology. This perspective allows midwives to reassure clients when common discomforts arise, while also developing the critical eye needed to recognize when a symptom falls outside the range of normal and may signal a complication.

Understanding these physiologic adaptations helps midwives educate clients, normalize their experiences, and strengthen trust in the body's wisdom. It also equips midwives to intervene appropriately when a client's condition requires more attention. In this way, knowledge of normal changes forms the foundation for safe, respectful, and holistic midwifery care.

CARDIOVASCULAR AND HEMATOLOGIC SYSTEM

During pregnancy, the cardiovascular system undergoes remarkable changes to meet the increased demands of both mother and fetus. The heart and blood vessels work harder in pregnancy than at any other time in life. These adaptations ensure adequate oxygen and nutrient delivery while preparing the body for blood loss at birth.

Mothers may feel a faster heartbeat, more shortness of breath, or swelling in their legs. Though often well tolerated, these changes can increase susceptibility to conditions such as anemia, edema, or thromboembolic disease. Understanding normal cardiovascular and hematologic changes helps midwives distinguish expected adaptations from pathology and provide safe, supportive care.

> **Key Vocabulary**
>
> - **Cardiac output:** The amount of blood the heart pumps in one minute, a product of heart rate and stroke volume.
> - **Plasma volume:** The liquid portion of blood (excluding blood cells) that expands significantly in pregnancy to support circulation.
> - **Physiologic anemia:** A dilutional anemia caused when plasma volume increases more than red blood cell mass, lowering hemoglobin concentration without true deficiency.
> - **Varicosities:** Dilated, twisted veins (often in legs, vulva, or rectum) caused by increased vascular pressure and hormonal effects in pregnancy.
> - **Supine hypotensive syndrome:** A drop in blood pressure that occurs when the pregnant uterus compresses the inferior vena cava while lying flat on the back.
> - **Hypercoagulability:** An increased tendency for blood to clot due to higher levels of clotting factors in pregnancy, which helps prevent hemorrhage but raises clot risk.

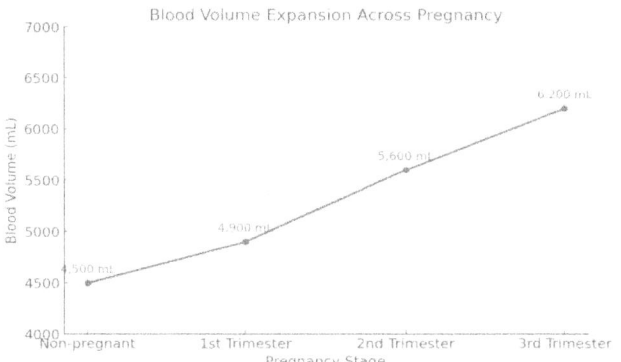

1. **Cardiac changes**
   - The heart increases in size by about 12%, with enlargement of the left ventricle and thickening of the ventricular wall.
   - Cardiac output rises by approximately 1.5 liters per minute at term (30–50% increase).
   - Resting heart rate increases from about 70 to 85 beats per minute.
   - Systemic vascular resistance decreases, which lowers diastolic blood pressure in mid-pregnancy.

- Systolic blood pressure remains largely unchanged; diastolic pressure gradually returns to pre-pregnancy levels by 26–28 weeks.

2. Blood Volume and Composition
- Plasma volume increases by 40–60%.
- Red blood cell (RBC) volume increases by about 30%.
- This mismatch produces physiologic anemia of pregnancy, with hemoglobin and hematocrit falling despite higher total blood volume.
- By 36 weeks, hematocrit is typically 5% lower than in the non-pregnant state.
- White blood cell count rises by about 8%, mainly from neutrophilia.
- Eosinophils, lymphocytes, and platelets remain unchanged.
- Overall erythrocyte count decreases.

> **Clinical Tip**
> Because pregnancy is a hypercoagulable state, mothers are at increased risk of blood clots. Encourage mobility, hydration, and awareness of warning signs.

3. Renal and Serum Changes
- Creatinine and blood urea nitrogen (BUN) decrease in the first trimester, stabilize in the second, and rise slightly near term.
- Serum cholesterol and lipids increase.
- Electrolyte changes:
    - Sodium and potassium decrease slightly.
    - Both ionized and non-ionized calcium decrease modestly.
    - Magnesium decreases by 10–20% in the first trimester.

4. Coagulation Factors
- Fibrinogen (Factor I) increases markedly.
- Factors VII, VIII, and X increase.
- Factors XI and XIII decrease at term.
- Antithrombin II is thought to be reduced.
- These changes create a hypercoagulable state—protective against hemorrhage at birth but raising the risk of thromboembolism.

> **Further Explanation**
> Clotting factors are proteins in the blood that help control bleeding. During pregnancy, these factors shift to protect the mother from hemorrhage at birth:
> - **Fibrinogen (Factor I)** and **Factors VII, VIII, and X** increase → making blood clot more easily.
> - **Factors XI and XIII** decrease → slightly reducing other clotting pathways.
> - **Antithrombin II** is thought to decrease → reducing the body's natural "brake" on clotting.
>
> These changes create a **hypercoagulable state**. This protects against dangerous bleeding during labor and birth but also increases the risk of blood clots (thromboembolism) in pregnancy and postpartum.

5. Vascular Changes
- Increased vascularity causes dilation of veins in the legs, vulva, and anus, leading to varicosities and hemorrhoids.
- Venous return is further obstructed by the enlarged uterus, especially in late pregnancy.
- Blood flow to the kidneys, skin, and mucous membranes increases.

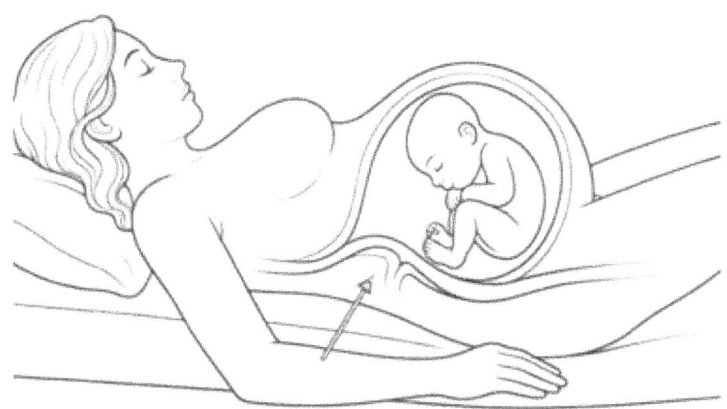

Pressure of Gravid Uterus on Vena Cava

Immune Adaptations

Pregnancy involves a carefully regulated transformation of the immune system, known as **immunomodulation**. This allows the body to tolerate the genetically distinct fetus while still defending against infection. Rather than full suppression, immunity shifts toward a selective and balanced response. As a result, pregnant women may be more susceptible to common infections such as colds or UTIs. A normal rise in white blood cell count, called **physiologic leukocytosis**, is especially common in the third trimester and should not be mistaken for pathology. Midwives interpret these changes when reviewing labs, provide reassurance, and emphasize preventive strategies such as rest and nutrition.

Midwifery Applications

Midwives play a central role in protecting clients from complications of hypertensive disorders in pregnancy. At every prenatal visit, they consistently track and interpret blood pressure readings, watching for early patterns of elevation. They provide counseling on hydration, balanced nutrition, mobility, and rest, all of which support healthy cardiovascular function. Midwives also explain normal immune shifts, reassuring clients that mild susceptibility to infections is expected while reinforcing prevention and wellness strategies.

CARDIOVASCULAR CHANGES

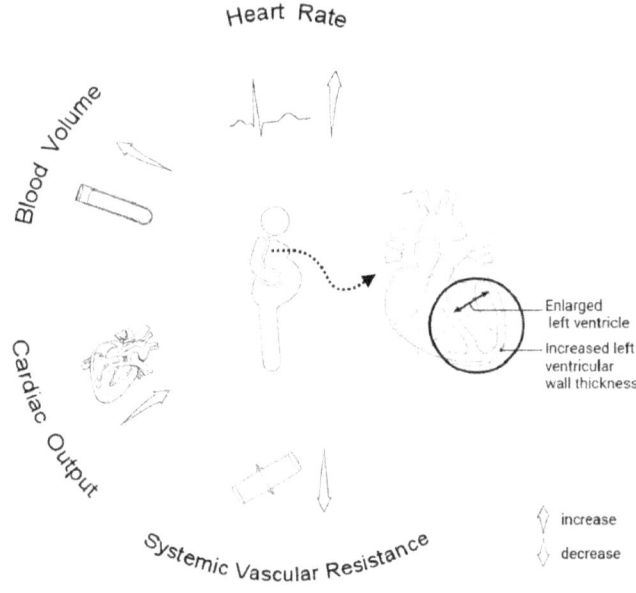

Exercise 7.6: Cardiovascular System
Answer the following:

1. State how blood viscosity is altered by pregnancy.

2. List factors that decrease the workload of the heart in pregnancy.

3. List factors that increase the workload of the heart during pregnancy.

4. Explain what is meant by *physiologic anemia*.

5. Describe how fluid is drawn back into the vascular space.

RESPIRATORY SYSTEM

During pregnancy, the respiratory system adapts in remarkable ways to provide enough oxygen for both mother and fetus. Many women notice they become short of breath more easily, even with mild activity. This sensation is normal and reflects an increase in tidal volume, elevation of the diaphragm, and changes in blood gases. Although the chest may feel compressed, the ribcage expands and the subcostal angle widens to help preserve lung capacity. These adjustments ensure that more oxygen is available for placental exchange, even as the growing uterus limits space in the thorax. Rising progesterone stimulates the brain's respiratory centers, increasing respiratory drive and tidal volume, which can lead to deeper breathing and a common sense of breathlessness in pregnancy. Nasal congestion and nosebleeds are more closely related to estrogen-driven vascular changes in the mucosa, and uncomplicated pregnancy does not appear to increase the risk of respiratory infections. Even so, these normal adaptations can contribute to fatigue or feeling "out of breath" during daily activities.

1. **Oxygen requirements**
   - Maternal oxygen needs increase by 15–20 percent due to higher metabolic activity and the oxygen demands of the uterus, placenta, and fetus.
   - This greater demand is met primarily by changes in ventilation rather than an increase in red blood cells.

2. **Breathing mechanics**
   - Tidal volume (air per breath) increases by about 30–40 percent, while respiratory rate remains relatively unchanged.
   - Minute ventilation rises primarily through deeper breathing, leading to a 20 percent increase in oxygen intake.
   - Many women describe this as "breathing for two," even though the rate of breathing stays almost the same.

3. **Diaphragm and thorax**
   - The diaphragm is displaced upward by as much as 4 cm as the uterus grows out of the pelvis.
   - Ribcage shape alters to allow for lung expansion despite reduced vertical space.
   - The subcostal angle widens, and anteroposterior and transverse chest diameters increase, helping maintain total lung capacity.

4. **Blood chemistry and gases**
   - Arterial pH remains stable at about 7.4–7.44 due to compensatory renal adjustments.
   - Mild respiratory alkalosis develops because of increased ventilation and reduced $PaCO_2$.
   - Partial pressure of oxygen (PaO_2) rises slightly, enhancing placental oxygen transfer.
   - Partial pressure of carbon dioxide ($PaCO_2$) falls to around 27–32 mmHg, creating a gradient that favors fetal CO_2 removal.

5. **Airway changes**
   - Hormonal influence causes nasal congestion, mucosal edema, and increased friability of airway tissues.
   - These changes make nosebleeds, sinus problems, and airway sensitivity more common in pregnancy.
   - Snoring and sleep-disordered breathing may increase, particularly in late pregnancy.

Key Vocabulary

- **Tidal Volume:** The amount of air inhaled or exhaled during a normal breath at rest.
- **Respiratory Alkalosis:** A mild rise in blood pH caused by lower carbon dioxide (CO_2) levels from increased ventilation.
- **Dyspnea:** The sensation of shortness of breath or difficulty breathing.
- **Diaphragmatic Elevation:** Upward displacement of the diaphragm caused by the enlarging uterus.

Key Fact

Pregnancy increases tidal volume by up to 40 percent. Women breathe more deeply, not faster.

Midwifery Applications

Midwives should monitor respiratory health throughout pregnancy, taking maternal reports of breathlessness seriously while also reassuring clients about normal adaptations. Counseling can include posture adjustments, pacing activities, and rest, since upright positioning often improves comfort.

Midwives should also remain alert for conditions such as asthma exacerbations, respiratory infections, or early signs of heart disease. Early recognition and referral safeguard both mother and fetus, while client education empowers women to distinguish normal changes from concerning symptoms.

> **Further Explanation**
>
> **Respiratory alkalosis** is a normal pregnancy adaptation. Deeper breathing causes women to exhale more carbon dioxide (CO_2), lowering CO_2 levels in the blood and slightly raising pH. The kidneys balance this by excreting more bicarbonate.
>
> **Why this matters:** Lower maternal CO_2 helps fetal CO_2 move into the mother's blood. Slightly higher maternal oxygen levels improve placental oxygen transfer.

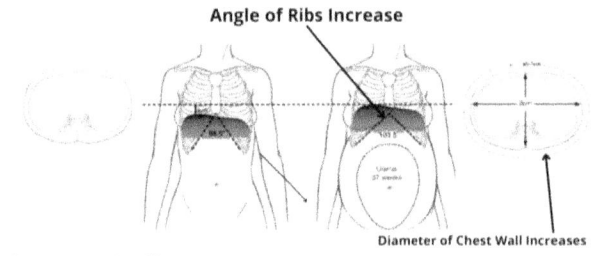

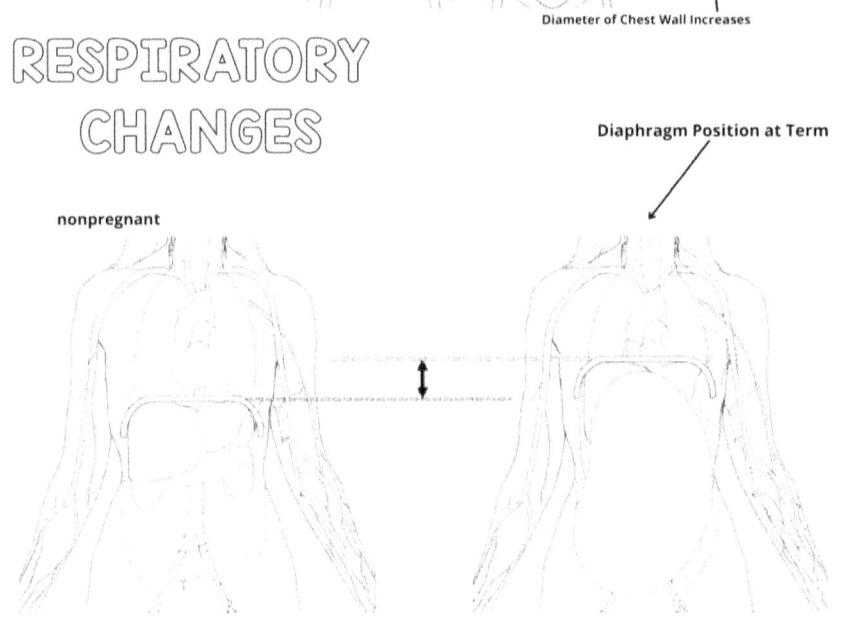

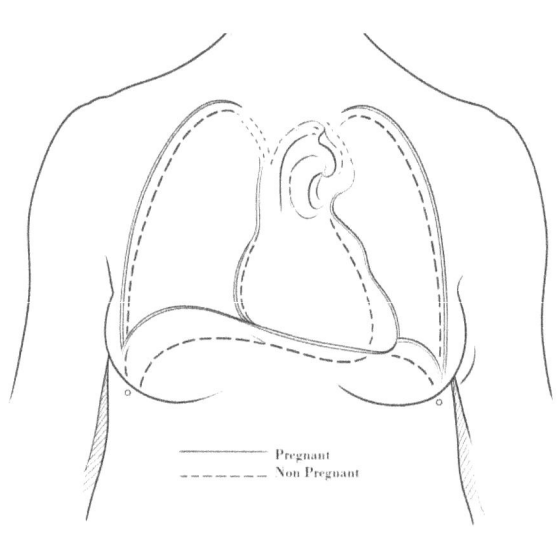

Exercise 7.7: Respiratory System

Answer the following:

1. List the factors that increase the body's need for oxygen during pregnancy.

2. State how the body's demand for oxygen alters during pregnancy.

3. Explain how the respiratory system meets this increased demand.

4. Describe the changes in tidal volume during pregnancy.

5. Explain how the ribcage is altered by pregnancy.

RENAL SYSTEM

During pregnancy, the renal system adapts significantly to meet the demands of maternal metabolism and fetal development. These changes increase kidney workload, alter solute handling, and modify fluid balance. While largely physiologic, they also raise the risk of urinary stasis and infection.

1. **Kidney and ureter changes**
   - Kidneys enlarge by about **1 cm** by mid-pregnancy.
   - Ureters dilate under the influence of progesterone, most noticeable after 16 weeks.
   - Right ureter is more dilated than the left due to uterine dextrorotation.

2. **Renal blood flow and filtration**
   - Renal plasma flow increases by 50–80% by 16 weeks, peaks around mid-pregnancy, and gradually declines near term (still above baseline).
   - Glomerular filtration rate (GFR) rises by about 50% by 12 weeks, remains elevated until late pregnancy, then declines slightly by 36 weeks.

> **Key Fact**
> Pregnancy transforms kidney function: blood flow and filtration both rise by about half, making urinary changes like mild glycosuria and increased UTI risk normal findings.

3. **Glucose and solute handling**
   - Increased GFR reduces tubular reabsorption capacity, leading to **physiologic glycosuria** in up to 70% of pregnant women.
   - Amino acids and water-soluble vitamins (e.g., vitamin C, B-complex) are also excreted in greater amounts.
   - **Persistent glycosuria** may indicate gestational diabetes.

4. **Electrolytes and fluid balance**
   - Sodium retention increases by 500–900 mEq over pregnancy, supporting plasma expansion.
   - Potassium retention also increases slightly, helping maintain blood volume.
   - Reduced excretion contributes to physiologic edema, especially after 28 weeks.

5. **Bladder and infection risk**
   - The bladder is displaced upward by the enlarging uterus, reducing capacity.
   - Ureteral dilation and urinary stasis appear after 16 weeks, increasing risk of urinary tract infection (UTI) and pyelonephritis.
   - A trace of protein may occur due to concentrated urine or contamination, but persistent proteinuria suggests preeclampsia.

6. **Endocrine activity**
   - Renin, angiotensin, and aldosterone levels rise, promoting sodium retention and blood volume expansion.
   - Erythropoietin production increases, stimulating red blood cell mass.
   - Activated vitamin D (calcitriol) rises by 50–100%, improving calcium absorption for fetal bone growth.

> **Clinical Tip**
> UTIs are more common in pregnancy because of ureteral dilation and urinary stasis. Even asymptomatic bacteriuria requires treatment, as it may progress to pyelonephritis and preterm labor.

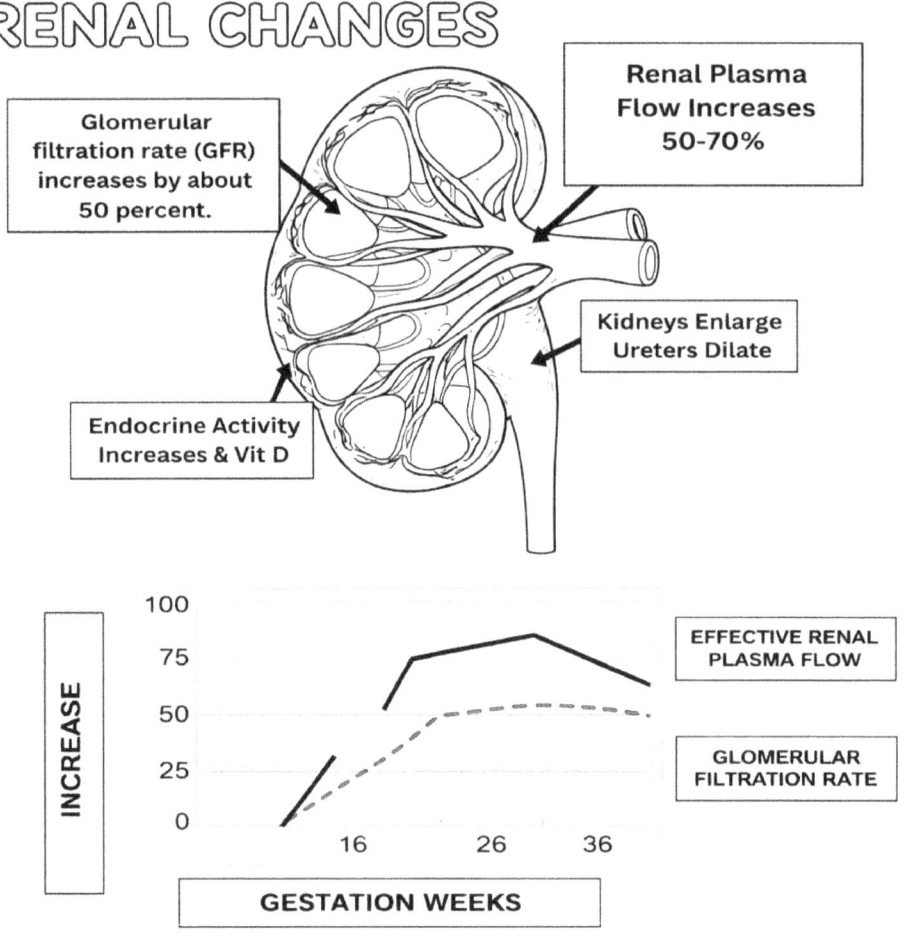

Exercise 7.8: Renal System
Answer the following:

1. Describe how pregnancy affects the body's retention of sodium and potassium.

2. Explain how renal blood flow changes during pregnancy.

3. Explain why urinary frequency is common in the first and last trimesters.

4. Describe why small amounts of glucose in the urine may be normal in pregnancy.

Gastrointestinal System

Pregnancy alters digestion and metabolism through both hormonal and mechanical changes. Progesterone relaxes smooth muscle, slowing gastrointestinal motility, while the enlarging uterus displaces the stomach and intestines upward. These adaptations improve nutrient absorption and ensure a steady supply of glucose, fat, and protein for fetal development. At the same time, the liver's workload increases to handle elevated hormone levels and metabolic by-products. While essential for pregnancy, these changes often contribute to heartburn, reflux, and constipation.

1. **Metabolic rate**
   - Basal metabolic rate (BMR) increases by **15–20%** during pregnancy, peaking in the **third trimester**.
   - This rise supports the energy demands of the fetus, placenta, and maternal tissues.
   - Extra protein (additional ~30 g/day) and iron are needed for fetal growth, maternal blood expansion, and uterine and breast development.

2. **Carbohydrate metabolism**
   - Insulin resistance increases progressively, especially after **20 weeks**, ensuring glucose availability for the fetus.
   - Fasting blood glucose is slightly lower, while post-meal blood glucose levels rise more sharply.
   - Some women develop **gestational diabetes** when pancreatic insulin production cannot keep pace.

> **Key Fact**
> Basal metabolic rate rises by up to **20%**, while intestinal transit time slows by nearly **50%**, ensuring nutrients reach the fetus but increasing the likelihood of constipation and heartburn.

3. **Fat metabolism**
   - In early pregnancy, fat is stored as an energy reserve.
   - By the **third trimester**, fat breakdown accelerates, providing maternal energy while sparing glucose for the fetus.
   - Circulating triglycerides can increase by 200–300% by late pregnancy.

4. **Protein metabolism**
   - Protein requirements increase steadily to support fetal growth, the placenta, and maternal tissue changes.
   - By term, total maternal protein deposition is about 500–900 g above non-pregnant levels.

5. **Digestive tract changes**
   - The intestines are displaced upward and laterally by the enlarging uterus by second trimester onward.
   - Progesterone slows peristalsis, extending intestinal transit time by 30–50%.
   - This promotes nutrient absorption but commonly results in **constipation**.

> **Key Fact**
> The microbiome is so vital to digestion, immunity, and pregnancy that some scientists consider it a separate body system, while others place it within the gastrointestinal system.

6. **Gastroesophageal changes**
   - Progesterone relaxes the lower esophageal sphincter from early pregnancy.
   - By the third trimester, uterine pressure on the stomach further increases reflux.
   - 30–50% of pregnant women report significant heartburn.

7. **Liver workload**
   - The liver processes elevated estrogen, progesterone, and other metabolic by-products.
   - Enzyme activity rises, but liver size remains unchanged.
   - Serum alkaline phosphatase levels may double due to placental production.

Gastrointestinal Function

Function / Measurement	Non-Pregnant Value	Pregnant Value (Typical Range)
Basal Metabolic Rate (BMR)	Baseline	↑ 15–20% (peaks in 3rd trimester)
Protein Requirement	~50 g/day	+30 g/day (total ~80 g/day)
Fat Metabolism	Stable triglycerides	Triglycerides ↑ 200–300% by late pregnancy
Carbohydrate Metabolism	Normal insulin sensitivity	Progressive insulin resistance after 20 weeks
Intestinal Transit Time	24–48 hours	Slowed by 30–50%
Heartburn/Reflux Incidence	5–10%	30–50% by 3rd trimester
Liver Enzymes (Alk. Phos.)	Normal range	Up to 2× baseline (placental source)

GASTROINTESTINAL CHANGES

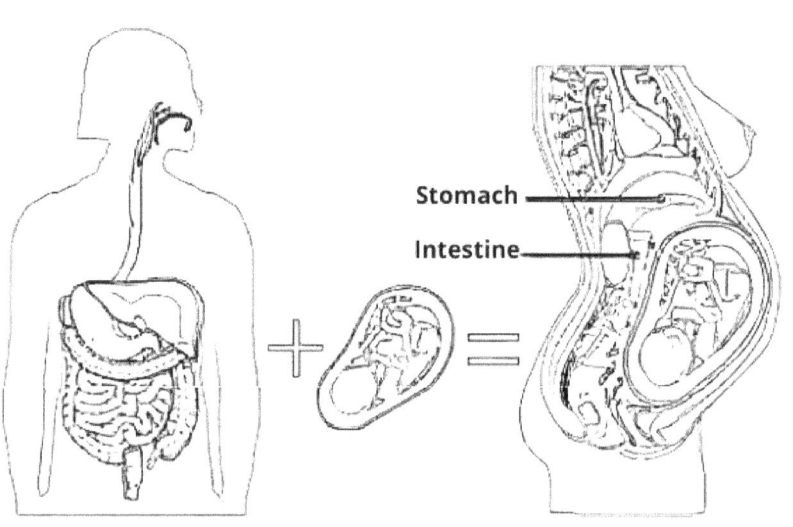

As the uterus enlarges, it rises up and out of the pelvic cavity displacing the the stomach, intestines and other adjacent organs.

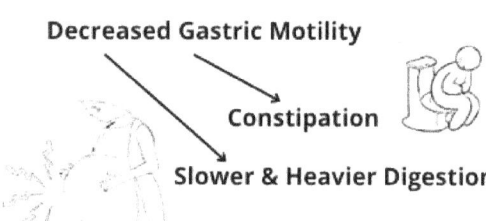

Decreased Gastric Motility → Constipation, Slower & Heavier Digestion

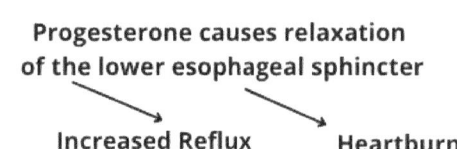

Progesterone causes relaxation of the lower esophageal sphincter → Increased Reflux → Heartburn

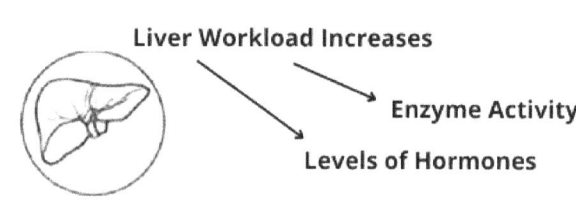

Liver Workload Increases → Enzyme Activity, Levels of Hormones

Exercise 7.9: Gastrointestinal System
Check the box in the correct column for each change that occurs in pregnancy.

Increases	Decreases
☐ Metabolic rate	☐ Gastric motility
☐ Insulin resistance	☐ Gastrointestinal sphincter tone
☐ Fat storage	☐ Gallbladder emptying
☐ Protein needs	☐ Gastric emptying
☐ Liver workload	☐ Bowel motility

NEUROLOGICAL SYSTEM

The neurological system undergoes subtle but meaningful changes during pregnancy, many of them driven by hormonal and vascular shifts. Pregnancy alters the brain as well as the body: rising levels of estrogen and progesterone influence neuroplasticity, neurotransmitters, and glial activity. These adaptations may support emotional bonding, stress regulation, and maternal behaviors.

Pregnant women often report symptoms such as "pregnancy brain," with forgetfulness, inability to concentrate, or fogginess. They also may experience dizziness, disrupted sleep, or headaches. While usually benign, these changes can affect daily function and quality of life. A clear understanding of normal neurological adaptations allows midwives to distinguish them from serious conditions such as preeclampsia, stroke, or neuropathies.

Common Neurological Changes
- **Cognitive fog**: A sense of mental cloudiness or forgetfulness.
- **Sleep disturbance**: Insomnia, disrupted rest due to hormonal shifts, discomfort, or frequent urination.
- **Tension headaches**: Often related to posture, dehydration, or stress.
- **Carpal tunnel syndrome**: Numbness, tingling, or pain in the hands caused by fluid retention and nerve compression in the wrist.
- **Sciatica** occurs when the large nerve in the lower back becomes compressed and sends intense pain radiating down the leg.

> **Key Fact**
> Pregnancy "rewires" the brain structure in small ways that can last for years after birth, reflecting long-term adaptations that support parenting.

Midwifery Applications
Midwives normalize benign symptoms—such as forgetfulness or poor sleep—while remaining alert for neurological red flags, including severe headaches, visual changes, or unilateral weakness. Education on posture, hydration, and ergonomic strategies can ease discomforts like tension headaches or carpal tunnel syndrome. This balanced approach provides reassurance, supports comfort, and promotes safe, attentive care.

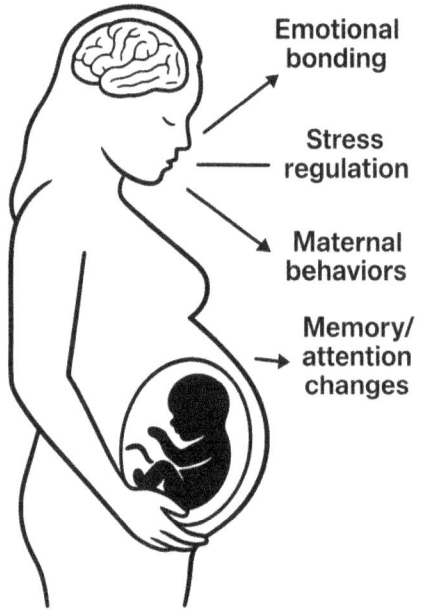

Pregnancy changes the brain
- Emotional bonding
- Stress regulation
- Maternal behaviors
- Memory/attention changes

Exercise 7.11: Neurological System
Answer the following:

1. How do hormonal changes during pregnancy influence the brain, and why might this be helpful for new parents?

2. Name two neurological symptoms that are common in pregnancy and explain how they typically affect daily life.

3. What warning signs should prompt a midwife to distinguish normal changes from serious neurological complications?

MUSCULOSKELETAL SYSTEM

Pregnancy alters the musculoskeletal system to support fetal growth and prepare the body for birth. The hormone **relaxin** loosens ligaments and joints, especially the sacroiliac joints and pubic symphysis, allowing the pelvis to widen for delivery. These changes, combined with the weight of the uterus, shift posture and strain the spine and lower limbs. Magnesium deficiency, electrolyte imbalance, or reduced circulation may contribute to cramping. While these changes are expected and usually temporary, they can interfere with comfort, movement, and daily activities. Midwives play a critical role in helping clients understand and manage these symptoms with reassurance, positioning guidance, and supportive therapies such as prenatal yoga, stretching, or aquatic exercise.

These musculoskeletal adaptations not only help the body carry the pregnancy but also prepare the pelvis and abdominal wall for birth. After delivery, many of these changes gradually resolve, though some women experience lingering effects such as **diastasis recti** or persistent back pain. Understanding both the temporary and long-term impacts helps midwives guide recovery as well as prenatal care.

1. **Joint and ligament changes**
   - Hormonal increased laxity may cause instability and a higher risk of sprains or joint discomfort.
   - **Round ligament pain**: a sharp or stretching pain in the lower belly or groin caused by the growing uterus pulling on its supporting ligaments.
   - **Diastasis recti:** separation of the abdominal muscles along the midline due to uterine growth, which may weaken core support.
   - **Limb symptoms:** eight gain and venous pressure may cause leg cramps, varicose veins, and edema.

2. **Spinal and postural adaptations**
   - **Lumbar lordosis:** an increased inward curve of the lower spine that develops in pregnancy to balance the weight of the growing uterus often resulting in backaches.
   - **Postural sway:** increased shifting of the body's weight during standing or walking, caused by changes in balance and coordination during pregnancy.
   - **Center of gravity:** the point in the body where weight is balanced; shifts forward in pregnancy, affecting posture and increasing the risk of falls.
   - **Pelvic girdle pain (PGP)**: pain in the lower back, hips, or thighs due to increased mobility and strain on the pelvis during pregnancy.

> **Clinical Tip**
> Prenatal yoga supports flexibility, balance, and relaxation. Gentle stretching and mindful breathing can reduce back pain, improve posture, and prepare the body for labor while also lowering stress and promoting emotional well-being.

Midwifery Applications

When a pregnant client reports hip or back pain, the midwife can explain how postural shifts and ligament laxity contribute to discomfort, the midwife normalizes the client's experience while remaining alert to signs that could indicate more serious concerns, such as preterm contractions. In this way, midwives balance empathy with clinical vigilance. Interventions might include recommending posture support devices, gentle stretching routines, or referral to prenatal yoga and aquatic therapy programs, all of which can improve comfort, mobility, and body awareness. Teaching proper body mechanics and encouraging regular movement empowers clients to adapt to the physical demands of pregnancy while reducing strain on the musculoskeletal system.

> **Cultural Tradition**
> Many Indigenous and traditional cultures encouraged daily walking, squatting, and carrying tasks during pregnancy. These movements supported flexibility, strength, and readiness for birth, while also keeping mothers active in community life.

MUSCULOSKELETAL CHANGES

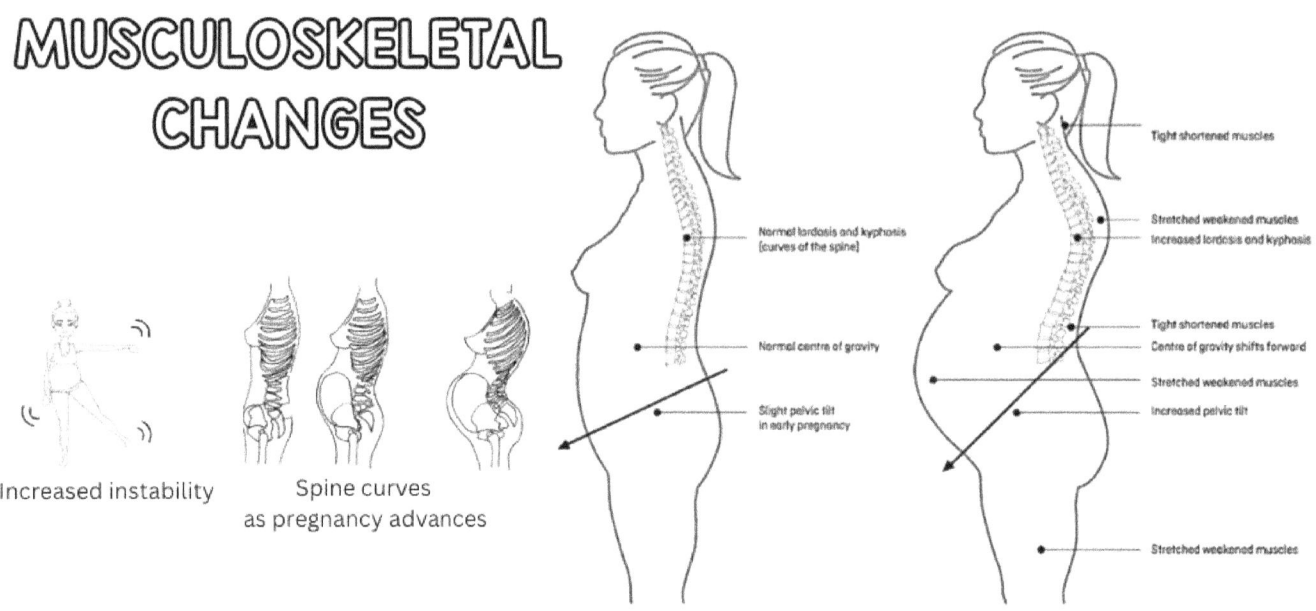

Exercise 7.12: Musculoskeletal System
Answer the following questions:
1. How does the weight of the pregnant uterus affect spinal curvature and posture?
2. Which hormones relax ligaments and increase joint mobility during pregnancy?
3. What are some possible causes of leg cramps in pregnancy?
4. What condition occurs when the abdominal muscles separate along the midline in pregnancy?
5. How can midwives help clients manage back or pelvic pain related to postural changes?

ENDOCRINE SYSTEM

During pregnancy, the endocrine system undergoes profound changes as multiple glands and the placenta adjust hormone production to support the growing fetus and prepare the mother's body for birth and lactation. Hormones rise dramatically, influencing metabolism, fluid balance, uterine growth, and breast development. The corpus luteum produces progesterone until about the 12th–14th week, when the placenta takes over as a major endocrine organ. Estrogen and progesterone rise dramatically, supporting implantation, maintaining uterine quiescence, and promoting growth of the uterus and breasts. These hormones also alter glucose metabolism, increasing insulin resistance to make glucose more available for the fetus.

1. **Reproductive Hormones**
   - Progesterone rises about 1,000-fold, first from the corpus luteum, then the placenta. It maintains the uterine lining, relaxes smooth muscle, and—together with estrogen—prevents further ovulation by suppressing LH and FSH.
   - Estrogen increases about 400-fold, supporting uterine growth, uterine blood flow, breast development, and fetal organ development. It also contributes to water and sodium retention.
   - Relaxin softens the cervix and loosens pelvic ligaments to prepare for birth.
   - Oxytocin is produced by the posterior pituitary, triggering uterine contractions during labor and milk let-down after birth.
   - Prolactin rises steadily to prepare the breasts for milk production.

2. **Placental Hormones**
   - Human chorionic gonadotropin (hCG) maintains the corpus luteum until the placenta takes
   - over hormone production at 8–10 weeks; it is the basis of pregnancy tests
   - Human placental lactogen (hPL) increases as the placenta grows, reducing maternal use of glucose so more nutrients are available for the fetus, and contributing to insulin resistance.

3. **Metabolic and Stress Hormones**
   - Insulin is essential for glucose uptake. During pregnancy, maternal tissues become more resistant, leading to lower fasting glucose and higher post-meal glucose—this ensures glucose supply for the fetus.
   - Cortisol increases to aid fetal lung development and shift maternal metabolism toward protein and fat use for energy.
   - Aldosterone and deoxycorticosterone rise to retain sodium and water, expanding maternal blood volume.

4. **Thyroid and Calcium Regulation**
   - Thyroid hormones (T3 and T4) increase to support maternal metabolism and fetal brain and nervous system development.
   - Parathyroid hormone (PTH) rises to mobilize calcium for the fetus.
   - Calcitonin helps balance calcium by promoting storage in bones.

5. **Pituitary gland**
   - Enlarges during pregnancy.
   - Secretes prolactin (stimulates breast development and postpartum milk production).
   - Increases oxytocin secretion near term to initiate labor.

6. **Thyroid and parathyroid**
   - T3/T4 increase basal metabolic rate.
   - Parathyroid hormone rises slightly to meet calcium demands; calcitonin helps regulate calcium balance.

7. **Adrenal changes**
   - Cortisol increases to support energy mobilization and immune modulation.
   - Aldosterone rises, promoting sodium and fluid retention to support increased blood volume.

Changes in Hormones During Pregnancy

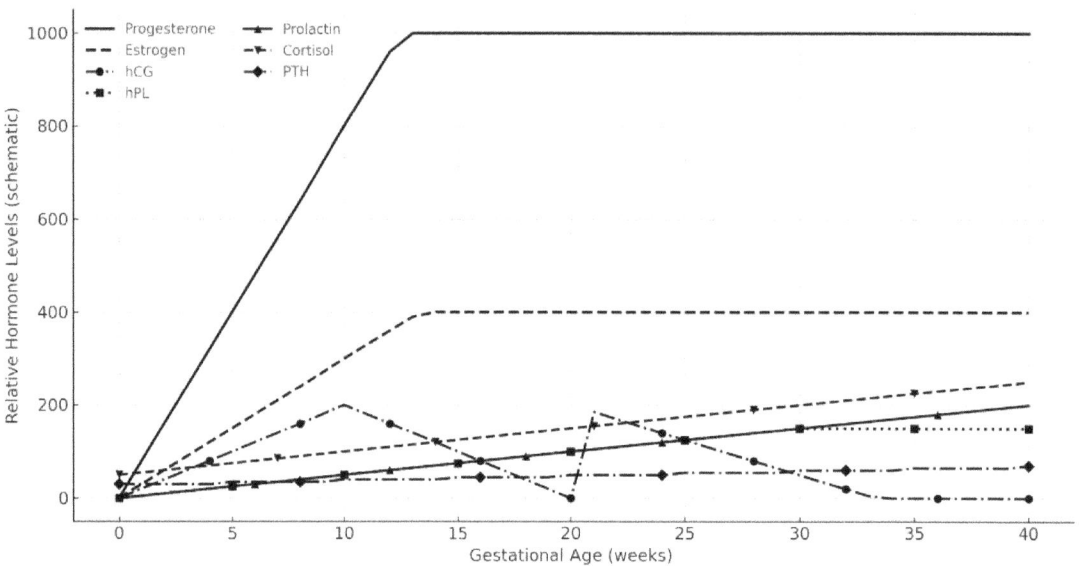

Use the graph to see overall patterns, and the table to review specific details.

Hormone	Early Pregnancy	Mid Pregnancy	Late Pregnancy	Primary Roles
Progesterone	Maintains implantation; suppresses LH & FSH	Uterine relaxation; supports placenta	Breast tissue prep for lactation	Prevents uterine contractions until term
Estrogen	Promotes uterine growth; vascular changes	Increases blood flow; ligament relaxation	Prepares cervix & breasts	Supports fetal growth and maternal adaptations
hCG	Maintains corpus luteum and progesterone	Declines after ~12–14 weeks	Minimal role late	Basis for pregnancy tests
hPL	Not yet active	Increases insulin resistance	Peaks; ensures glucose to fetus	Alters maternal metabolism to favor fetal needs
Relaxin	Softens uterine tissue; loosens joints	Pelvic ligament relaxation	Cervical softening	Prepares pelvis and cervix for birth
Prolactin	Rising levels prime breasts	Further gland development	High at term	Initiates milk production after birth
Oxytocin	Low baseline	Increases near term	Surge at labor	Stimulates uterine contractions and milk let-down

Midwifery Applications

When a client asks why their blood sugar seems to fluctuate more in mid-pregnancy, the midwife can draw on endocrine knowledge to explain the role of hPL in increasing insulin resistance. This normal physiological change ensures a steady supply of glucose to the fetus but also sets the stage for gestational diabetes in some clients. Understanding these shifts allows midwives to interpret laboratory values more accurately, screen for gestational diabetes at the right time, and provide individualized counseling on nutrition and lifestyle. By connecting hormone function with clinical decision-making, midwives can offer informed, compassionate care that bridges physiology and lived experience.

ENDOCRINE SYSTEM OF PREGNANCY

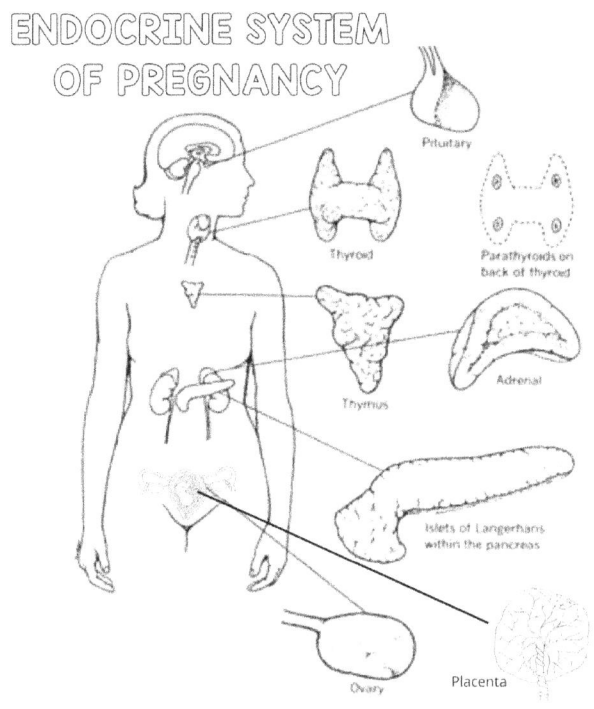

Exercise 7.13: Endocrine
Match each microbiome location with its primary role during pregnancy:

1. Reproductive hormones _____

2. Placental hormones _____

3. Metabolic and stress hormones _____

4. Thyroid and calcium regulation _____

A. Progesterone
B. hCG
C. Cortisol
D. Calcitonin
E. Estrogen
F. hPL
G. Thyroid hormones (T3, T4)
H. Prolactin
I. Aldosterone
J. Relaxin
K. Oxytocin
L. Parathyroid hormone (PTH)
M. Deoxycorticosterone
N. Insulin

INTEGUMENTARY SYSTEM

Pregnancy often brings noticeable changes to the skin, hair, and nails mainly driven by increased levels of estrogen, progesterone, and melanocyte-stimulating hormone, along with changes in blood flow and immune response. These changes may be highly visible and sometimes distressing to clients, especially when they appear suddenly or alter familiar features.

Hyperpigmentation, increased vascularity, and changes in skin elasticity are all normal and expected findings. While most are harmless and temporary, they can have a significant emotional impact. Some changes, such as the darkening of the areola or the development of a linea nigra, are so common they are considered normal signs of pregnancy.

> **Key Fact**
> Increased estrogen during pregnancy raises blood flow to the skin, which can make pregnant women feel warmer and sometimes leads to the "pregnancy glow."

Common Changes:
- **Pigmentation of the areola**: Darkening of the nipples and areola, usually more pronounced in women with darker complexions; may persist after birth.
- **Linea nigra**: A dark line running from the umbilicus to the pubis, caused by increased skin pigmentation.
- **Striae gravidarum (stretch marks)**: Pink, red, or purple streaks on the abdomen, thighs, breasts, and buttocks from skin stretching. They fade but rarely disappear completely.
- **Chloasma** (also called melasma, or the 'mask of pregnancy'): Irregular, blotchy facial pigmentation, especially on the forehead, cheeks, and nose. It often fades postpartum.
- **Vascular changes**: Spider angiomas (bright red, branching vessels) and palmar erythema (reddening of the palms) are common and usually resolve after birth.
- **Pruritic urticarial papules and plaques of pregnancy (PUPPP)**: Intensely itchy red papules, often in stretch marks late in pregnancy. Benign but uncomfortable; relieved by soothing measures or topical treatments.
- **Hair and nail changes**: Hair often appears fuller due to prolonged growth cycles, while nails may grow faster but can become softer or more brittle.

SKIN CHANGES OF PREGNANCY

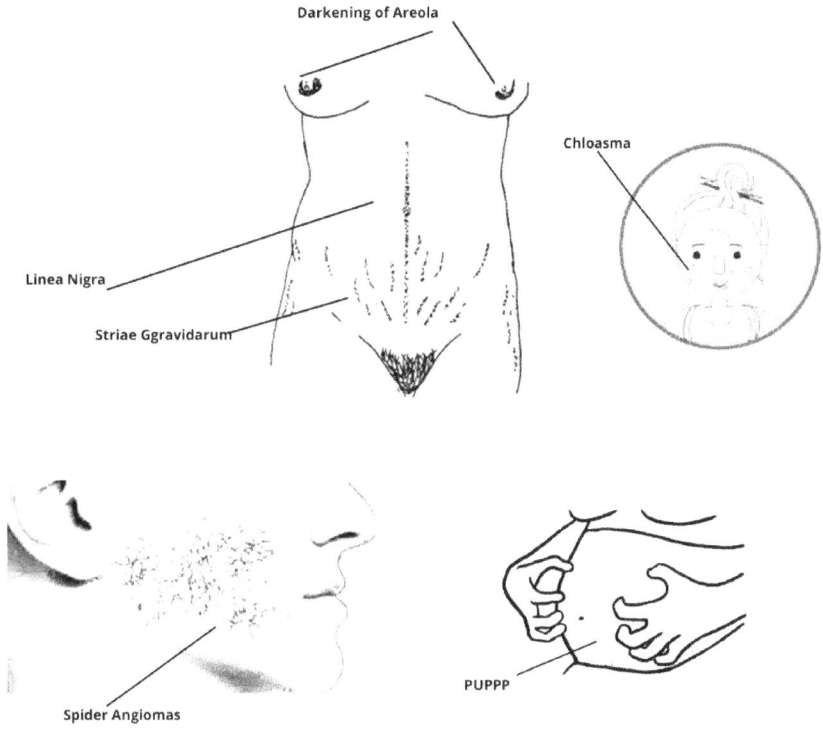

Midwifery Applications

When a client expresses distress about the sudden appearance of stretch marks, the midwife has an opportunity to provide both clinical information and emotional support. By explaining that striae gravidarum are a common and normal adaptation to skin stretching and that they often fade in color over time, the midwife can help reframe the experience as part of a healthy pregnancy. Midwives are uniquely positioned to discuss appearance changes respectfully, using inclusive and body-positive language that honors the client's lived experience. This includes normalizing pigmentation changes such as linea nigra or chloasma, affirming that these shifts vary widely and are influenced by individual skin tone and genetics. At the same time, midwives stay alert for rare but serious dermatologic conditions such as cholestasis-related rashes or PUPPP (pruritic urticarial papules and plaques of pregnancy), ensuring timely diagnosis and care when needed. By blending reassurance with clinical vigilance, midwives support both body trust and safe outcomes.

> **Clinical Tip**
> Encourage women to use sunscreen during pregnancy, since hormonal changes can make the skin more sensitive to sunlight and worsen chloasma.

Exercise 7.14: Integumentary System
Match the pregnancy-related integumentary change with its description:

1. ____Linea nigra	**A.** Irregular blotchy darkening of the face, often called the mask of pregnancy
2. ____Striae gravidarum	**B.** Dark pigmented line running from the umbilicus to the pubis
3. ____Chloasma	**C.** Itchy red papules and plaques appearing in stretch marks late in pregnancy
4. ____Spider angiomas	**D.** Small bright-red vascular lesions with radiating "legs" that usually resolve postpartum
5. ____PUPPP	**E.** Pink, red, or purple streaks caused by stretching of the skin

Reproductive System

During pregnancy, the reproductive system undergoes profound transformations that touch nearly every aspect of a mother's experience. Reproductive adaptations in pregnancy go beyond visible enlargement of organs. Increased vascularity, tissue remodeling, and hormonal influence alter how the body functions and feels. Hormonal shifts influence not only physical growth but also sensations such as breast tenderness, increased discharge, and changes in sexual response. These adaptations can be both reassuring signs of progress and sources of discomfort, reminding mothers that reproduction is a whole-body process.

Uterus
- Enlarges to seven to eight times its non-pregnant size.
- Becomes two to seven times wider.
- Capacity increases from about 10 mL to more than 5 liters.
- Weight increases from 50 grams to about 1,000 grams.
- Growth results mainly from hypertrophy of existing muscle fibers.
- In the first trimester, muscle fibers thicken by 1–2 cm.
- Fibroelastic tissue develops around muscle bundles, providing strength.
- By the third trimester, uterine walls thin to less than 0.5 cm.
- During labor, powerful contractions propel the fetus through the vagina.

> **Key Fact**
> The uterus grows from the size of small plum to the size of a watermelon during pregnancy, with its capacity increasing more than 500 times.

Cervix
- Cervical mucosa undergoes marked glandular changes.
- Endocervical glands expand to occupy about half the cervix at term.
- Increased secretions form the cervical mucus plug, which acts as a protective barrier against ascending bacteria.
- Increased vascularity and softening of the cervix occur (Goodell's sign).

Breasts
- Mammary glands enlarge due to stimulation by estrogen, progesterone, and prolactin.
- Ductal tissue proliferates and alveoli increase in size and number.
- Breasts become larger, heavier, and more vascular, often causing tenderness.
- Areolae enlarge and darken; Montgomery's glands become more prominent.
- Colostrum (a thick, yellowish fluid) may be secreted as early as the second trimester.

Vagina and Vulva
- Increased vascularity produces a bluish discoloration (Chadwick's sign).
- Vaginal mucosa thickens and secretions increase.
- Secretions become more acidic, creating protection against infection.
- Increased glycogen in epithelial cells supports lactobacilli growth, lowering pH further.

> **Clinical Tip**
> Increased vaginal discharge during pregnancy is normal. It is usually thin, white, and acidic, helping protect against infection.

Ovaries
- Ovulation ceases during pregnancy due to suppression by high estrogen and progesterone levels.
- The corpus luteum of pregnancy persists until about 10–12 weeks, producing progesterone until the placenta is capable of hormone production.
- After placental takeover, the corpus luteum gradually regresses.

REPRODUCTIVE CHANGES

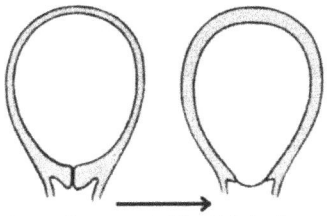
Uterine Walls Thicken

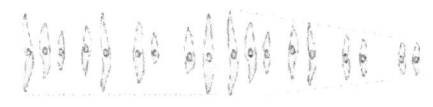
Uterine Muscle Fibers Grow

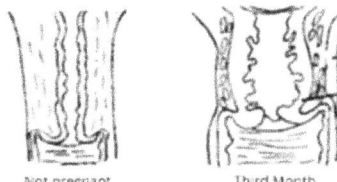
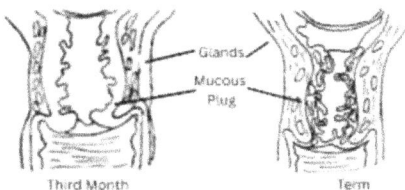
Endocervical Glands Create Mucus Plug

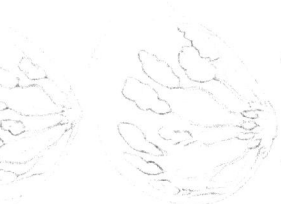
Breasts Grow & Change

Key Facts

- **Estrogen** levels rise nearly 1,000 percent during pregnancy, driving uterine growth, increasing blood flow, and supporting fetal development.

- **Progesterone** levels increase more than 1,000-fold during pregnancy, maintaining the uterine lining, preventing contractions, and supporting breast development for lactation.

Exercise 7.15: Reproductive System
Describe the changes to the following reproductive structures during pregnancy

1. Ovaries

2. Cervix

3. Vagina

4. Breasts

5. Uterus

Weight Gain During Pregnancy

While "normal" weight gain is often considered between 25–35 pounds, women may gain as little as 10 pounds or as much as 75 pounds and still be healthy depending on their pre-pregnant weight and overall condition. BMI is often used as a guideline, but it is a limited tool. It does not account for body composition, metabolic health, trauma history, or lived experiences. Emerging research shows that for women with higher BMIs, lower or even stable weight gain can be safe when paired with good nutrition and regular monitoring.

Weight gain in pregnancy is expected, but it can also bring up intense emotions. Many women have complex histories with food and body image, and for some, pregnancy reactivates past trauma, eating disorders, or experiences of fat shaming. Others may fear judgment from providers, family, or their own internalized beliefs about weight. Midwives must approach this subject with sensitivity, recognizing both the emotional and physiological realities of weight gain.

In a culture that idealizes thinness, many women struggle with body image and worry about gaining too much weight. Some may restrict food or diet during pregnancy, denying their baby essential nutrition. Others gain more than average but lose weight quickly with breastfeeding and increased activity. For some women, excess weight lingers, affecting their long-term health and self-esteem.

> **Guidelines by Pre-Pregnancy BMI**
>
> *According to the Institute of Medicine (IOM), weight gain goals vary by body mass index (BMI):*
>
> - **Underweight (BMI < 18.5):** 28–40 pounds
> - **Normal weight (BMI 18.5–24.9):** 25–35 pounds
> - **Overweight (BMI 25–29.9):** 15–25 pounds
> - **Obese (BMI ≥ 30):** 11–20 pounds
>
> These ranges are general guidelines. A midwife's individualized counseling is essential, considering the woman's health, diet, and activity level.

Risks and Concerns
- Underweight women face increased risks of preeclampsia and low-birth-weight infants.
- Overweight women who gain excessively may experience hemorrhoids, varicose veins, stretch marks, backache, fatigue, indigestion, and shortness of breath.
- Excessive weight gain that persists beyond the first postpartum year can contribute to long-term health challenges.

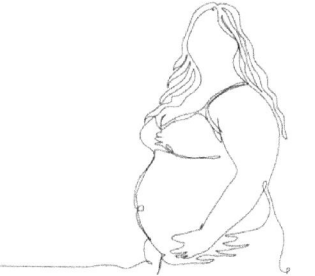

Many women feel discouraged when they weigh themselves weekly, even if their gain is normal. Midwives should reassure women that weight gain is both normal and necessary for pregnancy and breastfeeding, while also encouraging balance and moderation.

Because the midwife may be the only health care provider a woman sees, her guidance is a powerful influence on health choices. Pregnancy is often the time when women are most open to adopting new lifestyle patterns. Midwives can help clients use this opportunity to build lasting habits of mindful nutrition and regular activity that support health far beyond pregnancy.

If there is concern about excessive weight gain—most often in women who begin pregnancy overweight—the best advice is to support safe, moderate exercise. While good nutrition matters, exercise is often the most effective way to manage weight during pregnancy. When women express concern about their weight, encourage gentle, sustainable activities such as walking, yoga, or swimming. Emphasize the importance of continuing to eat nourishing food, and reassure them that with breastfeeding and regular movement, they are likely to return to a comfortable weight.

Average Weight Gain by Trimester:
- First trimester: 2–6 pounds
- Second trimester: 10–18 pounds
- Third trimester: 10–20 pounds, or about one pound per week in the last eight weeks

Average Weight Distribution at Term:
- Baby = 7–8 pounds
- Placenta = 1–2 pounds
- Amniotic fluid = 2 pounds
- Uterine enlargement = 2 pounds
- Maternal breast tissue = 2 pounds
- Maternal blood flow = 2 pounds
- Fluids in maternal tissue = 4 pounds
- Maternal fat stores = 7 pounds

> **Clinical Tip**
> Many midwives encourage women to keep a three-day food diary, writing down everything they eat and drink. Reviewing this at the next visit helps open conversations about nutrition, weight gain, and healthy habits.

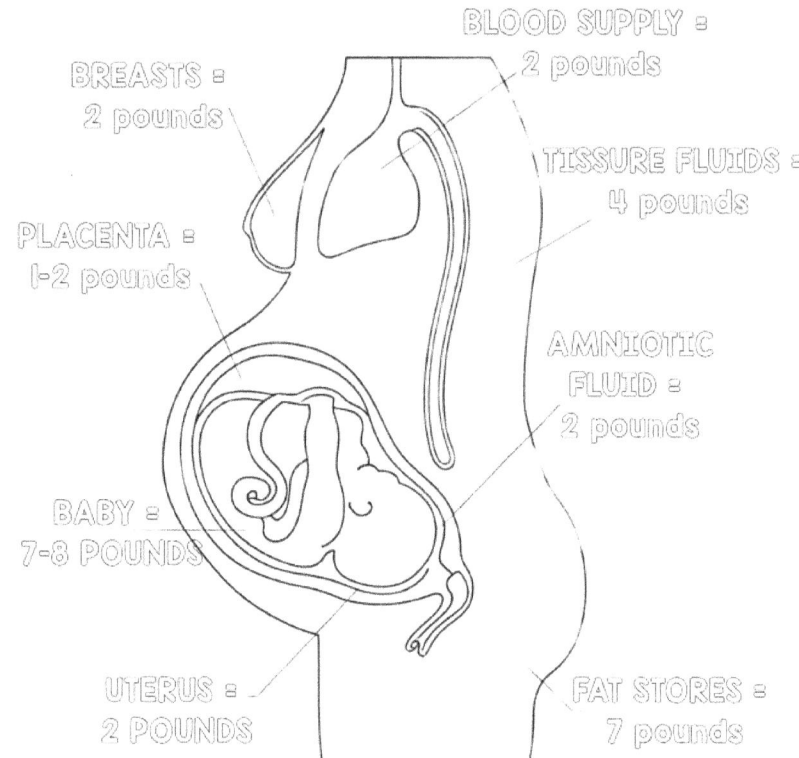

Exercise 7.16: Weight Gain
Answer the following questions:

1. Why is weight gain during pregnancy necessary for both the mother and the baby?

2. Many women worry about "gaining too much." As a midwife, how would you reassure a woman who feels anxious about her weight?

3. List two healthy nutrition recommendations you might give a woman to support appropriate weight gain.

4. Give examples of discussions about empty calories.

5. Why is pregnancy often considered a key opportunity to encourage long-term healthy habits?

Common Discomforts of Pregnancy

Normalizing the Spectrum of Discomforts

While pregnancy is often described as a time of joy and anticipation, it also brings with it a wide array of physical discomforts. These changes are largely the result of hormonal shifts, anatomical adaptations, and metabolic demands required to support the growing fetus. Discomforts are normal and expected, though their intensity and impact vary widely. By understanding the physiology behind common symptoms and offering evidence-based strategies for relief, midwives can provide reassurance, improve quality of life, and deepen trust with clients.

CIRCULATORY/VASCULAR DISCOMFORTS

Edema

Mild swelling of the ankles, feet, and hands is common in late pregnancy due to fluid retention and pressure on pelvic veins. It is usually normal but should be distinguished from edema linked to hypertension or preeclampsia. *Comfort measures include:* elevating the feet, lying on the left side, wearing supportive shoes or compression socks, and staying well-hydrated.

Varicose Veins

- Varicosities in the legs or vulva result from progesterone, uterine pressure, and venous congestion. They may be uncomfortable but rarely dangerous. *Do not massage directly over varicosities.*

Comfort Measures
- Wear compression stockings or support hose.
- Engage in regular gentle exercise (swimming is excellent).
- Elevate legs several times daily.

Respiratory Discomforts

Dyspnea

Shortness of breath is common in later pregnancy as the uterus presses against the diaphragm. This is usually benign but should be distinguished from sudden or severe breathlessness, which may indicate pathology. *Comfort measures include:* upright posture, pacing activity, reassurance, and rest.

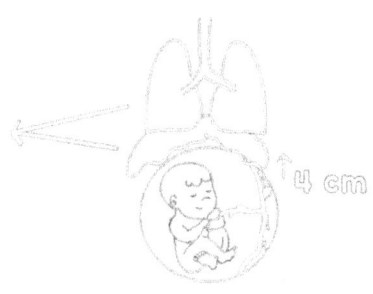

Digestive Discomforts

Morning Sickness

Nausea and vomiting in the first trimester are not confined to the morning and vary with each individual. About half of pregnant women experience morning sickness, and one third of those have both nausea and vomiting. Symptoms usually begin around the fourth week and may continue until the twelfth to fourteenth week.

Although widely studied, no single cause has been identified. Theories include hormonal changes (hCG, estrogen, progesterone), altered glucose metabolism, and slowed gastric emptying. Hypoglycemia often plays a role, especially after hours without food, and vitamin B6 deficiency may contribute. Studies show many women improve with vitamin B6 supplementation (20–50 mg per day, ideally as part of a B complex).

Comfort Measures
- Eat smaller, more frequent meals rich in complex carbohydrates and protein.
- Keep snacks such as crackers, nuts, or cheese on hand.
- Use acupressure wristbands "Sea Bands" available at boating supply stores for seasickness.
- Recommend cold or room-temperature foods if smells are triggering
- Peppermint, lemon balm, and other cooling herbs or ginger

Ptyalism (Sialorrhea)

Excessive saliva in pregnancy is uncommon and usually limited to the first trimester. Its cause is uncertain but may be linked with hormones and is often associated with nausea or hyperemesis gravidarum. *Comfort measures include:* gargling with salt water, using mild mouth rinses, or chewing sugar-free gum.

Heartburn (Pyrosis)

Heartburn presents as epigastric burning, belching, or acid regurgitation. Progesterone relaxes the valve at the top of the stomach, and the growing uterus adds upward pressure. Spicy or fatty foods, coffee, and tobacco can worsen symptoms.

Comfort Measures
- Eat smaller, more frequent meals.
- Avoid lying down after eating.
- Limit trigger foods and beverages.
- Elevate the head of the bed.
- Use chewable calcium tablets (e.g., Tums) **Avoid aluminum-containing antacids.**
- Eat yogurt or drink whole milk after meals.

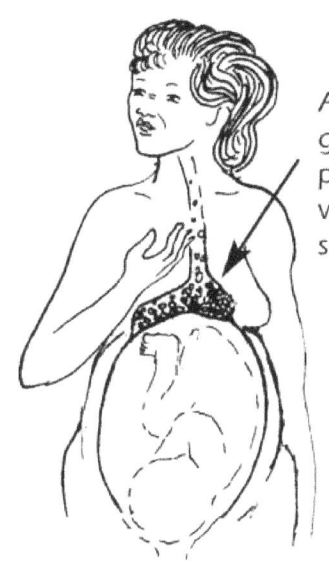

As the baby grows, he/she pushes the woman's stomach up.

Pica

Pica is the craving and ingestion of non-food substances such as ice, clay, starch, or dirt. It is often linked to iron deficiency anemia or other mineral deficiencies. *Comfort measures include:* nutritional assessment, iron and mineral supplementation, and counseling on the health risks of ingesting non-food substances.

Constipation

Progesterone slows bowel motility, the uterus displaces intestines, and iron supplements may harden stools. Stress, diet, and lack of exercise can worsen symptoms. Hemorrhoids often accompany constipation.

Comfort Measures
- Drink six to eight glasses of water daily.
- Eat fiber-rich foods, fruits, vegetables, and dried fruits.
- Use probiotics such as yogurt or kefir.
- Engage in daily gentle exercise.
- Try bulk-forming agents such as psyllium or flaxseed.
- Use a small footstool while on the toilet to mimic squatting.
- Avoid stimulant laxatives or frequent enemas.
- Encourage at least 28 grams of fiber daily
- Recommend flax, chia, or psyllium for gentle fiber support

> **Cultural Tradition**
> In Mexican tradition, *atole*—a warm corn-based drink—is often given during pregnancy to provide nourishment and ease digestion. This practice reflects the cultural view of food as both medicine and comfort, supporting the mother's strength and the baby's growth.

Hemorrhoids

Swollen rectal veins may cause pain, itching, or bleeding. Contributing factors include constipation, increased venous pressure, and hormonal relaxation of blood vessels.

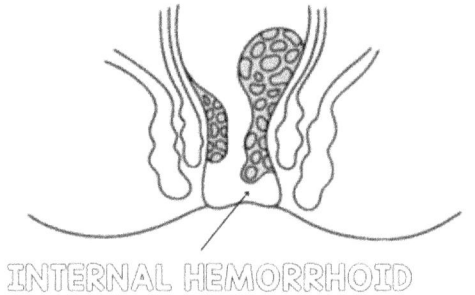
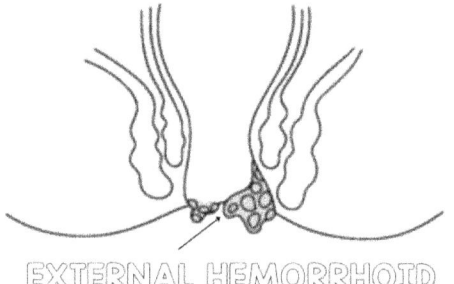

Comfort Measures
- Prevent constipation with hydration and fiber.
- Use witch hazel wipes or moist pads for cleansing.
- Take warm sitz baths.
- Consider stool softeners as needed.
- Do Kegel exercises to improve circulation.

NEUROLOGICAL/GENERAL DISCOMFORTS

Fatigue

Fatigue is common in the first and third trimesters due to hormonal fluctuations, increased metabolic demands, and disrupted sleep. *Comfort measures include:* adequate rest, balanced nutrition, gentle exercise, and screening for anemia or thyroid dysfunction if severe.

Insomnia

Difficulty sleeping occurs throughout pregnancy due to hormonal changes, physical discomfort, and frequent urination. Anxiety may also contribute. *Comfort measures include*: maintaining good sleep hygiene, taking warm baths before bed, using supportive pillows, and practicing relaxation techniques.

URINARY DISCOMFORTS

Urinary Frequency

Frequent urination is common in the 1st trimester due to hormonal changes and in the 3rd trimester as the enlarged uterus presses on the bladder. It is usually benign but should be distinguished from urinary tract infection if accompanied by pain or burning. *Comfort measures include:* limiting fluids before bedtime, practicing double-voiding, and reassuring clients that frequency is normal unless painful.

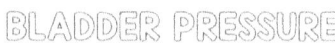
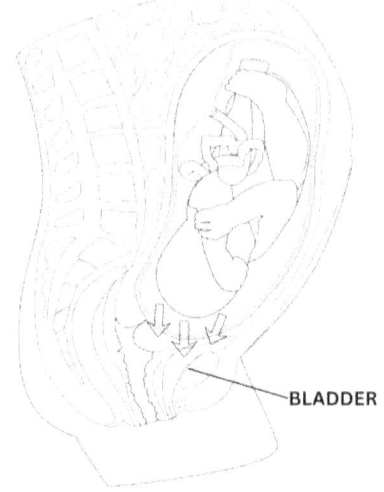

Musculoskeletal/Structural Discomforts

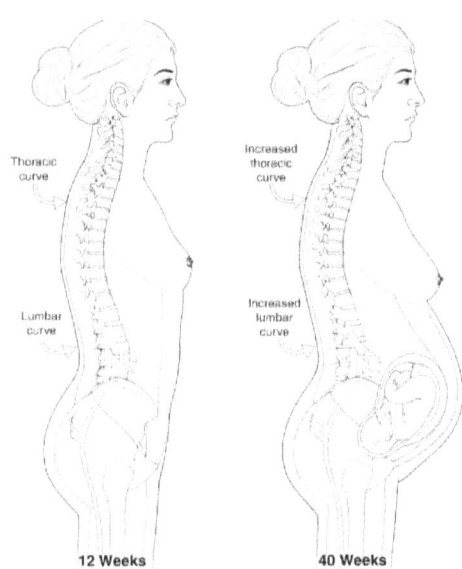

Back Pain
Back pain or backache is common in late pregnancy due to ligament laxity from relaxin, altered posture, and weight gain.

Comfort Measures
- Practice good body mechanics and change position frequently.
- Use supportive pillows while sleeping.
- Engage in prenatal yoga or swimming.
- Apply warm compresses.
- Differentiate from contractions when appropriate.

Round Ligament Pain
As the uterus grows, the round ligaments stretch, often causing sharp, brief pains in the lower abdomen or groin, especially with movement. This is most common in the 2nd trimester. *Comfort measures include:* changing position slowly, using warm compresses, wearing a support belt, and resting when discomfort is intense.

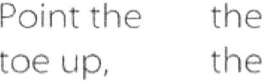

Leg Cramps
Often occurring at night in the calves, cramps may relate to circulatory changes or mineral deficiencies (calcium, magnesium, potassium, B6).

Comfort Measures
- Stretch daily and stay hydrated.
- Supplement calcium, magnesium, or B6 if deficient.
- Engage in gentle aerobic activity.
- If cramps occur: straighten the knee, flex the ankle, massage, and apply heat.

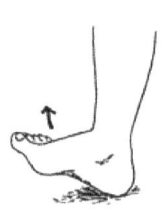 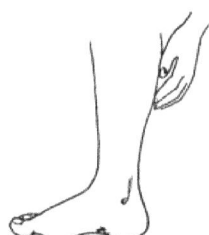

Integumentary/Breast Discomforts

Breast Tenderness
Caused by increased circulation and developing glandular tissue, especially in early pregnancy. *Comfort measures include:* wearing a well-fitting supportive bra and applying warm or cold compresses.

Bleeding Gums
Increased vascularity of mucous membranes during pregnancy often leads to gum bleeding. *Comfort measures include:* using a soft toothbrush, maintaining good oral hygiene, and continuing routine dental care.

Skin Changes (Chloasma, Linea Nigra, Striae)
Skin changes are common in pregnancy due to hormonal pigmentation and stretching of connective tissue. These are usually benign and fade postpartum. *Comfort measures include:* using emollients for skin comfort and sunscreen to reduce pigmentation changes.

COMMON DISCOMFORTS OF PREGNANCY

Discomfort	Trimester(s)	Cause	Comfort Measures
Nausea & vomiting	1st (peaks ~9 wks)	hCG, estrogen, slowed gastric emptying	Small frequent meals; ginger; B6; acupressure; avoid triggers
Heartburn (pyrosis)	2nd–3rd	Progesterone relaxes LES; uterine pressure	Small meals; avoid lying down; limit spicy/fatty foods; elevate head; calcium tabs/yogurt; avoid aluminum antacids
Constipation	All	Progesterone slows bowel; iron; uterine pressure	Hydration; fiber; dried fruit; prune juice; probiotics; exercise; psyllium/flax; footstool
Hemorrhoids	2nd–3rd	Venous pressure; constipation	Hydration; fiber; witch hazel pads; sitz baths; stool softeners; Kegels
Round ligament pain	2nd–3rd	Stretching ligaments as uterus grows	Slow position changes; warm compress; support belt; rest
Back pain	2nd–3rd	Relaxin → ligament laxity; posture; weight gain	Yoga; swimming; pillows; body mechanics; warm compress
Leg cramps	2nd–3rd	Circulatory changes; electrolyte imbalance	Stretch; hydrate; Ca/Mg/B6; massage; heat
Edema	3rd	Fluid retention; venous compression	Elevate feet; hydrate; left-side rest; compression socks
Dyspnea	3rd	Uterine pressure on diaphragm	Upright posture; pace activity; reassurance; rest
Insomnia	All	Hormones; discomfort; anxiety; urinary frequency	Sleep hygiene; warm bath; relaxation; pillows
Varicose veins	2nd–3rd	Venous congestion; progesterone relaxes veins	Compression stockings; elevate legs; swim; gentle exercise
Carpal tunnel syndrome	2nd–3rd	Fluid retention compresses median nerve	Wrist braces at night; cold compress; rest
Urinary frequency	1st & 3rd	Uterine pressure; ↑ renal blood flow	Limit fluids before bed; double-void; reassure unless painful
Breast tenderness	Early, may persist	↑ circulation; glandular growth	Supportive bra; warm/cold compress
Bleeding gums	All	↑ vascularity of mucous membranes	Soft toothbrush; oral hygiene; routine dental care
Skin changes (linea nigra, striae, chloasma)	2nd–3rd	Hormones; skin stretching	Emollients; sunscreen; reassure changes fade

Exercise 7.17: Common Discomforts Review
Answer the following:
Case 1: A client in the second trimester complains of sharp pains in her lower abdomen when she stands up quickly. 1. What is the likely cause? 2. What comfort measure could you suggest?
Case 2: A client in the third trimester reports nightly calf cramps that wake her from sleep. 1. What physiologic changes contribute to this discomfort? 2. What strategies can help prevent or relieve it?
Case 3: A client is worried about swollen ankles late in pregnancy and fears it may mean something is wrong with her baby. 1. When is edema usually normal? 2. What warning signs would prompt further evaluation?
Case 4: A client at 28 weeks reports burning in her chest after meals that sometimes keeps her awake at night. She worries her baby may be "too big." 1. What is the most likely cause of her discomfort? 2. What simple comfort measures could you recommend?
Case 5: A client in early pregnancy feels exhausted all the time and worries that something is wrong. 1. What physiologic changes explain her fatigue? 2. How can a midwife provide reassurance while also supporting healthy lifestyle strategies?

Midwifery Applications

Midwives support clients through the wide spectrum of normal pregnancy discomforts by combining clinical knowledge with practical, individualized care. When a client reports constipation, the midwife may explore diet, hydration, and supplement choices, offering simple strategies such as adding fiber-rich foods, gentle exercise, or probiotics. In cases where symptoms stem from iron supplements or other medications, midwives evaluate alternatives that protect both maternal comfort and fetal well-being.

Other discomforts, such as heartburn or edema, may raise anxiety for clients who fear something is wrong with their pregnancy. A midwife distinguishes between normal, hormonally driven changes and warning signs of pathology. For example, reflux that worsens with gestational age can be normalized with dietary guidance and positioning strategies, while persistent swelling is monitored carefully for signs of preeclampsia. This balance allows midwives to reassure clients while remaining attentive to early indicators of complication.

Equally important is the emotional dimension of discomfort. A client who expresses distress over varicose veins, disrupted sleep, or persistent fatigue may not only need a practical remedy but also validation that her experience is real and significant. Through empathetic listening and culturally appropriate strategies—whether suggesting safe herbal supports, posture adjustments, or relaxation techniques—midwives affirm the client's resilience and reinforce trust in the body's capacity to adapt. By meeting discomforts with both clinical skill and compassionate presence, midwives foster safety, comfort, and confidence throughout pregnancy.

Pregnancy Emotional Journey and Psychosocial Adaptation

Pregnancy is not only a physical event. It is also a profound psychological and emotional journey. As the body grows and hormones shift, so too does the pregnant woman's identity, sense of self, and relationships with others. Emotional experiences in pregnancy may include excitement, fear, ambivalence, anxiety, pride, grief, and joy—sometimes all within the same week or even the same day. Bursts of energy, changes in libido, mood swings, and crying spurts are also common, reflecting both hormonal influence and the magnitude of life transition.

These fluctuations are shaped not only by physiology but also by the woman's broader life context: her support system, relationship dynamics, cultural expectations, and financial or housing stability. Women in non-traditional or vulnerable situations, such as adolescents, single women, lesbian parents, or those with limited resources, may face additional stressors alongside normal pregnancy shifts. Some individuals feel an immediate bond with the pregnancy, while others may feel detached or overwhelmed until much later.

Midwives play a key role in normalizing this full range of emotions while remaining vigilant for signs of depression or psychosocial difficulty that may require referral. By holding space for ambivalence, joy, worry, or grief, midwives create a safe and affirming environment for psychosocial adaptation. This balance of empathy and clinical awareness allows midwives to validate lived experience while safeguarding mental health.

> **Cultural Tradition**
> In Lakota culture, pregnancy is sacred. Families speak only positive words around the mother, avoiding cursing so the baby hears good language. Songs and prayers may also be offered to strengthen and protect both mother and child.

Emotional adaptation also has practical effects on care. Mood shifts may influence a client's ability to rest, eat well, or follow through with prenatal care recommendations. Family dynamics and cultural traditions may shape how a woman experiences support, anxiety, or confidence in her pregnancy. Many cultures have rituals, taboos, or practices around pregnancy that affirm emotional change. Midwives can weave together evidence-based strategies with an awareness of these psychosocial layers, helping families integrate both ancestral wisdom and modern clinical guidance. These adaptations also prepare the ground for postpartum transitions, where emotional resilience and supportive care remain essential.

Maternal Role Attainment: Rubin and Mercer's Stages

The theory of maternal role attainment, developed first by Reva Rubin and later expanded by Ramona Mercer, describes the evolving psychological process of becoming a mother. While the original language of these stages is dated, the framework continues to help midwives understand and support the transitions of pregnancy and early parenthood.

- **Validation of Pregnancy**: accepting that pregnancy is real, often prompted by physical signs or confirmation from a provider. This may include sharing the news with others or noticing bodily changes.
- **Fetal Embodiment**: beginning to connect emotionally with the fetus as part of oneself, imagining what the baby looks like, talking to the fetus, or changing behaviors to protect it.
- **Fetal Distinction**: recognizing the fetus as a separate being with its own movements, temperament, and needs, deepening attachment and initiating separation.
- **Role Transition**: preparing to parent the baby by envisioning a new identity, reflecting on becoming a parent.

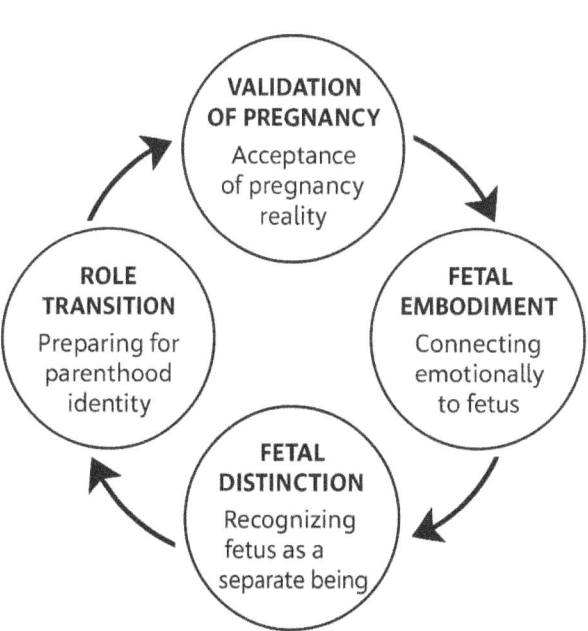

SUPPORTING EMOTIONAL WELL-BEING

Pregnancy may also surface deeper emotional challenges. Clients sometimes struggle with perfectionism, grief and loss, relationship stress, or feelings of not being good enough. These patterns do not necessarily indicate pathology, but they can heighten vulnerability during pregnancy. Awareness of these possibilities helps midwives provide sensitive, supportive care and make timely referrals when needed.

Midwives also play a role in screening for perinatal mood and anxiety disorders, which affect up to one in five women during pregnancy or postpartum. Distinguishing between normal mood fluctuations and signs of depression or anxiety is critical. Simple screening questions, active listening, and appropriate referrals to mental health providers strengthen safety nets for families. By collaborating with other professionals when necessary, midwives support both emotional well-being and physiologic health.

Across cultures, pregnancy has been recognized as a time of emotional transformation. Many cultures have rituals, taboos, or practices around pregnancy that affirm emotional change. Midwives can acknowledge these traditions alongside clinical care, reinforcing that the body and spirit are both engaged in preparing for new life. Whether through prayer, storytelling, song, or community gatherings, cultural traditions can help provide grounding, identity, and resilience during this transition.

Midwifery Applications

Midwives support clients through the wide range of normal pregnancy discomforts by combining reassurance with practical strategies. When constipation is distressing, a midwife may suggest hydration, fiber-rich foods, or adjustments to iron supplementation. For heartburn, clients may benefit from dietary guidance, positioning, and reassurance that reflux is usually a benign physiologic change. Symptoms such as edema, fatigue, or varicosities are normalized while still carefully screened to rule out warning signs of complications. This balance allows midwives to validate lived experience while staying alert to early indicators of pathology.

> **Key Fact**
> Up to one in five pregnant women experience significant anxiety or depression. Supportive midwifery care and timely referrals greatly improve outcomes for mothers and babies.

In addition to normal developmental stages, pregnancy may surface deeper emotional challenges. Clients may struggle with perfectionism, self-confidence, or feeling "not good enough." Others may experience grief and loss, relationship stress, or resurfacing trauma from the past. These patterns do not necessarily indicate pathology, but they can intensify vulnerability during pregnancy. Awareness of these possibilities helps the midwife provide sensitive, supportive care and make timely referrals when needed.

Compassionate listening is central to this work. Some clients may feel frustrated, anxious, or even fearful that common discomforts signal something wrong with the pregnancy. By listening attentively, asking reflective questions, and contextualizing symptoms within normal physiologic change, midwives provide both education and emotional relief. They also remain mindful of external stressors, such as housing, relationships, or trauma, that may intensify physical discomforts. In doing so, midwives uphold the model of whole-person care, weaving together clinical vigilance with empathy to foster safety, comfort, and trust.

Exercise 7.18: Maternal Role Attainment

Match each stage of maternal role attainment with its description:

1. _____ Validation of pregnancy	A. Begins to see fetus as separate from self
2. _____ Fetal embodiment	B. Accepts the pregnancy as real
3. _____ Fetal distinction	C. Begins imagining baby's personality or appearance
4. _____ Role transition	D. Begins thinking about self as a parent and making preparations

Sexuality During Pregnancy

Sexual Function, Safety, and Emotional Connection

Sexuality during pregnancy is a deeply individual experience, shaped by physical changes, emotional states, relationship dynamics, and cultural messages. Some people experience heightened libido and deeper intimacy, while others feel disconnected from their bodies or prefer cuddling and non-penetrative forms of intimacy. Desire can remain unchanged for some. These shifts are influenced by hormonal fluctuations, body image, fatigue, nausea, trauma history, and emotional needs.

Concerns about safety are common, especially in the first and third trimesters, but for most pregnancies without complications, sexual activity is safe. Orgasm stimulates oxytocin release, which can cause temporary Braxton-Hicks contractions — a normal physiologic response. Communication between partners may be enhanced or strained as needs and comfort levels change. Some partners worry about hurting the baby, even though the fetus is well protected as long as membranes are intact and no complications are present. Midwives play a central role in opening space for these conversations, dispelling myths, and helping clients navigate intimacy with sensitivity and respect.

> **Key Vocabulary**
>
> - **Libido**: Desire for sexual activity, which may increase or decrease during pregnancy due to hormonal or emotional factors.
> - **Dyspareunia**: Pain during intercourse, which may occur in pregnancy due to pelvic congestion, vaginal dryness, or positional discomfort.
> - **Consent**: Ongoing agreement to any sexual activity, essential at every stage of pregnancy.
> - **Trauma-informed care**: An approach that prioritizes emotional and physical safety, recognizing the possibility of past trauma.
> - **Inclusive language**: Words and communication that affirm diverse gender identities, sexual orientations, and relationships.

Physiologic and Psychosocial Contributors

Pregnancy brings a wide range of physical changes that may influence sexuality. Increased vascularity and blood flow to the pelvis can enhance sensitivity but may also cause discomfort. Nausea, fatigue, breast tenderness, and a growing abdomen can affect desire or comfort. Certain sexual positions may become uncomfortable in later pregnancy, and alternatives such as side-lying or rear-entry may improve comfort and reduce pressure.

Psychosocial factors such as stress, shifting identity, partner dynamics, and body image can also shape how a person experiences sexuality during pregnancy. Prior trauma may resurface, especially during physical exams or intercourse, requiring midwives to approach care with trauma-informed awareness. These layered experiences are normal and deserve open, affirming support.

Consent, Trauma-Informed Care, and Inclusive Language

Affirming sexual health in pregnancy requires a trauma-informed approach that centers consent and uses inclusive, respectful language. Midwives must assess comfort, safety, and history without assuming a client's gender, orientation, relationship structure, or previous experience. Asking permission before discussing sexual health or conducting exams, acknowledging that desire and comfort levels vary, and affirming that all feelings are valid help create a supportive space. Midwives can also use a client's pronouns and relationship terms, and avoid assumptions about who is present or involved in their intimate life. This inclusive approach fosters trust and dignity.

Midwifery Applications

A midwife who supports sexuality during pregnancy validates it as a normal and important part of health, while also respecting the deeply personal and varied ways it may be experienced. By initiating open, judgment-free conversations, the midwife can normalize fluctuations in desire, provide evidence-based reassurance about safety, and offer options for managing discomfort. Trauma-informed practice includes asking permission before exams, recognizing when a client's withdrawal or anxiety may relate to past experiences, and offering alternatives that preserve autonomy. Using inclusive language affirms diverse identities and relationships. In all cases, the midwife supports the client's right to define their own boundaries, desires, and needs throughout pregnancy, and honors sexuality as part of holistic care.

Exercise 7.19: Sexuality in Pregnancy	
Match each term to its definition:	
1. ____Dyspareunia 2. ____Trauma-informed care 3. ____Libido 4. ____Inclusive language	A. Acknowledges past experiences and centers emotional safety B. Pain during intercourse C. Sexual desire D. Communication that affirms diverse identities

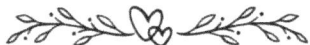

PHYSIOLOGY OF PREGNANCY ESSENTIAL TAKEAWAYS

Pregnancy is a normal physiologic process that transforms every major system of the body in order to support new life. These adaptations—whether in the cardiovascular system, the gastrointestinal tract, or the brain—reveal the body's remarkable capacity for balance and growth. While these changes may bring discomforts such as nausea, fatigue, or back pain, midwives help clients understand that most are temporary and benign. By offering reassurance, practical comfort measures, and guidance on when to seek further evaluation, midwives protect both safety and confidence.

Emotional and psychological adaptations are equally profound. Pregnancy is not only physical but also a time of shifting identity, relationships, and self-perception. Rubin and Mercer's model of maternal role attainment provides one framework for understanding how clients move from validating the pregnancy, to embodying and distinguishing the fetus, and finally to preparing for parenthood. Cultural traditions also shape these transitions, reminding us that pregnancy is embedded within community, spirituality, and ancestral wisdom. Midwives play a vital role in honoring these dimensions while also screening for mood disorders and offering timely support.

Sexuality during pregnancy highlights the diversity of human experience. For some, intimacy deepens and desire increases, while others experience discomfort, fear, or disconnection. All of these responses are normal. By using trauma-informed, inclusive approaches, midwives affirm sexuality as a meaningful part of health while dispelling myths about safety. Above all, holistic midwifery care weaves together physiology, psychology, culture, and intimacy, recognizing pregnancy as both a biological event and a transformative journey into parenthood.

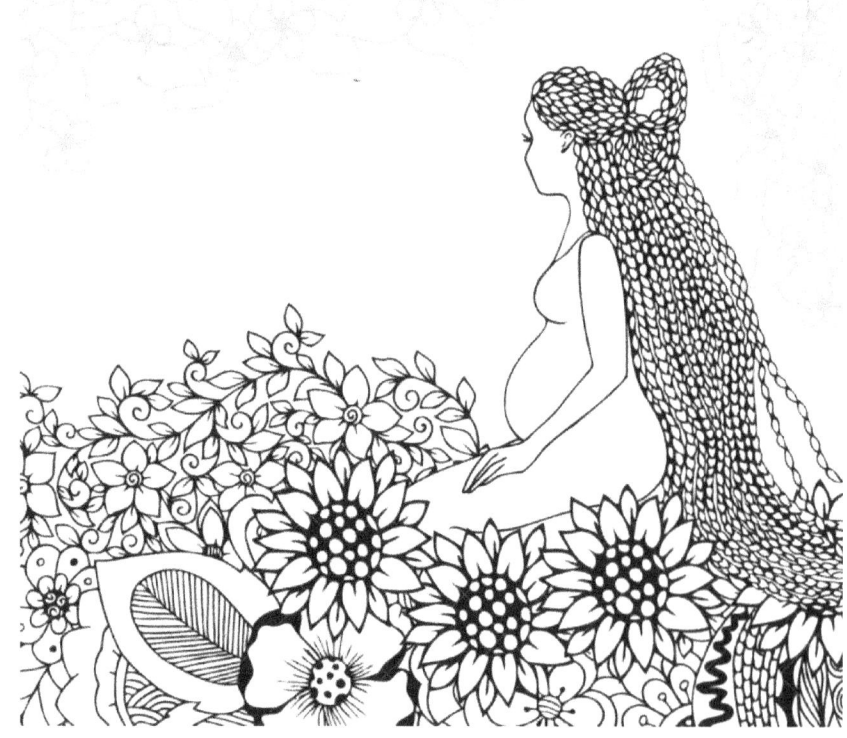

Chapter Seven: Self-Assessment

Multiple Choice

1. Which cardiovascular change is typical in pregnancy?
   a) Decreased cardiac output
   b) Increased blood volume
   c) Decreased heart size
   d) Decreased resting heart rate

2. Which of the following is not considered a normal emotional experience in early pregnancy?
   a) Ambivalence
   b) Joy
   c) Detachment
   d) Persistent delusions

3. Which respiratory adaptation helps meet the oxygen demands of pregnancy?
   a) Decreased tidal volume
   b) Increased respiratory rate
   c) Increased tidal volume
   d) Decreased oxygen uptake

4. Which renal change is common in pregnancy?
   a) Kidney size decreases
   b) Glomerular filtration rate increases
   c) Ureters shorten
   d) Bladder capacity decreases

5. Which endocrine hormone preserves the corpus luteum in early pregnancy?
   a) Estrogen
   b) Progesterone
   c) Human chorionic gonadotropin (hCG)
   d) Oxytocin

6. Which skin change is most likely to persist after pregnancy?
   a) Linea nigra
   b) Striae gravidarum
   c) Spider angiomas
   d) Pregnancy "glow"

7. Which musculoskeletal change contributes most to back pain?
   a) Increased bone density
   b) Relaxin-induced ligament laxity
   c) Decreased spinal curvature
   d) Increased joint stability

8. Which of the following gastrointestinal changes is normal in pregnancy?
   a) Increased peristalsis
   b) Slowed gastric emptying
   c) Decreased nutrient absorption
   d) Increased stomach acid production

9. What is one way a midwife can support psychosocial adaptation in pregnancy?
   a) Correcting emotional responses
   b) Reassuring the client that connection to the fetus will come in time
   c) Avoiding emotional topics during visits
   d) Referring all clients to psychiatry regardless of presentation

10. Which of the following statements is true regarding sexuality in pregnancy?
    a) Sexual activity is unsafe in all third-trimester pregnancies
    b) Libido may increase, decrease, or remain stable
    c) Clients should stop intercourse by 32 weeks gestation
    d) Orgasm always causes preterm labor

11. Which immune change is normal in pregnancy?
    a) Complete suppression of immune function
    b) Balanced immunomodulation
    c) Increased risk of all infections equally
    d) No change in immune activity

12. Which discomfort is most likely related to electrolyte imbalance?
    a) Back pain
    b) Heartburn
    c) Leg cramps
    d) Varicosities

13. Which midwifery response is most appropriate when a client fears sex will harm the baby?
    a) Avoid the discussion unless asked directly
    b) Offer reassurance that sex is generally safe in healthy pregnancies
    c) Recommend abstinence for all clients in the third trimester
    d) Dismiss the concern as unnecessary

Matching

14. Match the pregnancy milestones with their timing or finding:
    1. ____Fetal heartbeat detected by Doppler   A. 20 weeks
    2. ____Quickening in a first-time pregnancy   B. 12 weeks
    3. ____Fundus at the level of the umbilicus   C. 18–20 weeks
    4. ____Fetal movement observed on ultrasound   D. 12–13 weeks

15. Match each pregnancy milestones with their timing or finding:
    1. ____Maternal role attainment   A. Process of integrating the identity of "mother"
    2. ____Fetal distinction   B. Emotional incorporation of the fetus into self
    3. ____Role transition   C. Recognition that the fetus is separate with its own traits
    4. ____Fetal embodiment   D. Shift toward preparing for parenting and identity change

16. Match the discomfort with its primary physiologic cause:
    1. ____Progesterone slows GI motility   A. Hemorrhoids
    2. ____Uterine pressure on the diaphragm   B. Constipation
    3. ____Venous congestion in rectal veins   C. Heartburn
    4. ____Relaxed esophageal sphincter   D. Dyspnea

Fill in the Blank

17. The immune adjustment in pregnancy that balances tolerance of the fetus with defense against infection is called _____.

18. The rapid mood shifts common in pregnancy are called _____.

19. Increased vascularity in the pelvis can cause _____, which may heighten sensitivity or discomfort during sex.

20. The increased blood volume in pregnancy often leads to _____ anemia.

21. The hormone primarily responsible for stimulating uterine growth and increasing uteroplacental blood flow is _____.

True/False

22. _____ Carpal tunnel syndrome in pregnancy is primarily caused by fluid retention and nerve compression.

23. _____ Emotional lability during pregnancy is usually a sign of a serious mood disorder.

24. _____ Most common discomforts of pregnancy are benign, but persistent or severe symptoms may require further evaluation.

25. _____ Libido changes during pregnancy are highly variable and not predictive of relationship problems.

26. _____ Supine hypotensive syndrome is caused by pressure of the gravid uterus on the vena cava when lying flat.

27. _____ Progesterone contributes to relaxation of smooth muscle, which can increase constipation and heartburn.

28. _____ Estrogen promotes increased blood flow to the skin, which can contribute to the "pregnancy glow."

29. _____ The kidneys filter less blood in pregnancy because of increased vascular resistance.

30. _____ Linea nigra is a temporary pigmentation change that usually fades postpartum.

31. _____ Increased joint laxity during pregnancy is caused primarily by the hormone relaxin.

32. _____ The maternal immune system shifts toward tolerance of the fetus while still defending against pathogens.

33. _____ Varicose veins and hemorrhoids are often worsened by increased venous pressure in late pregnancy.

34. _____ Quickening typically occurs later in women who have previously been pregnant (multiparas) than in those pregnant for the first time (primigravidas).

35. _____ Supine hypotensive syndrome can usually be relieved by having the mother lie on her left side.

Increase/Decrease

36. Indicate whether the following cardiovascular changes normally **increase (↑)** or **decrease (↓)** during pregnancy:
    - A. _____ Heart size
    - B. _____ Resting heart rate
    - C. _____ Hematocrit
    - D. _____ Blood volume
    - E. _____ Cardiac output

37. Indicate whether following normally increase (↑) or decrease (↓) during pregnancy:
    - A. _____ Tidal volume
    - B. _____ Functional residual capacity
    - C. _____ Glomerular filtration rate (GFR)
    - D. _____ Bladder capacity
    - E. _____ Total body water
    - F. _____ Skin pigmentation changes (e.g., chloasma, linea nigra)
    - G. _____ Gastrointestinal motility
    - H. _____ Joint stability
    - I. _____ Immune tolerance
    - J. _____ Libido (average trend — though individual variation is wide)

Chapter Seven Reading & References

Recommended Reading: Physiology of Pregnancy

- Varney, H., Kriebs, J. M., & Gegor, C. L. (2014). ***Varney's Midwifery*** (5th ed.). Jones & Bartlett Learning. Comprehensive midwifery textbook that integrates physiology with management of pregnancy and birth.
- Miles, M. (2020). ***Textbook for Midwives*** (17th ed.). Elsevier. Classic midwifery reference, widely used in education, covering anatomy, physiology, and applied midwifery practice.
- Wylie, L. (2016). ***Essential Anatomy & Physiology in Maternity Care*** (2nd ed.). Churchill Livingstone/Elsevier. Accessible and student-friendly, directly connecting A&P with maternity care practice.
- Coad, J., & Dunstall, M. (2020). ***Anatomy and Physiology for Midwives*** (4th ed.). Elsevier. Written specifically for midwifery students, this text presents complex concepts in a clear, approachable format.
- Stables, D., & Rankin, J. (2010). ***Physiology in Childbearing with Anatomy and Related Biosciences*** (3rd ed.). Elsevier. Focused on applying physiology to childbearing, bridging science and practice in an accessible way.
- Hesperian Foundation. (2015.). ***Where There Is No Midwife.*** A practical community-based resource, emphasizing physiological understanding and supportive care in pregnancy.

References

Blackburn, S. T. (2017). *Maternal, fetal, and neonatal physiology: A clinical perspective* (5th ed.). Elsevier.

Cunningham, F. G., Leveno, K. J., Bloom, S. L., Dashe, J. S., Hoffman, B. L., Casey, B. M., & Spong, C. Y. (2018). *Williams obstetrics* (25th ed.). McGraw-Hill Education.

Fraser, D. M., & Cooper, M. A. (2021). *Myles' textbook for midwives* (17th ed.). Elsevier.

Hesperian Foundation. (2015). *Where there is no midwife*. Hesperian Health Guides.

Hoekzema, E., Barba-Müller, E., Pozzobon, C., Picado, M., Lucco, F., García-García, D., Soliva, J. C., Tobeña, A., Desco, M., Crone, E. A., Ballesteros, A., & Carmona, S. (2017). Pregnancy leads to long-lasting changes in human brain structure. *Nature Neuroscience*, 20(2), 287–296. https://doi.org/10.1038/nn.4458

International Forum for Wellbeing in Pregnancy. (n.d.). *Psychological changes during pregnancy*. https://www.ifwip.org/psychological-changes-during-pregnancy/

King, T. L., & Klass, C. S. (2017). *Varney's midwifery* (6th ed.). Jones & Bartlett Learning.

Lockwood, C. J., & Magriples, U. (2022). *Normal physiology of pregnancy*. UpToDate. Retrieved Month Day, Year, from https://www.uptodate.com

Merck Manual Professional Edition. (n.d.). *Physiology of pregnancy*. https://www.merckmanuals.com/professional/gynecology-and-obstetrics/approach-to-the-pregnant-woman-and-prenatal-care/physiology-of-pregnancy

Mor, G., & Cardenas, I. (2010). The immune system in pregnancy: A unique complexity. *American Journal of Reproductive Immunology*, 63(6), 425–433. https://doi.org/10.1111/j.1600-0897.2010.00836.x

National Center for Biotechnology Information. (2019). *Physiology of pregnancy*. https://www.ncbi.nlm.nih.gov/books/NBK539766/

Pairman, S., Tracy, S., Dahlen, H., & Dixon, L. (2019). *Midwifery: Preparation for practice* (4th ed.). Elsevier.

Physiopedia. (n.d.). *Physiological changes in pregnancy*. https://www.physiopedia.com/Physiological_Changes_in_Pregnancy

Sherwood, L. (2015). *Human physiology: From cells to systems* (9th ed.). Cengage Learning.

Soma-Pillay, P., Nelson-Piercy, C., Tolppanen, H., & Mebazaa, A. (2016). Physiological changes in pregnancy. *Cardiovascular Journal of Africa*, 27(2), 89–94. https://doi.org/10.5830/CVJA-2016-021

Stables, D., & Rankin, J. (2010). *Physiology in childbearing with anatomy and related biosciences* (4th ed.). Elsevier.

Wylie, L. (2016). *Essential anatomy and physiology in maternity care* (2nd ed.). Elsevier.

Chapter Eight:
Health Promotion for Midwives

Objectives
After completing this chapter, the student should be able to:
1. Comprehend the midwife's role in prenatal nutrition, education, and counseling.
2. Understand the role nutrition plays in the outcome of pregnancy.
3. Comprehend how to review a history for nutritional risk factors.
4. Identify nutritional risk factors in pregnancy.
5. Review nutritional requirements during pregnancy.
6. Explain the role of iron in pregnancy and how it is absorbed and utilized.
7. List foods high in necessary nutrients required during pregnancy.
8. Describe the functions of necessary nutrients during pregnancy.
9. Explain the physical and psychological benefits of prenatal exercise.
10. Discuss guidelines for exercising safely during pregnancy.
11. Identify conditions:
    - with contraindications for exercise during pregnancy;
    - that would gain additional benefit from prenatal exercise;
    - that would necessitate modifying or limiting prenatal exercise.
12. Describe several benefits of using herbs during pregnancy.
13. Explain why certain types of herbs are not recommended in pregnancy.
14. List specific herbs contraindicated in pregnancy.

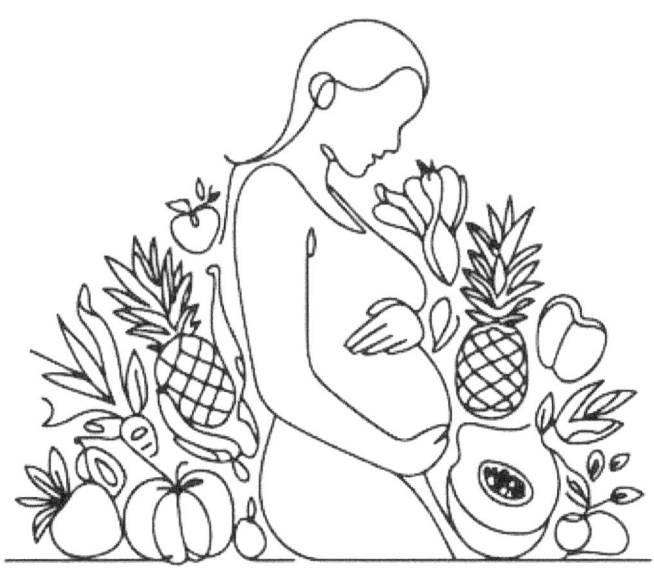

Introduction to Health Promotion in Pregnancy

The Midwife's Role

Midwives play a unique and powerful role as educators throughout the pregnancy journey. Pregnancy is often a time of reflection, motivation, and openness to change. Many clients improve their diet, begin exercising, or learn to manage stress because they want to give their baby the best start possible. These changes, though prompted by pregnancy, often lead to lasting improvements in the parent's health and well-being.

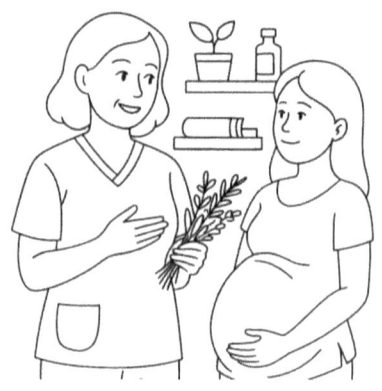

For midwives, becoming a trusted guide involves more than sharing facts. It means building relationships, communicating clearly, and offering information that respects a client's personal values and lived experience. A woman's ability to access good nutrition, safe exercise, or herbal care may be shaped as much by her circumstances as by her choices. Midwifery education is not about giving lectures; it is about listening deeply, validating knowledge, and providing information in ways that empower and respect autonomy.

Midwives help clients learn by:
- Validating their existing knowledge and lived experience
- Using clear, accessible, and nonjudgmental language
- Offering tools and resources rather than prescriptive advice
- Supporting decision-making instead of pushing an agenda

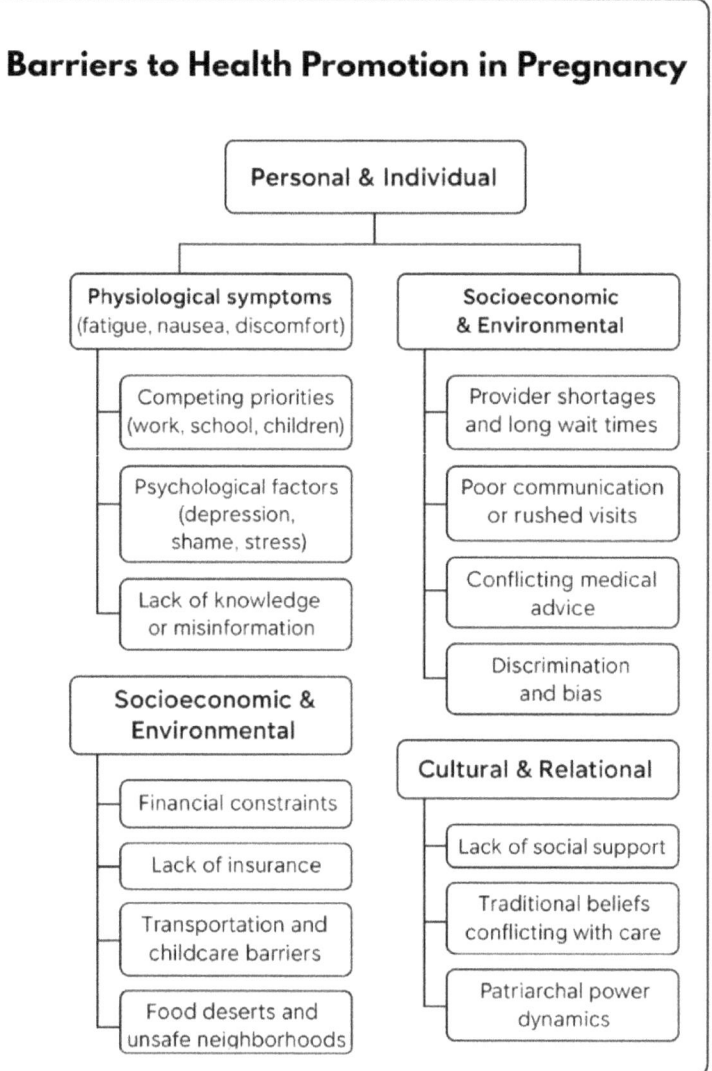

Pregnancy also brings more frequent contact with healthcare providers, creating repeated opportunities for education and encouragement. Midwives can use these touchpoints to introduce new ideas gradually, reinforce them over time, and build confidence.

At the same time, not all clients have equal access to the resources needed to make healthy changes. Intersectionality reminds us that multiple factors such as race, culture, income, immigration status, body size, education, and language interact with systems of power and privilege. These factors shape which recommendations feel realistic and how care is received. For instance, a client may know what foods are recommended but live in a food desert, or may feel conflicted between medical advice and family traditions. Midwives who understand these complexities can offer education that is compassionate, realistic, and grounded in the client's full context.

In practice, midwives often find that health promotion happens in small, meaningful moments. A gentle question during a blood pressure check, a follow-up from a previous visit, or a quiet word of encouragement can open the door to deeper conversations about nutrition, stress, relationships, and self-care. These interactions build trust, and trust allows clients to share what they are really experiencing.

Midwives learn to read body language and tone as well as words. A client may say, *"I'm fine,"* while clearly holding back tears. Asking, *"What's feeling heavy this week?"* or *"Is there anything taking up space in your mind?"* can create a safe opening for honest discussion. Not every topic will be addressed at every visit, and that is okay. Health promotion is a gradual process that unfolds over time.

Midwives quickly learn that pacing matters. Education offered in small, manageable pieces is easier to absorb and apply. A calm, respectful approach allows clients to feel supported rather than judged. Building a culturally grounded understanding of food and health beliefs, especially within Hispanic, African, Asian, and East Indian communities, can transform care. When midwives are familiar with traditional foods, home remedies, and postpartum healing customs, they can provide guidance that is relevant and respectful rather than contradictory.

Midwives should also be aware of the structural barriers clients face. Resistance to a recommendation may reflect deeper issues such as food insecurity, housing instability, language barriers, or past trauma. Understanding how racism, classism, or fatphobia affect health access helps midwives offer care that is compassionate and realistic. This begins by listening well, asking thoughtful questions, and trusting the client's innate capacity to know what is best for themselves and their baby. Health promotion in pregnancy goes beyond just nutrition or exercise. It includes the mental, emotional, social, and environmental factors that influence a person's well-being. Midwives have the opportunity to talk with clients about stress, sleep, relationships, body image, substance use, and other core areas that affect health. These conversations help clients feel heard and supported, and they build trust over time. They are also an opportunity to screen for risk factors and offer resources in a way that is respectful and nonjudgmental.

Exercise 8.1: Principles of Health Promotion	
Match each midwifery action with the principle it supports:	
1. _____ Asking open-ended questions	A. Cultural humility
2. _____ Learning about dietary traditions	B. Building trust through relevance
3. _____ Explaining one new health concept per visit	C. Avoiding overload
4. _____ Validating a client's existing knowledge	D. Respecting client experience

CORE HEALTH PROMOTION TOPICS

Stress Management

Pregnancy can be both exciting and overwhelming. Many clients carry stress related to work, finances, family dynamics, past trauma, or fear about birth. Chronic stress can affect sleep, digestion, blood pressure, and even fetal development. While stress is a normal part of life, high or unrelenting stress during pregnancy can be harmful.

Midwives do not need to eliminate stress for their clients, but they can offer helpful tools and referrals. These may include breathing exercises, journaling, therapy, mindfulness, movement, prayer, cultural or spiritual practices, and more. The goal is not to shame clients for feeling overwhelmed, but to normalize their experience and offer a path toward greater balance. Mental health screening should also be offered using the **Edinburgh Postnatal Depression Scale** (EPDS), even before birth.

Chronic stress can negatively impact pregnancy outcomes.
- Every client experiences stress differently.
- Supportive relationships, counseling, and simple grounding techniques can be helpful.
- Midwives can screen for stress and offer realistic, culturally appropriate options.

Self-Esteem and Body Image

Pregnancy often changes the way people feel about their bodies. Some feel powerful and proud, while others may struggle with weight gain, stretch marks, or feeling out of control. Past trauma, eating disorders, and cultural pressures can all shape a client's experience of their changing body.

Midwives can help by holding a neutral, affirming, and body-positive space. It is not the midwife's role to comment on appearance or weight unless clinically indicated, and even then, how it is framed matters. Language should be nonjudgmental and focused on function, strength, and health rather than size or aesthetics.

Pregnancy can affect how clients feel about their body and self-worth:
- Midwives should avoid appearance-based comments.
- Body neutrality or body positivity can support self-esteem.
- Clients with a history of disordered eating or trauma may need extra support.

Self-Care Behaviors

Clients often benefit from reminders to care for themselves in simple, consistent ways. This includes rest, hydration, movement, asking for help, setting boundaries, and nourishing routines. For many clients, especially parents of other children or those working multiple jobs, self-care may feel unrealistic or selfish.

Midwives can help reframe self-care as a survival tool, not a luxury. They can also help clients identify small daily actions that feel doable within their own life circumstances.

Self-care includes:
- Basic needs like rest, hydration, and asking for help.
- Barriers to self-care should be acknowledged without judgment.
- Midwives can help clients create realistic self-care goals that match their life context.

Healthy Relationships and Social Support

Pregnancy can bring relationship changes, both supportive and stressful. Some clients feel deeply nurtured by partners, family, or friends, while others feel isolated, controlled, or unsafe. Strong social support is linked to better outcomes in pregnancy, including lower rates of depression, anxiety, and preterm birth.

Midwives can gently ask about emotional and physical safety, as well as who helps the client feel supported.

> **Key Fact**
> Strong social support during pregnancy is linked to lower rates of depression, anxiety, and preterm birth. Having a trusted partner, friend, or community member can significantly improve outcomes for both mother and baby.

Social support improves outcomes for both parent and baby.
- Relationship strain or isolation may surface during pregnancy.
- Midwives can screen for safety and refer when needed.
- Culturally safe practices should be used when discussing family dynamics.

Pregnant women may find support and strength through a variety of community or spiritual connections, including:
- Faith-based gatherings such as church services, temple, mosque, synagogue, or prayer circles.
- Cultural or community events such as powwows, community feasts, naming ceremonies, or seasonal festivals.
- Supportive group activities such as prenatal yoga classes, childbirth education groups, talking circles, or peer support groups.
- Social and community connections such as volunteering, parent meetups, book clubs, women's circles, or neighborhood gatherings.

These connections lessen isolation, reinforce belonging, and strengthen resilience for both mother and family.

Intimate Partner Violence Screening

Midwives play a vital role in assessing both physical and emotional safety in a way that is supportive, nonjudgmental, and trauma-informed. All clients should be screened for intimate partner violence (IPV) during pregnancy in a private setting using validated tools and sensitive, trauma-informed approaches.

IPV affects an estimated **4% to 8% of pregnant women** in the United States, with higher rates in marginalized or under-resourced communities. Research shows that violence often **begins or intensifies during pregnancy**, and is associated with preterm birth, low birth weight, placental abruption, postpartum depression, and even homicide, which is one of the leading causes of death in pregnancy and the first postpartum year.

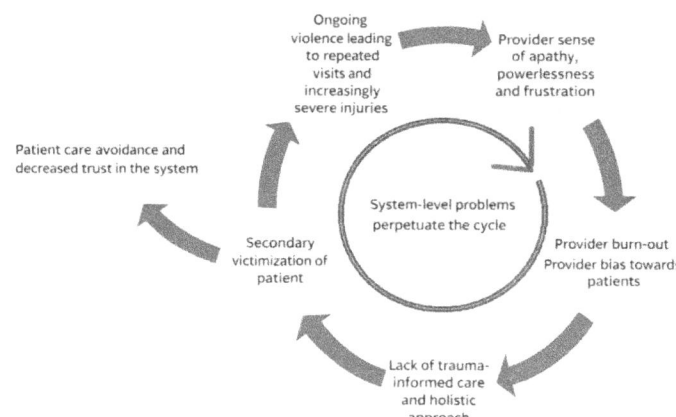

When Safety Is Missed:
Cycles Created by Unaddressed Intimate Partner Violence

Midwives should screen early and repeat screening throughout pregnancy and the postpartum period. Positive screening should be met with validation, reassurance, and practical support. Midwives should maintain an updated list of **local and national resources**—including shelters, hotlines, and advocacy programs—and know how to connect clients discreetly and safely.

- IPV screening is a standard of care and should be repeated throughout pregnancy and postpartum.
- Screening must be private and compassionate, never in the presence of a partner or family member.
- Always document findings objectively, using the client's own words when possible, and ensure confidentiality to the extent the law allows.

Lifestyle Safety Considerations

Environmental safety also includes common household and personal risks that can be minimized with awareness and support. Preventable injuries are a leading cause of harm during pregnancy and postpartum, particularly among those caring for young children, working physically demanding jobs, or living in under-resourced housing.

Basic home and lifestyle safety practices should be reviewed during prenatal care. These include functional smoke alarms and carbon monoxide detectors, hot water heaters set below 120°F, medications and chemicals stored safely out of reach, secure locks and adequate lighting, stable furniture, and clear walkways to reduce falls or tip-over injuries. Families should also consider whether they are prepared for common emergencies, such as power outages.

Movement and daily activity should also be addressed. Counsel clients on consistent seatbelt use (lap belt under the belly, shoulder belt between the breasts), supportive footwear with good traction, and caution on wet or uneven ground. Advise against climbing ladders or working on unstable surfaces. Encourage safe body mechanics for lifting and turning, and remind clients to pause activity if they experience dizziness, swelling, or fatigue.

Clients may not control their entire environment. Midwives can support them in assessing risks without blame or pressure. When available, home-visitor programs or community agencies may provide supplies such as smoke detectors, outlet covers, or bath thermometers.

Important to Remember

- Many pregnancy-related injuries are preventable with simple changes.
- Footwear, lighting, body mechanics, and environmental awareness matter.
- Midwives should offer respectful, realistic safety education.
- Clients in shared, transitional, or under-resourced housing may need tailored support.
- Reinforce seatbelt use and fall-risk awareness as pregnancy progresses.

Environmental Exposures in Pregnancy

Environmental exposures can affect pregnancy outcomes. Common concerns include lead, pesticides, workplace chemicals, mold, and infections from pets such as toxoplasmosis. Clients may also become more aware of the substances and environments they encounter daily; some carry clear risks, while others require individualized counseling.

Common Environmental Exposures
- Pesticides in food and on lawns
- BPA in plastics and food containers
- Phthalates and parabens in body products
- Lead from old paint or pipes
- Mercury in certain fish
- Formaldehyde in furniture or nail salons

Midwives play an important role in screening for environmental health risks by asking targeted questions about the home, workplace, and community, with attention to income, housing, food access, and cultural norms. Guidance should emphasize achievable changes rather than creating fear or shame. Although avoiding all exposures is unrealistic, midwives can help clients reduce unnecessary contact with known or suspected toxins through practical adjustments such as improving ventilation, using protective equipment, or avoiding certain tasks.

Important to Remember
- Many environmental chemicals are unregulated in the US and may affect reproductive health.
- Complete avoidance is not realistic, but reduction strategies can lower risk.
- Clients should not be shamed for exposures they cannot avoid.
- Avoid handling cat litter; wear gloves when gardening to prevent toxoplasmosis exposure.

Reducing Chemical Exposures

Exposure	Safer option
Pesticides on produce	Wash thoroughly or choose organic when possible
BPA in plastics	Use glass or stainless steel containers
Phthalates/parabens	Choose fragrance-free, low-toxicity products
Mercury in fish	Opt for salmon, sardines, or trout
Harsh cleaning chemicals	Use vinegar, baking soda, or castile soap
Air fresheners/fragrances	Ventilate rooms, simmer citrus or herbs
Chemical sunscreens	Use mineral-based sunscreen (zinc or titanium)
Hair/nail products with fumes	Choose low-toxicity brands; ventilate well
Dry cleaning chemicals	Air out clothes before wearing

Exercise 8.2: Reducing exposures

Answer the following questions:

1. List two environmental exposures that may affect pregnancy.

2. What are two practical strategies clients can use to reduce exposure at home?

3. How might a midwife introduce this topic without creating fear or shame?

Harm Reduction: Tobacco, Alcohol, Cannabis, and Substance Use

While many clients choose midwifery care because they are health conscious, midwives increasingly work in all kinds of settings with all types of clients. Some may enter care using tobacco, alcohol, cannabis, or other substances. They may be open to change, unsure, or fearful of being judged. Midwives can approach these conversations using a harm reduction model that centers dignity, relationship, and safety rather than punishment. When discussing substance use, avoid yes/no questions. Instead, ask open-ended questions like, *"What helps you relax when you feel stressed?"* This builds trust and may open the door to safer options and gradual change.

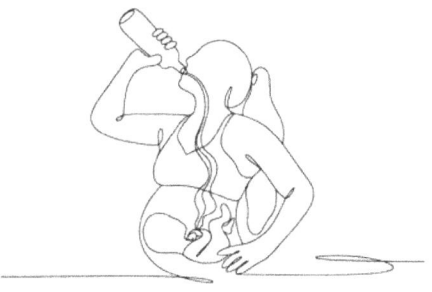

The goal is to understand the client's story, offer support and information, and help them reduce risk in ways that feel manageable. Building trust may lead to long-term change, even if it begins with small steps.

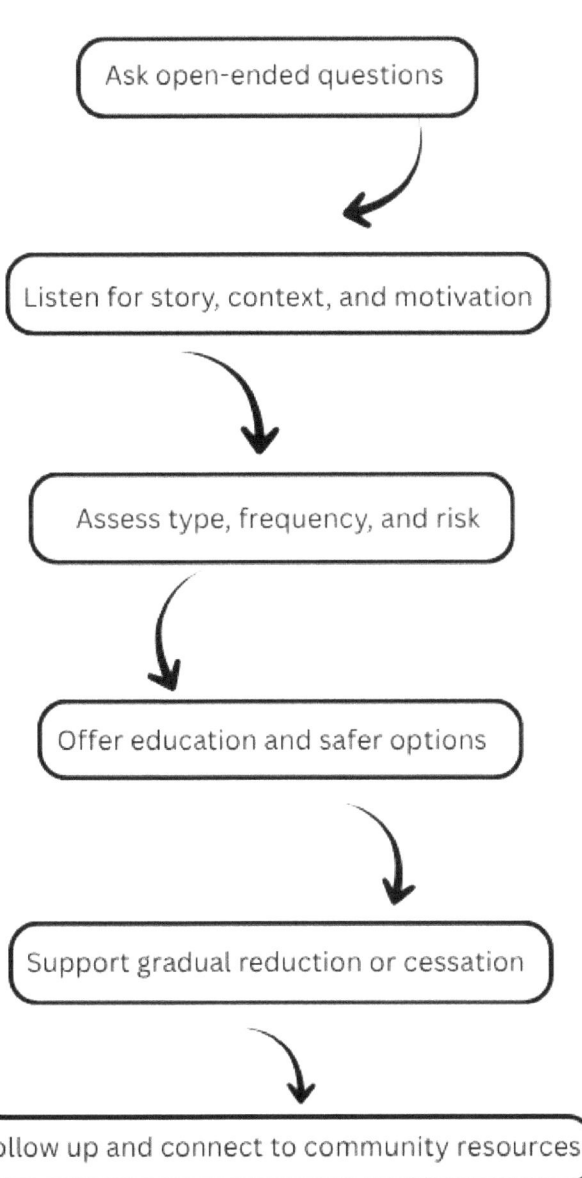

Midwife's Approach to Substance Use

- Ask open-ended questions
- Listen for story, context, and motivation
- Assess type, frequency, and risk
- Offer education and safer options
- Support gradual reduction or cessation
- Follow up and connect to community resources

Important to Remember

- **Tobacco** increases risks such as low birth weight, preterm birth, and placental problems; support nicotine replacement or gradual reduction if quitting feels overwhelming.
- **Alcohol** has no known safe level in pregnancy; emphasize complete avoidance while supporting clients with honesty and without shame.
- **Cannabis** current guidelines recommend avoiding it during pregnancy and lactation, but harm reduction may mean exploring reasons for use and safer alternatives.
- **Street drugs and prescription misuse** (opioids, stimulants, cocaine, sedatives, etc.) carry significant risks; apply harm reduction principles, connect clients with resources, and avoid punitive or shaming language.

Cannabis is sometimes framed as a natural alternative to prescription medications for nausea, pain, anxiety, or insomnia. Some clients report it improves appetite or relieves nausea. Others may have used cannabis regularly before pregnancy and are unsure whether to continue.

While cannabis is widely used and legal in many states, professional guidelines currently recommend avoiding cannabis use in pregnancy and lactation. Concerns include potential effects on fetal brain development, low birth weight, and preterm birth. Research is still emerging, and some clients may have limited access to safer alternatives.

Midwives should approach cannabis use in pregnancy with the same harm reduction framework. Rather than judging or warning clients, explore the reasons for use, frequency, and form. If the client relies on cannabis for symptom relief, offer safer or more targeted alternatives and follow up regularly. Discuss avoiding high-THC strains, synthetic cannabinoids, or concentrates. Support clients in cutting back or stopping use safely and respectfully when they are ready.

Exercise 8.3: Health Promotion Checklist

Check each area of health promotion that should be discussed or assessed during prenatal visits.

Health Promotion Focus	Midwifery Actions
Stress management	☐ Ask about stress sources and coping strategies. ☐ Offer grounding, breathing, or mindfulness options. ☐ Refer for counseling or therapy when needed.
Self-esteem and body image	☐ Use body-neutral language. ☐ Avoid appearance-based comments. ☐ Validate strength and function over size.
Self-care	☐ Encourage small, realistic self-care goals (hydration, rest, support). ☐ Normalize asking for help. ☐ Address barriers without judgment.
Healthy relationships and social support	☐ Ask who helps the client feel supported. ☐ Encourage social, cultural, or spiritual connections. ☐ Screen for isolation or control.
Intimate partner violence screening	☐ Use private, trauma-informed screening tools. ☐ Document in the client's words. ☐ Provide discreet referrals to hotlines or shelters.
Lifestyle and environmental safety	☐ Discuss home and work safety. ☐ Review seatbelt use, fall prevention, and emergency preparedness. ☐ Offer community safety resources.
Substance Use	☐ Review use of alcohol, tobacco, cannabis and street drugs. ☐ Assess type and frequency. ☐ Offer community resources.

Reflection

1. Which of these areas feel most natural for you to discuss with clients?

2. Which might require more practice, sensitivity, or supervision?

Nutrition in Pregnancy

Nutrition plays a central role in the health of the pregnant woman and the developing fetus. A balanced diet supports fetal growth, placental development, energy levels, and healthy weight gain throughout pregnancy. Adequate intake of protein, calories, vitamins, and minerals helps prevent complications such as anemia, low birth weight, and preterm birth.

In the late 20th century, British epidemiologist Dr. David Barker introduced what became known as the **Barker Hypothesis**, the idea that adult diseases often originate in the womb. His research showed that poor nutrition during pregnancy could permanently alter fetal development, increasing the child's risk for heart disease, diabetes, and stroke later in life. Barker's work challenged the belief that chronic illness begins only in adulthood and reframed maternal nutrition as a lifelong determinant of health.

One of the most striking examples came from the Dutch Hunger Winter of 1944–45, when pregnant women experienced severe famine during World War II. Decades later, studies of their children revealed higher rates of obesity, diabetes, and cardiovascular disease compared with those conceived after the famine. These findings supported Barker's theory that inadequate nutrition during critical periods of fetal growth can "program" the body's metabolism, blood pressure, and organ development for life.

For midwives, Barker's work underscores the importance of supporting balanced, nutrient-dense diets throughout pregnancy. Adequate maternal nutrition not only promotes healthy fetal growth but also lays the foundation for lifelong wellness in the next generation.

Nutrition, however, is more than nutrients. Food is deeply social and emotional. What people eat is shaped by culture, family, memory, income, trauma, community, and convenience. Education about nutrition during pregnancy is one of the most important roles of a midwife. Many clients enter pregnancy with limited nutrition education or with eating habits shaped by stress, poverty, trauma histories, or food insecurity.

Midwives are often the first providers to offer nutritional counseling, and their approach can make a lasting impact. Rather than offering rigid rules or idealized diets, midwives can help clients make meaningful improvements by starting with what they already eat, honoring what is important to them, and identifying small, sustainable changes that support nourishment and well-being. The key is to listen first and work with clients from where they are, not where you think they should be. Avoid pushing dietary dogmas or personal beliefs. Keep recommendations simple and practical. Some women may feel stressed if they cannot afford organic food, so keep budget in mind when making recommendations. Emphasize the importance of simple whole foods and of avoiding processed or fast foods whenever possible. One helpful guideline is the "flexitarian" diet: eat mostly plants, occasionally foods that eat plants, and avoid foods that are made in plants (factories).

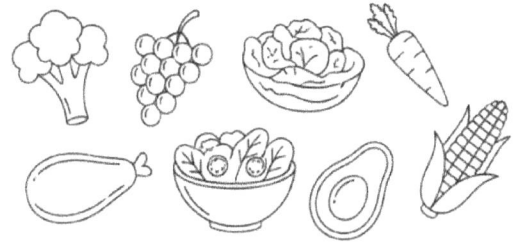

FLEXITARIAN DIET

EAT MOSTLY PLANTS

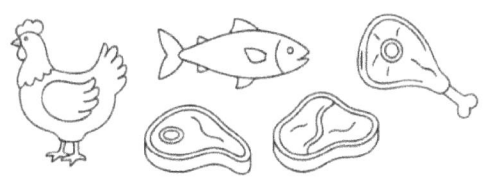

OCCASIONALLY THINGS THAT EAT PLANTS

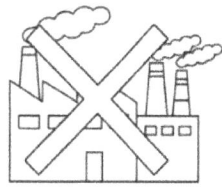

AVOID FOODS MADE IN PLANTS

Food, Culture, and Inclusion

Food is more than fuel; it is family, memory, survival, and love. Many clients come to pregnancy with eating patterns shaped by culture, religion, trauma, or tradition. Some follow vegetarian, vegan, halal, kosher, gluten-free, or intuitive eating practices, while others simply eat according to inherited or community foodways. These choices may reflect joy, belonging, or resource limitations influenced by colonization, migration, or poverty.

Midwives can promote dignity and trust by asking about each client's lived experience and affirming what already works in their diet. Build from, rather than replace, cultural foodways. For example, iron-rich foods may include lentils or blackstrap molasses for vegetarians, or organ meats and plantains in African or Caribbean traditions. Clients are more likely to make lasting changes when those changes respect their identity and values.

- Food is deeply tied to culture, memory, safety, and identity.
- Traditional foodways often include nutrient-dense ingredients that support pregnancy.
- Guidance is most effective when lived experience is respected.
- Midwives should ask open-ended questions and remain curious, not prescriptive.
- Counseling should consider the impact of trauma, colonialism, migration, and food access.

Food sovereignty is the right of people and communities to define their own food systems and maintain control over how food is grown, shared, and eaten. Originating in Indigenous and tribal movements to reclaim traditional foodways and land stewardship, it now extends to all efforts that restore local food production, cultural connection, and community self-reliance. Supporting food sovereignty strengthens both maternal nutrition and long-term community health.

Key Vocabulary	
• **Complex Carbohydrate**: Starches; digested slowly, steady energy. • **Simple Carbohydrate**: Sugars; quick energy. • **Carbohydrate Types** – • *Monosaccharide*: single sugar (glucose). • *Disaccharide*: double sugar (sucrose, lactose). • *Polysaccharide*: many sugars (starch, glycogen). • **Refined**: Processed food with nutrients removed. • **Fortified**: Extra nutrients added. • **Enriched**: Nutrients replaced after processing. • **Protein**: Made of amino acids; builds and repairs tissues. • **Amino Acids**: Building blocks of proteins. • **Essential Amino Acids**: Must come from diet. • **Complementary Proteins**: Foods combined to supply all essential amino acids (beans + rice).	• **Essential Fatty Acids**: Needed fats the body cannot make. • **Types of Fats** – • *Saturated*: solid at room temp; excess raises cholesterol. • *Monounsaturated*: olive oil, avocado; heart-healthy. • *Polyunsaturated*: includes omega-3 & omega-6. • **Fiber**: Undigested plant material; supports digestion. • *Soluble*: lowers cholesterol, regulates blood sugar. • **Antioxidant**: Protects cells from free radical damage. • **Minerals**: Inorganic nutrients (e.g., calcium, iron). • **Trace Minerals**: Needed in tiny amounts (zinc, iodine). • **Cholesterol Types** – • *LDL*: "bad" cholesterol; clogs arteries. • *HDL*: "good" cholesterol; clears LDL.

FOOD INSECURITY

Some clients live in settings where shopping, storing, or preparing food is difficult. Others may have limited access to fresh groceries due to income, transportation, or housing instability. Food insecurity is a recognized social determinant of health, and during pregnancy it may influence not only what someone eats, but also how they feel about eating. The stress of not knowing where the next meal is coming from can increase anxiety, affect sleep, and shape a person's overall experience of pregnancy.

Food insecurity can affect people from many different social and economic strata, though it is more common among those facing systemic inequities. With the recent increase in grocery prices, even families who were once stable may find themselves struggling. Many clients may feel reluctant to bring this up because of shame, fear of judgment, or past negative experiences with health care providers. For this reason, it is important that midwives ask in a compassionate, nonjudgmental way. Open-ended questions such as, *"What's been hard about eating well right now?"* or *"Do you ever find it difficult to get enough healthy food for yourself or your family?"* can open the door to honest conversations.

Clients experiencing food insecurity may eat whatever is available, rely heavily on convenience or fast foods, or skip meals entirely. These choices are often shaped by circumstances, not preference. A person may want to eat more fruits and vegetables but live in a "food desert" with limited access. Others may have to choose between buying food and paying rent, or may lack refrigeration or a working stove to store and prepare meals. Recognizing these realities helps midwives understand that food patterns are not always about knowledge or willpower.

Midwives can offer meaningful support by providing judgment-free guidance, validating the client's experience, and offering practical resources. Having an updated list of local food pantries, community kitchens, WIC offices, farmer's markets that accept food benefits, and culturally appropriate food programs can make a real difference. Even small suggestions, like connecting clients with community gardens or meal delivery programs, may help them feel supported.

It is not the midwife's role to "fix" food insecurity, but simply listening, normalizing the struggle, and offering gentle support can be powerful. Encouraging regular meals, reducing shame around food choices, and affirming the importance of nourishment in pregnancy can help clients feel more confident and cared for. By acknowledging the broader context of food access, midwives can empower clients to make the best possible choices within their circumstances and feel less isolated in the process.

Food Insecurity in Pregnancy

Barriers
- Facing rising grocery prices
- Lacking reliable transportation
- Experiencing housing instability
- Living in food deserts

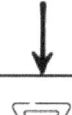

Impacts
- Skipping meals
- Experiencing stress and anxiety
- Having limited choices
- Relying on processed foods

Midwife Support
- Listening without judgment
- Normalizing the experience
- Encouraging regular meals
- Referring to resources

Exercise 8.4: Nutritional Counseling
Fill in the Blank:

1. Food is often tied to _____, _____, _____, and survival.

2. Some clients may eat irregularly due to _____, _____, or limited access to a kitchen.

3. The approach that supports hunger cues and body trust is called _____.

4. Emotional eating, bingeing, or restricting may be signs of _____ or trauma history.

5. Midwives can build trust by starting with what clients _____ _____.

Assessing Nutritional Needs

Some midwives offer advanced nutritional advice, have the client write a three-day diet diary, and some either through questionnaires or interview assess nutritional needs with this advice.

Nutrition-Related Risk Factors: Past Health History
1. **Anemia or significant blood loss** (heavy periods, IUD use, surgery, accidents). Blood loss can deplete iron, folate, copper, and vitamin B12.
2. **Frequent or recent infections.** May indicate increased needs for immune-supportive nutrients such as vitamins C and D or zinc, or problems with absorption.
3. **Slow clotting time.** May reflect low vitamin K or calcium.
4. **Liver disease** (hepatitis or other conditions). The liver is central to nutrient metabolism; damage may impair absorption and storage.
5. **History of alcohol or substance use.** May lead to liver damage and nutrient depletion.
6. **Underweight or history of eating disorders** (anorexia, bulimia). Often associated with poor nutrient reserves.
7. **Rickets or past nutritional deficiencies.** Suggests risk for vitamin D or calcium deficiency.
8. **Digestive disorders** (colitis, celiac disease, chronic diarrhea, or parasites). These can reduce nutrient absorption.
9. **Closely spaced pregnancies.** Short recovery time increases nutritional demands.
10. **Pregnancy while breastfeeding, or within 3 months of weaning.** Nutrient stores may already be low.
11. **Diabetes** (type 1, type 2, or gestational in prior pregnancy). Increases monitoring needs for blood sugar and diet quality.
12. **Family history of anemia or diabetes.** Suggests possible inherited risk.
13. **Pica.** Craving nonfood items (ice, dirt, clay, starch) may signal iron deficiency or other nutritional concerns.

> **Cultural Tradition**
> In many cultures, special pregnancy foods are believed to strengthen mother and baby. In Mexico, *caldo de pollo* (chicken soup) is often given. In parts of Asia, pregnancy is seen as a 'hot' state, so cooling foods may be restricted. Respecting these beliefs builds trust while supporting nutritional health.

Nutrition-Related Risk Factors: Current Pregnancy
If any of the following are present, the client may need more than standard prenatal nutritional support:
1. **Anemia**
2. **Smoking**
3. **Currently breastfeeding another child**
4. **Adolescent pregnancy (<19) or advanced maternal age (>35)**
5. **Strict vegetarian or vegan diet**
6. **Concern about or restriction of weight gain**
7. **Persistent nausea or vomiting (hyperemesis)**
8. **Bleeding gums or easy bruising** (possible vitamin C or K deficiency)
9. **Leg cramps** (possible calcium or magnesium deficiency)
10. **Vision changes** (night blindness, light sensitivity; possible vitamin A issue)
11. **Fatigue** (may suggest anemia, thyroid imbalance, or micronutrient deficiencies)
12. **Poor appetite**
13. **Skin rashes or conditions** (possible deficiencies in essential fatty acids, zinc, or other micronutrients)
14. **Frequent constipation**
15. **Upper right quadrant pain** (possible gallbladder or liver involvement)
16. **High physical demands** (athletes, physically strenuous jobs)
17. **Multiple pregnancy**
18. **Grand multiparity** (five or more pregnancies)
19. **Hypertension**

BASIC NUTRITIONAL REQUIREMENTS IN PREGNANCY

Calories

Calorie needs increase during pregnancy to support fetal growth and maternal tissue changes. Requirements vary by height, weight, age, and activity level.
On average:
- **First trimester:** No additional calories are generally needed.
- **Second trimester:** An additional ~340 calories per day is recommended.
- **Third trimester:** An additional ~450 calories per day is recommended.

This brings the average total intake for many pregnant women to about 2,200–2,800 calories daily, depending on activity. Adequate caloric intake is essential to protect protein from being used for energy and to ensure sufficient vitamins and minerals. Poor maternal weight gain is clearly linked to poor fetal growth and adverse outcomes.

Protein

Protein supplies the amino acids needed for tissue growth and maintenance. Uterine muscle, fetal organs, and connective tissues all depend on adequate protein intake. The current recommended dietary allowance (RDA) is about **71 grams per day** in pregnancy, beginning in the second trimester.
- **Good sources** include eggs, poultry, fish, lean meats, beans, lentils, nuts, seeds, and dairy products.
- Vegans and women with milk allergies an meet their needs with careful planning, emphasizing legumes, nuts, and combinations of grains and beans to create complete proteins.

> **Clinical Tip**
> It's entirely possible to reach 71 grams of protein on a vegan diet with planning and by combining plant sources:
> - 1 cup cooked **lentils** + 1 cup cooked **rice** ≈ 24 g protein
> - 1 cup **tofu** + ½ cup quinoa ≈ 30 g protein
> - 1 cup **black beans** + 2 **corn** tortillas ≈ 18 g protein
>
> *Add snacks such as nut butters, hummus, or fortified plant milks to meet daily needs.*

Fat

If calorie and protein needs are met, about 25–35% of total calories can safely come from fat. Emphasis should be on healthy fats, particularly omega-3 fatty acids, which support fetal brain and eye development.
- **Adequate Intake** (AI): ~13 grams/day of omega-6 and ~1.4 grams/day of omega-3 fatty acids.
- **Encourage fatty fish** (salmon, sardines, trout) 2–3 times per week.
- **Avoid** high-mercury fish such as shark, swordfish, king mackerel, and limit albacore tuna to 6 oz/week.
- **Plant** sources include flaxseed, chia seeds, walnuts, and canola oil.

Fiber

Fiber requirements are similar to those for non-pregnant women: about 28 grams per day. Adequate fluid intake is important, especially when fiber intake is increased, to prevent constipation.

Carbohydrates

Carbohydrates are the body's primary source of glucose, essential for both mother and fetus. The RDA in pregnancy is **175 grams per day**. Focus should be on complex carbohydrates such as whole grains, fruits, vegetables, and legumes.

Exercise 8.5: Daily Nutritional Requirements

Match each nutrient with its recommended daily intake during pregnancy:

1. _____ Calories (2nd trimester)	A.	175 grams per day
2. _____ Protein	B.	340 additional calories per day
3. _____ Fiber	C.	71 grams per day
4. _____ Carbohydrates	D.	28 grams per day
5. _____ Omega-3 fatty acids	E.	1.5 grams per day

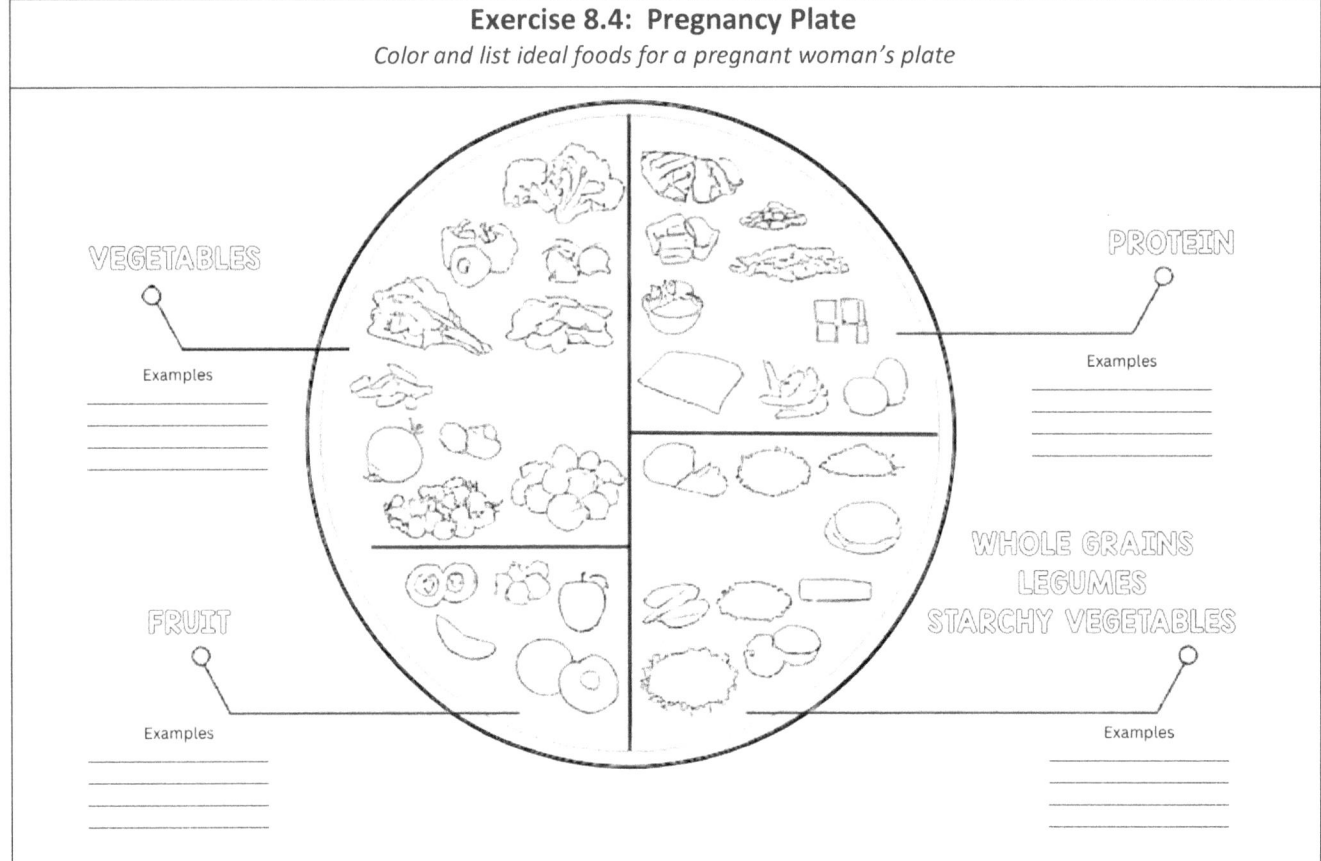

Micronutrients in Focus

While food should be the primary source of nutrients in a healthy pregnancy, many clients benefit from targeted supplementation to meet their changing needs. Even with a balanced diet, it can be difficult to obtain enough folate, iron, B12, iodine, choline, and vitamin D from food alone. Some clients may have higher requirements due to dietary choices, absorption issues, or medical conditions. Midwives should understand which micronutrients are essential, when supplementation is recommended, and how to individualize support for each client.

Prenatal supplements vary widely in quality and content:
- Not all essential nutrients are included in one formula.
- Midwives should help clients review labels and choose high-quality options.
- Additional testing or supplementation may be needed based on diet and lab values.

Vitamin A

Vitamin A is important for vision, especially in dim light, and for healthy skin and epithelial tissues. Deficiency can cause night blindness. However, excess intake (usually from high-dose supplements or liver products) can be toxic and has been linked to fetal malformations.
- Safe intake during pregnancy is **770 mcg (2,565 IU) RAE** per day.
- Avoid high-dose supplements or large amounts of liver.
- Emphasize food sources such as carrots, sweet potatoes, spinach, and fortified dairy.

Vitamin C and B Complex

Vitamin C supports collagen formation, vascular health, and immune defense. The RDA in pregnancy is **85 mg per day**, usually met with a diet rich in fruits and vegetables. Large doses are unnecessary and may cause rebound deficiency in the infant if used excessively in pregnancy.

The B complex vitamins support energy metabolism, red blood cell formation, and nervous system health. B6 may help reduce nausea and vomiting. B12 is especially important for vegetarians and vegans, as deficiency can cause anemia and neurological issues.

Calcium

Calcium supports bone and tooth development, blood clotting, muscle function, and blood pressure regulation. During pregnancy, calcium absorption increases, making intake more efficient.

An old saying claimed that *"for every child, a mother loses a tooth."* While not literally true, it reflects the real risk of maternal bone depletion if calcium intake is inadequate.

- The RDA is **1,000–1,200 mg/day** (1,300 mg/day for adolescents).
- Deficiency may contribute to leg cramps, headaches, bleeding gums, or bone loss.
- Dairy products are the most concentrated source; fortified plant milks, tofu, almonds, and leafy greens are vegetarian/vegan options.

> **Clinical Tip**
> Remind clients that calcium and vitamin D work together. Without enough vitamin D, the body cannot absorb calcium efficiently, even if intake is adequate.

Choline

- Recommended daily intake in pregnancy is **450 mg**.
- Supports brain development, memory, and neural tube health.
- Found in eggs, liver, fish, soy, and some legumes.
- Often missing from prenatal supplements.

> **Key Fact**
> Choline is essential for fetal brain development, but most prenatal vitamins do not contain it. Dietary sources such as eggs or targeted supplements may be needed.

Vitamin D

Vitamin D supports calcium absorption, bone health, immune function, and mood. Deficiency is common, especially in clients with limited sun exposure, darker skin, higher body weight, or those who live in northern climates. Testing may be considered in high-risk clients. Supplementation is often needed in addition to prenatal vitamins.

- Most prenatal vitamins contain only 400–600 IU of vitamin D.
- Optimal intake is closer to 1,000–2,000 IU per day for most clients.
- Deficiency may contribute to fatigue, low mood, or bone issues.
- Safe sun exposure and fortified foods are also helpful sources.

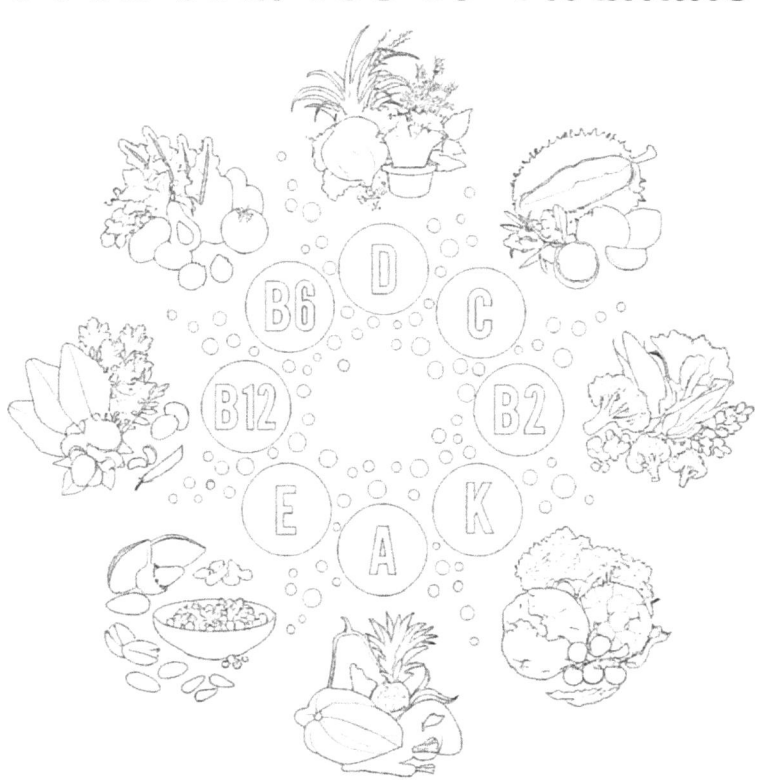

Food Sources of Vitamins

Folate and Folic Acid

Folate plays a critical role in early fetal development, particularly in closure of the neural tube. Synthetic folic acid is found in most prenatal vitamins and fortified foods, while natural folate is present in leafy greens and legumes. Supplementation is especially important in the first trimester and ideally should begin before conception. Clients with a history of neural tube defects, certain genetic conditions, or medications that interfere with folate metabolism may require higher doses.

- Folate is essential for preventing neural tube defects.
- The recommended intake is at least 400 mcg of folic acid per day.
- Begin supplementation ideally before conception or as soon as pregnancy is confirmed.
- Encourage dietary folate from foods like spinach, lentils, and avocado.

Iron

Iron needs increase significantly in pregnancy. Iron supports the expansion of blood volume, fetal growth, and placental development. The placenta actively transfers iron to the fetus, and the fetal liver stores iron to meet the infant's needs for the first six months. Low maternal iron in pregnancy has been linked to longer labors, increased pain from uterine muscle fatigue, postpartum depression, and higher infection risk. Deficiency can lead to anemia, fatigue, and increased risk of complications. Many clients benefit from iron-rich foods along with supplemental iron, especially in the second and third trimesters.

> **Clinical Tip**
> Iron supplements are not all the same. Ferrous sulfate is common but more likely to cause constipation. Ferrous gluconate, ferrous fumarate, or chelated forms such as iron bisglycinate are often gentler on digestion and may improve compliance.

- Daily intake should reach **27–30 mg** depending on diet and labs.
- Symptoms of deficiency include fatigue, dizziness, and shortness of breath.
- Choose gentle, food-based or chelated forms to reduce constipation.
- Monitor ferritin and hemoglobin as needed during prenatal care.
- Best absorbed with vitamin C; absorption is reduced by calcium, coffee, and tea.

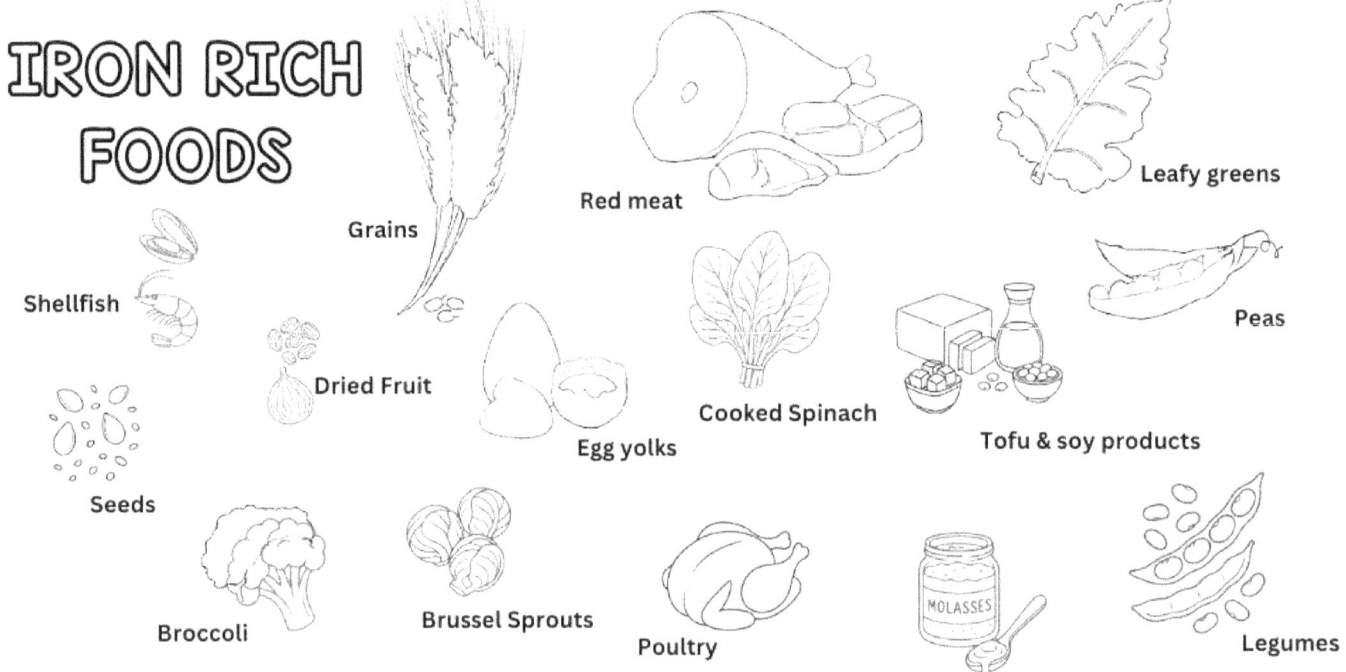

Minerals in Pregnancy

In addition to vitamins, minerals play critical roles in supporting maternal health and fetal development. *Some key minerals include:*

- **Zinc:** Supports cell growth, immunity, and wound healing. Deficiency may contribute to poor fetal growth and delayed wound healing postpartum.
- **Iodine:** Essential for thyroid function and fetal brain development. The RDA is **220 mcg/day** in pregnancy. Severe deficiency can cause goiter or developmental delays.
- **Copper:** Helps form red blood cells and connective tissue, and supports iron metabolism. Found in nuts, seeds, shellfish, and whole grains.
- **Potassium:** Important for fluid balance, blood pressure regulation, and muscle function. Found in fruits, vegetables, beans, and dairy products.

- **Magnesium and Calcium:** Already covered in detail, but both are central to bone health, muscle function, and blood pressure regulation.

Nutrition Quick Reference

Important vitamins and minerals in pregnancy and where to find them:
- **Vitamin A**–carrots, sweet potatoes, spinach, fortified dairy
- **Vitamin C**–citrus fruits, strawberries, bell peppers, tomatoes
- **Vitamin D**–sunlight, fortified milk, salmon, sardines, eggs
- **Vitamin E**–nuts, seeds, vegetable oils, leafy greens
- **Vitamin K**–kale, spinach, broccoli, cabbage
- **Folate/Folic Acid**–leafy greens, lentils, beans, fortified grains
- **Vitamin B6**–poultry, bananas, potatoes, fortified cereals
- **Vitamin B12**–meat, fish, eggs, dairy, fortified plant milks
- **Choline**–eggs, liver, soybeans, fish, legumes
- **Calcium**–milk, yogurt, cheese, fortified plant milks, almonds, tofu
- **Iron**–red meat, poultry, beans, lentils, spinach, fortified cereals
- **Iodine**–iodized salt, dairy, seaweed, fish
- **Zinc**–meat, poultry, beans, nuts, whole grains
- **Magnesium**–nuts, seeds, leafy greens, whole grains
- **Potassium**–bananas, oranges, potatoes, beans, dairy
- **Copper**–nuts, seeds, shellfish, whole grains

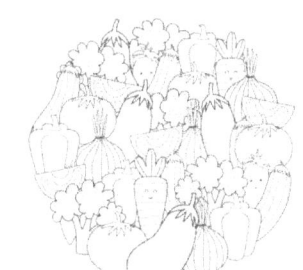

Exercise 8.6: Nutrition & Cultural Awareness

Match each term to its correct description:

1. _____ A religious dietary system observed in many Muslim households
2. _____ Traditions, rituals, and inherited eating patterns that shape what people eat
3. _____ An approach to eating that emphasizes body trust and responding to hunger and satisfaction cues
4. _____ Limited access to healthy food due to housing, transportation, or financial barriers
5. _____ The right of people and communities to define their own food systems and maintain control over how food is grown, shared, and eaten

A. Intuitive eating
B. Food insecurity
C. Halal
D. Food sovereignty
E. Cultural foodways

Exercise 8.7: Matching Nutrients and Roles
Match each micronutrient with its primary role in pregnancy:

1. _____ Supports neural tube closure and prevents birth defects
2. _____ Expands blood volume and prevents anemia
3. _____ Improves calcium absorption and immune function
4. _____ Supports brain and spinal cord development
5. _____ Promotes brain and visual development

A. Folate
B. Iron
C. Vitamin D
D. Choline
E. Omega-3 fatty acids

FOODS TO AVOID DURING PREGNANCY

Pregnant women are at higher risk of foodborne illness because hormonal changes can weaken the immune system and alter digestion. Even mild infections may pose greater risks during pregnancy, including dehydration, miscarriage, or preterm labor. Most foodborne illnesses can be prevented with careful food handling and preparation practices.

To reduce this risk:
- Wash all produce, even pre-washed items.
- Cook meats, poultry, and fish to safe internal temperatures (fish to 145°F until flaky and opaque; shellfish until clams and mussels open).
- Reheat leftovers and deli items until steaming hot.
- Avoid raw sprouts, unpasteurized dairy, and high-mercury fish.
- Avoid raw fish and shellfish such as sushi, sashimi, ceviche, and oysters.
- Avoid foods made with raw eggs, such as raw batter, hollandaise, or homemade Caesar dressing.
- Eat soft cheeses such as brie, feta, and blue cheese only if labeled "made with pasteurized milk."

Seafood and Mercury

Fish is an excellent source of protein and omega-3 fatty acids, which support fetal brain and eye development. However, larger and older fish tend to accumulate more mercury, which can affect the developing nervous system. Clients should avoid shark, swordfish, king mackerel, marlin, bigeye tuna, orange roughy, and tilefish. Safer options include salmon, sardines, trout, cod, shrimp, tilapia, catfish, and light canned tuna.

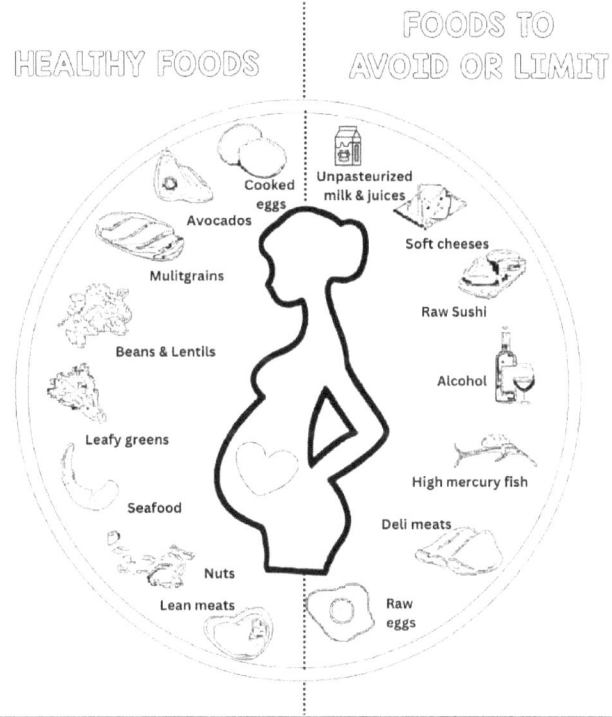

Exercise 8.8: Safe or Unsafe?
Circle whether each food is safe or unsafe to eat during pregnancy.

1. Salmon grilled to 145°F — **Safe / Unsafe**
2. Brie cheese made with unpasteurized milk — **Safe / Unsafe**
3. Light canned tuna — **Safe / Unsafe**
4. Homemade Caesar salad dressing with raw eggs — **Safe / Unsafe**
5. Fresh apple slices (washed) — **Safe / Unsafe**
6. Ham salad from the deli counter — **Safe / Unsafe**
7. Raw alfalfa sprouts — **Safe / Unsafe**
8. Shrimp cooked until opaque — **Safe / Unsafe**

Nutrition in Practice
- Respect cultural food traditions when giving nutritional advice. For example, in some cultures certain foods are avoided during pregnancy; understanding these beliefs builds trust.
- Encourage balanced meals rather than strict dietary rules. A plate with protein, complex carbs, vegetables, and healthy fats is usually sufficient.
- Address common issues like nausea, anemia, and constipation through diet first, using foods like yogurt, leafy greens, and fiber-rich fruits.
- Support clients in making realistic changes within their budget, such as choosing beans or lentils for affordable protein.
- Simplify supplement use to avoid duplication and excess; recommend one high-quality prenatal and only add extras if labs or history show a need.

Midwifery Applications

Clients often present with unique nutritional needs. For example, one vegetarian with fatigue and low ferritin improved after adding iron-rich foods and a gentle supplement. Another arrived with multiple supplements from friends; the midwife simplified her plan to avoid duplication. A third, feeling foggy and low, was assessed for B12 and vitamin D deficiency, with labs and follow-up arranged.

Exercise 8.9: Case Studies in Nutrition and Pregnancy

Answer the following:

Case 1: Julia
Julia is 16 years old, G1 T0 P0 Ab0 L0. She is still in high school, and her diet consists mainly of soda, potato chips, and pizza. At the beginning of pregnancy she weighed 190 lbs at a height of 5'2".

1. What was her BMI at the beginning of pregnancy? _____
2. What are some concerns you have for her nutritional health?

3. How would you encourage her to eat healthier?

4. How would you encourage healthy changes without making her feel lectured?

Case 2: Maya
Maya is 28 years old, G3 T1 P0 Ab1 L1. She works as a seamstress. Her child, now two years old, weighed 5 lbs 6 oz at term. She recently weaned her toddler. She is 5'7" and weighed 115 lbs prepregnancy. Maya follows a strict vegan diet.

1. By what percentage is she underweight? _____%
2. What concerns might you have for her nutritional status?

3. What changes would you recommend in her diet, and why?

4. How would you encourage a healthy pregnancy while respecting her veganism?

Prenatal Fitness & Exercise

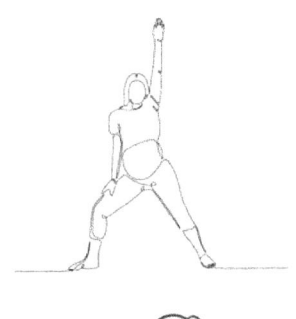

Giving birth, especially outside of the hospital, requires significant physical stamina. A first-time mother may labor for twenty-four hours or more, much of it spent walking, squatting, or changing positions. A woman's level of fitness during pregnancy can influence not only her birth experience but also her recovery. Research shows that women who engage in regular exercise during pregnancy often have shorter labors, fewer interventions, lower rates of cesarean section, and faster postpartum healing. They also experience less discomfort and report higher energy levels compared to those who remain sedentary.

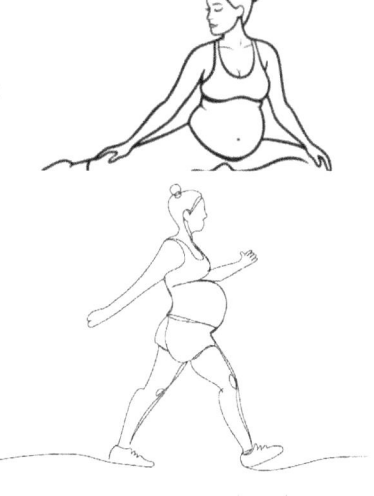

The benefits of exercise extend beyond labor and delivery. Regular activity strengthens the heart and lungs, improves circulation, enhances flexibility, and supports the body's ability to adapt to pregnancy changes such as increased weight and shifting posture. Exercise also boosts mood, lowers stress, and helps reduce the risk of complications such as gestational diabetes, hypertension, constipation, and excessive weight gain. For many women, movement is also a powerful tool for managing anxiety and improving sleep.

Not all women feel comfortable exercising, especially in public or fitness-oriented settings. Cultural expectations, modesty, body image concerns, or past trauma may influence how a person feels about movement. Midwives should approach these conversations with sensitivity, emphasizing function, comfort, and emotional well-being rather than appearance or weight. Encourage gentle, accessible movement—such as walking, stretching, gardening, or dancing at home—when structured exercise feels out of reach.

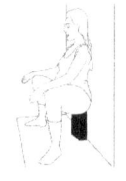
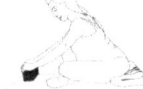

Pregnancy is not a time to train for marathons or to push the body to extremes, but most women can safely continue an active lifestyle with minor modifications. Walking, swimming, and low-impact aerobics remain excellent choices, as they improve endurance without placing undue stress on joints. Prenatal yoga is particularly beneficial: it builds strength and flexibility, improves posture, reduces back pain, and teaches breath awareness that can be applied in labor. Yoga also emphasizes relaxation and mindfulness, helping women feel more connected to their changing bodies. Studies suggest that women who practice yoga regularly during pregnancy may experience less stress, better sleep, and improved pain management in labor.

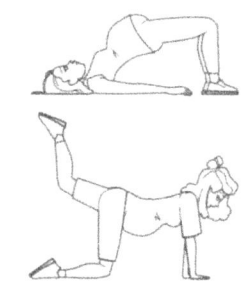

For women who were already physically active before pregnancy, many routines can be maintained with adjustments for safety. High-risk activities such as contact sports, long-distance running, scuba diving, or horseback riding should be avoided. Community programs, such as water aerobics or prenatal yoga classes, can offer safe exercise while also creating opportunities for social connection.

Some women should limit or avoid exercise unless cleared by a qualified provider. Contraindications include placenta previa, preterm labor, ruptured membranes, incompetent cervix, or preeclampsia. Exercise should also be modified or postponed in cases of severe anemia, significant heart or lung disease, uncontrolled hypertension, or multiple gestation with risk of preterm birth. Warning signs such as bleeding, chest pain, dizziness, or severe headaches mean exercise should stop immediately, with follow-up care as needed. Midwives should screen for contraindications early and revisit activity plans throughout pregnancy, adjusting recommendations as energy levels, trimester, and comfort change.

The guiding principle is balance: enough movement to build strength and stamina for birth, but not so much intensity that it risks injury or exhaustion. Even light activity performed regularly can make a meaningful difference in a woman's overall well-being and her birth outcomes. Midwives play an important role in encouraging safe activity, helping women set realistic goals, and tailoring exercise recommendations to fit each client's body, lifestyle, and preferences.

Exercise 8.10: Benefits of Prenatal Movement
Match each activity to its primary benefit:

1. _____ Builds endurance for labor
2. _____ Improves joint stability and reduces strain
3. _____ Enhances breath, balance, and flexibility
4. _____ Supports continence and postpartum recovery
5. _____ Regulates blood sugar and improves circulation

A. Swimming
B. Walking
C. Yoga
D. Strength training
E. Pelvic floor exercises

Clinical Tip

Group exercise classes such as prenatal yoga, water aerobics, or walking groups provide more than just physical benefits. They help women connect with peers who are also pregnant, building community and reducing isolation. These social ties often become informal support networks that continue into the postpartum period, supporting emotional health and confidence.

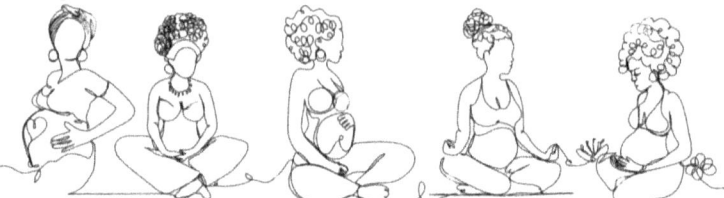

DO'S AND DON'TS OF PRENATAL EXERCISE

 Do's

- Warm up before and cool down after.
- Eat small, frequent meals and snacks to maintain energy.
- Stay well hydrated before, during, and after activity.
- Exercise in the aerobic zone for 15–30 minutes, 3–5 times per week.
- Vary your routine to work different muscle groups.
- Create realistic, gradual fitness goals.
- Choose safe, low-impact activities (walking, swimming, prenatal yoga, water aerobics).
- Stop exercising if cramps, pain, bleeding, or contractions occur.

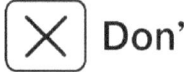 **Don'ts**

- Exercise to exhaustion or excessively vigorously.
- Exercise on slippery or uneven surfaces.
- Do vigorous upright exercise for more than 30 minutes continuously.
- Do exercises lying flat on the back for long periods.
- Stand in one position for extended periods.
- Do activities requiring balance that could lead to falls or abdominal injury.
- Ignore warning signs such as chest pain, dizziness, nausea, or fluid leakage.

Exercise 8.11: Prenatal Fitness Scenarios
Read each client description and answer the questions that follow.

Maria is 32 weeks pregnant and has always enjoyed jogging. She asks if she can continue running three miles a few times a week.

1. What advice would you give her about modifying her routine?

2. What warning signs should she watch for?

Jasmine is 24 weeks pregnant and recently joined a prenatal yoga class. She says she feels more relaxed afterward but wonders if it really benefits her pregnancy.

1. What are two specific benefits of prenatal yoga you can share with her?

2. How might participating in the class help her beyond physical fitness?

Aisha is 18 weeks pregnant and reports constipation and difficulty sleeping. She has no medical contraindications for exercise.

1. What type of physical activity might help relieve these discomforts?

2. How would you encourage her to begin safely?

Carla is 28 weeks pregnant and overweight. She is embarrassed to attend group classes and asks if walking is "enough."

1. How would you respond to her concern?

2. Suggest two realistic goals for her exercise routine.

Herbs in Pregnancy

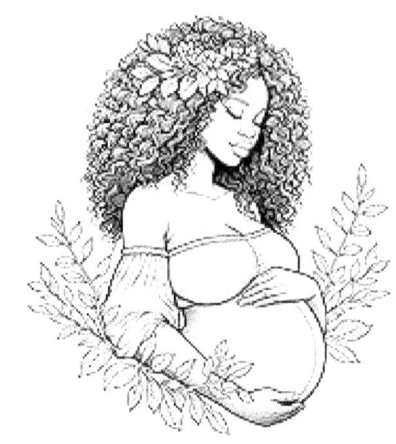

For as long as women have been giving birth, herbs have been among their closest allies. Across the world, midwives have turned to the plant people for nourishment, comfort, healing, and strength. Herbs are more than remedies; they are part of the fabric of life, woven into food, ceremony, and healing traditions.

In Ojibwe, the word for plants is sometimes translated as *"the ones who take care of us,"* expressing a worldview that recognizes plants not as resources to be used, but as relatives who nurture and protect us. This teaching echoes across many Indigenous cultures, where plants are understood to hold spirit, wisdom, and responsibilities within the great web of life. They feed us, clothe us, provide medicine, and help us remember our place in creation.

Pregnancy, perhaps more than at any other time in life, calls forth the nurturing role of herbs. Some plants can be taken daily as foods or teas, offering vitamins, minerals, and gentle support for the changing body. Others serve as remedies, easing nausea, calming heartburn, strengthening the kidneys, or soothing cramps. Still others are held in reserve, powerful medicines to be used sparingly at the right moment, whether to help labor along, prevent hemorrhage, or aid recovery after birth.

Yet it is precisely because herbs are powerful that they must be treated with respect. An herb that strengthens in one stage of pregnancy may endanger in another. A plant that heals in small doses may harm in larger ones. Midwives through the ages have repeated the same wisdom: *first, do no harm*. Care, caution, and discernment are as important as knowledge of recipes or plant names.

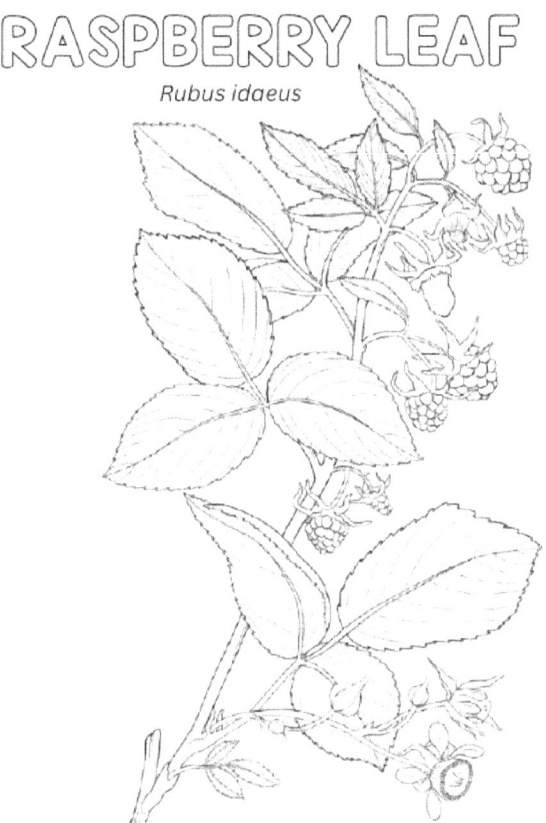

RASPBERRY LEAF
Rubus idaeus

Working with herbs also means working in relationship. Traditional teachings remind us that healing is not only about chemistry, but about connection. Before harvesting, many Indigenous healers pause to ask permission, to listen, and to make an offering. They take only what is needed, leaving enough for the plant to thrive and for others to benefit, and they always give thanks. These acts of reciprocity honor the spirit of the plants and help ensure that healing remains balanced and respectful.

In our modern world, it is easy to forget these ways. Plants are harvested for mass production, stripped of context, and turned into pills or powders on store shelves. As midwives and mothers reclaim herbal knowledge, we also reclaim the responsibility that goes with it: to use herbs wisely, to keep learning, and to hold gratitude for the plant relatives who care for us.

Cultural Tradition

Among the Diné (Navaho), juniper (*Juniperus monosperma*) branches are burned, and the sifted ash is mixed into blue corn mush. This ash is rich in calcium and minerals and has traditionally been given to pregnant and postpartum women to strengthen bones and support recovery, reflecting the Diné value of nourishment and balance during childbearing.

Ways to Use Herbs

Herbs can be prepared in many forms, each suited to different purposes.
- **Teas and Infusions:** Steep leaves, flowers, or stems in hot water. Nutritive and rich in vitamins/minerals (e.g., nettle, raspberry, alfalfa).
- **Decoctions:** Simmer roots, barks, or seeds to extract deeper properties (e.g., ginger, cramp bark).
- **Tinctures:** Concentrated extracts made with alcohol, glycerin, or vinegar. Typical doses are small (½ tsp a few times daily) and not harmful in pregnancy.
- **Capsules and Powders:** Not recommended. Potency and quality are unreliable compared to teas, tinctures, or fresh forms.
- **Syrups:** Tea or decoction with honey/sugar; soothing for children or coughs.
- **Salves/Ointments:** Herb-infused oil with beeswax for topical healing.
- **Poultices/Compresses:** Mashed herb applied directly to skin and wrapped.
- **Essential Oils:** Highly concentrated; avoid internal use. Safe externally in diluted form or a mister.

Herbal Preparations Overview

For detailed instructions on making herbal products, see Daphne Singingtree's *Eagletree Guide to Herbal Medicine Making* (Eagletree Press, 2024).

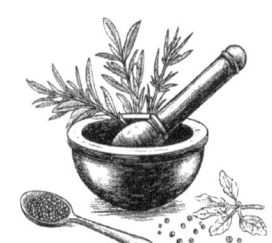

Infused Herbal Oils (Crock-Pot Method)

1. Use dried herbs. Lightly crumble and fill a clean quart jar about ½ full.

2. Cover herbs with oil (olive, coconut, sunflower) by 1–2 inches. Stir to release air bubbles and top up so herbs stay submerged.

3. Place a folded washcloth in the bottom of the Crock-Pot; set the jar on top.

4. Add water until it comes just below the jar's shoulder (deep enough to heat evenly).

5. Heat on LOW/WARM for 12–24 hours.

7. Check water level and top off with warm water as needed.

8. Strain warm oil through cheesecloth; store in dark glass in a cool place.

Making Tinctures

Alcohol tincture: For dried herbs, use a 1:4 ratio (¼ cup dried herb to 1 cup alcohol, usually vodka). For fresh herbs, use a 1:2 ratio (½ cup fresh herb to 1 cup alcohol

Glycerin tincture (glycerite): 1 part dry herb to 3 parts vegetable glycerin.

Method: Chop or crumble herbs. Place in jar. Completely cover with alcohol or glycerin. Cap and store 4–6 weeks in a cool dark place, shaking daily. Strain and bottle in dark glass.

Making Salves & Balms

1. Begin with strained infused oil.
2. Warm gently in a double boiler. Add 1 oz beeswax per 1 cup oil; stir until melted.
3. Use butters like cocoa butter for a richer balm, but reduce beeswax accordingly.
4. Take off heat. Add 1 teaspoon liquid vitamin E as preservative.
5. Add essential oils if used.
6. Pour into clean tins or jars; cool and cap.

Nutritive Herbs

Pregnancy is a time when the body is working constantly to build new life. The need for vitamins, minerals, and trace nutrients increases, and while food should always be the first source of nourishment, herbs can play an important role in filling those needs. Many herbs are so gentle and nutritive that they are best understood as food rather than medicine. These are the plants midwives return to again and again, offering daily support that is safe for both mother and baby

A traditional guideline is to notice the taste of an herb. Mild-tasting herbs are often nutritive, strengthening and nourishing the body when taken regularly. Bitter or acrid herbs are more likely to act as alteratives — stimulating or cleansing in ways that may not be safe during pregnancy. This is not a rigid rule, but it remains a useful guide: when an herb tastes like food, it often behaves like food.

- **Nutritive herbs** often taste mild, pleasant, or even sweet. These can usually be taken in larger amounts or as daily teas. They strengthen, tone, and nourish.
- **Alterative herbs** are more likely to taste bitter, sharp, or acrid. Because of their stronger effect, which sometimes acts like drugs on the body, pregnant women should be cautious when using them.

This is not an absolute rule; some mild-tasting herbs have strong actions, and some bitter herbs are safe in small amounts, but it offers a useful way to distinguish everyday allies from plants that require caution.

Common Nutritive Herbs in Pregnancy:

- **Alfalfa:** Rich in vitamins A, D, E, B6, and K; supports blood clotting, prevents hemorrhage, increases milk supply.
- **Borage:** Supports adrenal glands; provides trace minerals.
- **Ginger root:** Warming, aids digestion, and relieves morning sickness.
- **Hibiscus:** High in vitamin C and antioxidants; adds a tart, pleasant flavor.
- **Lemongrass:** Calms digestion and reduces stress.
- **Nettle:** Exceptionally nutritive, high in calcium, iron, magnesium, and potassium; strengthens kidneys and reduces cramps.
- **Peach leaves:** Traditional remedy for nausea.
- **Red clover:** Nutritive, contains calcium and phytoestrogens that balance the system.
- **Red raspberry leaf:** Rich in vitamins, tones pelvic muscles, prepares uterus for efficient labor.
- **Rosehips:** Excellent source of vitamin C and bioflavonoids.
- **Slippery elm:** Mucilaginous and calming to the digestive tract; safe as a tea.
- **Spearmint and peppermint:** Refreshing mints that ease digestion and help with nausea.
- **Strawberry leaves:** Mineral-rich, gentle tonic.
- **Watercress:** Rich in vitamins and minerals, especially calcium and iron.
- **Yerba Buena:** A traditional mint relative, soothing for digestion.

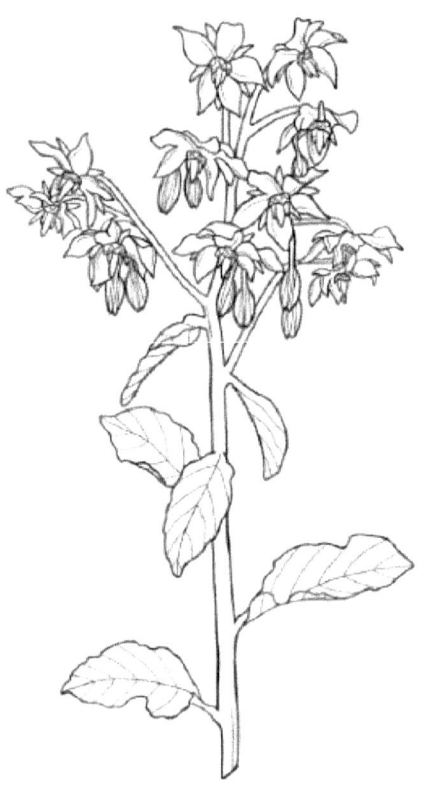

BORAGE
Borago officinalis

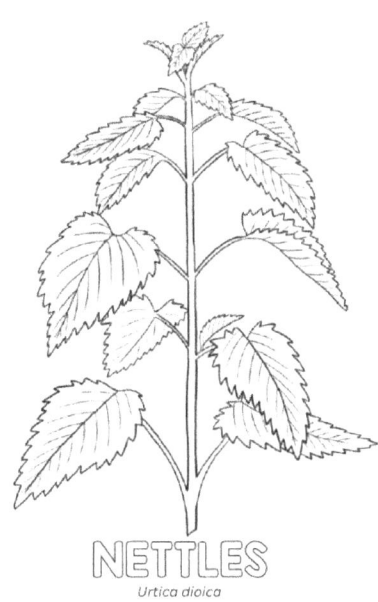
NETTLES
Urtica dioica

Pregnancy Tea Blend

One of the most common and effective ways to use nutritive herbs in pregnancy is through a daily tea. This tea not only provides daily nourishment but also strengthens and tones the body, preparing for labor and supporting recovery. NORA tea is a popular midwifery blend made from equal parts of nettle, oatstraw, red raspberry leaf and alfalfa. A smaller amount of spearmint or peppermint are popular additions.

Directions: Mix equal parts of dried herbs. Use ¼ cup per quart of boiling water. Steep until well-infused, strain, and drink several cups a day. It also make a good ice tea.

Red Raspberry (*Rubus idaeus*): The best-known pregnancy herb, rich in vitamins A, B, C, and E, as well as calcium and iron. Raspberry leaf contains an alkaloid called fragarine that tones the pelvic muscles, especially the uterus, supporting efficient contractions during birth and reducing the risk of complications.

Alfalfa (*Medicago sativa*) complements both raspberry and nettle. Known for its high vitamin K content, alfalfa helps prevent hemorrhage in both mother and baby. It also contains vitamins A, D, E, and B6, as well as iron and chlorophyll, which supports overall vitality. In the postpartum period, alfalfa is valued for its ability to increase milk supply.

Oatstraw *(Avena sativa)*: A gentle nutritive herb that supports the nervous system, helping to ease stress, irritability, and fatigue during pregnancy. Rich in calcium, magnesium, and B vitamins, oatstraw helps strengthen bones and muscles while promoting restful sleep and balanced moods. It is especially valued for calming anxiety and supporting resilience in times of physical and emotional change. With a mild, slightly sweet flavor, oatstraw blends well with other nutritive herbs such as nettle, raspberry leaf, and alfalfa. Safe for use throughout pregnancy and postpartum, it also supports healthy milk production.

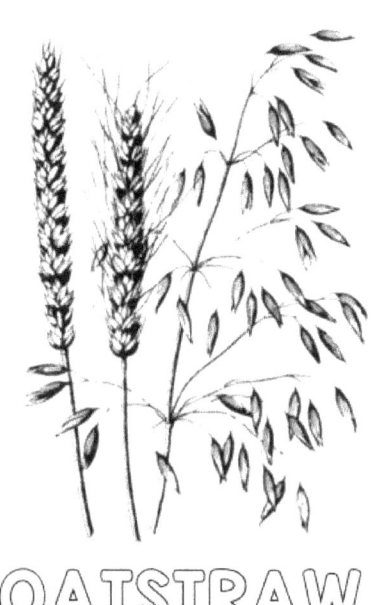
OATSTRAW
Avena sativa

Nettle (*Urtica dioica*): Known as one of the most nutritive herbs, containing high levels of vitamins A, C, D, and K, as well as calcium, iron, magnesium, and potassium. Nettles also support kidney function, reduce leg cramps, ease muscle spasms, and lower the risk of postpartum hemorrhage.

Herbs for Relief of Common Discomforts

Herbs can offer gentle relief when used with knowledge and care. These remedies, many of them centuries old, are often simple teas or external preparations that calm the body, ease digestion, and support rest. The goal is not to medicate every symptom, but to restore balance and comfort so the mother can carry her child with greater ease.

Morning Sickness

Nausea often resolves by the second trimester, the first weeks can feel long and exhausting. Herbal teas, when cooled, refrigerated, and served over ice, are often better tolerated than hot tea, and are convenient for sipping small amounts throughout the day.

- **Raspberry leaf** tones the uterus and soothes the stomach.
- **Peach leaves** have long been valued as a calming tea for nausea.
- **Peppermint or spearmint** are refreshing and gentle on the digestive tract.
- **Ginger root** is one of the most effective anti-nausea herbs used worldwide.
- **Nettles and strawberry leaves** are nutritive and calming to digestion.

Heartburn

Other safe aids include papaya enzymes, ice chips, carbonated water, and calcium carbonate tablets.
- **Peppermint** or **spearmint** to cool and calm.
- **Ginger** to support digestion.
- **Fennel** and **fenugreek** to ease gas and bloating.

Constipation

Avoid strong laxative or cathartic herbs such as senna, cascara, aloe, or rhubarb, but fiber- and mucilage-rich plants are safe and effective.
- **Psyllium:** bulking fiber that softens stools.
- **Chia seeds:** mucilaginous, soothing, and hydrating.
- **Flaxseeds:** rich in fiber and omega-3 fatty acids.
- **Oat bran:** gentle fiber, easy to incorporate into meals.
- **Marshmallow root:** mucilaginous herb that soothes the digestive tract.

Stretch Marks

While much of the tendency toward stretch marks is genetic, external care can help keep the skin supple. Herbal oils and salves provide nourishment and elasticity. A belly balm can be made with infused calendula oil, or with simple ingredients such as coconut oil, cocoa butter, shea butter, and vitamin E.

Leg Cramps

Leg cramps are often linked to mineral deficiencies, especially calcium and magnesium. Nutritive herbs provide these minerals in an absorbable form. Nettle and alfalfa teas are particularly effective.

Hemorrhoids

Herbs can bring relief through both addressing constipation and external application. An effective **Anti-Hemorrhoid Salve** can be made with infused yarrow and plantain leaves. **Witch Hazel Wipes:** Soak gauze pads in witch hazel extract and store in a small jar by the toilet for soothing wipes.

Vaginal Irritation

Increased vaginal discharge is normal in pregnancy. Unless accompanied by odor, burning, or irritation, it is not a sign of infection. Occasionally, however, irritation or itching may occur without infection. In these cases, aloe vera gel applied externally can soothe tissues. Calendula ointment is another option, reducing inflammation and irritation.

Herpes Outbreaks

External applications of lemon balm infused oil, St. John's wort oil, calendula ointment, aloe vera gel, or spirits of camphor can speed healing, reduce pain, and calm irritation. Internal support with lysine and zinc supplements, along with hydration, helps reduce duration and severity.

Colds & Coughs

Pregnant women, like everyone else, sometimes face seasonal colds. Herbs can support healing and comfort without harsh medicines.
- **General support:** Red clover, garlic, raspberry, nettle, rose hips, fenugreek, peppermint, chamomile, ginger, plantain, mullein.
- **Dry coughs:** Slippery elm, mullein, marshmallow, Yerba Buena, fennel, hops.
- **Mucus coughs:** Ginger, plantain, St. John's wort, raspberry, strawberry leaves.

Herbs for Labor and Birth

Labor is usually best left to unfold naturally, guided by the body's wisdom. In a healthy pregnancy with no complications, there is rarely a need for intervention. However, there are times when herbs can support the process — either by helping maintain a threatened pregnancy, encouraging contractions when overdue, or assisting the uterus during birth.

Because these herbs are strong in action, they should always be treated with respect and used only with careful assessment by an experienced practitioner. Misuse can lead to premature labor, uterine exhaustion, or harm to the baby. For this reason, midwives usually rely on nutritive and supportive herbs in pregnancy, reserving stronger remedies for when intervention is truly necessary.

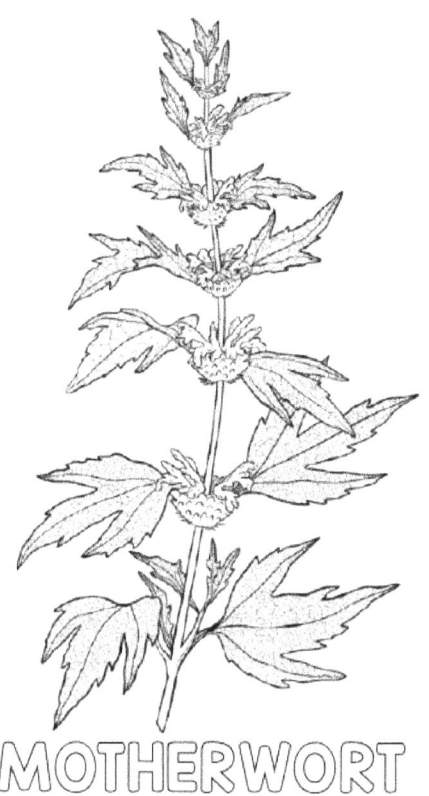

MOTHERWORT
Leonorus cardiaca

Herbs for Threatened Miscarriage

If spotting, cramping, or threatened miscarriage occurs in early pregnancy, traditionally herbs may help calm the uterus and reduce risk. Immediate evaluation for any spotting or cramping by a licensed clinician is recommended. These herbs are not guaranteed preventives, but they have been relied upon historically for support:

- **Alfalfa** *(Medicago sativa)*: High in vitamin K, builds blood, helps prevent hemorrhage.
- **Black haw** *(Viburnum prunifolium)*: Antispasmodic and uterine relaxant; useful in calming cramps.
- **False unicorn root** *(Chamaelirium luteum)*: Traditionally used as a uterine tonic, balancing hormones and preventing miscarriage.
- **Raspberry leaf** *(Rubus idaeus)*: Tones and supports uterine tissue, providing stability.
- **Wild yam** *(Dioscorea villosa)*: Antispasmodic and hormonal support, often paired with black haw.

Herbs as Uterine Stimulants

When a pregnancy is overdue, or when labor has stalled despite rupture of membranes or other readiness signs, certain herbs can stimulate the uterus. These are **strong remedies** and should only be used with careful assessment.

- **Birthroot** *(Trillium pendulum)*: Uterine stimulant, also helps prevent hemorrhage.
- **Black cohosh** *(Actaea racemosa)*: Encourages coordinated contractions; sometimes used in tincture form during labor.
- **Blue cohosh** *(Caulophyllum thalictroides)*: Potent uterine stimulant; used only in very small amounts due to potential toxicity.
- **Motherwort** *(Leonurus cardiaca)*: Mild uterine stimulant and calming nervine; sometimes used in transition stage.
- **Osha root** *(Ligusticum porteri)*: Stimulates uterine action and clears stagnation.
- **Partridge berry** (*Mitchella repens*): Traditionally used to prepare the uterus for birth.

Herbs During Active Labor

Some herbs can help strengthen contractions, relieve pain, or sometimes support rest:

- **Blue and black cohosh (with caution):** To encourage contractions when stalled.
- **Motherwort:** To calm fear and support uterine strength.
- **Shepherd's purse** *(Capsella bursa-pastoris)*: Not a labor stimulant, but a vital ally immediately postpartum to control bleeding.
- **Skullcap:** to help rest if trying to sleep when labor is on and off.

Postpartum Herbs

The postpartum period is a time of deep transformation. A mother's body shifts rapidly from pregnancy to lactation, with major changes in hormones, blood volume, and tissue recovery. Herbs can be invaluable allies during this transition, supporting healing, preventing complications, and nourishing the mother as she adjusts to caring for her newborn.

Preventing and Controlling Hemorrhage

Herbs are most effective as **preventatives**. Once heavy hemorrhage is underway, stronger measures are usually required, but starting herbs early can reduce risk and support uterine tone.

- **Alfalfa** *(Medicago sativa)*: High in vitamin K, supports blood clotting and prevents excessive bleeding.
- **Nettle** *(Urtica dioica)*: Builds iron and minerals, restores strength after blood loss.
- **Raspberry leaf** *(Rubus idaeus)*: Astringent and uterotonic, helps the uterus contract and stay firm.
- **Shepherd's purse** *(Capsella bursa-pastoris)*: One of the most important postpartum anti-hemorrhagic herbs.
- **Yarrow** *(Achillea millefolium)*: Astringent, reduces bleeding, and supports tissue healing.

> **Cultural Tradition**
> In Chinese and Korean traditions, **mugwort** is widely used in pregnancy and postpartum care. Dried mugwort is burned as "moxa" near acupuncture points, particularly on the little toe, to encourage a breech baby to turn. The leaves are added to postpartum baths or soups to restore warmth, circulate blood, and protect against "cold" entering the body. This reflect the importance of balancing hot and cold energies for recovery and long-term health.

Retained Placenta

If the placenta fails to deliver promptly, herbs, in addition to breastfeeding, may help:

- **Angelica** *(Angelica archangelica)*: Encourages uterine contractions and placental expulsion.
- **Birthroot** *(Trillium pendulum)*: Helps stimulate the uterus while also supporting hemostasis.

Afterpains

After the uterus begins to contract down, mothers often feel "afterpains." These can be especially strong in multiparas. Herbs with antispasmodic and pain-relieving properties can help:

- **Cramp bark** *(Viburnum opulus)*: One of the best antispasmodic herbs for uterine cramps.
- **Dong quai** *(Angelica sinensis)*: A traditional postpartum herb in Chinese medicine; not used during pregnancy but beneficial after birth.
- **Raspberry leaf:** Mild uterine tonic that can help ease the cramping process.
- **St. John's wort** *(Hypericum perforatum)*: Nervine and pain-relieving, calms both nerves and uterine discomfort.
- **Valerian** *(Valeriana officinalis)*: Strong nervine relaxant; use in tincture form for severe afterpains.

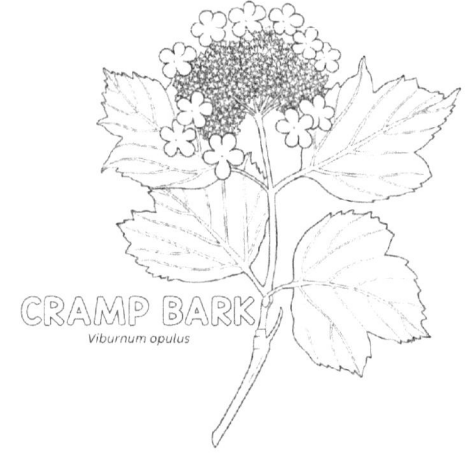
CRAMP BARK
Viburnum opulus

Healing Tears and Stitches

Herbs can help tissues knit and heal after perineal tears or surgical repair. Avoid powders or oils applied directly to stitches, as they can trap moisture and delay healing.

- **Peri rinse:** Use cooled tea made from comfrey and sage. Pour over the perineum after urination or bowel movements.
- **Sitz baths:** Combine sage, comfrey, uva ursi, and sea salt. Add to a shallow warm bath for 15–20 minutes to promote healing and reduce soreness.
- **Calendula** *(Calendula officinalis)*: Gentle antimicrobial and healer, can be added to rinses.

Supporting Breastfeeding

Some herbs act as **galactagogues** — plants that help increase milk supply. These are usually nutritive or aromatic herbs that support hormonal balance, digestion, and circulation.

Galactagogues:
- **Alfalfa** *(Medicago sativa)*
- **Anise** *(Pimpinella anisum)*
- **Blessed thistle** *(Cnicus benedictus)*
- **Dandelion** *(Taraxacum officinale)*
- **Fennel** *(Foeniculum vulgare)*
- **Fenugreek** *(Trigonella foenum-graecum)*
- **Goat's rue** *(Galega officinalis)*
- **Hops** *(Humulus lupulus)*
- **Moringa** *(Moringa oleifera)*
- **Nettle** *(Urtica dioica)*
- **Oatstraw** *(Avena sativa)*
- **Shatavari** *(Asparagus racemosus)*

Nursing Mother's Tea Blend
- 2 parts nettle
- 2 parts alfalfa
- 1 part blessed thistle
- 1 part fenugreek
- 1 part fennel
- 1 part goat's rue

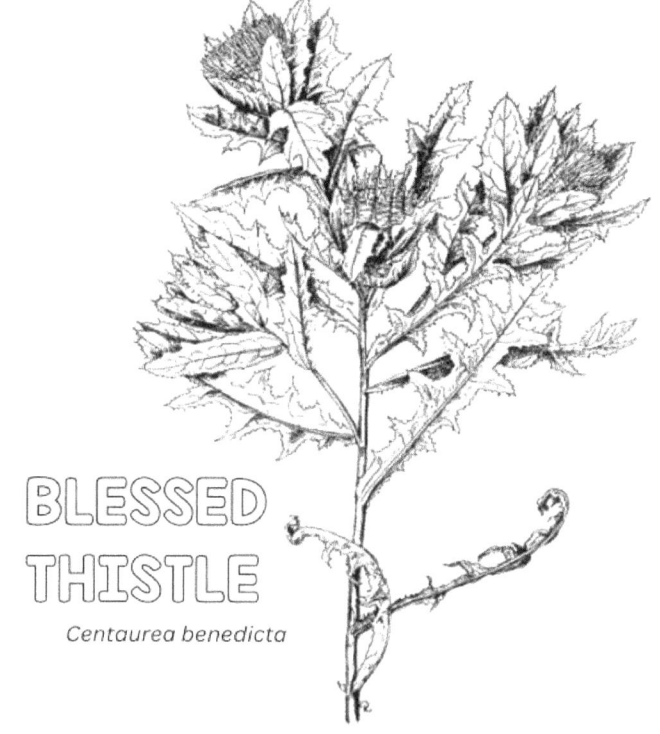

BLESSED THISTLE
Centaurea benedicta

Decreasing Milk Supply
For weaning, engorgement, or in cases of infant death or adoption, some herbs help reduce milk production:
- **Cornsilk** *(Zea mays)*
- **Parsley** *(Petroselinum crispum)*
- **Sage** *(Salvia officinalis)*
- **Yarrow** *(Achillea millefolium)*

Sore Nipples
Cracked or sore nipples are common in early breastfeeding and require prevention, such as proper positioning, as well as healing salves.
- **Poke root** *(Phytolacca americana)*: Used in ointments or salves for severe inflammation; apply sparingly.
- **Lanolin** (anhydrous, pure): Provides a protective, healing barrier.

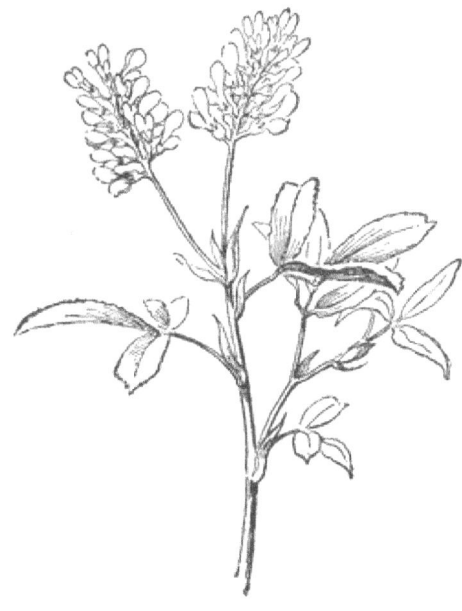

ALFALFA
Medicago sativa

POKE ROOT
Phytolacca americana

HERBS FOR BABIES

Midwives are health care providers for mother and baby during the first six weeks after birth. During this time, they are not only monitoring physical recovery and newborn growth, but also answering questions about breastfeeding, infant care, and maternal well-being. Herbs can be a valuable part of these conversations, as midwives help families choose safe, gentle remedies while reinforcing that healing takes time and support. Infants are delicate and highly sensitive to both foods and medicines. Because their systems are still developing, herbs should never be given internally during the first four months. Instead, herbs are best applied externally — through baths, compresses, washes, or in the mother's milk.

Herbal baths are especially effective, since babies absorb medicinal properties easily through their skin, and the warm water also soothes and relaxes them. Always strain baths thoroughly to prevent skin irritation from floating particles. Observe carefully for any signs of rash or sensitivity.

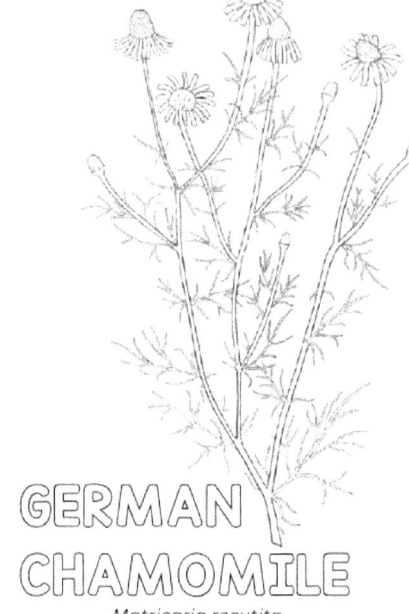
GERMAN CHAMOMILE
Matricaria recutita

General Herbal Bath Method
1. Place 1 ounce of dried herb (or 1–2 handfuls fresh) in a heatproof container.
2. Pour 1 gallon of boiling water over the herbs.
3. Cover and steep for at least 30 minutes.
4. Strain carefully to remove all plant matter.
5. Add the infusion to baby's bath once cooled to a safe temperature.

This method can be adapted for single herbs or blends.

Colic and Gas
Babies suffering from gas or colic may benefit from herbal baths that calm digestion and ease discomfort.
- **Anise** (*Pimpinella anisum*): Relieves gas and bloating.
- **Chamomile** (*Matricaria recutita*): Calms fussiness, relieves stomach upset.
- **Fennel** (*Foeniculum vulgare*): Aromatic seed, eases digestive spasms.
- **Fenugreek** (*Trigonella foenum-graecum*): Mildly warming, supports digestion.
- **Peppermint** (*Mentha piperita*): Cooling, relieves colic and cramping.

Fussy or Restless Babies
Sometimes babies are overtired, overstimulated, or simply fussy. Gentle nervine herbs can help them relax and rest more easily.
- **Chamomile** (*Matricaria recutita*): Perhaps the best-known baby herb, soothing both digestion and nerves.
- **Oatstraw** (*Avena sativa*): Mildly calming, nutritive, and safe.

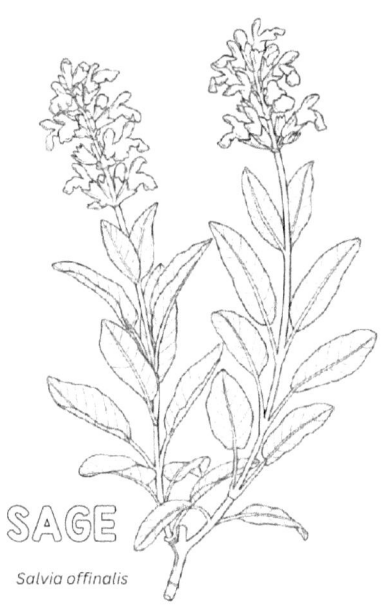
SAGE
Salvia offinalis

Colds and Congestion
For mild colds, congestion, or respiratory irritation, herbs can be used externally to soothe breathing passages. Local honey is sometimes used for coughs in older children, but it should **never** be given to babies under one year due to risk of botulism.
- **Eucalyptus** (*Eucalyptus globulus*): Strong decongestant; use sparingly and never directly on a baby's skin. Add a few drops of diluted infusion to bathwater or use nearby as steam.
- **Sage** (*Salvia officinalis*): Antimicrobial and astringent; can be added to baths to ease congestion and mild throat irritation.

Herbs in Pregnancy and Postpartum: Quick Reference			
Herb Name	**Stage Used**	**Primary Use or Benefit**	**Safety Notes**
Red raspberry leaf	Second–third trimester	Supports uterine tone and birth preparation.	Avoid in early pregnancy if there is a history of preterm labor or recurrent miscarriage.
Nettle leaf	All trimesters	Provides iron, calcium, and vitamin K.	Generally safe; use dried leaf rather than root.
Alfalfa	Second–third trimester	Provides vitamin K and supports blood building.	Monitor if the client has a clotting disorder; avoid with a history of lupus.
Lemon balm	First–second trimester	Relieves nausea and supports calm digestion.	Mild and well tolerated; use cautiously with hypothyroidism.
Chamomile	All trimesters	Supports sleep and digestive calm.	Avoid high doses; check for ragweed allergy.
Ginger	First trimester	Relieves nausea and supports digestion.	Safe in food or tea amounts; may worsen heartburn in some clients.
Slippery elm	All trimesters	Relieves heartburn and constipation.	Safe as a lozenge or tea; avoid internal powder from unknown sources.
Dandelion leaf	All trimesters	Acts as a gentle diuretic and supports liver and kidney function.	Leaf infusion is safe; root decoction is stronger and should be supervised.
Cramp bark	Late pregnancy, postpartum	Eases uterine irritability and afterpains.	Generally safe; use with guidance if uterine stimulation is a concern.
Blue cohosh	Labor only	Stimulates uterine contractions.	Not for casual use; supervised use only due to safety concerns.
Black cohosh	Late third trimester or labor	Supports cervical ripening and uterine toning.	Use is controversial; best reserved for experienced practitioners.
Fenugreek	Postpartum	Increases milk supply.	May cause infant gas or colic; avoid in pregnancy due to uterine stimulation.
Blessed thistle	Postpartum	Supports lactation.	Often used in tea with fenugreek or alfalfa.
Calendula	Postpartum	Heals perineal tissue and soothes skin.	Topical use only; gentle and effective.
Witch hazel	Postpartum	Reduces hemorrhoid swelling.	Topical use is safe; not for internal use.
Aloe vera (gel)	Postpartum	Soothes skin and promotes healing.	External use only in pregnancy; avoid internal latex or juice.
Garlic	All stages	Provides immune support and antimicrobial action.	Safe in food doses; avoid very high doses near birth due to bleeding risk.
Moringa	Postpartum	Provides dense nutrition and may support milk supply.	Best used postpartum; pregnancy safety data are limited.

HERBS TO AVOID DURING PREGNANCY

While many herbs are gentle allies, some can stimulate the uterus, interfere with hormones, or contain toxic compounds that may harm the mother or fetus. A few are safe in very small amounts as food seasonings but should be avoided as teas, tinctures, or medicinal doses. These herbs should **not** be used internally during pregnancy unless under the guidance of an experienced practitioner. Some may be considered safe postpartum or in food amounts.

Herbs That Stimulate the Uterus or May Cause Contractions
- **Angelica** (*Angelica archangelica, Angelica sinensis*)
- **Basil, large doses** (*Ocimum basilicum*)
- **Bayberry** (*Myrica cerifera*)
- **Beth root / Birth root** (*Trillium erectum, T. pendulum*)
- **Black cohosh** (*Actaea racemosa*)
- **Blue cohosh** (*Caulophyllum thalictroides*)
- **Bugleweed** (*Lycopus virginicus*)
- **Broom flowers** (*Cytisus scoparius*)
- **Catnip** (*Nepeta cataria*)
- **Clary sage** (*Salvia sclarea*)
- **Cottonwood root** (*Populus* spp.): sometimes used postpartum, not during pregnancy
- **Cramp bark** (*Viburnum opulus*): sometimes used postpartum, not during pregnancy
- **Devil's claw** (*Harpagophytum procumbens*)
- **Dong quai** (*Angelica sinensis*)
- **Ergot** (*Claviceps purpurea*)
- **Feverfew** (*Tanacetum vulgare*)
- **Gotu kola** (*Centella asiatica*)
- **Hops** (*Humulus lupulus*)
- **Juniper berry** (*Juniperus communis*)
- **Lady's mantle** (*Alchemilla xanthochlora*)
- **Maidenhair fern** (*Adiantum capillus-veneris*)
- **Mistletoe** (*Viscum album*)
- **Motherwort** (*Leonurus cardiaca*)
- **Mugwort** (*Artemisia vulgaris*, other *Artemisia* spp.)
- **Oregano** (*Origanum vulgare*): safe as seasoning; avoid medicinal doses or essential oil
- **Osha root** (*Ligusticum porteri*)
- **Passionflower** (*Passiflora incarnata*)
- **Pennyroyal** (*Mentha pulegium*): essential oil is highly toxic
- **Rosemary** (*Rosmarinus officinalis*): safe as seasoning; avoid medicinal doses or essential oil
- **Rue** (*Ruta graveolens*)
- **Sage** (*Salvia officinalis*): safe as seasoning; avoid medicinal doses or essential oil
- **Shepherd's purse** (*Capsella bursa-pastoris*): used postpartum, not in pregnancy
- **Skullcap** (*Scutellaria lateriflora*)
- **Spikenard** (*Aralia racemosa*)
- **Squaw vine** (*Mitchella repens*)
- **St. John's wort** (*Hypericum perforatum*): safe postpartum, not during pregnancy
- **Tansy** (*Tanacetum vulgare*)
- **Valerian** (*Valeriana officinalis*): nervine, but avoid in pregnancy
- **Vervain** (*Verbena officinalis*)
- **Wormwood** (*Artemisia absinthium*, other *Artemisia* spp.)
- **Yarrow** (*Achillea millefolium*)

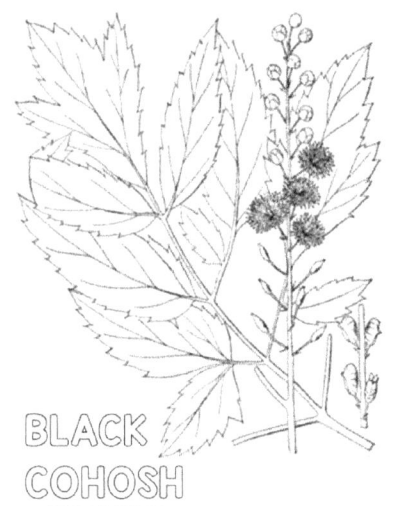

BLACK COHOSH
Actaea racemosa

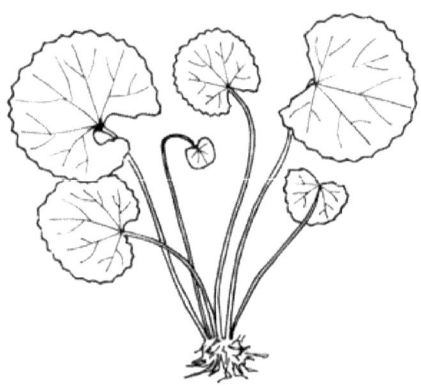

GOTU KOLA
Centella asiatica

Herbs Containing Toxic or Potentially Toxic Compounds
- **Aloe latex** (*Aloe vera, Aloe barbadensis*): topical gel is safe
- **Boldo** (*Peumus boldus*)
- **Buckthorn** (*Rhamnus purshiana*)
- **Chaparral** (*Larrea tridentata*)
- **Comfrey** (*Symphytum officinale*)
- **Datura/Jimsonweed** (*Datura stramonium*)
- **Goldenseal** (*Hydrastis canadensis*)
- **Lobelia** (*Lobelia inflata*)
- **Mandrake** (*Podophyllum peltatum*)
- **Male fern** (*Dryopteris filix-mas*)
- **Sassafras** (*Sassafras albidum*)
- **Senna** (*Senna alexandrina*)
- **White oak** (*Quercus alba*)
- **White willow bark** (*Salix alba*)
- **Wild lettuce** (*Lactuca virosa*)
- **Wintergreen** (*Gaultheria procumbens*)

Hormone-Mimicking or Hormone-Stimulating Herbs
- **Burdock** (*Arctium lappa*)
- **Damiana** (*Turnera diffusa*)
- **Ginseng** (*Panax ginseng, P. quinquefolius*)
- **Licorice root** (*Glycyrrhiza glabra*)
- **Sarsaparilla** (*Smilax* spp.)
- **Vitex / Chasteberry** (*Vitex agnus-castus*)
- **Wild yam** (*Dioscorea villosa*)

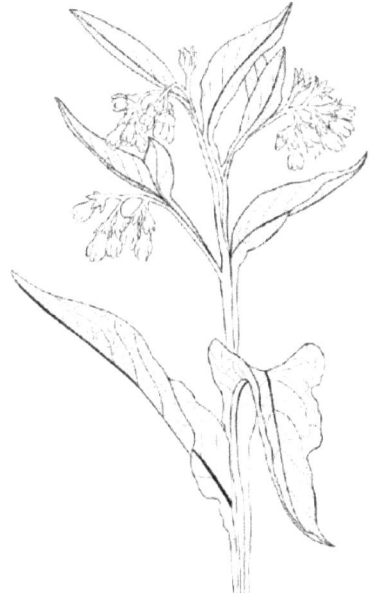
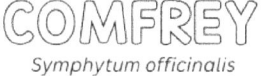
COMFREY
Symphytum officinalis

Laxatives to Avoid

Laxative herbs that act as strong purgatives can irritate the intestines and stimulate uterine contractions. Gentle laxatives based on fiber (chia, flax, psyllium, oat bran) are considered safe in pregnancy.
- **Aloe latex** (*Aloe vera, Aloe barbadensis*)
- **Buckthorn** (*Rhamnus purshiana*)
- **Cascara sagrada** (*Rhamnus purshiana var. sagrada*)
- **Goldenseal** (*Hydrastis canadensis*)
- **Oregon grape root** (*Mahonia aquifolium*)
- **Pokeweed** (*Phytolacca americana*)
- **Rhubarb root** (*Rheum* spp.)
- **Senna** (*Senna alexandrina*)

Diuretics to Avoid

Because the pregnant body is meant to hold extra fluid for blood volume and postpartum recovery, strong diuretic herbs should be avoided.
- **Buchu** (*Agathosma betulina*)
- **Cleavers** (*Galium aparine*)
- **Corn silk** (*Zea mays*): Safe postpartum, not during pregnancy
- **Cubeb berries** (*Piper cubeba*)
- **Dandelion** (*Taraxacum officinale*): Food amounts are safe, avoid strong diuretic use
- **Hops** (*Humulus lupulus*)
- **Parsley** (*Petroselinum crispum*): Safe as seasoning, avoid medicinal doses
- **Uva ursi** (*Arctostaphylos uva-ursi*)

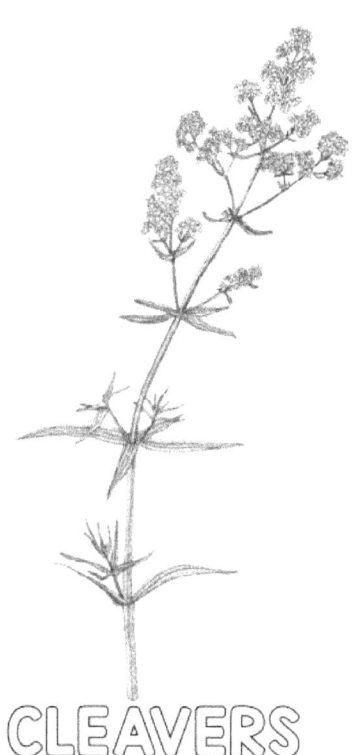
CLEAVERS
Galium aparine

Adaptogens

Herbs to help the body cope with stress by acting on the hypothalamic–pituitary–adrenal (HPA) axis and modulating cortisol and inflammation. Pregnancy is a physiologically pro-inflammatory state (important for implantation, placental development, and labor), so adaptogens that blunt or shift these responses, or that have hormonal effects, may interfere with normal processes, especially early in pregnancy.

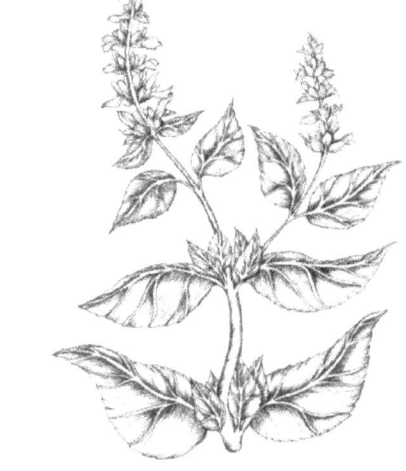

HOLY BASIL
Ocimum tenuiflorum

Common adaptogens:

- **Ashwagandha** (*Withania somnifera*)
- **Holy basil / Tulsi** (*Ocimum tenuiflorum* or *O. sanctum*)
- **Rhodiola** (*Rhodiola rosea*)
- **Eleuthero / Siberian ginseng** (*Eleutherococcus senticosus*)
- **Licorice root** (*Glycyrrhiza glabra*): avoid high-glycyrrhizin products; associated with elevated blood pressure and adverse outcomes
- **Panax ginseng** / Asian ginseng (*Panax ginseng*)
- **American ginseng** (*Panax quinquefolius*)
- **Schisandra** (*Schisandra chinensis*)
- **Astragalus** (*Astragalus membranaceus*)
- **Shatavari** (*Asparagus racemosus*)
- **Maca** (*Lepidium meyenii*)
- **Gotu kola** (*Centella asiatica*)

Exercise 8.12: Herbs to Avoid in Pregnancy			
Place a check mark for each herb:			
Herb	Safe for specific use	Safe with caution	Unsafe in any form
Ashwagandha			
Black cohosh			
Blue cohosh			
Broom flowers			
Cramp bark			
Comfrey			
Dandelion root			
Ginseng			
Goldenseal			
Licorice root			
Pennyroyal			
Rhodiola			
Rue			
Sage			
Shepherd's purse			
Valerian			
Yarrow			

Principles of Herbal Midwifery Practice

Herbs have been companions to midwives for as long as women have attended birth. They offer nourishment, comfort, and sometimes powerful medicine — but they also require knowledge, caution, and respect. A skilled midwife knows when a gentle tea is enough, when a tincture may be helpful, and when it is wiser to seek stronger measures.

- **Start with gentle allies.** Nutritive herbs such as nettle, raspberry, and alfalfa build blood and tone tissues over time.
- **Use stronger herbs with respect.** Uterine stimulants and anti-hemorrhagic herbs can save lives but carry risks if used without clear need.
- **Document everything:** the herb used, form, dosage, and outcome. This not only ensures accountability but adds to the shared body of knowledge among midwives.
- **Balance tradition and research:** many herbal uses come from oral tradition and midwives' experience, while new studies provide additional guidance.
- **First, do no harm.** In pregnancy and birth, the safest course is often patience and support, not intervention.

Example Contents of a Midwife's Herbal Kit

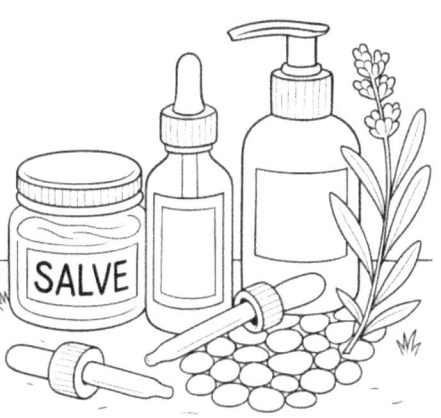

Nutritive Teas and Tonics
- Raspberry leaf, nettle, alfalfa, oat straw
- Rose hips for vitamin C
- Blended "Pregnancy Tea" for daily nourishment

Digestive and Comfort Aids
- Ginger root for nausea and digestion
- Peppermint and chamomile for stomach upset and relaxation
- Peach leaves for morning sickness

Nervines and Calming Herbs
- Lemon balm for gentle relaxation
- Chamomile for both mother and baby
- Valerian tincture (for severe afterpains or insomnia; cautious use)

Labor and Birth Allies
- Blue and black cohosh tinctures (skilled use only, to stimulate labor)
- Motherwort tincture (for calming and aiding transition)
- Shepherd's purse tincture (for postpartum hemorrhage prevention)

Postpartum Recovery
- Anti-hemorrhage tincture (shepherd's purse, birthroot, alfalfa)
- Cramp bark tincture for afterpains
- Herbs for sitz baths: sage, comfrey, uva ursi, calendula
- Nipple care: calendula oil, lanolin, poke root salve (sparingly)

Breastfeeding Support
- Galactagogues: alfalfa, fenugreek, fennel, goat's rue, nettle, blessed thistle, others as available
- Nursing Mother's Tea blend ready-made

Topical and First Aid Herbs
- Plantain and yarrow salves for skin and hemorrhoids
- Aloe vera for irritation and burns
- Witch hazel wipes for hemorrhoids or perineal soreness

> **Exercise 8.13: Herbal Scenarios**
> *Read each description and answer the questions that follow.*

1. **Morning sickness:** A pregnant woman in her first trimester is struggling with nausea. Which gentle herbs could she try, and why are they considered safe?

2. **Leg cramps:** A mother in her third trimester is waking at night with painful leg cramps. Which nutritive herbs would you recommend, and what minerals do they provide?

3. **Preparing for birth:** A mother asks how she can prepare her body naturally for labor. Which daily tea blend might you suggest, and how does it help the uterus?

4. **During Labor:** Labor is progressing slowly, everything is WNL, but there is concern the woman may be too tired to push effectively, what herbs would be recommended to gently increase contractions. What would you use and why?

5. **Postpartum recovery:** A new mother is tired and wants to rebuild her strength. Which herbs can support blood building and healing after birth?

> **Exercise 8.14: Client Scenarios**
> *Check all that apply*
>
> **1. A 24-year-old pregnant woman reports fatigue, nausea, and poor appetite.**
>   ☐ Encourage iron-rich foods
>   ☐ Suggest daily walking
>   ☐ Teach peppermint tea for nausea
>   ☐ Screen for intimate partner violence
>
> **2. A 32-year-old mother reports swollen ankles and leg cramps.**
>   ☐ Recommend nettle tea for minerals
>   ☐ Encourage calf stretches and hydration
>   ☐ Advise avoiding strong diuretics
>   ☐ Reinforce need for prenatal vitamins
>
> **3. A 19-year-old client has heartburn and asks if she should stop exercising.**
>   ☐ Suggest small, frequent meals
>   ☐ Reassure that walking is safe and helpful
>   ☐ Discourage all herbs until postpartum
>   ☐ Teach upright posture after eating

HEALTH PROMOTION FOR MIDWIVES ESSENTIAL TAKEAWAYS

Promoting health in pregnancy is about more than avoiding problems; it is about building strength, resilience, and confidence. Midwives support women by encouraging healthy habits while also screening for issues that can put mothers and babies at risk, such as intimate partner violence, substance use, or unmanaged medical conditions. Health promotion includes attentive listening, culturally respectful care, and practical strategies that empower women to protect their well-being throughout pregnancy.

Nutrition is one of the strongest foundations for a healthy pregnancy. Balanced meals rich in protein, complex carbohydrates, iron, folate, and other essential vitamins and minerals build strength for both mother and baby. Adequate hydration is equally important, supporting digestion, circulation, and amniotic fluid levels. Midwives can guide women toward food and drink choices that reflect both nutritional needs and cultural traditions, reinforcing that nourishment is an act of care for the whole family.

Exercise during pregnancy is not just safe for most women, it is beneficial. Regular movement supports circulation, improves mood, reduces discomfort, and prepares the body for labor. Walking, stretching, swimming, and prenatal yoga are all accessible forms of activity that adapt to different fitness levels. Even small amounts of daily movement provide meaningful benefits, and midwives can encourage women to find activities they enjoy and can sustain.

Herbs are not replacements for skilled clinical judgment or emergency medicine. Instead, they are partners offering strength, nourishment, and gentle medicine that supports the natural process of pregnancy and birth. Herbs remain important allies for nourishment and comfort in pregnancy when used with respect and knowledge. Herbal care is most effective when it balances traditional wisdom with modern safety knowledge, offering support without risk.

BIRTH ROOT
Trillium erectum

Chapter Eight Self-Assessment

Multiple Choice
1. What is a common side effect of traditional iron supplements?
   a) Rash
   b) Constipation
   c) Leg cramps
   d) Headache

2. Which food is highest in natural folate?
   a) Cheese
   b) Lentils
   c) Chicken breast
   d) White rice

3. Which of the following is NOT typically recommended for managing constipation?
   a) High-fiber foods
   b) Warm compresses
   c) Carbonated beverages
   d) Senna tea

4. Which mineral supports thyroid hormone production and fetal brain development?
   a) Magnesium
   b) Iodine
   c) Calcium
   d) Zinc

5. Which of the following is an example of culturally responsive care?
   a) Advising all clients to take daily bubble baths for self-care
   b) Learning traditional postpartum practices used by the client's community
   c) Using the same handout for every prenatal client regardless of background
   d) Avoiding discussion of trauma or emotions during visits

6. What is one possible reason for leg cramps during pregnancy?
   a) High iron levels
   b) Dehydration and poor circulation
   c) Low blood pressure
   d) Excessive protein intake

7. Which herbal remedies may help with nausea?
   a) Comfrey and goldenseal
   b) Peppermint and ginger
   c) Red clover and echinacea
   d) Burdock and dandelion

8. Which of the following best describes intersectionality?
   a) Teaching nutrition in group classes
   b) Focusing only on dietary intake during visits
   c) Understanding how multiple identities and systems affect health
   d) Encouraging clients to follow a weight-loss plan

9. Which exercise approach is generally recommended for most pregnant women?
   a) High-intensity interval training daily
   b) Gentle, regular activity like walking or swimming
   c) Bed rest for the entire third trimester
   d) Abdominal crunches to maintain muscle tone

10. Which herb is commonly used as a nutritive tonic and uterine support in pregnancy?
    a) Raspberry leaf
    b) Pennyroyal
    c) Blue cohosh
    d) Sage

11. Which vitamin is especially critical for preventing neural tube defects?
    a) Vitamin A
    b) Vitamin C
    c) Folate
    d) Vitamin K

12. Which of the following foods is an excellent source of omega-3 fatty acids during pregnancy?
    a) Flaxseed
    b) White bread
    c) Chicken breast
    d) Cheese

13. Which activity should generally be avoided during pregnancy?
    a) Swimming
    b) Hot yoga
    c) Walking
    d) Prenatal stretching

14. Which mineral is most often linked with preventing anemia in pregnancy?
    a) Magnesium
    b) Iron
    c) Zinc
    d) Calcium

15. Which of the following herbs is generally considered unsafe in pregnancy?
    a) Nettle leaf
    b) Red raspberry leaf
    c) Blue cohosh
    d) Peppermint

Fill in the Blank

16. Clients should be encouraged to eat _____ meals throughout the day to manage nausea.
17. To reduce heartburn, clients should remain in an _____ position after eating.
18. The herbal remedy _____ is often used for its soothing effect on the digestive tract.
19. A client who feels isolated or afraid in their relationship should be offered referrals to _____ and _____ resources.
20. During pregnancy, frequent contact with a midwife creates repeated opportunities for _____ and _____.
21. The recommended daily intake of iron in pregnancy is _____ mg.
22. Choline supports _____ development and is often found in _____.
23. _____ is a fat-soluble vitamin important for calcium absorption and immune function.
24. A deficiency in _____ can cause anemia and neurological symptoms, especially in vegans.

True or False

25. _____ Nausea usually resolves by the end of the first trimester.
26. _____ Ginger is effective for all clients experiencing nausea in pregnancy.
27. _____ Heartburn is uncommon in pregnancy and should be investigated as a red flag.
28. _____ Constipation can be worsened by iron supplements.
29. _____ Leg cramps are most often related to magnesium or calcium imbalance.
30. _____ Red raspberry leaf tea is considered a safe during all stages of pregnancy.
31. _____ Iron is better absorbed when taken with calcium.
32. _____ Folate is especially important in the first trimester.
33. _____ Vitamin D needs vary depending on sun exposure, skin tone, and body size.
34. _____ A client with a vegan diet may need to supplement with B12 and DHA.
35. _____ Chronic stress during pregnancy has no known impact on outcomes.
36. _____ Harm reduction is about helping people reduce risk without judgment.
37. _____ Clients with strong social support tend to have better mental health in pregnancy
38. _____ Midwives should only provide education when a client asks for it.
39. _____ Clients are often more open to changing health behaviors during pregnancy.
40. _____ Moderate exercise during pregnancy usually improves circulation and reduces discomfort.
41. _____ Pennyroyal tea is a safe option for nausea in pregnancy.
42. _____ Hydration supports both nutrient absorption and circulation during pregnancy.
43. _____ Unpasteurized cheeses are a safe and nutritious food in pregnancy if eaten in moderation.
44. _____ Poor maternal nutrition during pregnancy can increase the child's risk of chronic disease later in life.
45. _____ Herbs such as nettle and alfalfa are considered nutritive and can safely support iron and mineral intake during pregnancy.
46. _____ Gotu kola is a safe herbal remedy for use during pregnancy
47. _____ Food sovereignty only applies to Indigenous people.
48. _____ Clients are more likely to follow nutritional advice that respects their traditional foodways.
49. _____ Essential oils should never be ingested internally.

Matching

50. Match the nutrient to its primary function:
    1. ____ Supports brain and spinal cord development   A. Iron
    2. ____ Helps regulate thyroid hormones and fetal brain growth   B. Vitamin D
    3. ____ Needed for red blood cell formation and oxygen delivery C. Iodine
    4. ____ Aids in muscle relaxation, digestion, and sleep   D. Choline
    5. ____ Supports bone strength and immune health   E. Magnesium

51. Match the discomfort with its recommended support:
    1. ____ Magnesium, hydration, calf stretches   A. Nausea
    2. ____ Calcium carbonate, upright posture   B. Constipation
    3. ____ Peppermint, small frequent meals   C. Heartburn
    4. ____ Flaxseed, fiber, fluids   D. Leg cramps

52. Match the activity or practice to its primary health benefit:
    1. ____ Improves circulation and helps regulate blood sugar   A. Walking
    2. ____ Supports fetal oxygen transport and prevents anemia   B. Swimming
    3. ____ Enhances breath awareness, balance, and flexibility   C. Prenatal yoga
    4. ____ Builds joint stability and reduces strain on the back and pelvis   D. Mindful eating
    5. ____ Supports emotional balance during meals   E. Iron-rich foods

Chapter Eight: Reading & References

Recommended Reading Health Promotion for Midwives
- Bowden, J. (2016). ***Health Promotion in Midwifery*** (4th ed.). Routledge. Focuses on the role of midwives in promoting health, addressing both practical and theoretical aspects of care.
- Clapp, J. F. III. (2012). ***Exercising Through Your Pregnancy*** (2nd ed.). Addicus Books. Evidence-based resource by a physician and researcher, highlighting the safety and benefits of exercise for both mother and baby.
- Guyett, A. (2017). ***The Herbalist's Guide to Pregnancy, Childbirth and Beyond.*** Aeon Books. Provides safe and practical guidance on herbal support during the childbearing cycle, integrating traditional and clinical perspectives.
- Nichols, L. (2018). ***Real Food for Pregnancy: The Science and Wisdom of Optimal Prenatal Nutrition.*** Comprehensive, evidence-based guide to prenatal nutrition that bridges modern science with practical application.
- Romm, A. (2014). ***The Natural Pregnancy Book: Your Complete Guide to a Safe, Organic Pregnancy and Childbirth with Herbs, Nutrition, and Other Holistic Choices*** (3rd ed.). Ten Speed Press. A handbook for those seeking a safe, eco-friendly, and integrative approach to pregnancy, featuring updated herbal and nutritional guidance.
- Singingtree, D. (2024). ***The Eagletree Guide to Herbal Medicine Making.*** Eagletree Press. A practical, accessible resource for creating tinctures, salves, teas, and other herbal preparations, emphasizing safety and empowerment in plant medicine.
- Weed, S. (1986). ***Wise Woman Herbal for the Childbearing Year.*** Ash Tree Publishing. A classic text offering traditional herbal knowledge and practical applications for pregnancy, birth, and postpartum care.

References

American College of Obstetricians and Gynecologists. (2020). *Physical activity and exercise during pregnancy and the postpartum period* (Committee Opinion No. 804). *Obstetrics & Gynecology, 135*(4), e178–e188. https://doi.org/10.1097/AOG.0000000000003772

Barker, D. J. P. (2008). *Nutrition in the womb: How better nutrition during development will prevent heart disease, diabetes, and stroke*. CRC Press.

Gholami, F., Neisani Samani, L., Kashanian, M., Naseri, M., Hosseini, A. F., & Hashemi Nejad, S. A. (2016). Onset of labor in post-term pregnancy by chamomile. *Iranian Red Crescent Medical Journal, 18*(11), e19871. https://doi.org/10.5812/ircmj.19871

Guyett, A. (2017). *The herbalist's guide to pregnancy, childbirth and beyond*. Aeon Books.

Kennedy, D. A., Lupattelli, A., Koren, G., & Nordeng, H. (2013). Herbal medicine use in pregnancy: Results of a multinational study. *BMC Complementary and Alternative Medicine, 13*, 355. https://doi.org/10.1186/1472-6882-13-355

Kennedy, D. A., Lupattelli, A., Koren, G., & Nordeng, H. (2016). Safety classification of herbal medicines used in pregnancy in a multinational study. *BMC Complementary and Alternative Medicine, 16*, 102. https://doi.org/10.1186/s12906-016-1079-z

Louik, C., Gardiner, P., Kelley, K., & Mitchell, A. A. (2010). Use of herbal treatments in pregnancy. *American Journal of Obstetrics and Gynecology, 202*(5), 439.e1–439.e10. https://doi.org/10.1016/j.ajog.2010.01.055

Marcian, M. (2013, July 9). *Alkaloids*. The Naturopathic Herbalist. https://thenaturopathicherbalist.com/plant-constituents/alkaloids/

Nichols, L. (2018). *Real food for pregnancy: The science and wisdom of optimal prenatal nutrition*. Blue Poppy Press.

Picciano, M. F. (2003). Pregnancy and lactation: Physiological adjustments, nutritional requirements, and the role of dietary supplements. *Journal of Nutrition, 133*(6), 1997S–2002S. https://doi.org/10.1093/jn/133.6.1997S

Terzioglu Bebitoglu, B. (2020). Frequently used herbal teas during pregnancy: Short update. *Medeni Medical Journal, 35*(1), 55–61. https://doi.org/10.5222/MMJ.2020.69851

University of Texas at El Paso. (2021). *Herbs to avoid during pregnancy*. Herbal Safety. https://www.utep.edu/herbal-safety/populations/herbs-to-avoid-during-pregnancy.html

Zeisel, S. H. (2006). Choline: Critical role during fetal development and dietary requirements in adults. *Annual Review of Nutrition, 26*, 229–250. https://doi.org/10.1146/annurev.nutr.26.061505.111156

Chapter Nine
Infection, Immunity, & Midwifery Practice

Objectives
After completing this chapter, the student should be able to:
1. **Describe** how the maternal immune system adapts during pregnancy and explain the concept of immune tolerance.
2. **Identify** the key infections of concern in pregnancy and outline prevention and screening measures (including TORCH, GBS, and others).
3. **Explain** the mechanism and prevention of Rh incompatibility.
4. **Discuss** the role of the microbiome in immune health and infection prevention.
5. **Recognize** the importance of immunizations during pregnancy and describe which vaccines are safe or contraindicated.
6. **Explain** the midwife's role in infection control.
7. **Demonstrate** correct handwashing technique and proper glove removal.
8. **Explain** Standard and Transmission-Based Precautions and apply them to midwifery practice.
9. **Identify** modes of infection transmission and describe ways to interrupt each link in the chain of infection.
10. **Differentiate** between cleaning, disinfection, and sterilization, and match equipment to the appropriate processing level.
11. **Outline** steps for safe instrument processing, including low-resource sterilization techniques.
12. **Apply** infection control principles to home birth and clinical settings, balancing safety with respect for family and environment.

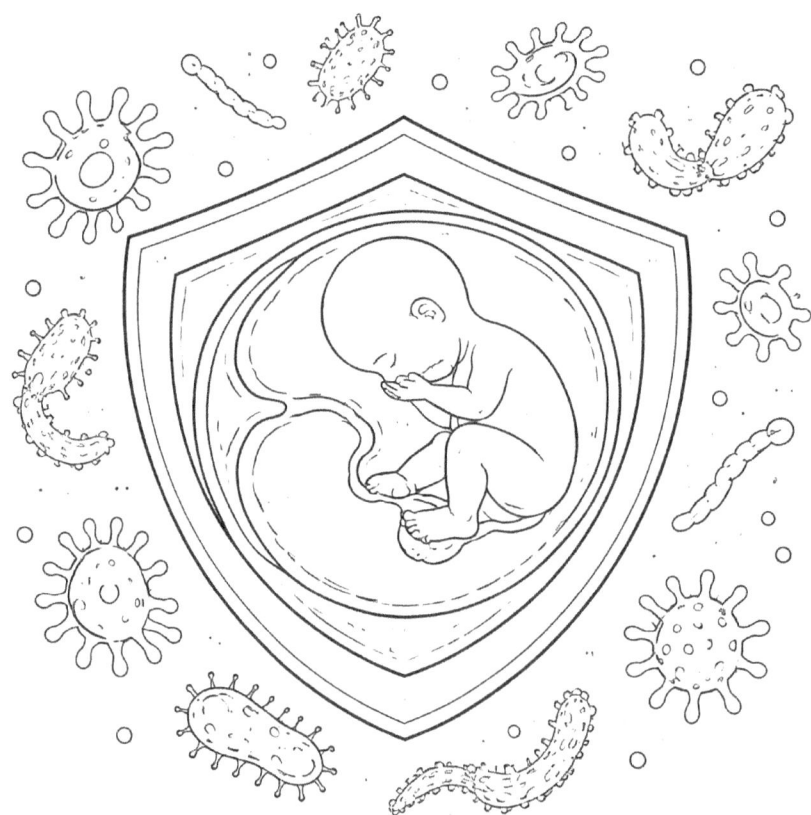

Pregnancy, Immunity & Infection Prevention

Pregnancy requires a remarkable balance. The mother's immune system must tolerate the growing fetus, which carries different genetic material, while continuing to protect both from harmful pathogens. At the same time, the body's microbiome, the community of helpful bacteria, fungi, and other microorganisms that live within and on the body, plays an essential role in digestion, immunity, and birth outcomes. Supporting these natural defenses is as important as preventing infection.

The immune system also remembers past exposures. During pregnancy, this memory can influence how the body responds to future pregnancies. Studies suggest immune cells retain information from previous pregnancies, shaping the body's tolerance and protection in later ones. Rh incompatibility is one example, where the mother's immune system may recognize and react to fetal blood cells as foreign if they differ in Rh type. Understanding how immune tolerance, sensitization, and memory work helps midwives anticipate and prevent complications before they arise.

Midwives care for pregnant women and newborns in diverse settings where infection risk is present yet often preventable. A solid understanding of how immunity adapts in pregnancy allows midwives to promote resilience while protecting against illness. When immune balance or microbial health is disrupted, infection or inflammation may occur. Midwives play a key role in recognizing early signs of imbalance, supporting immune strength, and teaching practical strategies that prevent infection and promote health.

> **Key Vocabulary**
>
> - **Pathogen:** A microorganism capable of causing disease.
> - **Colonization:** When microorganisms live on or in a body surface without causing illness.
> - **Virulence:** The degree to which a pathogen can cause disease.
> - **Host:** A person or organism that harbors a microorganism.
> - **Antibody:** A protein produced by the immune system that recognizes and helps neutralize specific pathogens.
> - **Antigen:** Any substance that triggers an immune response, such as parts of bacteria, viruses, or other foreign cells.
> - **Vector:** A living carrier, such as a mosquito or tick, that transmits infection between hosts.
> - **Fomite:** An inanimate object or surface, such as linens or instruments, that can transfer pathogens.
> - **Droplet Transmission:** Spread of infection through respiratory droplets produced when coughing, sneezing, or talking; droplets travel short distances and fall quickly.
> - **Airborne Transmission:** Spread of pathogens through tiny particles that remain suspended in air and can travel long distances.
> - **Nosocomial Infection:** An infection acquired within a healthcare setting, also known as a healthcare-associated infection (HAI), and one that midwives work hard to prevent.

Ways Midwives Support Immune Health
- Encourage balanced nutrition and hydration
- Promote rest, stress management, and emotional well-being
- Support healthy gut and vaginal microbiota through diet and gentle herbal care
- Monitor Rh status and discuss antibody screening as part of prenatal care
- Reduce unnecessary antibiotic use and help clients restore microbial balance
- Provide culturally sensitive education about natural immune support

Ways Midwives Prevent Infection
- Teach effective hand hygiene to clients and birth support people
- Practice and model clean or sterile technique as appropriate
- Recognize early signs of infection such as fever, uterine tenderness, or unusual discharge
- Educate clients on food safety and reducing exposure to toxoplasmosis or listeria
- Maintain proper disinfection, sterilization, and waste disposal procedures

The Maternal Immune System in Pregnancy

Pregnancy is a state of finely tuned immune adaptation. The mother's body must protect against infection while tolerating the presence of the fetus, which carries genetic material from both parents. Rather than weakening the immune system, pregnancy reorganizes it, shifting toward tolerance in some areas and heightened defense in others.

The immune system protects the body through two closely linked processes:

- **Innate Immunity** is the body's rapid, first line of defense. It includes barriers such as the skin and mucous membranes, inflammation, and white blood cells like macrophages and neutrophils that attack invaders non-specifically.
- **Adaptive Immunity** is slower but more specialized. It relies on lymphocytes (B and T cells) that recognize specific pathogens, remember prior exposures, and generate antibodies for lasting protection.

During pregnancy, both systems adjust in complex ways through a process called **immune modulation**. In early gestation, innate immune activity increases to protect implantation and the developing embryo. Later, adaptive immunity shifts toward tolerance to prevent rejection of the fetus while maintaining defense against disease. Specialized white blood cells, including **T regulatory cells (Tregs)**, help the immune system recognize the fetus as safe, while hormones such as progesterone and estrogen calm inflammation and support placental development.

The **placenta** serves as both a barrier and a communication bridge. It prevents direct contact between maternal and fetal blood while allowing oxygen, nutrients, and antibodies to cross safely. Immune cells at the maternal–fetal interface continuously exchange chemical messages to regulate inflammation and maintain healthy pregnancy function.

The immune system also develops a form of **immune memory** during pregnancy. Cells that recognize paternal antigens from the fetus may persist in the mother's body for years, influencing how her immune system responds in future pregnancies. This memory can help promote faster adaptation but also explains why Rh incompatibility sometimes occurs in subsequent pregnancies.

Because immune balance can be influenced by stress, nutrition, and infection, midwives play a vital role in supporting immune health. Encouraging rest, good nutrition, and emotional well-being, as well as reinforcing infection-prevention measures such as hand hygiene and timely treatment of urinary or vaginal infections, helps maintain immune stability. Understanding these mechanisms enables midwives to interpret common pregnancy changes, such as mild nasal congestion, fatigue, or increased susceptibility to certain infections, as part of normal immune modulation while remaining alert for warning signs that indicate illness.

> **Did You Know?**
> During pregnancy, a small number of fetal cells can cross the placenta and remain in the mother's body for decades. This phenomenon, called **microchimerism**, means that traces of each pregnancy may persist long after birth. Researchers are studying how these cells might influence immune function, tissue repair, and autoimmune disease. Although the full significance is not yet understood, it reminds us of the deep biological connection that continues between mother and child.

The maternal immune system is designed to protect both mother and baby, recognizing which cells belong and which do not. However, this system of tolerance is not perfect. In some cases, the mother's immune system reacts to fetal blood cells as foreign and produces antibodies against them. This process, known as **Rh incompatibility**, represents a special kind of immune response that can affect future pregnancies if not carefully managed.

BLOOD TYPES AND RH FACTOR

Understanding blood types and Rh compatibility is essential to safe pregnancy care. Midwives play an important role in recognizing potential incompatibilities, educating families, and ensuring that appropriate testing and preventive treatment occur.

Blood Types

There are four basic blood types in humans: **O, A, B, and AB.**

Blood Type	Frequency	Key Features
O	46% (universal donor)	Lacks both A and B antigens
A	41%	Has A antigens, produces anti-B antibodies
B	9%	Has B antigens, produces anti-A antibodies
AB	4% (universal recipient)	Has both A and B antigens and no antibodies

(Percentages are approximate as they population-specific and vary widely by ethnicity and region).

Each blood type is defined by **antigens** on the surface of red blood cells. Antigens are proteins that can trigger the formation of **antibodies**, which protect the body from foreign substances.

- Type **A** blood has A antigens and anti-B antibodies.
- Type **B** has B antigens and anti-A antibodies.
- Type **O** has neither antigen but both antibodies, allowing it to donate to all other types.
- Type **AB** has both antigens and no antibodies, allowing it to receive from any type.

The Rh Factor

The **Rh factor** (Rhesus factor) is another antigen that may be present on red blood cells.

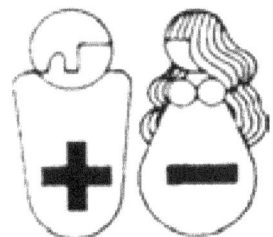

- **People with the Rh antigen are Rh positive (Rh⁺).** Among people of European descent, approximately 85 percent are Rh positive. Rh incompatibility occurs less frequently among people of African or Asian descent.
- **Those without the Rh antigen are Rh negative (Rh⁻).** Among people of European descent, approximately 15 percent are Rh negative.

If blood from an Rh-positive person enters the bloodstream of someone who is Rh negative, the immune system recognizes the Rh antigen as foreign and forms antibodies against it. This process is called **isoimmunization** or **sensitization**.

During pregnancy, an **Rh-negative woman** carrying an **Rh-positive baby** may be exposed to small amounts of fetal blood. This can occur during birth, miscarriage, abortion, abdominal trauma, or procedures such as amniocentesis. The first pregnancy is usually unaffected, but once sensitized, the mother's immune system "remembers" the Rh antigen and produces antibodies more rapidly in later pregnancies. These antibodies can cross the placenta and destroy fetal red blood cells, causing hemolytic disease of the newborn. Routine Rh screening and timely Rhogam administration have made Rh disease rare in modern midwifery practice. Midwives ensure prevention by identifying Rh-negative clients early, providing clear education, and coordinating care for antibody monitoring or specialist referral when needed. Rh incompatibility occurs only when an Rh-negative mother carries an Rh-positive baby. If both parents are Rh negative, no incompatibility exists.

How Rh Disease Develops

1. Fetal red blood cells from an Rh-positive baby enter the bloodstream of an Rh-negative mother.
2. The mother's immune system responds by forming **anti-Rh antibodies**.
3. These antibodies remain in her blood after pregnancy.
4. In a future Rh-positive pregnancy, antibodies cross the placenta and attack fetal red blood cells.

This immune reaction can cause fetal anemia, jaundice, or severe complications such as **hydrops fetalis** (fetal heart failure caused by anemia).

How Rh Disease Develops

Rh negative mother / **Rh positive father**

- **DURING PREGNANCY**: Rh negative mother with Rh positive baby
- **AT DELIVERY**: Rh positive baby's blood enters mother's bloodstream
- **MONTHS LATER**: Maternal immune system forms Rh antibodies that remain after pregnancy
- **LATER PREGNANCY**: In later pregnancies, maternal antibodies cross the placenta and destroy fetal red blood cells

Other Blood Group Sensitivities

While the Rh factor is the most clinically significant, other antigens can also cause sensitization:

- **Du factor**: A weak form of the Rh antigen. Women who are Rh negative but Du positive are rarely at risk and are considered Rh positive for practical purposes.
- **Kell factor**: Found in about 9% of the population. Kell-positive babies can sensitize a Kell-negative mother similarly to Rh sensitization.
- **C, E, and Duffy** factors: Less common but occasionally associated with hemolytic disease.

Prevention and Testing

Rhogam (Rh Immune Globulin) is a preventive injection containing anti-Rh antibodies that protect the mother's immune system from reacting to Rh-positive fetal cells.

- Given at **28 weeks gestation** and again within **72 hours after birth**, miscarriage, abortion, or any event involving maternal–fetal blood exchange.
- Also administered after trauma, amniocentesis, or vaginal bleeding.

Routine **antibody screening** (Indirect Coombs test) is done early in pregnancy and repeated at 28 weeks for all Rh-negative clients.

- If antibodies are found, further testing (Antibody Identification and Direct Coombs) determines the type and level of sensitivity.
- Rising **antibody titers** above 1:16 suggest increased risk for fetal hemolysis and require specialist consultation.

Midwives play a key role in ensuring timely administration of Rh immune globulin, monitoring antibody titers, and documenting all Rh-related results in prenatal charts. These preventive steps are simple yet lifesaving. Rhogam prevents sensitization but does not remove existing antibodies. Once antibodies form, Rhogam is no longer effective. Regular antibody screening helps detect sensitization early so appropriate follow-up and referral can occur.

> **Key Fact**
> Routine Rh screening and timely Rhogam administration have made Rh disease extremely rare in the developed world. However, in areas where medical resources or Rhogam are unavailable, hemolytic disease of the newborn from Rh incompatibility may still occur.
>
> Access to screening and preventive care remains the most effective way to eliminate this condition worldwide.

Rh Testing and Rhogam Administration

Timing	Purpose	Action / Notes
First prenatal visit	Determine maternal Rh type and antibody status	Perform ABO/Rh typing and Indirect Coombs test
28 weeks gestation	Prevent sensitization during pregnancy	Administer Rhogam to all Rh-negative, unsensitized clients
After any potential blood exchange	Prevent sensitization	Give Rhogam after miscarriage, abortion, trauma, amniocentesis, or bleeding
After delivery	Protect future pregnancies	Administer Rhogam within 72 hours postpartum if baby is Rh positive
If antibody screen is positive	Monitor sensitization	Perform Antibody ID and monitor titers; refer if levels rise or remain high

---

Exercise 9.1 Rh Prevention
Complete the sentences using the correct term or phrase.

1. The _____ screens for antibodies in an Rh-negative client early in pregnancy.
2. Rhogam should be given routinely at _____ weeks gestation and again within _____ hours after delivery.
3. Rh incompatibility occurs only when an _____-negative mother carries an _____-positive baby.
4. Once antibodies are formed, _____ is no longer effective.
5. Rising antibody _____ above 1:16 may indicate a need for specialist referral.

Infection in Pregnancy

The placental barrier provides an important level of protection by filtering many potential pathogens, but it is not impenetrable. Certain viruses, bacteria, and parasites such as **cytomegalovirus (CMV), rubella, toxoplasmosis,** and **syphilis** can cross into the fetal circulation and cause serious complications. The effects of infection depend on the type of microorganism, the stage of pregnancy, and the health of both mother and baby.

Infections during pregnancy can affect:
- **Maternal health:** Increased risk of complications such as preterm labor, fever, or sepsis.
- **The fetus:** Some pathogens cross the placenta and may lead to miscarriage, congenital infection, or birth defects affecting the brain, heart, or other organs.
- **Pregnancy outcome:** Depending on timing and type, infections can increase risks of stillbirth, low birth weight, or premature delivery.

Early identification and appropriate treatment of infections are essential parts of prenatal care. Midwives play a key role in prevention by teaching hygiene, nutrition, and safe food handling practices, as well as ensuring timely testing and referrals. Good infection control protects not only the mother and baby, but also the birth team and community.

Postpartum and Newborn Considerations

After birth, the newborn's immune system remains immature and relies heavily on passive immunity from the birthing parent, particularly through antibodies transferred across the placenta during pregnancy and through breastfeeding. Infections during the postpartum period can affect both mother and baby, making early detection and careful follow-up especially important. Supporting good hand hygiene, clean cord care, and breastfeeding can significantly reduce the risk of illness in the early weeks of life.

Understanding how infections begin helps midwives recognize risks, interpret early symptoms, and provide effective prevention strategies, an important foundation for protecting both mother and child.

Chapter Nine: Infection, Immunity, & Midwifery Practice

What is Infection?

Infection occurs when a harmful microorganism overcomes the body's natural defenses and begins to multiply. This can disrupt normal function and trigger symptoms such as fever, swelling, pain, or fatigue. Infections can be mild or severe, acute or chronic, localized or systemic. Not all microorganisms cause disease, and many are part of the body's normal flora.

Some microorganisms—like those in the gut and on the skin—play essential roles in digestion, immune regulation, and pathogen defense. This beneficial community is called the microbiome.

Types of Pathogens

A. BACTERIA Single-celled organisms that may cause urinary tract infections (UTIs), Group B Strep colonization, or chorioamnionitis.

B. VIRUSES Require host cells to replicate. Examples include influenza, COVID-19, and herpes simplex virus.

C. FUNGI Include yeasts like *Candida*, which can cause vaginal or oral thrush.

D. PARASITES Organisms like *Toxoplasma gondii*, which may be transmitted via undercooked meat or cat feces and can affect the fetus.

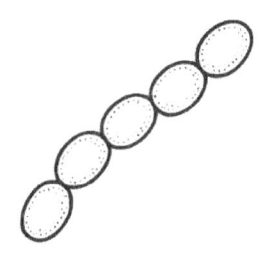
A: Bacterium
Group B Streptococcus

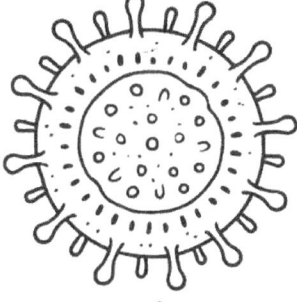
B: Virus
Cytomegalovirus

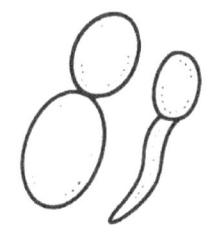
C: Fungus
Candida albicans

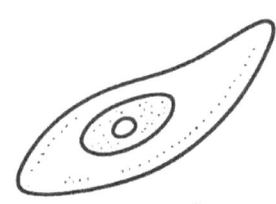
D: Parasite
Toxoplasma gondii

Common Infections in Pregnancy

While many infections are mild, certain pathogens are especially important in pregnancy because they can affect fetal development. These are often remembered by the acronym **TORCH**, which stands for:

T – Toxoplasmosis: Caused by *Toxoplasma gondii*, often transmitted through undercooked meat or cat feces. May lead to miscarriage, stillbirth, or neurological effects.

O – Other infections: Includes **syphilis**, **varicella (chickenpox)**, and **parvovirus B19**. These can cause stillbirth, fetal anemia, or congenital abnormalities.

R – Rubella: Also known as German measles; can cause congenital rubella syndrome with heart, eye, or hearing defects if infection occurs early in pregnancy.

C – Cytomegalovirus (CMV): Usually mild in adults but may cause congenital infection, hearing loss, or developmental delays in the fetus.

H – Herpes simplex virus (HSV): May cause neonatal herpes if transmitted during birth; suppressive antiviral therapy may be recommended near term.

The **TORCH** group provides a useful framework for remembering infections that can cross the placenta and cause congenital disease. However, modern midwifery and infectious disease care now recognize several additional infections that can also pose risks. These include **HIV**, **hepatitis B and C**, and **Zika virus**, which are sometimes grouped with TORCH under the expanded term **TORCHES** or **TORCH-Z**. While the term TORCH is still used informally, the trend is towards specific diagnostic testing. Each requires preventive screening, counseling, and appropriate treatment or referral as part of comprehensive prenatal care. Midwives play an essential role in recognizing risk factors, supporting preventive education, and ensuring testing and treatment when indicated.

Along with screening and education, immunization is another key tool in preventing infection-related complications during pregnancy.

Group B Streptococcus (GBS)

Group B Streptococcus (GBS) is a common bacterium found naturally in the digestive and genital tracts. Many healthy women carry GBS without symptoms, but during pregnancy or birth, it can pass to the baby and cause serious infection such as sepsis, pneumonia, or meningitis. GBS is a leading cause of newborn infection, but most cases are preventable through screening and treatment during labor.

Screening for GBS colonization is usually performed at **35–37 weeks** with a vaginal and rectal swab. If results are positive, antibiotics in labor help prevent newborn infection.

Midwives play a key role in education, explaining that GBS is not sexually transmitted or a sign of poor hygiene, but a normal bacterium that can temporarily overgrow. Discussing the benefits and timing of antibiotics, as well as alternative approaches when appropriate, supports informed, family-centered care.

Types of Infections in Pregnancy

Infection	Cause / Type	Transmission	Risks in Pregnancy	Prevention / Midwifery Focus
Toxoplasmosis	*Toxoplasma gondii* (parasite)	Undercooked meat, cat feces, soil	Miscarriage, stillbirth, congenital infection	Wash hands, cook meat thoroughly, avoid cat litter
Other (Syphilis, Varicella, Parvovirus B19)	Bacteria or virus	Sexual contact or respiratory droplets	Fetal death, anemia, congenital infection	Routine screening, safe sexual practices, prenatal testing
Rubella	Rubella virus	Airborne droplets	Birth defects, deafness, heart and eye abnormalities	Vaccinate before pregnancy, avoid exposure
Cytomegalovirus (CMV)	CMV virus	Saliva, urine, or bodily fluids	Congenital hearing or vision loss, growth restriction	Hand hygiene after contact with young children; avoid sharing utensils
Herpes Simplex Virus (HSV)	Herpes virus type 1 or 2	Direct contact with lesions	Neonatal herpes during birth	Antiviral therapy, avoid contact with active lesions
Group B Streptococcus (GBS)	*Streptococcus agalactiae* (bacterium)	Vaginal or rectal colonization at birth	Neonatal sepsis, pneumonia, meningitis	Routine screening at 35–37 weeks, intrapartum antibiotics
Bacterial Vaginosis (BV)	Imbalance of vaginal flora (*Lactobacillus* loss)	Overgrowth of anaerobic bacteria (not STI)	Preterm birth, PROM, postpartum infection	Support vaginal microbiome health; treat symptomatic cases
Listeria	*Listeria monocytogenes* (bacterium)	Contaminated food (unpasteurized dairy, deli meats)	Miscarriage, stillbirth, neonatal sepsis	Avoid high-risk foods, refrigerate properly
Zika Virus	Flavivirus (mosquito-borne)	Mosquito bites, sexual contact	Microcephaly, developmental delays	Mosquito control, repellents, avoid travel to affected regions
Hepatitis B	Hepatitis B virus	Bloodborne, sexual, or perinatal	Maternal liver disease, neonatal infection	Universal screening, vaccination, newborn prophylaxis
HIV	Human immunodeficiency virus	Bloodborne or sexual	Maternal illness, perinatal transmission	Antiretroviral therapy, in some cases avoid breastfeeding
Varicella (Chickenpox)	Varicella-zoster virus	Airborne, contact with lesions	Maternal pneumonia, congenital varicella syndrome	Preconception vaccination, avoid exposure

Pathways of Perinatal Infection

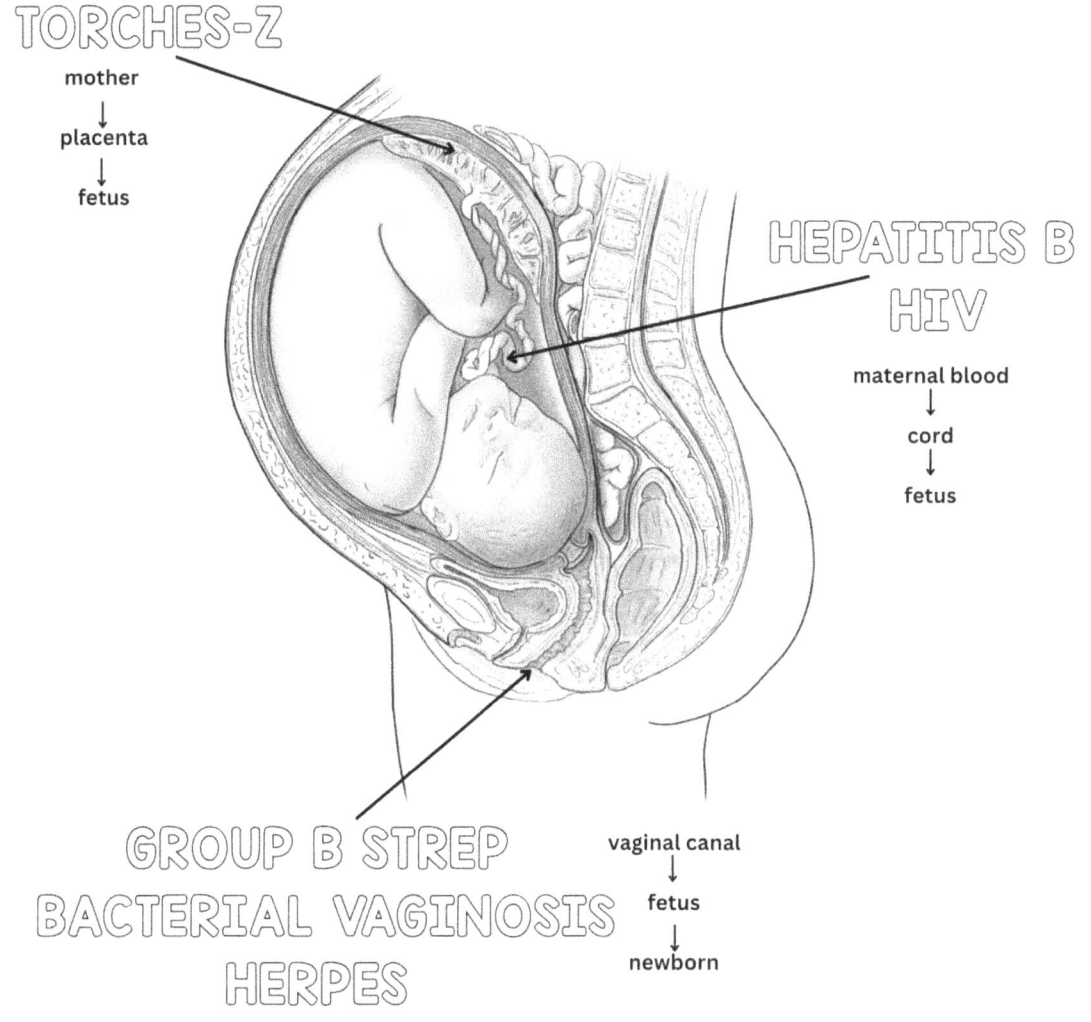

Exercise 9.2: Recognizing Infection Risks
Match each infection to its description or route of transmission.

1. _____ Rubella 2. _____ Cytomegalovirus 3. _____ Toxoplasmosis 4. _____ Syphilis 5. _____ Group B Streptococcus 6. _____ Varicella (Chickenpox) 7. _____ Herpes Simplex Virus 8. _____ Zika Virus	**A.** Spread by mosquitoes; may cause severe birth defects including microcephaly **B.** Caused by *Toxoplasma gondii*; spread through cat feces or undercooked meat **C.** Can cause congenital hearing and vision problems **D.** Preventable through vaccination before pregnancy **E.** Crosses the placenta and can cause stillbirth or congenital infection **F.** May be passed to baby during labor and cause newborn sepsis **G.** Primary infection in pregnancy may cause congenital varicella syndrome **H.** Can be transmitted to the newborn during birth and cause neonatal herpes

Immunizations During Pregnancy

Vaccinations during pregnancy aim to protect both mother and baby from preventable diseases. Certain vaccines can safely strengthen maternal immunity and provide antibodies that cross the placenta, offering protection to the newborn during the first months of life. Midwives support clients in making culturally sensitive, well-informed choices about vaccination. This includes discussing timing, safety, and community considerations, and respecting personal or cultural beliefs while providing clear, evidence-based guidance. Some clients may decline certain or all vaccinations; their choices should be respected while ensuring they receive balanced information to support autonomous decision-making.

Commonly recommended vaccines include:

- **Tdap (Tetanus, Diphtheria, Pertussis):** Recommended in each pregnancy, ideally between 27 and 36 weeks, to protect newborns from whooping cough.
- **Influenza:** Safe in any trimester; helps prevent severe maternal illness and protects infants after birth.
- **COVID-19 (if applicable):** Current guidelines support vaccination when benefits outweigh risks, especially for clients at higher risk of exposure or complications.

Live vaccines such as MMR (measles, mumps, rubella) and Varicella are **contraindicated** during pregnancy because they may pose a risk to the fetus. These should be given before conception or postpartum if needed.

Microbiome and Infection Prevention

The microbiome acts as a natural defense system during pregnancy. These beneficial microorganisms protect against infection, support digestion, and strengthen immunity for both mother and baby. Hormonal and immune shifts can alter microbial balance, sometimes increasing vulnerability to infection. Maintaining a healthy microbiome is a vital strategy for infection prevention during pregnancy and postpartum.

Prebiotics and **probiotics** work together to create a supportive environment for balanced immunity, digestion, and overall wellness during pregnancy and postpartum.

- **Prebiotics** enhance the survival of probiotics and promote long-term microbiome stability for both mother and baby.
- **Probiotics** can help reduce risks of vaginal infections, improve digestion, and support healthy immune function.

The maternal microbiome, particularly in the vagina, gut, and skin, helps seed the infant's microbiome and supports immune and digestive development. Research also suggests that the placenta may have its own microbiome, influencing early immune priming. A balanced microbiome depends on good oral health, a healthy vaginal environment, and nutrition that supports beneficial bacteria.

Practical Tips for Supporting the Microbiome

- **Eat a rainbow:** Variety supports microbial diversity.
- **Avoid unnecessary antibiotics;** they can disrupt healthy flora.
- **Use gentle soaps;** harsh antibacterial products strip the skin microbiome.
- **Spend time outdoors;** soil microbes strengthen immune balance.
- **Breastfeed when possible;** these early exposures seed lifelong immunity.

> **Did You Know?**
> The composition of a mother's microbiome can change from early to late pregnancy, often increasing in diversity. This shift helps prepare the body for birth and early milk production, showing how dynamic and responsive the microbiome truly is.

Supporting and Protecting the Developing Microbiome
1. **Oral Health**
   - Pregnancy hormones can lead to gum inflammation and bleeding, creating pathways for infection.
   - Periodontal disease has been linked to preterm birth and low birth weight.
2. **Vaginal Protection**
   - *Lactobacillus* dominates during pregnancy, producing lactic acid that maintains an acidic environment hostile to harmful bacteria.
   - Disruptions, such as bacterial vaginosis, increase risks of preterm labor, miscarriage, and postpartum infection.
3. **Infant Microbiome Seeding**
   - Vaginal birth exposes newborns to maternal microbes that colonize the gut and support immune development.
   - Babies born by cesarean may have different microbial patterns, often resembling skin or hospital flora.
   - Antibiotic use, mode of birth, and breastfeeding all influence microbial inheritance.
4. **Gut Health Support**
   - During pregnancy and postpartum, maintaining a healthy gut through balanced nutrition—including prebiotic and probiotic foods—helps sustain the microbiome for both mother and baby.

Prebiotics

Prebiotics are non-digestible fibers and plant compounds that feed the beneficial bacteria already living in the gut. By nourishing probiotics, prebiotics help those microbes thrive and improve the overall resilience of the microbiome.

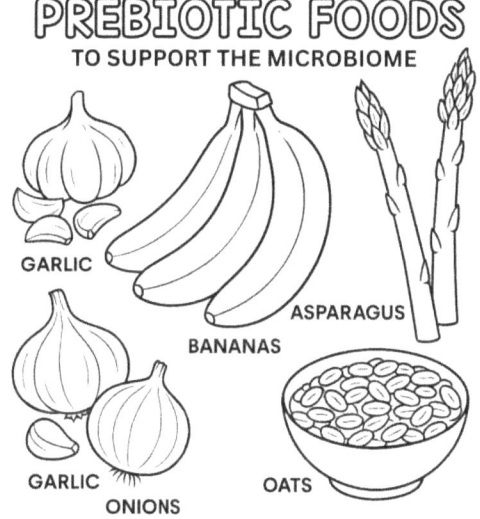

Examples of Prebiotic Foods:
- **Garlic:** contains inulin, a prebiotic fiber.
- **Onions:** rich in fructooligosaccharides (FOS).
- **Asparagus**: high in inulin and other prebiotic fibers.
- **Bananas:** slightly green bananas contain resistant starch.
- Oats: provide beta-glucan and resistant starch.

Probiotics

Probiotics are live microorganisms that, when consumed in adequate amounts, support health by strengthening the body's natural microbiome. They help balance "good" and "bad" bacteria in the digestive tract, improve digestion, and may reduce infection risk.

Examples of Probiotic Foods:
- **Yogurt**: cultured dairy with live active cultures.
- **Kefir:** fermented milk drink rich in diverse bacteria and yeasts.
- **Kombucha:** fermented tea with beneficial microbes.
- **Apple cider vinegar:** raw, unpasteurized versions contain acetic acid bacteria.
- **Miso:** fermented soybean paste used in soups and sauces.
- **Tempeh:** fermented soybeans with a firm, nutty flavor.

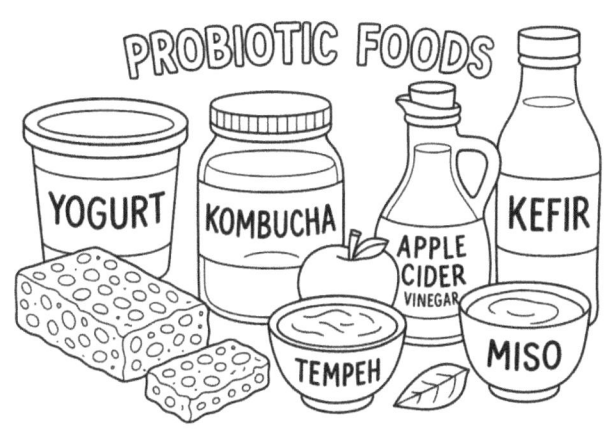

Exercise 9.3: Infection, Immunity, and the Microbiome
Match each term with the correct definition:

1. ____ Colonization
2. ____ Infection
3. ____ Innate immunity
4. ____ Adaptive immunity
5. ____ Prebiotics
6. ____ Probiotics

A. Live microorganisms that support health when consumed in adequate amounts.
B. Non-digestible fibers that feed beneficial microbes in the gut.
C. When microbes are present but not causing illness.
D. When pathogens invade and cause illness.
E. First line of defense, fast but non-specific (skin, inflammation).
F. Specific and slower immune response involving antibodies and memory cells.

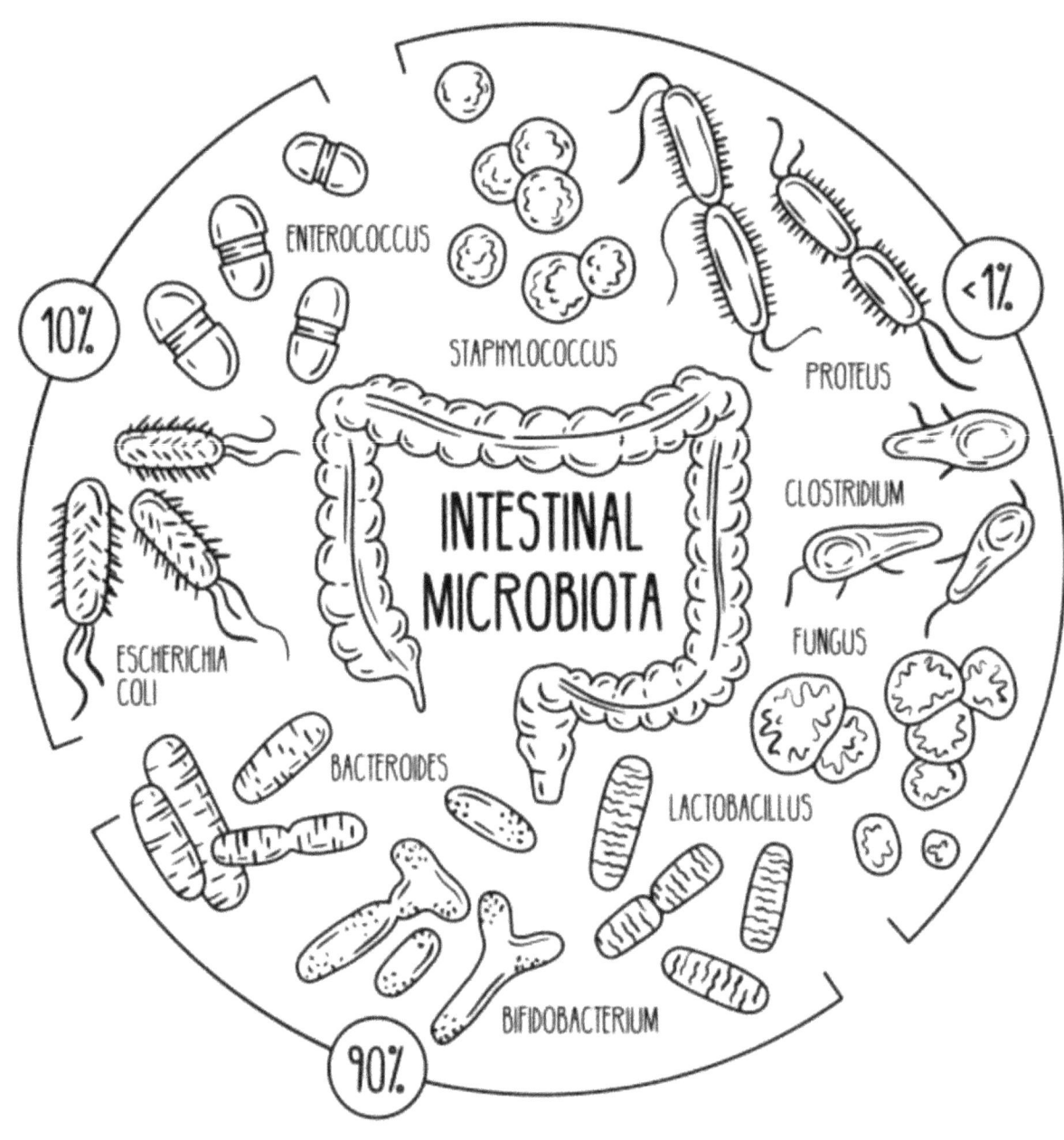

INFECTION CONTROL FOR MIDWIVES

Effective infection control protects mothers, newborns, and families while preserving the warmth and trust that define midwifery care. Whether at home, in a clinic, or in a birth center, infection prevention depends on both knowledge and presence: understanding how pathogens spread and modeling calm, consistent hygiene practices that empower families to do the same.

Midwives are responsible for creating and maintaining safe clinical environments. Infection control includes visible actions such as wearing gloves and disinfecting tools, but also requires awareness of unseen risks and daily habits. From the moment a midwife enters a client's home or opens the clinic for the day, every surface, tool, and interaction holds the potential for either contamination or protection.

Good infection control begins with presence and intention. It involves being grounded in the birth space, anticipating needs, and ensuring each client feels safe. It also includes reflection: What has this space been exposed to? What needs to be cleaned, covered, or prepared before hands-on care begins?

Midwives integrate safety into the rhythm of care without disrupting the intimacy of birth or the sacredness of postpartum. By blending sterile technique with calm presence and helping clients understand the "why" behind each practice, midwives promote both safety and empowerment.

A midwife's habits model best practices for families. Consistent, mindful infection control reinforces education, prevents outbreaks, and fosters a sense of shared responsibility for health.

How Infection Spreads

To prevent infection, midwives must understand how pathogens move from one person or surface to another. This knowledge guides practical strategies: for example, droplet-borne illnesses may require masks and eye protection, while surface contamination calls for handwashing or glove use.

Prevention also includes thoughtful clinical design, family education, and visible modeling of hygiene. Teaching clients how to protect themselves during flu season, why shared items should be disinfected, or how to prevent hand-to-genital transmission begins with a clear understanding of transmission pathways.

Because midwives work in varied environments—homes, clinics, and birth centers—they are uniquely positioned to recognize risks and reinforce effective hygiene practices. Through calm consistency and open communication, midwives build trust and strengthen community health.

Standard Precautions

Standard Precautions are the foundation of infection control in all health care settings. Formerly known as *Body Substance Isolation (BSI)* or *Universal Precautions (UP)*, these guidelines now form a single, unified protocol for all health care providers, including midwives. They protect both caregivers and clients from pathogens transmitted through blood, body fluids (except sweat), non-intact skin, and mucous membranes.

Standard Precautions apply to all clients, regardless of known infection status, and include:
- Performing hand hygiene before and after every client contact
- Wearing gloves when in contact with body fluids, performing vaginal exams, or providing wound care
- Using personal protective equipment (PPE), protective clothing, and eye protection when exposure risk is present.
- Cleaning and sterilizing instruments and surfaces between clients
- Handling and disposing of sharps safely and immediately after use
- Maintaining distinct clean and contaminated zones in birth spaces
- Practice proper handling of laboratory specimens
- Properly dispose of biohazards such as anything contaminated with birth fluids

Chain of Infection

Infection spreads when a pathogen finds a way to move from one host to another. The "chain of infection" includes six links:

1. **INFECTIOUS AGENT** bacteria, viruses, fungi, or parasites

2. **RESERVOIR** where the organism lives (people, surfaces, equipment)

3. **PORTAL OF EXIT** how the organism leaves the reservoir (e.g., blood, saliva)

4. **MODE OF TRANSMISSION** how it travels (contact, droplets, airborne)

5. **PORTAL OF ENTRY** how it enters a new host (e.g., broken skin, mucous membranes)

6. **SUSCEPTIBLE HOST** anyone whose defenses are lowered (pregnant women, newborns)

Breaking any link—through hand hygiene, barriers, or disinfection—prevents infection.

Different transmission routes helps midwives choose the right prevention strategies.

- **Direct contact:** Spread by physical touch or exposure to blood and body fluids.
  Examples: herpes simplex, hepatitis B.
  Midwifery relevance: frequent during hands-on care at birth and postpartum.

- **Indirect contact (fomites):** Spread via contaminated surfaces, instruments, or linens.
  Examples: MRSA, norovirus.
  Midwifery relevance: proper cleaning and sterilization prevent cross-contamination.

- **Droplet:** Large respiratory droplets from coughing, sneezing, or talking.
  Examples: influenza, RSV, COVID-19.
  Midwifery relevance: consider masks during outbreaks or illness in family members.

- **Airborne:** Tiny particles that remain suspended in air and travel long distances.
  Examples: measles, tuberculosis, varicella.
  Midwifery relevance: rare but serious; ensure proper ventilation in clinics or birth centers.

- **Vector-borne:** Transmitted by living carriers such as mosquitoes or ticks.
  Examples: Zika virus, malaria, Lyme disease.
  Midwifery relevance: Zika virus is a key pregnancy concern due to congenital risks.

- **Foodborne:** Spread through contaminated food.
  Examples: listeria, salmonella, E. coli.
  Midwifery relevance: teach food safety and avoidance of unpasteurized or undercooked foods.

- **Waterborne:** Spread by contaminated water.
  Examples: cholera, Giardia.
  Midwifery relevance: ensure proper disinfection of tubs used for water birth.

- **Bloodborne:** Spread via infected blood or sharps injuries.
  Examples: HIV, hepatitis B, hepatitis C.
  Midwifery relevance: use gloves and puncture-proof sharps containers consistently.

Handwashing Is the Most Effective Way to Prevent the Spread of Infection

Thorough, consistent hand hygiene protects mothers, newborns, and families in both clinical and home birth settings. Midwives model this essential skill by washing hands before and after every client contact, after glove removal, and whenever moving between clean and contaminated tasks. Regular handwashing reduces the spread of bacteria and viruses that can cause complications for mothers, newborns, and families.

Education is equally important. Midwives can model and encourage good handwashing habits among family members and visitors to create a safe home environment and reinforce shared responsibility for infection prevention.

Soap, warm running water, and friction for at least 20 seconds are key elements of effective handwashing. Alcohol-based hand sanitizers may be used when water is unavailable, but visible dirt or organic material must always be washed off with soap and water.

Consistent hand hygiene protects both families and care providers and helps prevent infection in every birth setting.

Everyone involved in birth and postpartum care should wash their hands:
- **Before and after** all client contact or newborn care
- **Before** performing sterile or clean procedures (e.g., vaginal exams, cord care, perineal care
- **After** contact with blood, body fluids, or contaminated items
- **After** removing gloves or other protective equipment
- **Before and after** eating, food preparation, or breastfeeding
- **After using the bathroom** or assisting someone else with toileting
- **After** diaper changes
- **After** coughing, sneezing, or touching the face
- **After** cleaning or handling soiled linens, instruments, or waste

10 Steps for Proper Handwashing

1. REMOVE rings, watches, and jewelry before washing.

2. RINSE hands and wrists with clean, warm (not hot) water.

3. APPLY soap or sanitizer generously to cover all surfaces.

4. RUB palms together to build a good lather.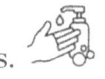

5. SCRUB the backs of hands and between fingers.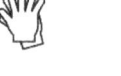

6. CLEAN under nails and around thumbs with firm friction.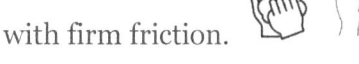

7. WASH wrists and lower forearms.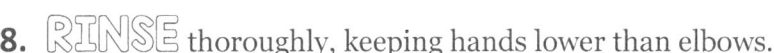

8. RINSE thoroughly, keeping hands lower than elbows.

9. DRY with a clean towel or disposable paper towel.

10. TURN off the faucet with a towel and enjoy clean hands!

Glove Use and Safety

Gloves protect both midwives and clients by preventing direct contact with blood, body fluids, and contaminated surfaces. Perform hand hygiene before donning and after removing gloves. Choose the correct size, inspect for tears, and put them on in a clean area—touching only the cuffs and avoiding non-essential surfaces; change immediately if torn or heavily soiled. Clean, single-use exam gloves are appropriate for most midwifery tasks such as vaginal exams, birth support, and general contact with mucous membranes. Sterile gloves are required for invasive procedures involving open skin (e.g., suturing or wound care) and must be used with sterile technique. Remove gloves by turning them inside out without touching the outer surface and dispose of them in an appropriate waste container. Gloves do not replace handwashing; they are an additional barrier that works best with consistent hygiene and attention to clean vs. contaminated zones.

1. GRASP the outside of one glove near the wrist, being careful not to touch your bare skin.

   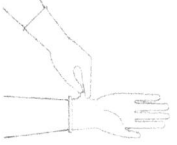

2. PEEL the glove away from your hand, turning it **inside out** as you pull it off.

   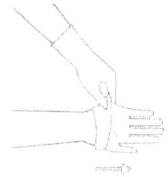

3. HOLD the removed glove in your still-gloved hand.

4. SLIDE two fingers from your ungloved hand under the wrist of the remaining glove.

   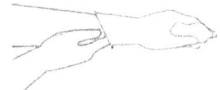

5. PEEL the second glove off from the inside, turning it inside out and trapping the first glove inside.

   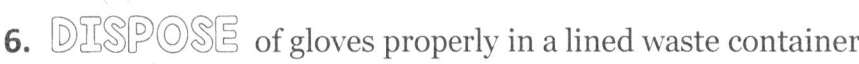

6. DISPOSE of gloves properly in a lined waste container.

7. WASH your hands thoroughly with soap and water or use hand sanitizer.

   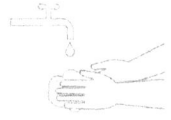

Home Birth Infection Control

Home birth is not a less safe place to give birth in terms of infection risk, but it does require intentional planning, respect for the family's space, and skillful navigation of hygiene within a shared environment. Unlike a clinical setting, the home environment is not fully controlled by the midwife. However, it is populated by the family's own familiar microbes, to which the birthing parent and newborn are already acclimated. This reduces exposure to unfamiliar or hospital-acquired pathogens but still calls for careful preparation and ongoing infection awareness throughout care.

While infection control includes visible practices such as handwashing and glove use, it also depends on awareness of unseen risks and silent habits. From the moment a midwife enters a client's home, every surface, tool, and interaction holds potential for either cross-contamination or protection.

Good infection control begins with presence and intention. It involves being grounded in the birth space, thinking ahead, and considering what each family needs to feel safe. Reflection is equally important: What has this space been exposed to? What needs to be cleaned, covered, or prepared before hands-on care begins?

Midwives practice infection control in ways that preserve the intimacy of birth and the sacredness of postpartum. By integrating sterile technique into calm, confident care—and by explaining the "why" behind each practice—midwives promote both safety and empowerment. A midwife's habits model best practices for clients; through consistent action and communication, midwives reinforce education, prevent infection, and foster a sense of shared responsibility for health.

Home birth infection control focuses on adapting professional standards to the realities of a client's space. Clear communication is essential. Families and support people benefit from calm, compassionate guidance that empowers them to take an active role in maintaining safety.

Practical considerations:
- Remind the birth team to avoid bringing contaminants from outside. Clothes and shoes are common vectors; use clean clothing and footwear reserved for the birth space.
- Bring all necessary PPE, hand sanitizer, and disinfectants.
- Designate separate clean and contaminated work surfaces.
- Establish a clear system for handling soiled linens and sharps disposal.
- Use portable sharps containers and disposable barriers.
- Ask about pets, smoking, or recent illness in the household.
- Provide anticipatory guidance on newborn hygiene and umbilical cord care.

Infection control is not impersonal or disconnected from the rhythm of care. It is protective, thoughtful, and intentionally woven into daily practice. It starts with clean hands and includes clear protocols for laundry, cleaning, sterilization, and trash removal. Midwives educate clients about infection control as part of collaborative care.

- Perform hand hygiene before and after every client interaction
- Wear gloves when handling bodily fluids, vaginal exams, or wound care
- Use PPE appropriately when exposure risk is present
- Sterilize or disinfect tools and surfaces between each use
- Dispose of sharps immediately into approved containers
- Maintain clean birth environments (home, clinic, birth center)
- Educate families on postpartum hygiene and newborn infection prevention

Midwives apply infection control principles across a wide range of client interactions, from intake assessments and prenatal exams to birth support and postpartum care.

- Setting up sterile birth trays in the birth center
- Teaching families how to clean a peribottle or use a sitz bath
- Safely cleaning and reusing Dopplers and other equipment
- Managing linens contaminated with body fluids.

Instrument Cleaning, Disinfection, and Sterilization

Proper instrument care is the foundation of infection control in midwifery practice. Every tool that touches blood, tissue, or mucous membranes can carry microorganisms that cause infection. Cleaning, disinfection, and sterilization are distinct steps in the process, each with a specific purpose. Understanding these differences ensures that midwives choose the right method for each situation, balancing safety, resources, and practicality in home and birth-center settings.

1. **Cleaning** removes visible debris, such as blood or tissue, using water and detergent. This is the first and most critical step because sterilization cannot occur if instruments are not completely clean.
2. **Disinfection** destroys most microorganisms on surfaces and instruments but may not eliminate bacterial spores. It is used for items that contact intact skin, such as thermometers or blood pressure cuffs.
3. **Sterilization** destroys all microorganisms, including spores, and is required for instruments that contact blood, mucous membranes, or sterile body tissues.

Each step builds on the last, creating a layered defense against infection. Skipping or shortening one step can compromise the entire process.

What Needs Disinfection and What Needs Sterilization

Midwives can group equipment into three main categories based on how each item is used:
- **Non-critical**: touches intact skin. Clean plus low-level disinfection.
- **Semi-critical**: touches mucous membranes or non-intact skin. High-level disinfection at minimum; sterilization preferred when feasible.
- **Critical**: enters sterile tissue or the vascular system. Sterilization required.

LEVELS OF CLEANING AND STERILIZATION

Process	Purpose	What It Does	Examples / Midwifery Use
Cleaning	Removes visible dirt and organic material	Uses soap and water or detergent to prepare items for disinfection or sterilization	Wash instruments, birth tubs, reusable equipment before disinfection
Disinfection	Kills most pathogens (not all spores)	Uses chemical or heat methods to reduce microbes	Wiping Doppler probes, blood pressure cuffs, or surfaces with 70% alcohol or approved disinfectant
High-Level Disinfection (HLD)	Kills all pathogens except some spores	Used for items contacting mucous membranes	Soaking specula or reusable suction bulbs in high-level disinfectant such as glutaraldehyde or 6–7.5% hydrogen peroxide
Sterilization	Destroys all microorganisms including spores	Uses steam, dry heat, or chemicals under pressure	Autoclave or pressure cooker for scissors, hemostats, forceps, amniotomy hooks
Antisepsis	Prevents infection on living tissue	Uses antimicrobial solutions safe for skin	Hand sanitizer, surgical scrub, cleaning perineum before procedures

QUICK GUIDE TO COMMON MIDWIFERY EQUIPMENT

Item	Classification	Required Process	Method at a Glance	Notes
Gloves	Noncritical	Disinfection	Use disposable or wash reusable with detergent; air dry	Inspect for damage before use
Doppler / Fetoscope	Noncritical	Disinfection	Wipe with 70% alcohol	Avoid soaking electronics
Blood Pressure Cuff	Noncritical	Cleaning	Wipe with detergent or alcohol	Keep cuff dry
Thermometer	Semicritical	High-Level Disinfection	Soak in alcohol or 6% hydrogen peroxide	Rinse and air dry
Speculum	Semicritical	High-Level Disinfection	Boil 20 min or soak 20 min in disinfectant	Rinse with warm water
Scissors / Forceps	Critical	Sterilization	Steam under pressure (autoclave or pressure cooker)	Dry and store wrapped
Cord Clamp	Critical	Sterilization	Steam 20 min or boil 20 min	Single-use preferred
Birth Bowl / Basin	Noncritical	Cleaning	Wash with detergent and rinse	Dry before reuse
Suction Bulb	Semicritical	High-Level Disinfection	Boil 20 min or soak in disinfectant	Ensure air passage is clear
Towels / Linens	Noncritical	Cleaning	Wash with detergent, rinse, and dry in sun or hot dryer	Use clean for each client

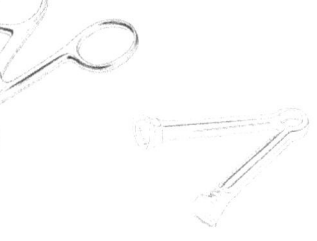 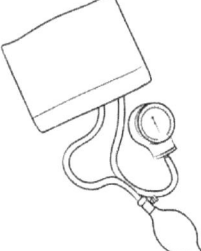 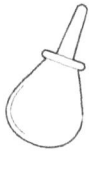 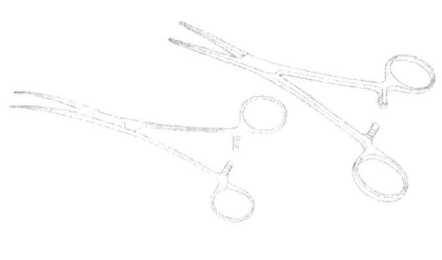

Exercise 9.4: Matching—Clean, Disinfect, or Sterilize
Match each item with the correct level of processing required.

1. _____Vaginal speculum	**A.** Clean
2. _____Cord scissors	
3. _____Doppler probe	**B.** Disinfect
4. _____Suturing needle	
5. _____Thermometer	**C.** Sterilize
6. _____Urine dipstick cup	
7. _____BP Cuff	
8. _____Fetoscope	
9. _____Linens	
10. _____Birth bowl/basin	

Step-by-Step Instrument Processing

1. **Preparation:** Immediately after use, rinse instruments under **warm, not hot, running water** to remove blood and organic material. Avoid hot water, which can cause proteins in blood and tissue to coagulate, making residue harder to clean and reducing the effectiveness of sterilization later.
2. **Cleaning:** Use a soft brush and mild detergent or enzymatic cleaner. Scrub while instruments are submerged to prevent splashing. Open hinges and joints to clean all surfaces. Rinse thoroughly and dry completely.
3. **Disinfection (if sterilization is not required):** Soak in an approved disinfectant (e.g., 70% alcohol, diluted bleach, or hydrogen peroxide 6%–7.5%) for the recommended time, then rinse with sterile or distilled water.
4. **Packaging:** Place clean, dry instruments into sterilization pouches, wraps, or metal trays. Use indicator tape or strips to confirm exposure to sterilizing conditions.
5. **Sterilization:** Process using the appropriate method (autoclave, pressure cooker, or other approved system) at the correct time, temperature, and pressure.
6. **Storage:** After sterilization, allow items to cool before handling. Store in sealed, dry containers or wrapped packages until use.
7. **Documentation:** Record sterilization date, method, and initials of the person responsible. Replace or re-sterilize any packs that become wet, torn, or older than 30 days.

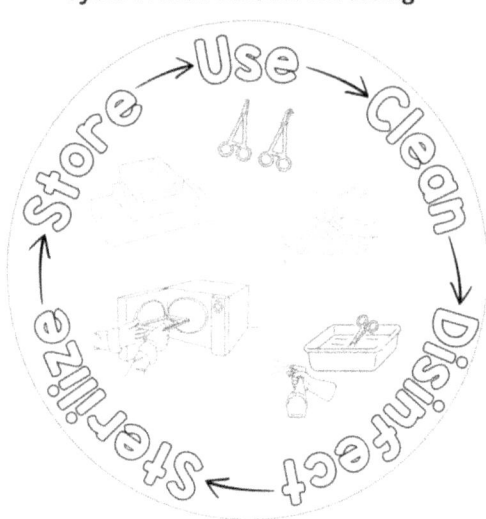

Cycle of Instrument Processing

Methods of Sterilization

Method	Process	Temp/Time	Advantages	Limitations
Autoclave (Steam Under Pressure)	Uses pressurized steam to sterilize metal, glass, and heat-resistant tools.	121°C (250°F) for 15–30 minutes	Gold standard; reliable and efficient	Requires power and drying cycle
Dry Heat Sterilization (Specialized Unit Only)	Used for glassware or non-hinged metal instruments.	160–170°C (320–340°F) for 1–2 hours	Useful when steam unavailable	Not effective for most instruments; not for home ovens
Pressure Cooker (Low-Resource Steam Sterilization)	Steam sterilization using a home pressure cooker.	~121°C for 20–30 minutes	Effective in low-resource or emergency settings	Must dry instruments afterward; confirm pressure gauge accuracy
Chemical Sterilization (High-Level Disinfection)	Immersion in glutaraldehyde, peracetic acid, or hydrogen peroxide (6%–7.5%) for 20–45 minutes.	Variable, depends on product	Useful when power or heat unavailable	Requires ventilation and thorough rinsing; toxic residues possible
Boiling (for Emergency Disinfection)	Boil instruments completely submerged in water.	≥100°C (212°F) for ≥20 minutes	Simple, low-cost method	Does not destroy all spores; short-term use only
Chemical + Heat Hybrid	Clean tools boiled, then soaked in alcohol or bleach if reused soon.	N/A	Appropriate for low-resource conditions	Temporary measure; must re-sterilize if stored

Low-Resource Sterilization

In settings without electricity or access to an autoclave, midwives can still maintain safety through careful adaptation and consistent technique.

Steam under pressure remains the most reliable method of sterilization. When autoclaves are unavailable, a pressure cooker (the kind used for canning) can achieve comparable conditions, reaching about 121°C (250°F) under pressure for 20–30 minutes. Instruments should be arranged loosely to allow steam circulation and should not touch the sides or lid. Pressure-cooker sterilization is effective only when instruments are cleaned first and steam reaches every surface. Because pressure cookers do not include a drying cycle, instruments must be dried afterward in a clean oven set to low heat (below sterilizing temperature) or air-dried in a covered sterile field. This drying step prevents rusting and recontamination, but it does not contribute to sterilization.

After the cycle, pressure must be released completely before opening, and instruments should remain covered until cooled.

- **Boiling or chemical disinfection** can be used temporarily when no pressure vessel is available, but these methods do not destroy all spores and should only be used for emergency or short-term care.
- Always use **clean, covered containers** for storage, label with the date and method, and reprocess any pack that becomes wet or older than 30 days.
- Whenever possible, confirm effectiveness with **sterilization indicator strips or spore tests.**
-

INFECTION, IMMUNITY, AND MIDWIFERY PRACTICE ESSENTIAL TAKEAWAYS

Pregnancy transforms the immune system into a finely balanced network of protection and tolerance. Midwives play a key role in safeguarding this balance—supporting immune health, preventing infection, and maintaining trust through careful, compassionate practice. From understanding immune modulation and Rh incompatibility to recognizing common infections in pregnancy, midwives integrate science with presence.

Infection control is more than sterile tools and gloves—it is a mindset of mindfulness and respect. Clean hands, proper disinfection, and clear communication protect not only mothers and babies but entire communities. Every action, from handwashing to sterilization, reinforces shared responsibility for health.

By combining knowledge of the maternal immune system, infection prevention, and practical hygiene, midwives uphold both safety and the sacredness of birth.

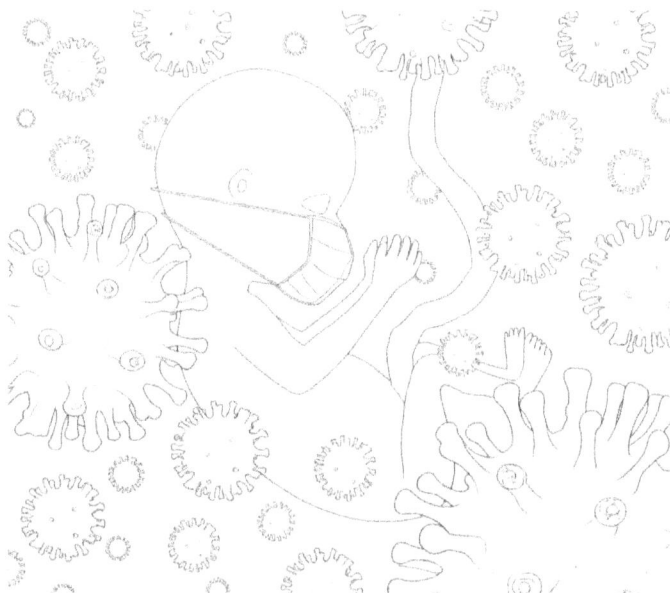

Chapter Nine: Self-Assessment

Multiple Choice

1. Which of the following best describes innate immunity?
   a) Produces antibodies specific to a pathogen
   b) Provides immediate, non-specific defense
   c) Depends on vaccination for activation
   d) Is only active during pregnancy

2. Which infection is preventable through preconception vaccination?
   a) Toxoplasmosis
   b) Rubella
   c) Cytomegalovirus
   d) Group B Streptococcus

3. The most effective way to prevent infection transmission in birth settings is:
   a) Wearing gloves at all times
   b) Using alcohol-based sanitizer only
   c) Frequent and thorough handwashing
   d) Avoiding all client contact

4. The Rh factor is found on:
   a) White blood cells
   b) Red blood cells
   c) Platelets
   d) Plasma proteins

5. Which instrument requires sterilization rather than disinfection?
   a) Blood pressure cuff
   b) Doppler probe
   c) Cord scissors
   d) Thermometer

6. Which statement best describes adaptive immunity?
   a) It acts immediately and non-specifically.
   b) It relies on antibodies and memory cells to recognize pathogens.
   c) It involves only physical barriers like skin and mucous membranes.
   d) It disappears during pregnancy to protect the fetus.

7. What is the primary function of Rhogam?
   a) To eliminate Rh-positive fetal cells from maternal circulation
   b) To prevent the mother's immune system from forming antibodies against Rh-positive blood
   c) To treat anemia in the fetus
   d) To increase maternal antibody production after birth

8. Which of the following is considered a *vector-borne* infection?
   a) Cytomegalovirus
   b) Zika virus
   c) Listeria
   d) Group B Streptococcus

9. When using an autoclave or pressure cooker for sterilization, the key factor for effectiveness is:
   a) Boiling for at least 10 minutes
   b) High temperature and pressure with adequate steam penetration
   c) Allowing instruments to dry in open air before sterilizing
   d) Using bleach solution before each use

10. Which of the following should be cleaned but does **not** require sterilization?
    a) Forceps
    b) Speculum
    c) Blood pressure cuff
    d) Cord scissors

11. Which practice helps maintain a healthy vaginal microbiome during pregnancy?
    a) Frequent douching
    b) Using antibacterial soaps
    c) Supporting Lactobacillus balance
    d) Taking broad-spectrum antibiotics

12. What is the safest method for preventing Group B Streptococcus infection in newborns?
    a) Administering antibiotics during labor
    b) Giving antivirals before birth
    c) Avoiding all vaginal exams
    d) Using herbal rinses before delivery

13. Which food carries the greatest risk for listeria infection in pregnancy?
    a) Fresh fruits and vegetables
    b) Unpasteurized soft cheese
    c) Baked chicken
    d) Frozen vegetables

14. Which statement about the microbiome is true?
    a) It only develops after birth.
    b) It increases infection risk in pregnancy.
    c) It supports immunity, digestion, and disease prevention.
    d) It should be eliminated through antibiotics in late pregnancy.

15. Which is an example of proper home birth infection control?
    a) Reusing gloves between tasks
    b) Keeping clean and contaminated zones separate
    c) Air-drying instruments after use
    d) Avoiding handwashing if gloves are used

Matching

16. ____ Can cause congenital hearing or vision loss.
17. ____ Transmitted through undercooked meat or cat feces.
18. ____ Preventable through vaccination before pregnancy.
19. ____ Spread by direct contact with lesions, especially during birth.
20. ____ Linked to foods such as unpasteurized dairy or deli meats.

A. Toxoplasmosis
B. Rubella
C. Cytomegalovirus
D. Listeria
E. Herpes Simplex

Fill in the Blank

21. The _____ test screens for antibodies in an Rh-negative client early in pregnancy.

22. Live vaccines such as _____ and _____ are contraindicated during pregnancy.

23. The bacterium _____ can be transmitted to the fetus during birth and cause neonatal sepsis.

24. A _____ is an inanimate object or surface that can transfer pathogens between hosts.

25. When using a pressure cooker for sterilization, instruments must later be _____ to prevent rusting and recontamination.

26. The _____ serves as both a barrier and a bridge between the maternal and fetal circulations.

27. During pregnancy, _____ cells help the immune system tolerate the fetus while preventing infection.

28. The most reliable method of sterilization is steam under pressure, also known as an _____.

29. _____ are beneficial bacteria that support digestion, immunity, and infection prevention.

30. The bacterium _____ can be found in unpasteurized dairy and deli meats and may cause stillbirth or neonatal sepsis.

True or False

31. _____ Pregnancy weakens the immune system, making all infections more dangerous.
32. _____ The placenta serves as both a barrier and a bridge between mother and baby.
33. _____ Innate immunity provides the body's first line of defense against infection.
34. _____ Adaptive immunity produces antibodies and immune "memory."
35. _____ Rh incompatibility can occur even when both parents are Rh-negative.
36. _____ Routine administration of Rhogam has made Rh disease extremely rare in modern midwifery practice.
37. _____ TORCH infections are primarily transmitted through contaminated food.
38. _____ Group B Streptococcus is a common cause of newborn infection but can be prevented by antibiotics in labor.
39. _____ Bacterial vaginosis (BV) is a sexually transmitted infection.
40. _____ The microbiome helps protect against infection by maintaining a healthy balance of microorganisms.
41. _____ Prebiotics are live microorganisms that support gut and immune health.
42. _____ Handwashing is the single most effective way to prevent the spread of infection.
43. _____ Gloves replace the need for proper hand hygiene.
44. _____ Sterilization destroys all microorganisms, including bacterial spores.
45. _____ Midwives must report certain communicable diseases to public health authorities according to local regulations.
46. _____ Hand sanitizer works equally well on visibly dirty hands.
47. _____ The placenta completely blocks all pathogens from reaching the fetus.
48. _____ Sterile gloves are required for invasive procedures such as suturing or wound care.
49. _____ Clients should always receive live vaccines, such as MMR or varicella, during pregnancy.
50. _____ Pressure cookers can serve as low-resource alternatives to autoclaves when used with proper cleaning and drying techniques.

Chapter Nine Reading & References

Recommended Reading: Infection, Immunity, and Midwifery Practice
- Ayliffe, G. A. J., & English, M. P. (2003). ***Hospital Infection: From Miasmas to MRSA***. Cambridge University Press. A concise history and practical foundation for modern infection control principles applied in healthcare settings.
- Blackburn, S. T. (2017). ***Maternal, Fetal, and Neonatal Physiology: A Clinical Perspective***. Elsevier. Explains the physiological and immunological changes that occur during pregnancy, birth, and the postpartum period.
- Garland, S. M. (Ed.). (2018). ***Infection Prevention in Maternal and Neonatal Care***. Springer. Focused specifically on infection control in maternity and neonatal settings, integrating microbiology with applied clinical prevention strategies.
- Lynne, C. M., & Brooker, C. (2010). ***Infection Prevention and Control: Theory and Practice for Healthcare Professionals***. Wiley-Blackwell. Comprehensive text on evidence-based hygiene, sterilization, and infection control, relevant to midwifery environments.
- Ravel, J., & Brotman, R. M. (2016). ***The Human Vaginal Microbiome in Health and Disease***. Springer. Research-based text on vaginal microbiota and implications for immunity, infection prevention, and preterm birth.
- World Health Organization. (2016). ***Core Components for Infection Prevention and Control Programmes***. WHO Press. Foundational guide to implementing infection prevention protocols in all health care and community birth settings.

References

American College of Obstetricians and Gynecologists. (2020). *Guidelines for infection prevention and control in obstetric care*. Obstetrics & Gynecology, 135(3), e100–e110. https://doi.org/10.1097/AOG.0000000000003709

Ayliffe, G. A. J., & English, M. P. (2003). *Hospital infection: From miasmas to MRSA*. Cambridge University Press.

Billingham, R. E., Brent, L., & Medawar, P. B. (1998). Immunological memory in pregnancy: Persistence of tolerance to paternal antigens. *The Lancet, 352*(9122), 1192–1195. https://doi.org/10.1016/S0140-6736(98)22023-X

Blackburn, S. T. (2017). *Maternal, fetal, and neonatal physiology: A clinical perspective* (5th ed.). Elsevier.

Centers for Disease Control and Prevention. (2023). *Guidelines for infection prevention in healthcare settings*. https://www.cdc.gov/infectioncontrol

Garland, S. M. (Ed.). (2018). *Infection prevention in maternal and neonatal care*. Springer.

Hesperian Foundation. (2019). *A book for midwives: Care for pregnancy, birth, and women's health*. Hesperian Health Guides.

Koren, O., Goodrich, J. K., Cullender, T. C., & Ley, R. E. (2012). Host remodeling of the gut microbiome during pregnancy. *Cell Host & Microbe, 12*(3), 277–288. https://doi.org/10.1016/j.chom.2012.08.003

Knight, R., & Ma, J. (2019). The pregnancy microbiome: Implications for health and disease. *Nature Medicine, 25*(3), 358–366. https://doi.org/10.1038/s41591-019-0375-0

Lynne, C. M., & Brooker, C. (2010). *Infection prevention and control: Theory and practice for healthcare professionals*. Wiley-Blackwell.

Ontario Association of Midwives. (2019). *Midwifery equipment cleaning tips: Infection prevention and control protocols*. https://www.ontariomidwives.ca

Ravel, J., & Brotman, R. M. (2016). *The human vaginal microbiome in health and disease*. Springer.

Roberts, C. M., & Andersson, M. (2017). Infection prevention and control in maternity and neonatal care: Global perspectives. *Midwifery, 53*, 15–22. https://doi.org/10.1016/j.midw.2017.07.005

Seale, H., & Leask, J. (2021). Vaccine communication in maternity care: Balancing risk, trust, and choice. *Vaccine, 39*(25), 3347–3352. https://doi.org/10.1016/j.vaccine.2021.04.016

World Health Organization. (2016). *Core components for infection prevention and control programmes*. World Health Organization.

Young, V. B. (2017). *The microbiome and health*. ASM Press.

Chapter Ten
Prenatal Care

Objectives
After completing this chapter, the student should be able to:
1. **Explain** the difference between good prenatal care and great prenatal care.
2. **Explain** the benefits of prenatal care.
3. **Describe** what HIPAA is and how it applies to midwifery practice.
4. **Explain** the importance of charting and give examples of charting rules.
5. **Define** a SOAP and SBAR and give examples.
6. **Describe** what is involved in writing practice guidelines/protocols.
7. **Describe** how to take a complete medical history, including:
   a) Communication techniques
   b) Family history
   c) Past medical and obstetric history
   d) Sexual history taking
   e) Current pregnancy
8. **Describe** what the first prenatal visit involves.
9. **Describe** how to give a complete head-to-toe physical exam.
10. **Explain** why physical exam skills are important for midwives to learn.
11. **List** information taken and charted on subsequent prenatal exams.
12. **Demonstrate** prenatal exam skills, including:
    a. Measuring fundal height.
    b. Taking vital signs and knowing the normal ranges.
    c. Listening to Fetal Heart Tones.
    d. Palpation using the steps of Leopold's maneuver.
13. **Describe** the rationale for pelvimetry, and how to perform it.
14. **List** the prenatal tests and when they are recommended.
15. **Describe** how Rh and other blood incompatibilities can affect pregnancy outcomes.
16. **List** purposes for the following antenatal tests and procedures:
    a. Amniocentesis.
    b. AFP testing.
    c. Chorionic Villi Sampling.
    d. Biophysical profile.
    e. Fetal movement counting.
    f. Ultrasound.
    g. Non-stress test and contraction stress test.

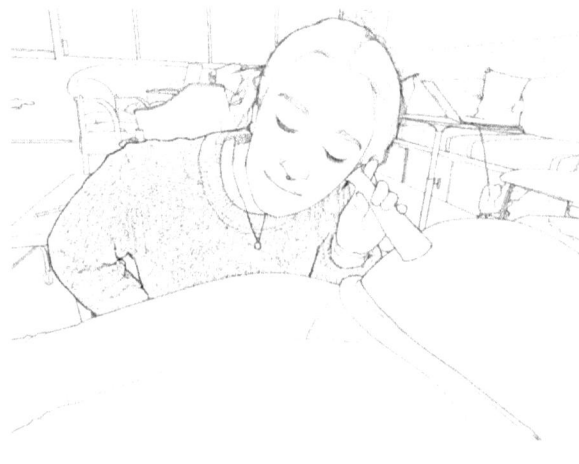

Prenatal Care

Midwives have a unique opportunity during prenatal care to support each pregnant client in understanding their body, exploring choices, and navigating pregnancy as a normal physiologic process. Rather than approaching care as a checklist of medical tasks, midwives cultivate health literacy, reduce fear, and build trust through relationship-centered care.

Prenatal visits create space to listen, educate, assess, and empower. Midwives spend time getting to know the whole person—their preferences, goals, and lived experiences. This connection allows for individualized care, responsive decision-making, and the development of mutual trust over time.

Midwives use their hands, eyes, and intuition to stay grounded in the physiology of pregnancy. Palpating a growing belly, listening to fetal tones, and observing subtle shifts across visits help them assess well-being without overreliance on technology. This direct engagement also supports the client's confidence, helping them experience pregnancy as a normal and healthy process rather than a condition to be managed.

Communication is central to this work. The way information is offered can shape how it is received. Midwives provide clear, balanced education and support informed decision-making without judgment or pressure. They also remain attentive to tone, pacing, and emotional cues—adjusting how information is shared to foster understanding and trust.

By centering the client's experience and honoring the normal physiology of pregnancy, midwives offer care that is both clinically sound and emotionally supportive. Relationship is the foundation that makes safe, individualized care possible.

The First Prenatal Visit

The first prenatal visit establishes the foundation for the care relationship. It is a time to build trust, gather information, and invite the client into shared decision-making. While many tasks may be completed—such as history, lab work, and physical assessment—this visit is also a chance to listen deeply and understand the person behind the chart.

Approaches vary depending on practice setting, resources, and philosophy of care. In some practices, testing and exams are completed at this first visit; in others, the focus is on conversation, education, and planning. Regardless of structure, the goal remains the same: to begin a collaborative, respectful partnership that supports both the physiology and the lived experience of pregnancy.

History Taking

Taking a thorough and sensitive history is the foundation of individualized prenatal care. Midwives approach this process not as a checklist, but as a conversation—one that builds trust, centers the client's lived experience, and honors the full story of body, mind, and community.

While many practices use paper forms or EMR templates to guide intake, these tools cannot replace genuine human connection. Listening deeply helps reveal patterns and meaning beyond data points. Midwives often describe this process as hearing a client's *herstory*—recognizing that every pregnancy carries a backstory shaped by identity, culture, and circumstance.

History-taking is an ongoing process, not a single event. Clients may need time to feel safe, reflect, or decide how much to share. Sensitive topics often emerge gradually and should never be rushed. Midwives create safety by explaining why questions are asked, framing them in terms of support, and adapting to each client's comfort level.

Trauma-informed care begins with presence and consent. Pay attention to verbal and nonverbal cues, allow space for emotion, and obtain permission before every touch or exam. Clients should always know they can pause or decline. In this way, even the act of gathering history becomes an expression of midwifery care—listening with empathy, documenting with accuracy, and respecting each person's story.

The Five Questions of History Taking

Who

- The client, who brings their health narrative, cultural background, values, and vulnerabilities
- The midwife, who brings curiosity, skill, cultural humility, and a trauma-informed presence
- Interpreters or support persons, when needed, to ensure language access and emotional safety

What

- Medical conditions, medications, family history, and mental health
- Obstetric, gynecologic, and sexual history
- Social, relational, and emotional experiences
- Cultural or spiritual factors influencing care
- The client's own words and interpretations of their health

Where

- In the exam room during intake or prenatal visits
- In the home, at community visits, or via telehealth
- Across multiple appointments, especially when trust is still forming

When

- A complete history does not need to be finished at the first visit
- Sensitive or complex topics may take time to emerge or feel safe to share
- Questions can be returned to later as trust develops
- Clients may choose to disclose personal information gradually, in their own time
- Revisiting topics later may offer clearer insight or updated context

Why

- Provide clinically appropriate, individualized care
- Identify factors that may affect pregnancy, birth, or postpartum
- Prevent triggers or re-traumatization
- Build a trusting and collaborative care relationship
- Respect the client's identity, values, and safety needs

The Story of Care

WHO

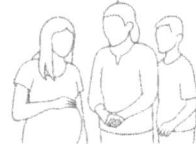

Build the relationship

WHAT

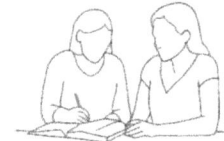

Gather the story

WHERE

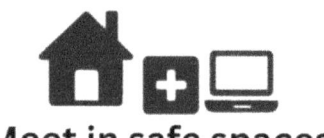

Meet in safe spaces

WHEN

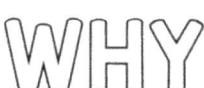

Unfolds over time

WHY

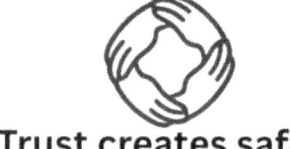

Trust creates safety

Trauma and History Taking

Many clients enter pregnancy care with personal histories that shape how they experience their bodies, relationships, and interactions with healthcare providers. Trauma may stem from childhood abuse, sexual assault, intimate partner violence, birth trauma, systemic racism, immigration stress, or previous negative medical encounters. These experiences are often unspoken but can strongly influence how someone feels during history taking, exams, and discussions of care.

Midwives practicing trauma-informed care begin with the understanding that trauma may be present even if it is not disclosed. Rather than assuming everything is fine unless told otherwise, trauma-informed care creates an environment where clients feel physically and emotionally safe. This approach builds trust over time and protects against re-traumatization.

Trauma-informed midwifery includes:
- Assuming a trauma history is possible, even if not disclosed
- Prioritizing emotional and physical safety in every encounter
- Offering choice, control, and consent at every step
- Listening without judgment or interruption
- Being aware of nonverbal cues like tone, body language, and pacing
- Avoiding unnecessary or invasive questions or exams
- Creating clear boundaries and predictable routines

It is important for clients to know that they are always in control. Midwives should clearly communicate that clients can skip any question, say no to any part of the exam, and revisit topics later if needed.

Clients should always be reminded:
- They have the right to decline questions or exams
- They can pause, take breaks, or slow down
- They do not have to disclose anything they are not ready to share
- They can change or update their responses over time

Using clear and affirming language helps reinforce this sense of safety. Even simple phrases can help reduce anxiety and build trust.

> **Compassion and Consent**
> Every assessment should begin with consent and respect. Compassionate, trauma-informed care builds trust as surely as clinical skill does.

Phrases that support trauma-informed care:
- "Some of these questions are sensitive, and you can always skip anything you don't want to talk about."
- "Take your time, there's no rush."
- "Let me know if anything feels uncomfortable or overwhelming."
- "Your comfort matters just as much as your health."

Not all trauma is visible, and not all healing happens quickly. A respectful, flexible, and relationship-based approach allows the client to feel seen, heard, and supported—whether or not they ever choose to share their story.

History Taking

A comprehensive prenatal history helps uncover both clinical concerns and personal context. The following categories are commonly used, but may be gathered over multiple visits. Forms and templates are useful, but should always be supplemented with open-ended conversation.

Ask questions such as, "How have you been feeling since you found out you were pregnant?" or "Can you tell me about your previous birth experiences?" These invite storytelling, build trust, and reveal details that may not surface through checklists alone.

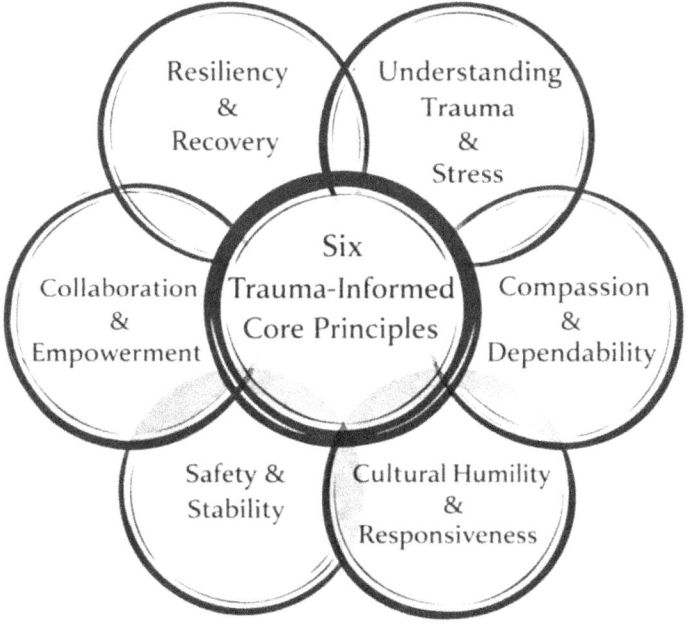

CATEGORIES OF HISTORY TAKING

Medical History
- Chronic conditions such as diabetes, hypertension, or thyroid disorders
- History of hospitalizations, surgeries, or general anesthesia
- Medication allergies or adverse drug reactions
- Current use of medications, supplements, or herbs
- History of blood transfusion
- Mental health conditions, past or present

Obstetric History
- All previous pregnancies, losses, and births
- Type of delivery (vaginal, cesarean, assisted)
- Gestational age, birthweight, and outcomes
- History of postpartum hemorrhage, retained placenta, or infections
- History of preterm or post-dates birth

Gynecologic History
- Age of menarche and menstrual patterns
- History of abnormal Pap smears or HPV
- Sexually transmitted infections or pelvic infections
- Surgeries such as LEEP, ablation, or laparoscopy
- Menstrual management and birth control use

Sexual and Relationship History
- Current sexual activity and partnerships
- History of painful sex, pelvic pain, or vaginismus
- History of sexual trauma or assault
- Domestic violence, coercion, or relationship instability
- Gender identity, sexual orientation, and comfort with exams

Family and Genetic History
- Major health conditions in immediate family members
- Genetic disorders such as Tay-Sachs, thalassemia, or cystic fibrosis
- Inheritable mental health or developmental conditions

Social History
Living situation and caregiving roles including:
- Support systems and stress levels
- Substance use, past or present
- Access to food, housing, and transportation
- Employment, education, and daily routine
- Immigration status or language access needs

Nutritional and Lifestyle Factors
- Typical eating patterns and any dietary restrictions
- Access to safe, culturally appropriate food
- Exercise habits and physical activity
- Sleep, rest, and recovery
- Cultural or religious practices affecting care

Emotional and Trauma History
- Past experiences of trauma, including abuse, violence, or medical mistreatment
- Coping strategies, mental health support, and resilience factors

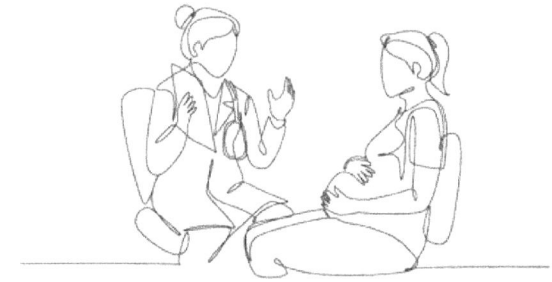

Using Motivational Interviewing and Open-Ended Questions

Motivational interviewing (MI) is a client-centered communication style that supports self-awareness, autonomy, and behavioral change. Midwives may use MI when discussing complex topics such as nutrition, substance use, prenatal testing, or stress.

Core skills include asking open-ended questions, offering affirmations, practicing reflective listening, and summarizing to clarify understanding. These tools allow clients to share at their own pace and uncover concerns that might not emerge through structured forms or checklists.

Examples of open-ended questions include:
- "Can you tell me about your last birth experience?"
- "What's important to you when it comes to this pregnancy?"
- "How are you feeling emotionally these days?"
- "What are some things that are helping you cope right now?"

Exercise 10.1: Matching Principles and Purposes of History Taking
Match each statement to its purpose.

1. _____History-taking is a process that unfolds over multiple visits.	**A.** Builds trust and allows sensitive topics to surface gradually
2. _____The midwife explains why each question is being asked.	**B.** Reduces anxiety and fosters transparency
3. _____Clients may decline questions or exams.	**C.** Supports autonomy and emotional safety
4. _____Open-ended questions and reflective listening are used.	**D.** Encourage meaningful dialogue and collaboration
5. _____Silence and incomplete answers are accepted.	**E.** Respects individual pacing and readiness
6. _____Consent is ongoing and can be withdrawn anytime.	**F.** Reinforces control and bodily integrity
7. _____Cultural and spiritual factors are explored.	**G.** Promotes culturally responsive care

Exercise 10-2 Comprehensive History-Taking Checklist
Check each area based on a simulated client case, role play, or clinical scenario.

Category	Completed	Needs Follow-Up	Not Applicable
Who — Identified client, midwife, and support persons; ensured language access and emotional safety	☐	☐	☐
What — Discussed medical, obstetric, gynecologic, and psychosocial history; documented client's own words	☐	☐	☐
Where — Determined safe and accessible setting (clinic, home, telehealth); adapted as needed	☐	☐	☐
When — Deferred sensitive topics respectfully; revisited information over time	☐	☐	☐
Why — Clarified purpose of each question; emphasized individualized care and trust	☐	☐	☐
Trauma-Informed Approach — Offered choice, consent, and control; validated client's comfort level	☐	☐	☐
Motivational Interviewing — Used open-ended questions, affirmations, reflective listening, and summaries	☐	☐	☐
Cultural Awareness — Recognized cultural or spiritual influences on care; used culturally appropriate communication	☐	☐	☐
Documentation — Recorded information accurately, respectfully, and in the client's own words	☐	☐	☐

Risk Assessment for Out-of-Hospital Birth

Risk assessment is a continuous, adaptive process in prenatal care. Midwives integrate clinical findings with personal context such as medical history, current symptoms, emotional health, and life circumstances to evaluate how a pregnancy is unfolding. Risk is not a label but a guide for care and collaboration.

Midwifery risk assessment is individualized. Its goal is not to exclude clients but to support informed decision-making, determine appropriate birth settings, and ensure access to consultation or co-management when needed.

Baseline and Cumulative Risk

- **Baseline risk** is assessed at the first prenatal visit using clinical history, physical findings, and psychosocial screening.
- **Cumulative risk** refers to how risk evolves over time as new information becomes available. This includes changing medical conditions, emerging stressors, or newly disclosed history.
- Risk assessment is **dynamic and ongoing**. It should be formally revisited at each trimester, again at the 36-week visit, and throughout the postpartum period, especially if complications, life changes, or new concerns arise.
- **Substance use** (such as cannabis) does not automatically indicate risk or require transfer. The clinical concern arises when use affects safety, decision-making, or fetal health. Use a harm reduction framework and assess impact, not just presence.

Risk and Responsibility in Out-of-Hospital Birth

Attending out-of-hospital births with higher risk factors can be a complex and deeply personal decision. Some midwives attend breech, twin, or other higher-risk births when they have appropriate training, informed consent, and collaborative medical support. As midwives, we strive to honor parents' freedom of choice, even when their decisions differ from those we might make for ourselves. Practice approaches vary widely and are influenced by experience, available resources, and the quality of hospital collaboration and backup.

It is important to remember that families rely on a midwife's expertise and judgment to safeguard the lives of both mother and child. The loss of a child is among the most devastating experiences imaginable. Thorough risk assessment, honest discussion, and timely collaboration are essential to prevent avoidable tragedy.

Always refer to local laws, licensing regulations, and organizational protocols when determining eligibility for home or birth center care. While some guidelines may seem overly restrictive, loss of licensure or insurance coverage can ultimately limit access to midwifery care for many families.

> **Principles of Risk Assessment**
>
> - Risk assessment is **ongoing** and should evolve with new information.
> - Decisions should balance client autonomy and safety.
> - **Collaboration** with medical or community resources strengthens outcomes.
> - Use risk tools to support, not replace, clinical judgment and relationship-based care.
> - **Documentation** of findings and communication protects both client and midwife.
>
> *Remember: Tools assist wisdom; they do not define it.*

Many experienced midwives remind clients that home birth is a philosophy, not merely a place. The goal is always the healthiest and safest outcome for mother and baby. When circumstances arise before or during labor that make hospital birth the safer option, a timely transport is an act of good judgment—not failure. It is always better to transport complications, not crises.

Assessing risk factors with honesty and diligence is an essential part of safe, ethical out-of-hospital midwifery care.

RISK AND RESILIENCE SCORING TOOLS

Risk Factor Scoring Tool	
Category & Risk Factor	**Score**
Obstetric History	
– Previous cesarean	1
– Postpartum hemorrhage	1
– Preterm birth or second trimester loss	2
– Grand multiparity (≥5 prior births)	1
Medical History	
– Chronic hypertension	2
– Diabetes (Type 1 or 2)	2
– Autoimmune or thyroid disorder	1
– BMI > 40 at intake	1
Current Pregnancy	
– First trimester bleeding	1
– Abnormal ultrasound (e.g., fibroids, low placenta)	1–2
– Gestational diabetes	2
– Hypertension or preeclampsia	2–3
Psychosocial Factors	
– IPV or domestic violence	2
– Substance use disorder	1–2
– Depression, anxiety, or trauma history	1
– ACES score ≥ 4	1–2
– Food, housing, or income insecurity	1
– Language or communication barrier	1
Logistics and Access	
– Missed ≥2 visits without contact	1
– Unstable transportation or no phone	1
Interpretation	
0–2 points → Routine prenatal care	
3–4 points → Enhanced prenatal care with increased support	
5+ points → Co-management or consultation recommended	

Resiliency and Protective Factor Scoring Tool	
Protective Factor	Score
Strong family or community support	1
Stable housing and access to healthy food	1
Regular use of coping tools (journaling, prayer, etc.)	1
Counseling or peer mental health support	1
Cultural, spiritual, or faith-based connection	1
Prior full-term, uncomplicated birth	1
Motivation for shared decision-making	1
Early and consistent prenatal care	1
Doula support during pregnancy or postpartum	1
Enrollment in childbirth education classes	1
Co-care with another provider (OB, MFM)	1
Interpretation	
0–2 points → Minimal buffer	
3–5 points → Moderate resilience	
6+ points → Strong protective framework	

Marginalization as a Risk Factor for Poor Maternal–Child Health Outcomes

Certain populations experience consistently worse maternal and infant outcomes, not because of their identity, but because of the ways systems treat them. **Marginalization** is a more accurate term than "race" for understanding how chronic stress, inequitable care, and structural barriers lead to harm.

Why marginalization matters:
- Black and Indigenous women face significantly higher rates of pregnancy-related mortality, even with similar income, education, and health status.
- These disparities reflect systemic racism, implicit bias, and structural inequities in housing, education, and healthcare.
- Chronic exposure to discrimination can lead to toxic stress, early aging, and increased vulnerability.
- Marginalized people may experience dismissal, under-treatment, or delayed care.
- Other forms of marginalization, such as disability, queer identity, immigration status, or language exclusion, may compound these risks.

Midwifery response:
- Use identity markers as prompts for deeper inquiry, not as diagnoses.
- Ask about past discrimination, access barriers, and previous care experiences.
- Consider marginalization as a factor that may amplify other risk indicators.
- Provide trauma-informed, culturally safe, relationship-centered care.

Contraindications to Midwifery Care and Community-Based Birth

Some clinical conditions may require consultation, co-management, or transfer of care. However, what constitutes a true contraindication can vary by location, credentialing body, and available backup systems. Midwives should always refer to their scope of practice, state regulations, and site-specific policies when making decisions. When risk factors arise, documentation of reasoning and consultations is essential. Clear records protect clients, strengthen communication, and demonstrate professionalism during peer or regulatory review.

Risk is not a label; it is a conversation. Midwives integrate patterns, context, and clinical knowledge while honoring each person's lived experience. Risk assessment should never remove the client from their care—it should bring the care closer to them.

Contraindications to Midwifery Care		
Condition	Midwifery Care	Community Birth
Uncontrolled diabetes or hypertension	✗ Not appropriate	✗ Not appropriate
Severe cardiac or renal disease	✗ Not appropriate	✗ Not appropriate
Seizure disorder uncontrolled by medication	✗ Not appropriate	✗ Not appropriate
HIV with high viral load	May consult	Varies by jurisdiction and scope
Placenta previa, accreta, or percreta	✗ Not appropriate	✗ Not appropriate
Breech presentation at term	May consult	Varies by jurisdiction and scope
Twins or higher-order multiples	May consult	Varies by jurisdiction and scope
Severe preeclampsia or eclampsia	✗ Not appropriate	✗ Not appropriate
Post-dates pregnancy > 42 weeks without labor	May consult	Varies by jurisdiction and scope
Inability to consent to care	✗ Not appropriate	✗ Not appropriate
No access to emergency transport	May consult	✗ Not appropriate
Active substance use (when impairing care, safety, or infant well-being)	✗ Not appropriate	✗ Not appropriate

Collaborative Care with Supportive Providers

When risk factors emerge, midwives do not always need to transfer care. Many clients benefit from **co-management** with an obstetric or medical provider, while maintaining the continuity, presence, and advocacy of a midwife. Clients benefit most when communication is clear, transitions are smooth, and all members of the care team respect the midwifery model of care. Support, education, trust, and resilience matter just as much as lab values. With respectful collaboration and adaptive planning, midwives can support excellent outcomes even when risk factors are present.

Collaborative care may include:
- Alternating prenatal visits with a physician or specialist
- Planning for hospital birth with midwife present for labor support
- Shared documentation and care plans
- Coordinated safety planning and postpartum follow-up

Exercise 10.2 Integrating Risk Assessment in Midwifery Care
Answer the following questions:

1. A new client enters care with a history of gestational diabetes and stable housing, strong family support, and early entry into care.
    a. Which **risk factors** and **protective factors** apply?

    b. How might these balance one another in your assessment?

2. During a prenatal visit, a client discloses prior trauma and reports elevated blood pressure at 30 weeks.
    a. What steps would you take using a **trauma-informed approach**?

    b. What type of consultation or co-management might be appropriate?

3. A client with chronic hypertension wishes to plan a home birth.
    a. Using the **Contraindications to Midwifery Care** table, what discussion should take place?

    b. How could you document shared decision-making and consultation?

4. Reflect on your own developing comfort level with risk assessment.
    a. Which areas feel clear and confident?

    b. Where might you need additional mentorship or supervision?

Vital Signs and Measurements

Vital signs are among the first assessments in prenatal care, including temperature, pulse, respirations, and blood pressure—key indicators of how the body adapts to pregnancy. They offer a snapshot of current health and valuable insight into trends over time. In midwifery, vital signs are interpreted within the context of each client's physiology and experience, not as isolated numbers. Patterns over time matter more than single readings.

When values fall outside expected ranges, midwives pause, reassess, and ask questions. Elevated blood pressure, persistent tachycardia, or low oxygen saturation may signal emerging complications, while smaller variations may reflect stress, dehydration, or discomfort.

Midwives are skilled observers who listen with their ears, eyes, and presence. Clinical accuracy matters, but so do kindness, privacy, positioning, and choice. When performed thoughtfully, even routine assessments can strengthen trust and communicate: *I see you, I respect you, and I am paying attention.*

BLOOD PRESSURE

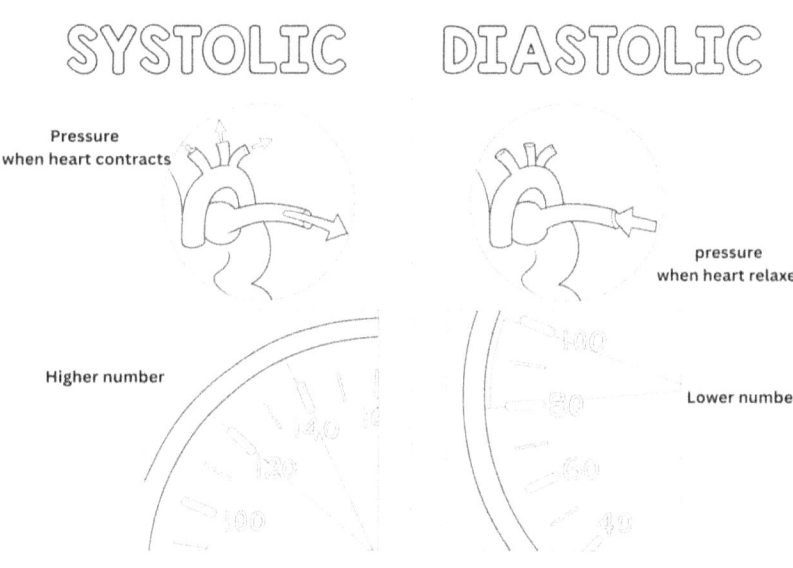

Blood pressure reflects how well the heart and blood vessels work together. **Systolic pressure** is the top number, showing the force of blood when the heart contracts. **Diastolic pressure** is the bottom number, showing the pressure when the heart relaxes. In pregnancy, blood pressure helps identify risk for hypertensive disorders such as preeclampsia. A normal pattern shows a slight drop in the second trimester followed by a return to baseline in the third. Even mild elevations or sudden increases from baseline can be clinically significant. Orthostatic changes may indicate dehydration or vascular instability.

Accurate measurement and consistency are essential. Use the same type of equipment and technique at each visit, and recheck after rest if a reading seems abnormal.

Follow these steps for taking blood pressure reliable readings:
1. Have the client rest quietly for 3–5 minutes before measuring.
2. Seat the client with back supported, feet flat, and legs uncrossed.
3. Use a cuff that matches the arm's circumference; a too-small cuff may give a falsely high reading.
4. Support the arm so cuff is level with the heart.
5. Place the cuff on bare skin when possible.
6. Center the cuff bladder over the brachial artery, about 2 cm above the antecubital crease.
7. For **manual readings**, place the stethoscope over the brachial artery. Inflate the cuff about 30 mmHg above the point where the radial pulse disappears. Slowly release the air (2–3 mmHg per second), listening to the first clear sound (systolic) and the point when sounds disappear (diastolic).
8. For **digital readings**, follow the manufacturer's instructions.
9. Avoid talking or movement during measurement.
10. Document results carefully, comparing them to the client's baseline rather than population averages.

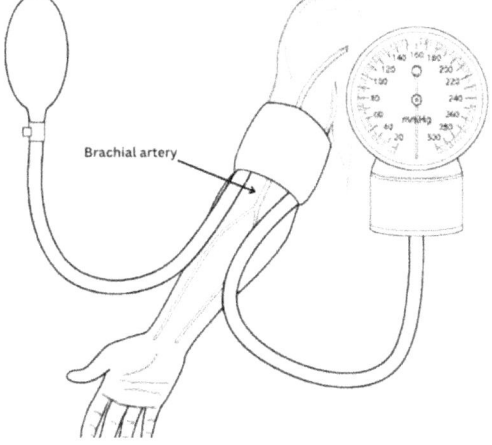

Blood Pressure Classification (Pregnant Woman)		
Category	Systolic (mmHg)	Diastolic (mmHg)
Normal	90–139	60–89
Mild hypertension	140–159	90–99
Moderate hypertension	160–179	100–109
Severe hypertension	180–209	110–119
Crisis hypertension	≥210	≥120

PULSE RATE

The pulse reflects how well the heart is pumping and how effectively blood circulates through the body. In pregnancy, a mild increase in rate is expected due to higher blood volume and metabolic demand. Normal adult pulse ranges from **60–100 beats per minute (bpm)**. Persistent **tachycardia** (above 100 bpm) may indicate anxiety, dehydration, infection, anemia, or other stressors. **Bradycardia** (below 60 bpm) may occur in well-conditioned individuals and is not always abnormal. In emergencies such as shock or postpartum hemorrhage, a rapid or faint pulse may indicate circulatory collapse. If the radial pulse is difficult to palpate, assess the carotid pulse and initiate emergency protocols.

How to Measure

1. Have the client seated and relaxed.
2. Locate the **radial pulse** on the thumb side of the wrist using your index and middle fingers. Avoid using your thumb, as it has its own pulse.
3. Press lightly until you feel the pulse.
4. Count for **30 seconds and multiply by two** if regular, or for a full **60 seconds** if irregular. Counting for a full minute also helps you gain skill and sensitivity through practice.
5. Note the **rate, rhythm, and strength** of the pulse:
   - **Regular:** evenly spaced beats that may vary slightly with breathing.
   - **Regularly irregular:** generally consistent pattern with occasional skipped beats.
   - **Irregularly irregular:** no consistent pattern; rhythm difficult to measure accurately.
6. Record your findings, including rate and rhythm, and report any sustained irregularities or unusually high or low results.

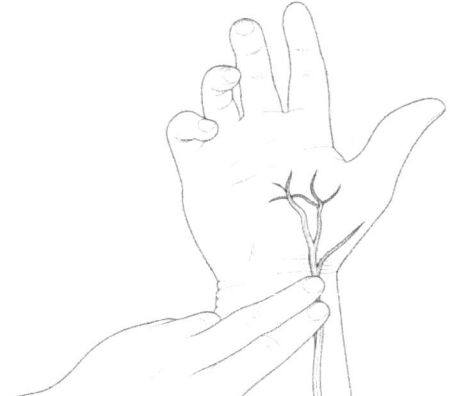

Developing Skill and Sensitivity

In many traditional systems, such as Chinese medicine, pulse assessment is a highly developed diagnostic art that reflects the state of balance and function throughout the body. Midwives can apply this same attentiveness by learning to *feel* rather than simply count. The more you take pulses, the better your fingers become at recognizing subtle qualities like speed, depth, tension, and tone. Over time, you will intuitively sense what a normal pulse feels like, so that abnormalities stand out clearly.

Factor	Possible Effect on Vital Signs
Stress or anxiety	↑ Pulse, ↑ BP, ↑ Respirations
Dehydration	↑ Pulse, ↓ BP
Ambient temperature	↑ or ↓ Temperature
Position change	Orthostatic variation in BP
Recent activity	↑ Pulse and Respirations

Respiratory Rate

Respiratory rate reflects how efficiently oxygen moves through the body. In pregnancy, breathing often becomes more shallow or slightly faster due to pressure from the growing uterus and hormonal changes that increase oxygen demand. An elevated rate may indicate infection, anxiety, asthma, or other pulmonary issues. The normal adult respiratory rate is **14–20 breaths per minute (rpm).**

How to Measure
1. After taking the pulse, continue holding the client's wrist as if still counting the pulse to avoid drawing attention to breathing.
2. Observe the rise and fall of the chest or abdomen **without announcing** that respirations are being measured, since awareness can alter breathing patterns.
3. Count for **30 seconds and multiply by two**, or for a full **60 seconds** if breathing is irregular.
4. Note the **rate, rhythm, depth, and character** of each breath, including any sighing, labored, or shallow patterns.
5. Repeat after exertion or conversation if needed for accuracy.
6. Record findings, noting any irregularities or signs of distress.

Temperature

Body temperature helps screen for infection, inflammation, or systemic stress. In pregnancy, metabolic rate increases slightly, and the baseline temperature may be a little higher than average, but any fever should be investigated. Normal adult temperature is approximately **98.6°F (37°C)**, though normal ranges vary slightly depending on the route and device used.

> **Patterns**
> Vital signs show more than numbers—they reflect the body's ongoing conversation with itself. Patterns, not single values, tell the real story. Always ask what may have changed in the client's day, body, or emotions before labeling a finding "abnormal."

How to Measure
1. Use the same route and type of thermometer for each visit to ensure consistency. Common routes include oral, temporal (forehead), and tympanic (ear).
2. Wait at least 15 minutes after eating, drinking, smoking, or exercising before taking an oral temperature.
3. Follow the manufacturer's instructions for electronic or infrared thermometers, ensuring the probe is clean and properly placed.
4. Avoid axillary (underarm) readings unless other routes are not possible, as this method is less accurate.
5. Record both the temperature and the route used (for example, *98.4°F oral* or *99.1°F temporal*).
6. Recheck if results are inconsistent with the client's symptoms or seem unusually high or low.

Pulse Oximetry (SpO₂)

SpO2 measures how much oxygen is circulating in the blood. While not routine in all prenatal visits, it is useful when clients report shortness of breath, chest pain, dizziness, or have conditions such as asthma or anemia. A healthy range is typically **95 percent or higher** at sea level, though slightly lower values may occur at higher altitudes.

How to Measure
1. Make sure the client's hands are warm and free of nail polish or artificial nails.
2. Place the probe on a still finger with good circulation.
3. Wait for a **steady reading and waveform** before recording.
4. Ask the client to remain still and quiet during measurement to avoid motion artifact.
5. Record the **SpO2 reading and probe location** (for example, finger, toe, or earlobe).
6. Repeat if the value seems unusually low or inconsistent with the client's overall appearance.
7. If low readings persist, check for equipment error and evaluate for respiratory or circulatory compromise.

WEIGHT AND HEIGHT

Tracking height and weight over time helps monitor nutritional status, fluid retention, and fetal growth. Weight should always be interpreted with care—**trends, not single numbers, are most useful.** Discussions should remain respectful, and care should never be restricted based on body mass index (BMI).

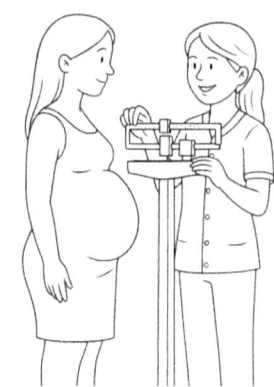

How to Measure
1. Measure height at the first visit.
2. Use a consistent, calibrated scale for weight.
3. Have the client remove heavy clothing and shoes.
4. Record weight in the same units at each visit.
5. Review trends together when appropriate.
6. Avoid framing weight changes as "good" or "bad."

Exercise 10.3: Vital Sign Matching	
Match each term:	
1. ____ Blood Pressure Measurement	A. Temperature above normal
2. ____ Febrile	B. Beats per minute
3. ____ Orthostatic change	C. Blood pressure shifts with position
4. ____ SpO₂	D. Upper number of BP
5. ____ Trend	E. Percentage of oxygen in the blood
6. ____ Systolic	F. Pattern of values across multiple visits
7. ____ Diastolic	G. Lower number of BP

Prenatal Laboratory Testing

Laboratory testing supports safe prenatal care by identifying infections, underlying conditions, and risk factors that may need monitoring or treatment. Some tests are considered routine; others are based on personal history, regional norms, or informed choice.

Not all lab tests must be completed during the first visit, but early identification of potential risks allows for timely referrals, health education, and planning. Labs are most useful when the midwife understands not only what to order but also what the results mean and how to discuss them with clients.

Informed Consent and Client Communication

Before discussing specific tests, midwives should explain how laboratory testing supports pregnancy health and ensure that clients understand their right to accept, decline, or delay any test. Informed consent is a continuing conversation, not a single signature.

When introducing testing, midwives might say: "I'd like to review which tests are available and why they might be recommended. You always have the choice to decide which ones feel right for you."

Public Health Reporting and Mandatory Action Reports (MARs)

Some prenatal lab results—especially those for infectious diseases—are *reportable conditions*. When a test result is positive, the lab or provider must report it to the local or state public health department. The purpose is to prevent outbreaks, offer treatment and partner follow-up, and maintain surveillance data. Reportable infections often include: Chlamydia, Gonorrhea, Syphilis, HIV, Hepatitis B & C.

Clients should be informed about this process before testing, especially for STIs or blood-borne pathogens, as it may influence their comfort or decision-making. Midwives might explain:

"If certain tests come back positive—like chlamydia, gonorrhea, or HIV—we're required by law to notify the public health department. They'll help make sure people get treatment and follow-up, and we'll always support you through that process.

ROUTINE FIRST-TRIMESTER LABS

Test Name	What It Tells You	Normal Result / Range
Blood type and Rh	ABO group and Rh factor	A, B, AB, or O; Rh positive or negative
Antibody screen	Detects unexpected antibodies (e.g., Rh sensitization)	Negative
Hemoglobin (Hgb)	Oxygen-carrying protein in red blood cells	≥ 11.0 g/dL (first trimester)
Hematocrit (Hct)	Red blood cell volume in blood	≥ 33 percent (first trimester)
White blood cell count	Screens for infection or immune response	4,000–11,000 per mm^3
Platelet count	Blood-clotting capacity	100,000–450,000 per mm^3
Rubella titer	Immunity to rubella (German measles)	Immune (IgG positive)
Hepatitis B (HBsAg)	Active hepatitis B infection	Negative
Hepatitis C antibody	Past or current hepatitis C infection	Negative
Syphilis (RPR or VDRL)	Screens for syphilis	Nonreactive
HIV antibody test	HIV status (offered with consent)	Negative
Thyroid (TSH)	Thyroid function	0.1–4.0 mIU/L
Urinalysis	Protein, glucose, leukocytes, nitrites, blood	Negative or trace
Urine culture	Asymptomatic urinary tract infection	No growth or < 10^5 CFU/mL
Gonorrhea and chlamydia	STI screening (urine or swab)	Negative

Blood (venipuncture)–used for:
- Blood type and Rh, antibody screen
- CBC (Hgb, Hct, WBC)
- Rubella, hepatitis B/C, HIV, syphilis
- TSH, NIPT, MsAFP

Urine–used for:
- Routine urinalysis (clean catch)
- Urine culture (clean catch)
- Gonorrhea/chlamydia NAAT (dirty catch preferred for best sensitivity)

Swabs (vaginal or cervical): swabs may be provider- or client-collected. Some require a speculum; others do not. Used for:
- Gonorrhea/chlamydia (if not using urine)
- Pap smear (requires speculum)
- Wet prep, HSV culture, GBS swab (36–37 weeks)

Other methods
- Saliva or buccal swab (carrier screening)
- Blood-based NIPT (fetal DNA)
- Amniotic fluid (by referral for diagnostic testing)

Urinalysis by Dipstick: Done Every Visit

Dipstick urinalysis is a quick, inexpensive screening tool used to detect potential concerns such as infection, dehydration, or elevated glucose. Although not diagnostic, it can prompt further investigation. Clients should provide a clean-catch midstream sample. The midwife briefly dips the test strip into the urine and interprets results according to the timing guide on the package. Document results and interpret in the context of the full clinical picture.
- Use a clean-catch midstream sample.

- Test promptly for accuracy.
- Screen for proteinuria, glucose, ketones, leukocytes, and nitrites.
- Trace values may be normal; 1+ or greater often requires follow-up

Screening vs. Diagnostic Tests

Screening tests look for the *possibility* of a condition; diagnostic tests confirm whether it is actually present. Think of it like a smoke detector. A screening test is like smelling smoke. It might mean there's a fire, or it might not. A diagnostic test is how we check to see what's really happening.

Clients should understand what each test looks for, how results are used, and what next steps may be recommended.

Tests That Usually Require Explicit Consent

Test	Why Consent Is Important
HIV antibody test	May require documented consent; affects confidentiality and care coordination.
Hepatitis B and C	May have legal or social implications depending on context.
NIPT	Optional; screens for chromosomal conditions. Follow-up may involve invasive testing.
Carrier screening	May influence partner or fetal testing decisions.
Fetal Rh via NIPT	Optional; may reduce need for Rhogam but is not standard everywhere.
Reflexive carrier testing	May be included in expanded NIPT; can reveal unexpected information.
Genetic screening (MsAFP, quad screen)	Optional and time-sensitive; can lead to further testing and complex decisions.

Midwives should document consent or refusal and offer ongoing opportunities for questions or discussion.

Noninvasive Prenatal Testing (NIPT)

NIPT is a blood test that analyzes cell-free DNA from the placenta. It screens for:
- Trisomy 21 (Down syndrome)

- Trisomy 18 and 13
- Sex-chromosome conditions
- Fetal sex (optional)
- Fetal Rh status (for Rh-negative clients)
- Reflexive carrier screening if a parental variant is identified

NIPT is most accurate after **10 weeks' gestation.** It is a *screening* test, not diagnostic; abnormal results should be confirmed by chorionic villus sampling (CVS) or amniocentesis.

Maternal Serum Alpha-Fetoprotein (MsAFP)

MsAFP is typically offered between 15 and 20 weeks. It screens for:

- Open neural-tube defects (e.g., spina bifida)
- Abdominal-wall defects
- Some chromosomal anomalies (as part of a quad screen)

Clients who decline NIPT may choose the quad screen instead. Clients who accept NIPT may still need MsAFP, since NIPT does not detect open neural-tube defects.

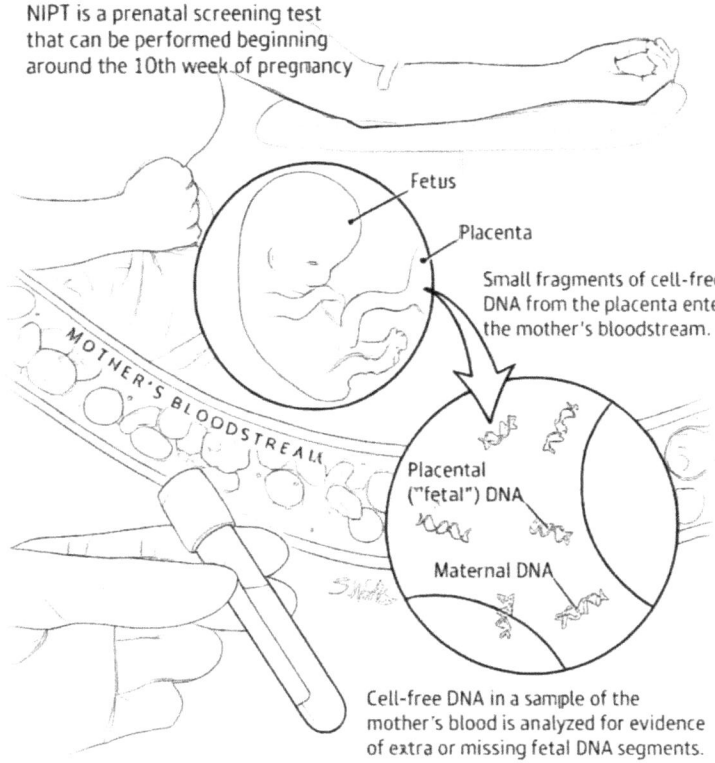

Ultrasound in Prenatal Care

Ultrasound uses high-frequency sound waves to create an image of the developing fetus and surrounding structures. It is considered a standard part of modern prenatal care, but like all procedures, it has both benefits and limitations.

Common Indications

- Confirm gestational dating when last menstrual period is uncertain
- Confirm viability in early pregnancy
- Assess pregnancy location (rule out ectopic)
- Identify multiple gestation
- Evaluate fetal anatomy (18–22 weeks)
- Assess fetal growth, amniotic fluid, placenta
- Determine fetal position late in pregnancy
- Follow up on concerning signs or symptoms

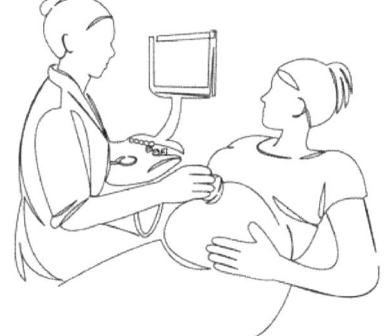

Risks and Limitations

- Not diagnostic in all cases; may prompt further testing.
- False positives and negatives can occur.
- Routine ultrasound has not been proven to improve outcomes in all low-risk pregnancies.
- Use only when medically indicated, not for entertainment or reassurance alone.
- Although no long-term harm has been shown, the precautionary principle supports minimizing unnecessary exposure.

Types of Ultrasound

- **Transvaginal** (early pregnancy or cervical assessment)
- **Transabdominal** (second and third trimesters)
- **Targeted** or level II (for suspected anomalies)
- **Biophysical profile** (BPP)–uses ultrasound plus NST

Benefits
- Confirms pregnancy details such as viability, location, and fetal number
- Detects many—but not all—structural anomalies
- Guides management in higher-risk cases
- Can reassure clients about fetal growth and development

Limitations
- Cannot detect every abnormality or guarantee a normal outcome
- False-positive and false-negative findings may occur
- Routine ultrasound has not been shown to improve outcomes in all low-risk pregnancies
- Although no long-term harm has been demonstrated, unnecessary exposure should be avoided

Informed Consent

Ultrasound should always be performed with informed consent. Clients should understand:
- Why the study is being recommended
- What it can and cannot show
- What follow-up may be needed based on results
- That declining is an option in most cases

Midwives might say: "Ultrasound can give us helpful information about your baby's size, position, or anatomy, but it's not perfect. Sometimes it raises questions that turn out not to be problems. Let's talk about what the test might show, how we'd follow up, and how you feel about getting that information."

Ultrasound at a Glance

Timing	Purpose	Common Use	Considerations
6–10 weeks	Confirm pregnancy, location, viability, number of fetuses	Dating, viability, ectopic rule-out	Often transvaginal; may not detect heartbeat if too early
11–14 weeks	Nuchal translucency (if part of early genetic screen)	Optional with early aneuploidy screening	Combined with blood tests; requires trained provider
18–22 weeks	Full anatomy scan	Standard anatomy ultrasound	May detect anomalies; false positives/negatives possible
28 + weeks	Growth scan, fetal position, fluid level	Follow-up for high-risk pregnancies or concerns	Less accurate for dating; assesses well-being
36–40 weeks	Position check, placenta recheck, growth if indicated	Late-pregnancy planning, VBAC, malpresentation	Informs birth planning but does not predict labor readiness

Midwifery Perspective: Ultrasound and the Art of Hands-On Care

While ultrasound is now a routine part of modern prenatal care, it is important to remember that midwives practiced for generations without it. Ultrasound is an invaluable tool that can reveal crucial information about fetal health, position, and anatomy—sometimes even saving lives. Yet its widespread use has also changed how practitioners engage with their clients.

Relying on ultrasound at every visit, particularly to determine fetal position or size, can lead to a loss of manual assessment skills. Palpation—learning the baby's lie, presentation, and movement through gentle touch—builds both clinical accuracy and connection.

Maintaining and refining this tactile skill remains essential, especially for midwives practicing in low-resource environments or during emergencies when technology may not be available. A skilled pair of hands is one of the most reliable diagnostic tools in any setting.

Exercise 10.4: Prenatal Lab Tests

Match each laboratory test to its primary purpose or key finding:

1. _____Blood type and Rh
2. _____Rubella titer
3. _____Syphilis (RPR or VDRL)
4. _____Hepatitis B (HBsAg)
5. _____HIV antibody test
6. _____Urinalysis
7. _____Hemoglobin and hematocrit
8. _____NIPT
9. _____Urine culture
10. _____Gonorrhea and chlamydia
11. _____MsAFP
12. _____Thyroid-stimulating hormone (TSH)

A. Detects antibodies that could cause hemolytic disease of the newborn
B. Checks immunity to a viral infection that may cause birth defects
C. Screens for a sexually transmitted infection that can cross the placenta
D. Detects a virus transmitted through blood and body fluids
E. Identifies immune status and supports perinatal infection prevention
F. Screens for protein, glucose, or infection in urine
G. Assesses oxygen-carrying capacity and risk for anemia
H. Screens fetal DNA for chromosomal conditions such as trisomy 21
I. Evaluates thyroid function and potential impact on metabolism and pregnancy
J. Detects asymptomatic urinary tract infection
K. Screens for sexually transmitted infections that can cause neonatal eye or respiratory infection
L. Screens for open neural-tube or abdominal-wall defects

Physical Exam

The physical exam is an essential part of the first prenatal visit or in well-woman care. It establishes a clinical baseline, supports individualized risk assessment, and helps build rapport through attentive, respectful care. For many clients, the midwife may be the only clinician they see during pregnancy, making this exam a vital opportunity to assess overall health, nutrition, and well-being.

Midwives should approach the exam as a collaborative, consent-based process. Explain what it includes, invite questions, and ask permission before each step. Allow the client to remain covered as much as possible, and offer a chaperone or support person if desired. Trauma-informed care means creating safety, maintaining communication, and allowing the client to pause or decline any part of the exam. The midwife might say, "I'd like to do a head-to-toe physical exam today so I can get a full picture of your health and how your body is adapting to pregnancy. I'll explain each part before I do it, and you're always welcome to pause, skip, or ask questions."

A well-performed physical exam is an act of presence as much as procedure. Through skilled hands and quiet observation, midwives learn to recognize the body's language—its texture, temperature, tone, and subtle signs of wellness or imbalance. These skills develop through practice, grounding students in the art of touch that lies at the heart of midwifery care.

Purpose of the Physical Exam
- Establish a baseline for physical findings and general health
- Detect variations that may influence pregnancy management
- Screen for chronic or previously undiagnosed conditions
- Determine whether additional testing or referral is needed
- Provide education on normal body changes in pregnancy

Equipment Needed
Stethoscope, blood pressure cuff, thermometer, light source, reflex hammer, gloves, and watch with a second hand. Otoscope and ophthalmoscope use may be optional depending on scope and training.

Head-to-Toe Exam Overview
- **General Appearance:** Observe posture, mobility, comfort level, hygiene, and emotional affect.
- **Skin, Hair, and Nails:** Inspect for pallor, jaundice, bruising, pigmentation changes, or rashes. Check skin *turgor* by gently pinching the skin to assess hydration; note brittleness or dryness that may indicate nutritional deficiency.
- **Head and Neck:** Palpate lymph nodes and thyroid for enlargement or tenderness. Observe for goiter, facial asymmetry, or edema.
- **Eyes, Ears, Nose, Throat:** Inspect conjunctiva for pallor, sclera for jaundice, and oral cavity for lesions or dental concerns. Nasal congestion or gum bleeding may be normal in pregnancy but should still be noted.
- **Chest and Lungs:** Observe chest symmetry and respiratory effort. Auscultate for clear breath sounds and note any wheezing or rales.
- **Heart:** Auscultate at the point of maximal impulse; note rhythm, rate, or murmurs. Some soft murmurs may be normal in pregnancy, but new or loud ones require evaluation.
- **Breasts:** Inspect for symmetry, tenderness, discharge, or skin changes. Palpate for lumps and offer education on normal breast changes and self-exam techniques.
- **Abdomen:** Inspect for scars or distension. Palpate for tenderness, liver edge, or diastasis recti. Auscultate bowel sounds and palpate uterine size if appropriate for gestation.
- **Spine and Musculoskeletal:** Observe alignment, mobility, and gait. Ask about back or joint pain.
- **Extremities:** Assess for edema, varicosities, pulses, and capillary refill. Check reflexes at the patella and Achilles and grade them 0–4+. Note presence of clonus if seen.
- **Neurologic:** Observe coordination and strength. Abnormal reflexes or clonus may suggest hypertensive complications.

Exercise 10.5: Physical Exam Findings
Match each component with its purpose or key consideration:

1. ____Palpation of CVA	A.	Detect kidney tenderness
2. ____Speculum exam	B.	Visualize cervix and assess vaginal health
3. ____Auscultation of lungs	C.	Listen for rales, wheezes, or diminished breath sounds
4. ____Fundal palpation	D.	Assess uterine size, position, and tone
5. ____Asking before touching	E.	Supports trauma-informed, consent-based care
6. ____Rectovaginal exam	F.	Assess posterior structures when indicated

PELVIC EXAM

Pelvic exams are not routinely required at prenatal visits unless indicated by history or if will guide care decisions. They may be appropriate if the client is due for a Pap smear, requires STI testing that cannot be done by urine, or if clinical findings suggest a need for further evaluation.

Pelvic exams should always be performed with full informed consent. The client should know why the exam is being recommended, what will happen, and how the findings will be used. Offer the option to pause or decline at any point, and provide clear, step-by-step explanations throughout. A chaperone or support person should be available if desired. The procedure offers valuable information about anatomy, tone, and health but must always be balanced with the client's comfort and autonomy. Sensitivity, clear communication, and respect transform this clinical task into an act of care.

Inspection of the Vulva and Perineum: The vulva should appear pink and moist without lesions, swelling, warts, varicosities, inflammation, or irritation. Vestibular glands should be free of redness or swelling. Observe for signs of infection, trauma, or scarring from previous births or surgeries.

Vaginal Examination: Inspect for color, moisture, and tone. The vaginal mucosa should be pink to bluish-purple in pregnancy (Chadwick's sign) and free from lesions or ulcerations. Discharge should be clear to cloudy, thin, and nonirritating. Note perineal tone, elasticity, and the presence of any old episiotomy scars. Observe for prolapse, cystocele, or rectocele. Ask the client to tighten the pelvic floor muscles to assess tone and offer education on Kegel exercises if appropriate.

Cervical Assessment: The cervix should appear pink or bluish and soft, with the os possibly slightly dilated in multigravid clients. Note any lesions, polyps, or white patches. A Pap smear or STI swabs may be performed if indicated. If the client is due or overdue for cervical screening, it may be completed safely during the first prenatal visit. If recent screening is up to date, it can be deferred until the postpartum period. Observe the client's face and check for discomfort throughout the exam.

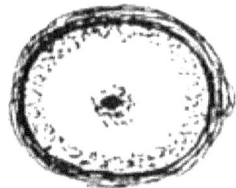 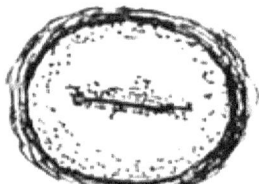 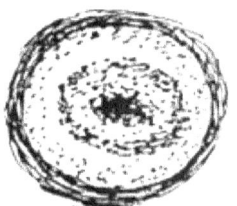

Nulliparous Cervix   **Multiparous Cervix**   **Cervical Erosion**

Bimanual Examination: Palpate the uterus to assess size, position, and tenderness. The uterus should feel enlarged and soft if consistent with early pregnancy. Adnexa (ovaries and fallopian tubes) should be non-tender, and no masses should be felt.

Rectal and Perineal Observation: Inspect the anus and rectum for rashes, tenderness, or hemorrhoids. No lumps or fissures should be present.

SPECULUM EXAMINATION

A speculum exam allows direct visualization of the cervix and vaginal walls and is performed only when clinically indicated and with full informed consent. Common reasons include cervical cancer screening (Pap smear), STI specimen collection, or evaluation of abnormal discharge or bleeding.

Midwives approach this procedure as both a technical skill and a moment of care. A calm presence, clear explanation, and attention to comfort transform what can be an anxious experience into one of trust and collaboration. Many clients have a history of medical trauma or discomfort with pelvic exams; sensitivity, warmth, and ongoing consent are essential. Always remind the client that they can pause or stop the exam at any time.

Preparation:
1. Explain the procedure clearly, including why it is needed and what it will involve.
2. Let the client know that some pressure or mild discomfort is normal, but pain is not expected.
3. Provide a gown and sheet for privacy, and ensure the room is warm and well lit.
4. Invite the client to lie on their back, bring their heels toward their buttocks, and relax their knees apart.

Gather all necessary supplies:
1. A speculum of appropriate size, gloves, a light source, and water-soluble lubricant.
2. Have specimen collection materials ready if performing a Pap smear or STI testing.
3. Warm the speculum with tap water.
4. Apply a small amount of lubricant to the outer sides of the blades, avoiding the tip if collecting a Pap smear sample.
5. Before beginning, reconfirm consent and ensure the client is ready.

Insertion:
1. Perform a brief external inspection, noting any lesions, inflammation, or discharge.
2. With your non-dominant hand, gently part the labia.
3. Hold the speculum with the blades closed and insert it at a slight angle—usually sideways at the 3 or 9 o'clock position.
4. Advance it slowly along the posterior vaginal wall, avoiding pressure on the urethra.
5. Once fully inserted, rotate the handle to face upward and open the blades slowly until the cervix is visible.
6. Lock the speculum in place to free one hand.

Inspection and Specimen Collection:
1. Observe the cervix for color, position, and the appearance of the os. Note any inflammation, lesions, or abnormal discharge.
2. If indicated, use sterile swabs or a cytology brush to collect specimens for Pap smear or STI testing
3. As you withdraw the speculum, observe the vaginal walls for color, tone, and any signs of lesions or atrophy.

Removal and Conclusion:
1. Loosen the locking mechanism and slowly close the blades while withdrawing the speculum.
2. Rotate slightly to the side as you remove it to prevent discomfort.
3. Offer tissues to remove any lubricant and allow privacy for the client to dress.
4. Explain that minor spotting can occur and provide reassurance as needed.
5. Document the procedure, findings, and client's tolerance of the exam.

Pelvimetry

Pelvic assessment, or pelvimetry, is becoming a lost art as imaging and trial of labor are more often used instead. Elder Midwives believe that estimating the size and shape of the bony pelvis by hand deepens understanding of how labor may progress for each individual woman. Although many factors influence labor outcomes, hands-on knowledge remains a valuable clinical skill. When performed with skill, consent, and gentleness, pelvimetry helps the midwife understand pelvic variation, anticipate potential challenges, and assess progress during labor.

Purpose
- Establish a baseline understanding of pelvic type and dimensions.
- Identify any deformities, masses, or limitations that may affect fetal descent.
- Support individualized birth planning and consultation when concerns arise.
- Strengthen the midwife's anatomical understanding of pelvic landmarks and variability.

Preparation and Consent

Before beginning, review pelvic anatomy and normal dimensions. Measure your own hand in centimeters—width of fist, span between thumb and forefinger, and distance between the tips of the index and middle fingers—to create a personal reference scale. Explain the procedure in detail, answer all questions, and obtain explicit informed consent. Let the client know they may pause or stop the exam at any time. A model of the pelvis is paced on the abdomen, allowing good visualization and used as a teaching moment for the mother. Pelvimetry should never be forced or painful; gentleness and communication are essential.

Technique

1. **Diagonal Conjugate (Inlet)** is measured from the lower border of the **symphysis pubis** to the **sacral promontory** and is usually about 12.5–13 cm. The true (obstetric) conjugate extends from the upper border of the symphysis pubis to the sacral promontory, cannot be measured directly, and is approximately 11–11.5 cm.

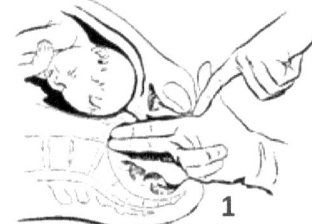

2. **Interspinous (Midpelvis):** withdraw slightly and locate the **ischial spines**. The distance between them—the *interspinous* or *bispinous diameter*—should exceed **10.5 cm**. Note whether the spines feel blunt or prominent.

3. **Sacrococcygeal (Outlet, Front-to-Back):** palpate to the **sacrococcygeal joint** and measure to the lower symphysis—about **11.5 cm**. Note sacral curve, coccyx mobility, and any tenderness.

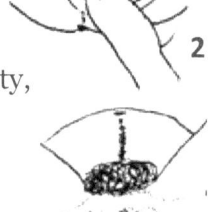

4. **Pubic Arch (Outlet, Lateral):** as you withdraw, assess the **pubic arch**. A normal angle is about **90 degrees**; a narrower angle suggests limited outlet space.

5. **Bituberous Diameter (External Outlet):** place a relaxed fist externally between the **ischial tuberosities**. The *bituberous diameter* should be over **10.5 cm**—your fist should fit easily between the bones.

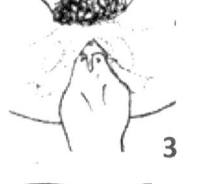

Documentation and Clinical Integration

Record findings descriptively (for example, "adequate," "borderline," "narrow outlet") rather than as pass/fail measurements. The most reliable "test" of pelvic adequacy is labor itself; descent and rotation over time reveal how well the pelvis accommodates the fetus. Observation, touch, and trust—rather than numbers alone—guide safe, individualized midwifery care. While pelvimetry can be one of many assessment tools, evidence does not support it as a reliable predictor of labor outcomes, and there is wide individual variation.

Prenatal Skills and Fetal Assessment

Prenatal visits are an opportunity for the midwife to build rapport while using hands-on skills to assess both the pregnant person and the developing fetus. Over time, clinical findings reveal trends in fetal growth, position, movement, and overall well-being. Skillful assessment allows the midwife to detect early signs of deviation from normal and to intervene or refer when needed. These skills are built through repetition, supervision, and integration of both touch and clinical reasoning.

Fundal Height Measurement

Measuring fundal height is a simple, reliable way to estimate gestational age and monitor fetal growth over time. After about 20 weeks, the fundal height in centimeters generally corresponds to the number of weeks of pregnancy. This low-tech method is quick and effective when performed consistently and documented accurately.

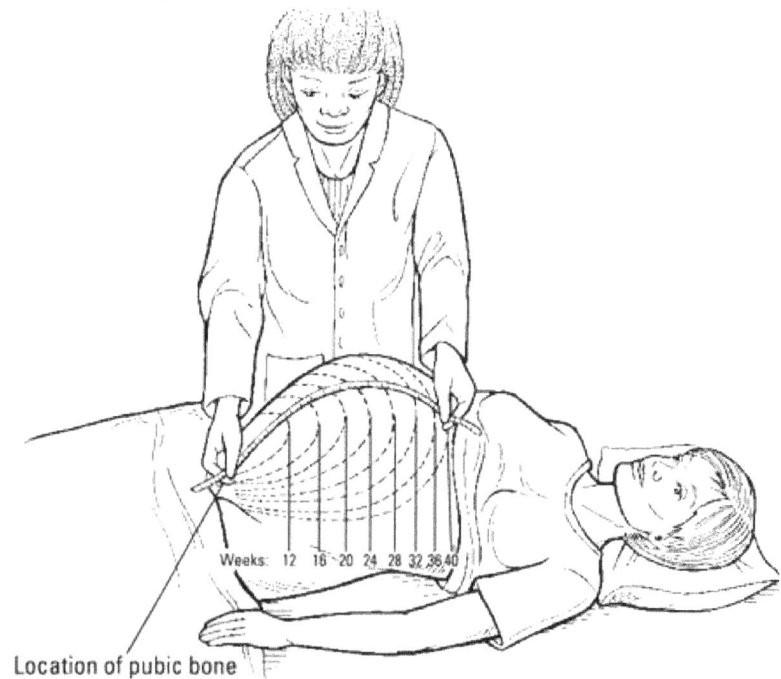

How to Measure: Have the client empty her bladder and lie in a semi-reclined or supine position. Using a flexible, non-stretch measuring tape, place the zero end at the midline of the upper border of the symphysis pubis. Stretch the tape over the abdomen to the top of the uterine fundus, using the edge of your other hand to locate the highest point of the uterus.

Tips for Accuracy:
- Keep the client in the same position each time, with the abdomen relaxed.
- Use the same examiner whenever possible for consistency.
- A difference of 1–2 cm between examiners is common.
- Between 18 and 36 weeks, fundal height usually corresponds to gestational age (for example, 24 cm ≈ 24 weeks).
- Normal variation is ± 1–2 cm; larger or sudden changes may warrant further evaluation.
- Record measurements carefully and watch for a steady growth pattern rather than absolute numbers.

Factors Affecting Measurement: Maternal body habitus, examiner pressure, fetal position, multiple pregnancy, amniotic-fluid volume, and bladder fullness can all influence results. The goal is not a single perfect number but a consistent curve of growth over time. Some midwives use disposable paper tapes and write the measurements directly on them as a keepsake for the client after birth. Others prefer reusable cloth or vinyl tapes for durability. Whatever the method, consistency is key to meaningful comparison across visits.

Exercise 10.5: Fundal Height Measurement
Fill in blanks of the following questions:

1. The fundus is at the level of the symphysis pubis at approximately _____ weeks.
2. The fundus is midway between the symphysis pubis and the umbilicus at approximately _____ weeks.
3. The fundus is at the level of the umbilicus at approximately _____ weeks.
4. The fundus is midway between the umbilicus and the xiphoid process at approximately _____ weeks.
5. The fundus reaches the level of the xiphoid process at approximately _____ weeks.
6. List three possible causes for a fundal height **greater** than expected:
   _____
7. List three possible causes for a fundal height **less** than expected:
   _____

Leopold's Maneuvers

Leopold's maneuvers are four specific palpation techniques used to determine fetal **lie**, **presentation**, **position**, and **engagement**. These are typically performed after 28 weeks of pregnancy, when the fetus is large enough to be easily assessed through the abdominal wall. In skilled hands, these maneuvers can provide highly accurate information about fetal orientation and descent. As ultrasound has become commonplace, hands-on assessment of fetal position is increasingly a lost art.

Preparation:

Have the client lie on a firm, flat surface in a semi-reclined or supine position with knees slightly bent. Ensure the bladder is emptied. Warm your hands and explain each step before beginning. Always maintain communication with the client to promote relaxation and comfort.

1. First Maneuver: Fundal Grip

Purpose: Identify which fetal pole (head or breech) occupies the uterine fundus.
Technique:
- Stand facing the client's head.
- Place both hands on the top of the fundus and gently curve the fingers around it.
- Assess the **shape, size, consistency,** and **mobility** of the part felt.
- The head will feel firm, round, and movable; the breech feels softer and less defined.

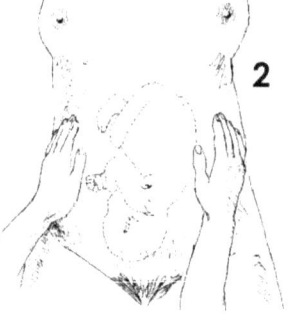

2. Second Maneuver: Lateral Grip

Purpose: Locate the fetal back and small parts (limbs).
Technique:
- With both hands on the sides of the uterus, apply gentle pressure with one hand to steady the fetus while palpating with the other.
- Slide your palpating hand from the midline outward toward the flank, using smooth, firm, rotary movements.
- The fetal back feels broad and firm; the small parts feel nodular and irregular.
- Reverse hand positions to palpate the opposite side.

3. Third Maneuver: Pawlik's Grip

Purpose: Identify the presenting part and determine whether it is engaged.
Technique:
- Place your thumb and fingers of one hand just above the symphysis pubis.
- Grasp the lower portion of the uterus between your thumb and fingers, pressing gently but firmly to feel what lies between them.
- If the presenting part is not engaged, it will move freely; if engaged, it will feel fixed.
- The fetal head is hard and round; the breech is softer and irregular.

4. Fourth Maneuver: Second Pelvic Grip

Purpose: Determine fetal engagement and attitude (flexion or extension).
Technique:
- Turn to face the client's feet.
- Place both hands on the sides of the uterus, with fingertips directed toward the symphysis pubis.
- Press deeply with the fingertips toward the pelvic inlet.
- If the head is flexed, the cephalic prominence will be felt on the opposite side from the fetal back. If extended, it will be on the same side as the back.
- Note whether the presenting part is engaged by how deeply it can be palpated.

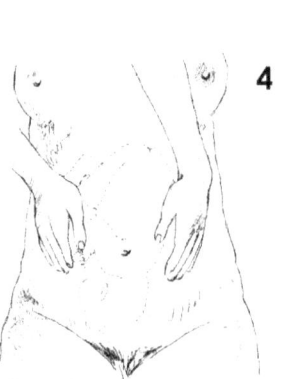

Interpretation
- **Fetal lie:** Longitudinal, transverse, or oblique
- **Presentation:** Cephalic (head down) or breech (buttocks down)
- **Position:** Location of the fetal back relative to the maternal abdomen (left, right, anterior, or posterior)
- **Engagement:** How far the presenting part has descended into the pelvis

---

Exercise 10.6: Leopold's Maneuvers
Fill in blanks of the following questions:

1. _____ maneuver identifies which fetal part is in the fundus.
2. _____ maneuver locates the fetal back and small parts.
3. _____ maneuver determines the presenting part and whether it is engaged.
4. _____ maneuver assesses fetal engagement and attitude.
5. These maneuvers are typically performed after _____ weeks of pregnancy

---

FETAL MOVEMENT AND CLIENT PERCEPTION

Fetal movement is a simple, noninvasive indicator of fetal well-being. Most clients begin to perceive movement between 16 and 22 weeks. By the third trimester, a recognizable pattern is expected, and changes from that individual baseline may signal concern.

Midwives should ask about fetal movement at every visit and listen for any departure from the client's usual pattern. Encouraging clients to tune in to their baby's typical rhythms builds connection and supports early recognition of potential problems. Decreased or absent movement should always be taken seriously and followed with appropriate evaluation.

- Ask open-ended questions such as *"How is your baby moving?"*
- Expect a regular pattern after 28 weeks.
- Emphasize awareness of the client's own baseline rather than comparisons with others.
- If movement seems decreased, further assessment may include non-stress testing (NST), ultrasound, or transfer of care as indicated.

When Further Evaluation May Be Needed
- No perceived movement during a period when the baby is usually active.
- Fewer than **ten movements in up to two hours** during a focused count ("count-to-ten" method).
- A sustained reduction from the client's normal pattern, especially if risk factors such as hypertension, diabetes, or growth concerns are present.
- After trauma or when accompanied by additional symptoms, such as vaginal bleeding, fluid leakage, or severe abdominal pain.

Teaching Notes for Clients
- Babies have sleep cycles lasting about 20–40 minutes; encourage rest, hydration, and quiet observation before counting.
- Track movement at roughly the same time each day for consistency.
- Advise clients to contact the midwife promptly if any worrisome change occurs; they should not wait until the next appointment.
- Remind clients that home Dopplers or mobile applications are **not** substitutes for clinical assessment.

Partnership in Care
When midwives invite clients to notice fetal movement and body changes, they nurture shared responsibility and strengthen confidence in the pregnancy process.

Edema Assessment

Edema is the abnormal accumulation of fluid in body tissues and is common in pregnancy, especially during the third trimester. While mild swelling in the lower extremities may represent a normal physiologic change, sudden or asymmetric edema can signal underlying complications that require further evaluation.

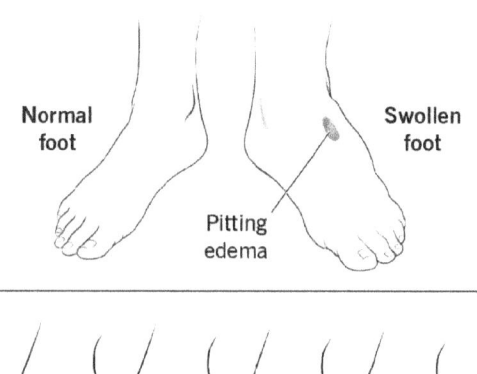

Assessment includes inspection and palpation of the ankles, lower legs, hands, and face. To check for **pitting edema**, press gently but firmly into the skin—typically over the shin or ankle—for about five seconds, then observe whether a depression remains. The presence, severity, and distribution of swelling should be documented, especially if it is new, one-sided, or accompanied by additional symptoms.

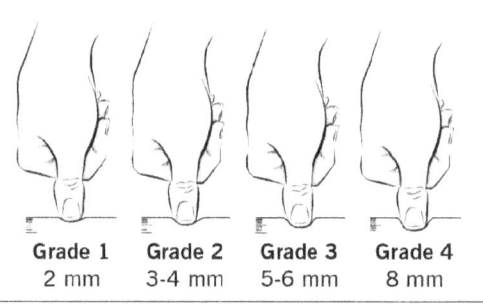

- Inspect for swelling in the hands, face, and lower extremities.
- Ask about changes in the tightness of rings, socks, or shoes.
- Press gently over the tibia or ankle to check for pitting (graded 1+ to 4+).
- Document the location, symmetry, and severity of edema.
- Follow up if swelling is sudden, localized, or worsening.

Assessing the Fetal Heartbeat

Assessing the fetal heartbeat is one of the most meaningful and useful skills in midwifery care. Listening to and measuring the fetal heart provide real-time information about fetal well-being and often create an emotional point of connection for families.

The term "fetal heart tones" (FHTs) is traditionally used in midwifery to describe listening to the baby's heartbeat, while "fetal heart rate" (FHR) is the preferred clinical term in current medical documentation. This practice blends **clinical skill and relational care**. For midwives, assessing the fetal heartbeat is both diagnostic and emotionally meaningful. Mastery of Doppler and fetoscope techniques ensures flexibility across home, clinic, and birth-center settings. Intermittent auscultation supports physiologic birth while providing adequate fetal surveillance. Integrating heart-rate findings with other indicators—such as fetal movement and fundal height—builds a complete, compassionate picture of fetal health.

When to Listen

Fetal heart activity is usually audible with a **Doppler** by **10–12 weeks** and with a **fetoscope** by **18–20 weeks**.

- A **Doppler** uses ultrasound waves to detect motion and amplify sound.
- A **fetoscope** functions like a stethoscope, requires no batteries or ultrasound, and is often preferred in low-intervention or out-of-hospital settings.

Types of Fetoscopes

Several styles of fetoscopes are used in midwifery, including the **Pinard horn**, the **Leffscope**, and **headband-style fetoscopes** that allow hands-free listening. Using a manual fetoscope is an acquired skill—the fetal heartbeat is often faint and subtle; it takes 'listening beyond listening.' This sensitivity develops through patience, repetition, and learning to distinguish the quiet, rhythmic fetal pulse from the maternal and placental background sounds.

Dopplers are easier for clients or family members to listen, which can deepen emotional connection. As with all forms of auscultation, a calm environment, gentle persistence, and attentive presence are essential.

Types of Fetoscopes

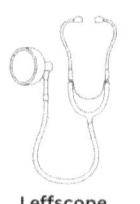
Leffscope

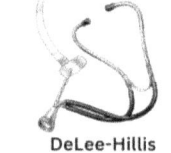
DeLee-Hillis

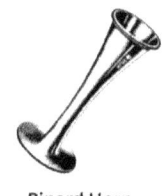
Pinard Horn

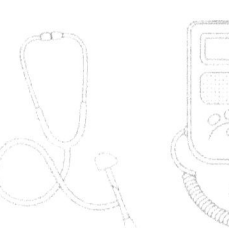
Allan fetoscope

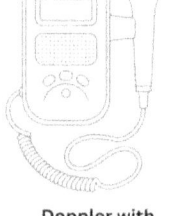
Doppler with digital readout

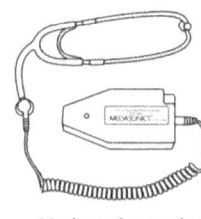
Medasonics analog Doppler

Locating the Fetal Heartbeat

The location of the fetal heartbeat often corresponds with fetal position: tones heard low in the pelvis suggest a **cephalic** (head-down) presentation, while tones heard higher on the abdomen often indicate **breech** presentation. Heart tones are usually clearest over the fetal back. In the most common left occiput anterior (LOA) position, they are best heard in the lower left quadrant of the abdomen.

Knowing fetal position through **Leopold's maneuvers** guides where to place the Doppler or fetoscope for the clearest tones. The fetal heartbeat is best heard where the fetal back lies closest to the abdominal wall. To locate it systematically, move the device in a slow **semicircular sweep** across the lower abdomen, beginning near the midline and extending outward in small arcs until the sound is strongest. Adjust the angle and pressure as needed, covering all quadrants if necessary.

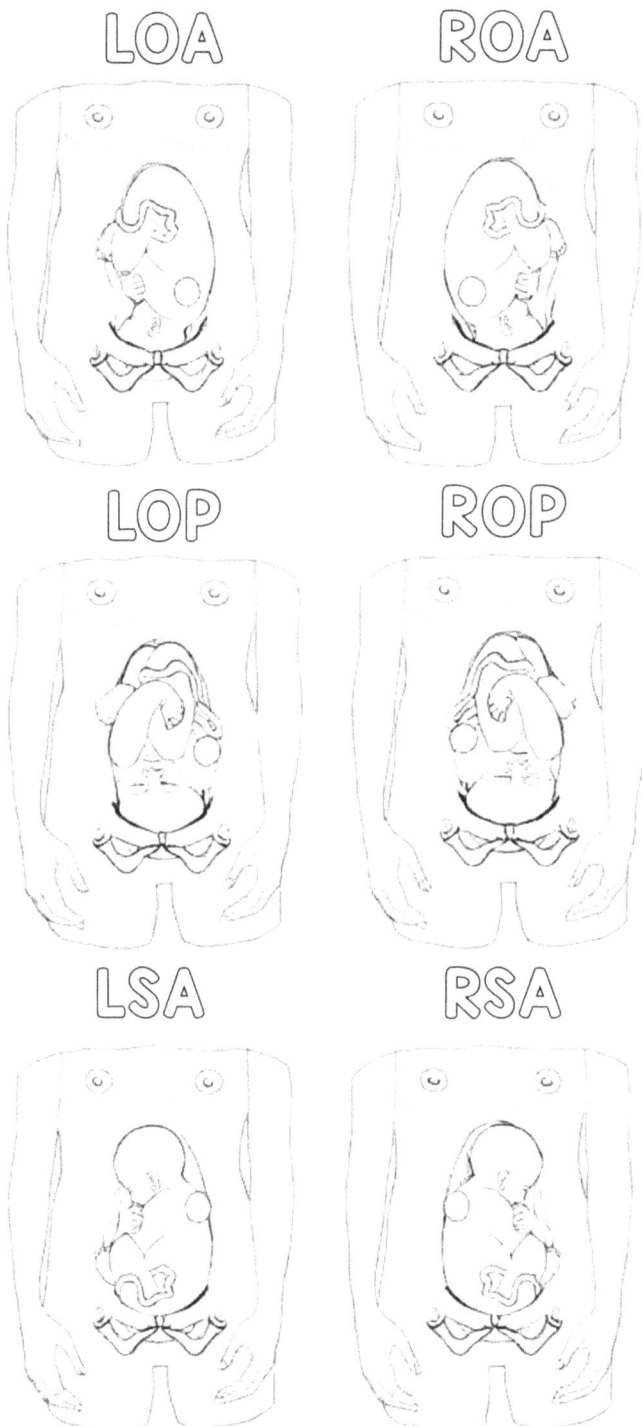

How to Assess

1. **Explain the procedure** and obtain consent. Apply a small amount of ultrasound gel or conductive jelly to the Doppler.
2. **Palpate the maternal radial pulse** before beginning to avoid confusing maternal and fetal heartbeats.
3. **Early pregnancy (10–16 weeks):**
   - Begin at the midline just above the pubic bone.
   - Tilt the Doppler slowly upward toward the umbilicus, as though shining a flashlight beam beneath the surface.
   - Maintain firm contact but do not press too hard, as excess pressure can reduce sound transmission.
4. **Second trimester (16–24 weeks):**
   - Use either a Doppler or a fetoscope.
   - Move systematically across the lower abdomen, about 2–3 cm at a time, listening carefully.
   - If no heartbeat is heard in the lower abdomen, repeat the process in the upper quadrants.
5. **After 24 weeks:**
   - Palpate to identify the fetal back (using Leopold's maneuvers) and place the device where tones are clearest.
   - If the fetal back cannot be located easily, begin at midline between the umbilicus and the pubic bone and move outward in a semicircle.
   - Identify where the heartbeat is heard in relation to fetal position and lie.

Provide clear explanations throughout the process and reassure the client if tones are not immediately located. Patience and calm communication build trust and reduce anxiety.

Counting and Interpreting

- A **"swooshing" sound**, called the *uterine souffle*, reflects maternal blood flow through uterine arteries and matches the maternal pulse.
- If the heartbeat is difficult to locate, **recheck position, angle, and pressure**, or return later after fetal movement changes the baby's orientation.
- If tones are irregular or absent, verify technique, reassess after repositioning, and refer for further evaluation as needed. Remain calm and reassuring; clients may experience anxiety if tones are not immediately heard.

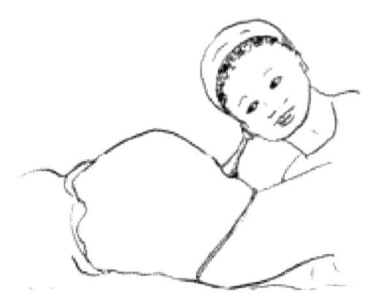

Once the fetal heartbeat is heard:
- Count for a full **60 seconds** for accuracy.
- In time-sensitive settings, use the **six-second rule** (count beats for six seconds and add a zero), though this is less precise and may miss irregularities.
- The **normal fetal heart rate** ranges from **110 to 160 beats per minute**.
- Note any **accelerations, decelerations,** or **irregular rhythms.**
- A gradual increase in rate with fetal movement and return to baseline afterward is a reassuring sign.
- When interpreting findings, consider all aspects of the clinical picture—fetal activity, gestational age, and maternal health—rather than isolated numbers.

Exercise 10.7: Fetal Heart Auscultation
Match each component with its purpose or key consideration:

1. _____Intermittent auscultation	A.	Listening to FHTs at intervals rather than continuously
2. _____Doppler	B.	Handheld device using ultrasound to detect FHTs
3. _____Fetoscope	C.	Acoustic tool for auscultation without electronics
4. _____6-second rule	D.	Quick method to estimate heart rate
5. _____Baseline fetal heart rate	E.	Average bpm in absence of changes

Midwifery Perspective Fetal Heart Auscultation

Fetal heart tone assessment is a powerful blend of clinical skill and emotional presence. For midwives, this practice is a routine yet deeply relational moment of care. Mastery of both the Doppler and fetoscope allows flexibility across settings, including home, clinic, and birth center care.

Intermittent auscultation supports physiologic birth while providing adequate fetal surveillance.

Midwives must use both technical skill and intuition to recognize when fetal heart tones are concerning and to counsel families with clarity and calmness. Integrating fetal tone assessment with other findings, such as fetal movement and fundal height, strengthens the clinical picture and supports safe, person-centered care.

Exercise 10.8: Routine Prenatal Care
Match each component with its purpose or key consideration:

1. _____Fundal height measurement	A.	Determine fetal lie and position
2. _____Leopold's maneuvers	B.	Assess fetal growth over time
3. _____Fetal heart tone monitoring	C.	Evaluate fetal well-being and rhythm
4. _____Urinalysis Dipstick	D.	Screen for glucose or proteinuria
5. _____Edema check	E.	Monitor for fluid retention and swelling

Subsequent Prenatal Visits

After the first prenatal visit, midwifery care continues with a series of scheduled follow-up visits that provide structure, surveillance, and support throughout the pregnancy. These visits offer ongoing opportunities to assess maternal and fetal well-being, build trusting relationships, and respond to changing needs. While a standard visit schedule is typically followed, individual visit timing may vary depending on testing, referrals, or emerging clinical factors.

Midwives must balance consistency with flexibility, tailoring care to each client's circumstances. Understanding the structure and purpose of ongoing prenatal visits allows midwives to be intentional about care planning. It's not just about showing up every two or four weeks—it's about what each visit adds to the larger picture of pregnancy.

> **Hands and Heart**
> The midwife's hands are diagnostic tools and instruments of reassurance. Touch used with skill and respect turns assessment into relationship.

Midwives must anticipate clinical needs, stay ahead of testing deadlines, and respond to emerging concerns in real time. Building continuity and trust over time means returning to the same client with deeper insight and sharper awareness at each encounter. When visits are guided by clinical insight, flexibility, and relationship, prenatal care becomes both safer and more meaningful.

Visit Frequency

The standard prenatal visit schedule follows a general rhythm based on gestational age:
- Every 4 weeks until 28 weeks
- Every 2 weeks from 28 to 36 weeks
- Every week from 36 weeks until birth

This structure supports regular surveillance of fetal growth, maternal adaptation, and early signs of complication. It also provides predictable opportunities for relationship-building and education. However, many factors may require midwives to adjust this schedule.

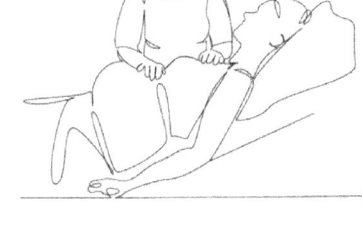

Some visits are scheduled specifically around time-sensitive testing, such as:
- **11–14 weeks:** Nuchal translucency ultrasound and early genetic screening
- **16–18 weeks:** Quad screen
- **18–22 weeks:** Anatomy scan
- **24–28 weeks:** Glucose tolerance testing, CBC, Rh screen
- **35–37 weeks:** Group B Strep culture

Referrals to specialists, such as Maternal–Fetal Medicine, nutrition counseling, or behavioral health, may also necessitate additional visits or coordination.

In addition, the client's personal needs or life circumstances may affect how care is structured. A client navigating transportation barriers, chronic conditions, or emotional stress may benefit from more frequent check-ins. Others may request fewer in-person visits with added virtual communication.

Midwives must maintain clinical vigilance while honoring the values of client-centered care. This means regularly revisiting the care plan, communicating clearly about testing timelines, and adjusting visit frequency as needed. At each visit, the midwife updates the cumulative clinical picture, reviews the plan of care, and reassesses risk and resilience.

Core Components of Each Visit

While every pregnancy and practice setting is unique, certain components form the backbone of prenatal assessment. These routine evaluations provide essential information for monitoring maternal and fetal well-being and detecting early signs of concern.

> **Clinical Integration**
> Prenatal assessment is more than measurement—it's interpretation. Midwives integrate observation, touch, and client insight to form a complete picture of pregnancy health.

Quick Reference: Every Prenatal Visit Should Include

Assessment	Key Points
Gestational age	Confirm weeks, update chart and EDD.
Weight	Track steady gain; note sudden changes (possible fluid retention or nutritional imbalance).
Blood pressure	Compare with baseline; monitor for rise ≥30 systolic or ≥15 diastolic; watch for preeclampsia symptoms.
Fundal height	Should roughly match gestational age (±2 cm after 20 weeks).
Fetal heart rate (FHR)	Normal 110–160 bpm; note rhythm and location.
Fetal movement/position	Ask about movement; palpate for lie and presentation as appropriate.
Urine dipstick	Screen for protein, glucose, ketones, and infection indicators.
Education and updates	Address discomforts, review labs/referrals, answer questions.
Documentation	Record all findings, education, and client choices clearly.

Closing the Visit

Closing the first prenatal visit is not just a formality. It is an opportunity to reinforce the care relationship, clarify the next steps, and ensure the client leaves feeling seen, supported, and informed. After completing assessments, labs, and education, the midwife should summarize the visit, provide anticipatory guidance, explain the plan for follow-up, and document clearly. A thoughtful closing creates a strong foundation for the visits that follow.

Clients often leave the first prenatal visit with a lot of new information. Taking a few extra minutes to review what was done and what to expect next helps build confidence and reduce overwhelm.

Start with a brief verbal summary: "Today we reviewed your medical and pregnancy history, completed your exams, listened to the baby, drew labs, and made a plan for your next visit." Let the client know when and why to return, and how to reach out if questions arise.

At this stage, tailor anticipatory guidance to early pregnancy. Common topics include nutrition, hydration, managing nausea, safe activities, and what symptoms warrant follow-up. Written handouts or summaries can help support retention.

If referrals are made for ultrasound, bloodwork, MFM, nutrition, behavioral health, or other services, clarify why the referral is being made and how it will be coordinated. Clients should leave knowing whether they or the clinic will make the appointment, and what to expect from that visit.

Shared decision-making continues at this point. Midwives should make space for client questions and ask, "Is there anything else on your mind today?" or "What questions do you still have?" This models collaboration and respect. The midwife may briefly reference the overall flow of prenatal care while letting the client know that the visit schedule and testing-based adjustments will be explained more fully over time.

Finally, ensure thorough and timely documentation. Chart what was discussed and done, what education was provided, what referrals were made or planned, and any follow-up instructions or agreements. If the client declined anything offered, such as labs, exams, or referrals, that should be noted clearly and without judgment.

Closing Reminders:
- Offer a brief summary of what was done at the visit
- Clarify the immediate next step and date of next visit
- Tailor anticipatory guidance to the trimester and client needs
- Clarify and document referrals and how they will be managed
- Make space for questions, emotional processing, or clarification
- Provide contact information for how to reach the clinic between visits
- Chart thoroughly, including all assessments, refusals, education, and the plan of care
- Close the visit with warmth and clarity. Example: "It was so good to meet you. We are looking forward to walking through this pregnancy with you."

The way a visit ends can shape how a client feels about the entire experience. When a midwife takes time to summarize, explain next steps, and answer questions, it reinforces trust and connection. Clear communication and documentation protect both client and provider while supporting continuity of care. Closing the visit with respect and warmth upholds the core values of relationship-centered care and lays the groundwork for the rest of the prenatal journey.

Exercise 10.8: Subsequent Prenatal Visits

Fill in blanks of the following questions:

1. The standard prenatal schedule shifts from every 2 weeks to weekly visits beginning at ____ weeks.
2. Visits scheduled to align with specific blood work or imaging are considered _____-based.
3. Flexibility in visit frequency should always be grounded in _____ and shared planning.
4. A detailed _____ of care should be updated at every visit.
5. Clients receiving care from multiple providers are participating in _____ care.

Charting and Documentation

Good charting is a cornerstone of professional midwifery practice. Accurate, timely records reflect the quality of care provided, support communication among providers, and protect both client and midwife. Whether written or electronic, clear charting ensures continuity, accountability, and trust.

> **Good Charting = Good care**
> Accurate charting is not just about compliance—it is a reflection of care. Every note tells the story of a relationship grounded in respect, skill, and accountability.

Paper and Electronic Charting

Midwives may document care using paper charts, electronic health records (EHRs), or a combination of both. When using **paper charts**, follow the format recommended by your state licensing body, professional organization, or educational program. Standardized prenatal and birth charts are available commercially, but customized layouts can create challenges when transferring records to hospitals or collaborating providers. Aligning documentation fields with local hospital or referral systems helps ensure smooth communication and prevents loss of critical information.

Electronic charting has become increasingly common in birth centers and community midwifery practices. EHR systems designed specifically for midwives—such as *Maternity Neighborhood* and *Mobile Midwife EHR*—allow for legible, time-stamped entries, secure data storage, and efficient sharing of lab results and consultation notes. These systems must be protected by strong passwords, encrypted backups, and user training to remain compliant with HIPAA and state privacy regulations.

Some midwives choose a **hybrid approach**—maintaining paper notes during home or low-resource births while entering summaries into an electronic system afterward. In emergency situations, paper documentation remains the most reliable and immediate option. Notes made in real time should later be scanned or transcribed into the permanent record to maintain continuity and legal protection.

Purpose of Charting

Charting is both a clinical and relational skill. Every note reflects the midwife's attention, accuracy, and respect for the client's story.

Charting:
- Preserves essential details and timelines of care.
- Communicates clearly between midwives and other professionals.
- Identifies trends, such as shifts in fetal growth or blood pressure.
- Provides documentation for licensing, accreditation, and quality review.
- Supports reimbursement, peer review, and research.
- Offers legal protection—complete, contemporaneous notes are the best defense in any review or inquiry.

HIPAA and Client Privacy

The Health Insurance Portability and Accountability Act (HIPAA) protects the privacy of health information for all clients. Every midwife, regardless of practice size, must follow HIPAA standards for storage, transmission, and disclosure of client data.

Key responsibilities include:
- Inform clients of their privacy rights and obtain acknowledgment.
- Use secure systems for both paper and electronic records.
- Train any staff or assistants in confidentiality practices.
- Designate one person responsible for HIPAA compliance.
- Limit access to records to those directly involved in care.

Midwives can meet these requirements through clear communication and simple, consistent systems. Always explain what information is recorded, how it is stored, and who can access it.

Charting Principles

Modern charting reflects both professionalism and compassion. Whether digital or handwritten, all entries should be:

- **Timely:** Chart as soon as possible after care is provided.
- **Accurate and objective:** Record observable facts and client statements, not interpretations or assumptions.
- **Legible and organized:** Use consistent headings and clear formats.
- **Respectful:** Avoid judgmental or speculative wording (for example, replace *"uncooperative"* with *"declined exam after discussion"*).
- **Complete:** Document assessments, education, client questions, and all instances of informed consent or refusal.
- **Secure:** Keep paper charts in locked storage and digital files password-protected.
- **Traceable:** Sign each entry with your name, credentials, and date/time.

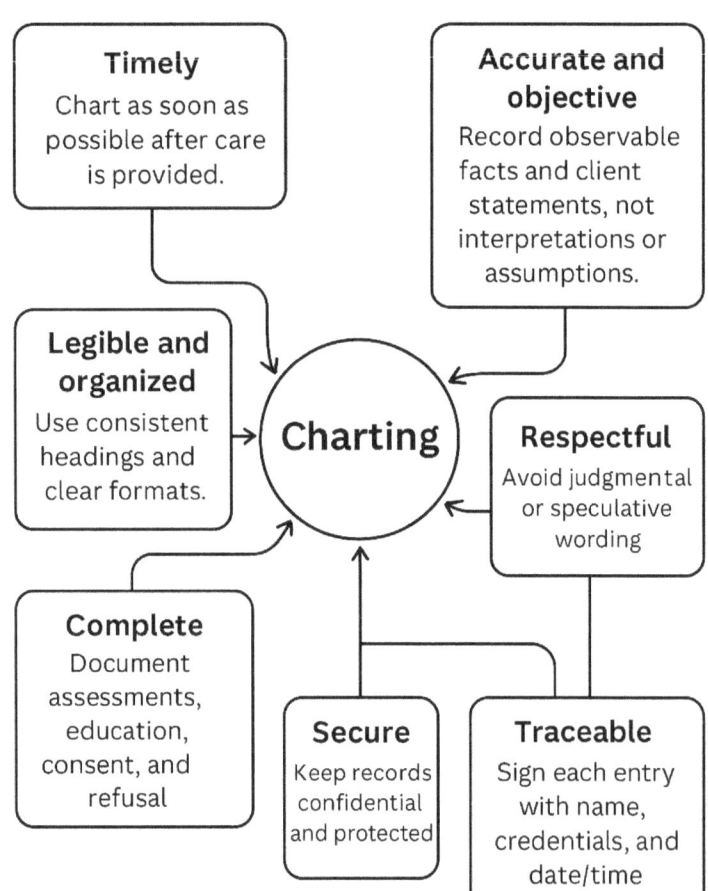

Additional documentation safeguards:
- Record relevant phone calls, emails, or electronic messages related to care or decision-making.
- Avoid copying and pasting previous notes in electronic records; update information each visit to maintain accuracy.
- If using paper charts, fill or strike through blank spaces to prevent later additions.
- When correcting an entry, draw a single line through the error (do not erase it), label it "error," add your initials and the date, and then write the correct information nearby. This ensures accuracy, accountability, and legal protection.
- For late entries, use the current date and time, explain the delay briefly, and link the note to the original event.

Documentation of Consent and Refusal

Informed consent is an ongoing process, not a single form. Chart discussions, questions, and the client's stated understanding.

When a client declines a recommendation, document:
- The information provided, including potential risks and alternatives.
- The client's stated reasoning or concerns.
- The midwife's acknowledgment of the client's autonomy.

Clear, neutral documentation protects the client's right to choose and demonstrates professional accountability.

SOAP Notes

SOAP charting organizes information in a concise, logical format used throughout health care.

S: Subjective–What the client reports (symptoms, concerns, feelings).
O: Objective–Observable findings, exam results, and lab data.
A: Assessment–Interpretation of findings or possible diagnosis.
P: Plan–Recommended actions, tests, follow-up, or referrals.

Some practices expand SOAP for ongoing care:
I: Implementation–What was done and by whom.
E: Evaluation–Client's response and effectiveness of care.
R: Reassessment–Updated findings or next steps.

Example:
S: Client reports dizziness and fatigue for five days, worsened this morning. Admits inconsistent use of prenatal vitamins.
O: BP 90/58, pulse 86, pale mucosa, Hct 32%, FHR 130 bpm.
A: Mild anemia causing orthostatic symptoms.
P: Encourage iron-rich foods, resume supplements, increase hydration, repeat CBC in two weeks, review if symptoms persist.

SBAR Communication

The SBAR format—**Situation, Background, Assessment, Recommendation**—is ideal for concise, professional communication during handoffs or hospital transfers.

S: Situation–Briefly describe what is happening now.
B: Background–Summarize relevant history and findings.
A: Assessment–State your impression or concern.
R: Recommendation–Specify what is needed or suggested next.

Using SBAR promotes clarity and consistency, especially in urgent or interprofessional settings.

Risk Management Note

Accurate documentation protects both client and midwife. Avoid judgmental or speculative language, copying previous notes, or leaving blank spaces. Record all care-related communications, including phone or electronic messages. For late entries, document the date, reason for delay, and link the note to the original event. These habits strengthen professional credibility and legal defensibility.

Exercise 10.9: Charting Variations in Care

Answer the following questions using the correct charting language and include date, time, and initials where appropriate.

1. **Late Entry Scenario:** You completed a home visit yesterday but forgot to chart your postpartum assessment until today. The client was one week postpartum, vital signs were stable, lochia normal, and breastfeeding going well. Write a short entry that documents the care provided while explaining why the note is being entered now.

Date and time of entry:
Description of care provided (from memory or notes):

Reason for delay:

Signature or initials:

2. **Correction Scenario:** While reviewing a prenatal record, you notice that you accidentally wrote "Fundal height 24 cm" instead of "34 cm" in a 34-week visit note. Write an *addendum or correction* that amends the record appropriately. Do **not** erase or overwrite the original entry:

Current date and time:
Correction statement:

Signature or initials:

3. **Refusal of Care Scenario:** At a 36-week prenatal visit, the client declines the recommended Tdap (tetanus, diphtheria, and pertussis) vaccination. She explains that she prefers to wait until after the birth. The midwife reviews the purpose of the vaccine, current recommendations, and the risks of newborn pertussis exposure. The client states she understands and still wishes to decline. Write a short documentation note that records the conversation, the client's decision, and her understanding of potential risks.

Client declined:
Reason stated:

Counseling provided:

Client response:

Follow-up plan:

Signature or initials:

Practice Guidelines and Protocols

Every midwifery practice should have written practice guidelines and protocols that describe how common clinical situations are managed. These documents support consistency, safety, and clear communication within the team. Written protocols keep midwifery practice safe, consistent, and transparent. They reflect the unique blend of skill, evidence, and accountability that defines professional midwifery care.

Having written protocols is also a key part of accountability and liability protection. They show that your practice provides care within a clearly defined, evidence-informed framework. In short:
Say what you do, and do what you say you do.

When writing protocols:
- Keep them realistic for your setting and scope of practice.
- Outline step-by-step actions, including when to consult, transfer, or refer.
- Use simple "if/then" algorithms.
- Be specific about labs, medications, or thresholds for concern.
- Review and update regularly as standards evolve.
- Document all deviations with clinical reasoning.

Protocols should always be based on:
- **Scope of practice:** what your license or certification legally allows you to do
- **Training and experience:** the skills you have been properly trained and tested in.
- **Transparency:** In short: say what you do, and do what you say you do.
- **Comfort level** with specific clinical presentations: for example, a midwife who does not attend breech births or VBACs should clearly state that in writing
- **Current best practices** and evidence: national guidelines, peer-reviewed literature, and state regulations should guide your clinical choices

These foundations help ensure that your protocols are both realistic and defensible, aligned with what you can safely and legally provide.

Why they matter:
- Promote safe, consistent care for every client
- Clarify when to consult, refer, or transfer care
- Provide legal and professional protection if care is reviewed
- Demonstrate that decisions are based on sound judgment, not personal preference
- Writing and using protocols:
- Keep them simple and action-based, using "if/then" statements
- Be specific about thresholds, labs, medications, and warning signs
- Review and update regularly as standards evolve
- Document any deviation from protocol with clear reasoning

Example Protocol: Elevated Blood Pressure

If blood pressure is ≥140/90 mmHg on two readings at least 15 minutes apart, then:

1. Have the client rest quietly for 15–20 minutes and repeat the measurement.
2. If the repeat remains ≥140/90, collect a urine sample to check for protein.
3. Assess for additional signs or symptoms (headache, visual changes, right upper quadrant pain, sudden swelling).
4. If symptoms are present, or diastolic pressure exceeds 100 mmHg, notify the collaborating provider or arrange medical consultation.
5. Document all findings, client symptoms, and communications in the chart.
6. Recheck blood pressure within 24 hours or sooner as indicated.

If readings return to normal and no symptoms are present, continue routine surveillance at each visit.

Example Protocol: Postpartum Hemorrhage (Emergency Response)

If postpartum bleeding appears excessive or estimated blood loss exceeds 500 mL for a vaginal birth, then:

1. **Call for help** and initiate emergency procedures.
2. **Massage the uterus** firmly until it is contracted.
3. **Assess tone, tissue, trauma, and thrombin** (the four Ts).
4. **Administer uterotonic medications** per standing orders or protocol (e.g., oxytocin, misoprostol, or methergine if no hypertension).
5. **Check for retained tissue** and inspect for lacerations if bleeding persists.
6. **Establish IV access** with large-bore catheter and begin fluids (normal saline or Ringer's lactate).
7. **Monitor vital signs** every 5 minutes and estimate ongoing blood loss.
8. **Notify or transfer to higher level of care** if bleeding does not subside promptly. Document all findings, interventions, medication doses, and response to treatment.

This protocol emphasizes calm, organized action and clear documentation. The midwife's ability to follow a rehearsed sequence under pressure is key to safety and effective response.

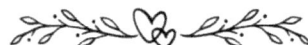

Prenatal Care Essential Takeaways

Prenatal care is the foundation of midwifery practice, a partnership that nurtures both physical and emotional well-being throughout pregnancy. Each visit offers an opportunity not only to assess the body but also to listen deeply, build trust, and strengthen confidence in the natural process of birth. Through ongoing assessment, education, and compassionate communication, the midwife supports adaptation, health, and self-knowledge.

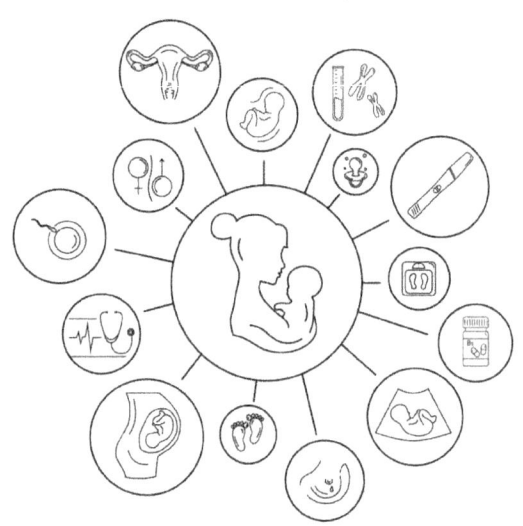

Effective prenatal care blends art and science. It includes careful attention to vital signs, fundal height, fetal growth, and fetal heart tones, yet extends beyond numbers and charts. Observation, intuition, and relationship are as essential as stethoscopes and measuring tapes. Midwives recognize that every mother carries her own story, culture, and circumstances, and that care must be individualized, flexible, and grounded in respect.

Barriers to care such as transportation, cost, discrimination, language, and systemic inequities can influence outcomes as powerfully as any physical condition. The midwife's role includes identifying these challenges and helping families navigate them with dignity and support. Collaboration, advocacy, and cultural humility are as vital as clinical expertise in ensuring safety and continuity of care.

Prenatal visits also provide time for teaching and reassurance, encouraging families to participate actively in their own care. Nutrition, rest, emotional health, and social connection are central to well-being and influence both pregnancy and postpartum recovery. By creating space for open dialogue and reflection, midwives help mothers prepare not only for birth but also for the transformation of parenthood.

The heart of prenatal care lies in presence, steady, attentive, and without judgment. Through partnership and trust, midwives safeguard the physiologic and emotional foundations of birth. In this way, prenatal care becomes more than a series of appointments; it becomes a model of compassionate, community-based health care that honors each family's strength, story, and sovereignty.

Chapter Ten: Self-Assessment

Multiple Choice
1. Which of the following testing windows typically requires a scheduled visit?
   a) 10–12 weeks for anatomy scan
   b) 35–37 weeks for glucose testing
   c) 24–28 weeks for glucose tolerance and Rh screen
   d) 30–32 weeks for GBS

2. A client receiving additional ultrasounds or specialist referrals might require:
   a) Fewer prenatal visits
   b) Earlier discharge from care
   c) Coordination of testing and visit timing
   d) All care to shift to the specialist

3. The primary reason for increasing visit frequency in the third trimester is to:
   a) Collect more urine samples
   b) Monitor fetal growth and maternal adaptation more closely
   c) Perform more pelvic exams
   d) Offer childbirth education

4. Which tool uses ultrasound waves to detect fetal heart motion?
   a) Fetoscope
   b) Doppler
   c) Pinard horn
   d) Stethoscope

5. The purpose of confirming the maternal pulse before listening for fetal heart tones is to:
   a) Determine if the fetus is breech
   b) Ensure the heart tones aren't being confused with maternal rate
   c) Estimate gestational age
   d) Rule out twins

6. Which of the following fetal heart rates would be considered within the normal range?
   a) 98 bpm
   b) 165 bpm
   c) 125 bpm
   d) 170 bpm

7. The third Leopold's maneuver helps determine:
   a) The location of the fetal back
   b) The engagement of the fetal head
   c) What part of the fetus is in the pelvis
   d) Whether fetal movement is adequate

8. Which of the following findings is most likely to require repeat urinalysis or lab follow-up?
   a) Trace ketones
   b) 1+ protein
   c) Clear urine with no odor
   d) Negative leukocytes

9. Which of the following signs may indicate concerning edema?
   a) Mild swelling in both feet at the end of the day
   b) Pitting edema only after standing for long periods
   c) Sudden swelling of one leg with calf tenderness

d) Slight puffiness in the fingers in warm weather

10. When auscultating the heart during a physical exam, the apical pulse is best heard at which location?
    a) Second intercostal space, right sternal border
    b) Midline above the umbilicus
    c) Fifth intercostal space, midclavicular line
    d) Left lower quadrant of the abdomen

11. Which statement best reflects trauma-informed pelvic exam practice?
    a) The exam is quick and not worth explaining unless there's a concern
    b) Only clients with a history of trauma require consent
    c) Offer control and options, including declining any part of the exam
    d) Assume all clients are comfortable once they've signed intake forms

12. Which of the following is part of correct blood pressure technique?
    a) Measuring over clothing
    b) Talking during the reading
    c) Supporting the arm at heart level
    d) Having the client stand during the reading

13. Which of the following might indicate orthostatic change?
    a) Blood pressure is higher when lying down
    b) SpO$_2$ rises after standing
    c) Client feels dizzy when standing and BP drops
    d) Pulse becomes slower during movement

14. The presence of 2+ protein on dipstick in the third trimester may indicate:
    a) Anemia
    b) Dehydration
    c) Hypertensive disorder
    d) Infection

15. Which of the following is an appropriate way to end a prenatal visit?
    a) "You're good to go."
    b) "We'll let you know if anything is wrong."
    c) "It was great to meet you. Please reach out if anything comes up before our next visit."
    d) "You do not need to follow up unless you feel like it."

16. What information should be included in documentation of the visit?
    a) All procedures and assessments
    b) Education given and referrals made
    c) Client questions and concerns
    d) All of the above

17. Which statement best describes the role of HIPAA in midwifery practice?
    a) HIPAA applies only to hospital-based care
    b) HIPAA ensures privacy and confidentiality of all client health information
    c) HIPAA requires verbal consent only
    d) HIPAA regulations are optional for small practices

18. Which best describes a "living document" in midwifery practice?
    a) A signed consent form
    b) A static copy of the prenatal chart
    c) A practice guideline or protocol that evolves with experience and evidence
    d) An archived patient record

19. The most reliable "test" of pelvic adequacy is:
    a) Ultrasound imaging
    b) Pelvimetry measurement
    c) Trial of labor
    d) Fetal head circumference

20. Which of the following represents a key principle of risk assessment?
    a) Risk is a label used to exclude clients from care
    b) Risk assessment is continuous and should evolve with new information
    c) Risk tools replace clinical judgment
    d) Once risk is determined, it does not change

True or False

21. _____ All prenatal clients should follow the same visit schedule regardless of testing or referrals.
22. _____ Weekly visits typically begin at 36 weeks gestation.
23. _____ The 28-week visit often includes time-sensitive lab testing.
24. _____ Flexibility in scheduling is a hallmark of client-centered midwifery care.
25. _____ Prenatal visit timing should never be adjusted based on individual risk level.
26. _____ A normal fetal heart rate falls between 110 and 160 bpm.
27. _____ Midwives should always confirm maternal pulse before listening to fetal heart tones.
28. _____ Trace protein on a dipstick may be normal in pregnancy.
29. _____ Pitting edema in both legs is always considered pathologic.
30. _____ Clients have the right to skip any question or exam during history-taking.
31. _____ A trauma history should be assumed unless clearly ruled out.
32. _____ A single elevated blood pressure reading should always be interpreted in context.
33. _____ Closing a prenatal visit warmly supports trust and continuity.

Fill in the Blank

34. The method of counting fetal heartbeats for six seconds and multiplying by ten is called the _____ method.
35. A _____ is a non-electronic tool used to listen to fetal heart tones.
36. The average number of beats per minute in the absence of changes is called the _____.
37. Leopold's maneuvers help determine fetal _____, _____, and _____.
38. The typical fetal heart rate range is _____ to _____ beats per minute.
39. The two numbers in a blood pressure reading are called _____ and _____ pressure.
40. The _____ conjugate estimates the pelvic inlet by measuring from the sacral promontory to the underside of the symphysis pubis.
41. The normal pubic arch angle is approximately _____ degrees.
42. Risk assessment in midwifery should be viewed as a _____ rather than a label.
43. Documentation should include any _____ of care, referrals, or declined services.
44. Providing _____ guidance helps clients know what is normal and what is not.
45. The midwife's written _____ and _____ outline consistent steps for common clinical situations.
46. HIPAA requires that midwives train all _____ and ensure records are stored securely.

Chapter Ten Reading & References

Recommended Reading: Prenatal Care

- American College of Nurse-Midwives. **Core Competencies for Basic Midwifery Practice** (Latest ed.). The national framework outlining essential knowledge, skills, and behaviors for midwives.
- Davis-Floyd, R., & Cheyney, M. **Birth Models That Work** (2nd ed.). Explores global maternity systems emphasizing relationship-centered and evidence-informed care.
- Frye, A. **Holistic Midwifery, Volume I: Care During Pregnancy**. Comprehensive reference on physiologic and clinical foundations of prenatal care from a midwifery perspective.
- Jordan, R. G., Farley, C. L., & Grace, K. T. **Prenatal and Postnatal Care: A Woman-Centered Approach** (2nd ed.). Integrates physiology, research, and practical application for individualized pregnancy care.
- Myles, M. F., Fraser, D. M., & Cooper, M. A. **Myles Textbook for Midwives** (17th ed.). The foundational global midwifery text offering in-depth coverage of anatomy, physiology, prenatal care, and professional practice standards.
- Pairman, S., Pincombe, J., Thorogood, C., & Tracy, S. **Midwifery: Preparation for Practice** (4th ed.). Comprehensive international text covering midwifery philosophy, prenatal care, and contemporary professional issues.
- Raynor, M. D., Marshall, J. E., & Sullivan, A. **The Midwife's Labour and Birth Handbook** (3rd ed.). A detailed guide to intrapartum and prenatal assessment skills, combining evidence-based practice with midwifery intuition.
- Simkin, P., Whalley, J., Keppler, A., Durham, J., & Bolding, A. **Pregnancy, Childbirth, and the Newborn** (6th ed.). Practical, evidence-based guide for pregnancy and birth education
- Sweet, B. R., & Oates, J. **Anatomy and Physiology for Midwives** (4th ed.). Clear explanations and visuals that link foundational science to midwifery practice.
- Varney Burst, H., et al. **Varney's Midwifery** (6th ed.). Core professional text covering the full scope of midwifery practice with detailed prenatal care chapters.
- Walsh, D., & Devane, D. **Critical Midwifery Practice: Core Concepts for Safe and Sustainable Care** (2nd ed.). Challenges conventional models of care and promotes relational, evidence-informed midwifery.

References

American College of Obstetricians and Gynecologists. (2021). *Prenatal care: Routine tests and procedures.* https://www.acog.org

Billingham, R. E., Brent, L., & Medawar, P. B. (1998). Immunological memory in pregnancy: Persistence of tolerance to paternal antigens. *The Lancet, 352*(9122), 1192–1195. https://doi.org/10.1016/S0140-6736(98)22023-X

Centers for Disease Control and Prevention. (2023). *Group B Streptococcus (GBS): Prevention and screening guidelines.* https://www.cdc.gov/groupbstrep

Centers for Disease Control and Prevention. (2023). *Prenatal testing and screening.* https://www.cdc.gov/pregnancy

Health Insurance Portability and Accountability Act of 1996, Pub. L. No. 104–191, 110 Stat. 1936.

Hesperian Foundation. (n.d.). *A book for midwives: Care for pregnancy, birth, and women's health.* Hesperian Health Guides. https://en.hesperian.org/hhg/A_Book_for_Midwives

Jordan, R. G., Farley, C. L., & Grace, K. T. (2019). *Prenatal and postnatal care: A woman-centered approach* (2nd ed.). Wiley-Blackwell.

National Center for Trauma-Informed Care. (2020). *Trauma-informed approach: Key principles and assumptions.* Substance Abuse and Mental Health Services Administration. https://www.samhsa.gov/nctic

National Institute for Health and Care Excellence. (2021). *Antenatal care for uncomplicated pregnancies* (NG201). https://www.nice.org.uk/guidance/ng201

U.S. Department of Health and Human Services. (2023). *Summary of the HIPAA Privacy Rule.* Office for Civil Rights. https://www.hhs.gov/hipaa

World Health Organization. (2016). *WHO recommendations on antenatal care for a positive pregnancy experience.* https://www.who.int/publications/i/item/9789241549912

Chapter Eleven
Labor & Birth

Objectives
After completing this chapter, the student should be able to:
1. **Explain** how "Four P's" of labor interact to influence the progress and outcome of labor.
2. **Identify** and describe the major features of the fetal skull, and explain why flexion reduces the presenting diameter.
3. **Define** fetal lie, presentation, position, attitude, station, and engagement, synclitism, and asynclitism and describe how each is assessed during labor.
4. **Describe** the anatomy of the maternal pelvis, including the pelvic inlet, midpelvis, and outlet, and summarize how pelvic shape and mobility affect fetal rotation and descent.
5. **Describe** the cardinal movements of labor and the stages and phases of labor.
6. **Recognize** normal signs that labor is beginning and differentiate common pre-labor changes from the onset of true labor.
7. **Describe** how uterine contractions develop and change, and the formation and function of the bag of waters.
8. **Summarize** the maternal physiologic responses to labor
9. **Describe** normal fetal physiologic responses to labor.
10. **Identify** reassuring fetal heart rate findings and explain when a fetal heart rate pattern becomes concerning and requires further evaluation.
11. **Describe** effective intrapartum midwifery care during the first stage, transition, and second stages of labor.
12. **Describe** step-by-step methods for a normal vaginal birth including protection of the perineum, assessment and management of a nuchal cord.
13. **Explain** the immediate newborn care after birth, and the importance of delayed cord cutting and skin-to-skin contact.
14. **Articulate** the midwife's role as protector of physiologic birth: balancing patience with vigilance, recognizing normal variation, supporting movement and coping, supporting the partner's role, and remaining prepared to respond if complications emerge.

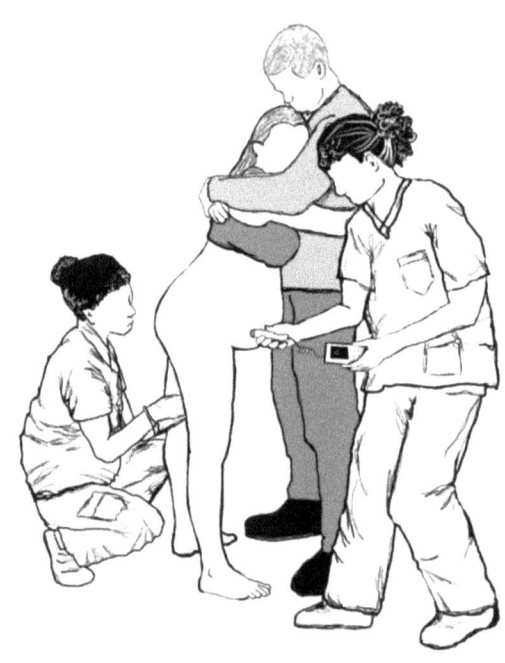

Mechanics of Normal Labor

For midwives to support birth safely and effectively, they must understand the mechanics of labor—the intricate relationship between the uterus, pelvis, and baby that allows birth to unfold. Every movement of this process reflects a precise balance between structure and physiology, a homeostatic dance in which both mother and baby play active roles.

Learning the mechanics of labor begins with studying the pelvis and the fetus's journey through it. Student midwives should spend time with a model pelvis and doll, tracing the cardinal movements and feeling how subtle shifts in position create space for descent and rotation. This tactile knowledge deepens awareness of how anatomy and movement interact, preparing the midwife to observe, assess, and respond skillfully in real time. Understanding these mechanics transforms clinical care. It enables midwives to recognize normal variations, support physiologic progress, and advocate confidently for freedom of movement during labor. By mastering the fundamentals of how the body and baby work together, the midwife becomes not only a guardian of safety but also a translator of the language of birth.

The Four P's of Labor

Labor is a finely balanced interaction between the birthing woman and her baby. While hormones and physiology create the conditions for birth, the actual progress of labor depends on how several key factors work together. These are known as the **Four P's of Labor**: the **Passenger**, **Passage**, **Powers**, and **Psyche**. Each plays a vital role: the baby and placenta (Passenger) must navigate the pelvis and soft tissues (Passage), propelled by contractions and maternal effort (Powers), within an environment that supports confidence, calm, and emotional readiness (Psyche). Understanding how these elements interact helps midwives assess labor effectively and respond with skill, patience, and trust in the process.

Four P's of Labor:

- PASSENGER: the baby, membranes, and placenta
- PASSAGE: the maternal pelvis and soft tissues
- POWERS: the uterine contractions, maternal position and pushing effort
- PSYCHE: the mother's emotional and psychological state and the birth environment

Each of these elements interacts constantly. A change in one may influence the others, either supporting smooth progress or creating challenges. Midwives observe and respond to these relationships, offering physical and emotional support to promote balance and effective labor.

PASSENGER: THE BABY

Fetal Size and Proportion: The fetal head is usually the largest and least compressible part of the body. A well-flexed head presents the smallest diameter, while extension increases the size of the presenting part. Shoulder width and overall fetal tone also influence descent. A smaller or premature baby may descend easily but rotate unpredictably, while a larger baby may require more molding or positional adjustment.

Fetal Skull: The fetal skull is made up of several bones connected by fibrous membranes, which allow flexibility during labor and birth. This flexibility lets the bones overlap slightly—a process called *molding*—which helps the head fit through the maternal pelvis.

The main bones of the fetal skull are:

A. One OCCIPITAL bone, located at the back of the head
B. Two PARIETAL bones, forming the sides of the skull
C. Two FRONTAL bones, forming the forehead

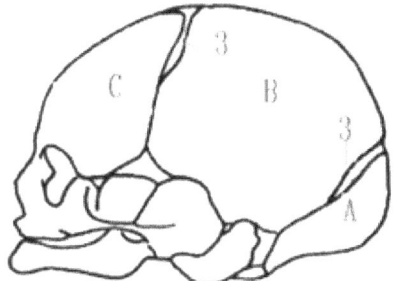

Sutures are the spaces between these bones, covered by thin membranes that permit movement:

1. FRONTAL **suture:** between the two frontal bones
2. CORONAL **suture:** between the frontal and parietal bones
3. LAMBDOID **suture:** between the occipital and parietal bones
4. SAGITTAL **suture:** between the two parietal bones, dividing the skull into left and right halves

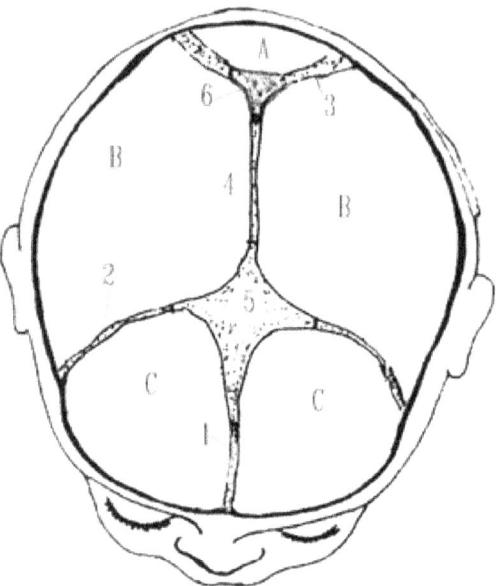

Fontanelles are wider spaces where two or more sutures meet:

5. ANTERIOR FONTANELLE **(bregma):** diamond-shaped; located at the junction of the frontal and parietal bones; closes by 18 months
6. POSTERIOR FONTANELLE **(lambda):** triangular; located where the sagittal and lambdoid sutures meet; closes by 6–8 weeks

During labor, sutures and fontanelles can be palpated during vaginal examination and used as landmarks to assess fetal position and orientation in the pelvis.

Head Molding and Caput Formation

Molding is the temporary reshaping of the fetal head caused by pressure from the uterus, cervix, and pelvic bones. During labor, the unfused cranial bones shift slightly over one another at the sutures, decreasing the presenting diameter and helping the head adapt to the pelvis.
Molding is most noticeable along the sagittal suture and resolves within one or two days after birth.
Caput succedaneum is a soft swelling of the scalp from pressure during descent. It often accompanies molding and usually disappears within 24–48 hours.

Fetal Tone and Flexion

Optimal flexion, with the chin tucked toward the chest, allows the smallest head diameter (the suboccipitobregmatic, about 9.5 cm) to present. Deflexion or extension widens the presenting diameter, often slowing progress or increasing discomfort. A flexed, relaxed baby adapts efficiently to contractions and maternal movements.

Fetal Lie and Attitude

The **fetal lie** describes the relationship between the long axis of the fetal spine and the long axis of the mother's spine. The baby's lie and attitude together determine which part of the fetus presents first and how easily the head and body can adapt to the maternal pelvis during labor.

- A **longitudinal lie**, in which the fetal spine is parallel to the mother's spine, is the most common and can result in either a **vertex (head-down)** or **breech (buttocks-down) presentation.**
- A **transverse lie**—in which the fetal spine lies across the uterus—or an **oblique lie**, at an angle, are uncommon and often indicate that the baby cannot be delivered vaginally unless the position corrects spontaneously or with an external cephalic version (ECV) at ≥36–37 weeks. Persistent transverse lie usually requires cesarean birth to prevent complications such as cord prolapse or uterine rupture.

Fetal attitude refers to the posture of the fetal head and limbs in relation to the body. A **flexed attitude**, in which the chin rests on the chest and the arms and legs are folded inward, is ideal for birth and allows the smallest possible diameters to present. An **extended attitude**, in which the head tilts backward and the limbs are stretched, increases the presenting diameter and may result in a **brow or face presentation**, which can complicate vaginal delivery.

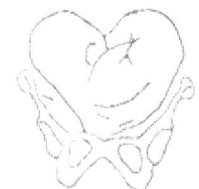

Longitudinal lie

Transverse lie

Fetal Denominator

The denominator is a specific bony landmark on the presenting part of the fetus used to describe fetal position within the maternal pelvis.
- In **vertex presentations**, the denominator is the **occiput**.
- In **brow or face presentations**, the denominator is the **chin (mentum)**.
- In **breech presentations**, the denominator is the **sacrum**.
- In **shoulder presentations**, the denominator is the **acromion process** (shoulder tip).

Understanding the denominator helps midwives accurately describe and document fetal position. For example, **Left Occiput Anterior (LOA)** means the occiput—the denominator—is directed toward the mother's left front side.

Fetal Presentation and Position

Presentation describes which part of the fetus enters the pelvic inlet first. **Position** refers to how that part is oriented within the maternal pelvis.

Midwives identify these through Leopold's maneuvers, auscultation, and vaginal examination or imaging when indicated.

Cephalic (Head-First) Presentations

Most common and favorable for vaginal birth.
- **Vertex:** head well flexed, occiput leading.
- **Occiput anterior (OA):** most favorable; head facing maternal sacrum, occiput toward symphysis. LOA most common.
- **Occiput posterior (OP):** occiput toward maternal sacrum; may cause longer labor but often rotates anteriorly.
- **Occiput transverse (OT):** occiput toward maternal hip; transitional position that may rotate spontaneously.

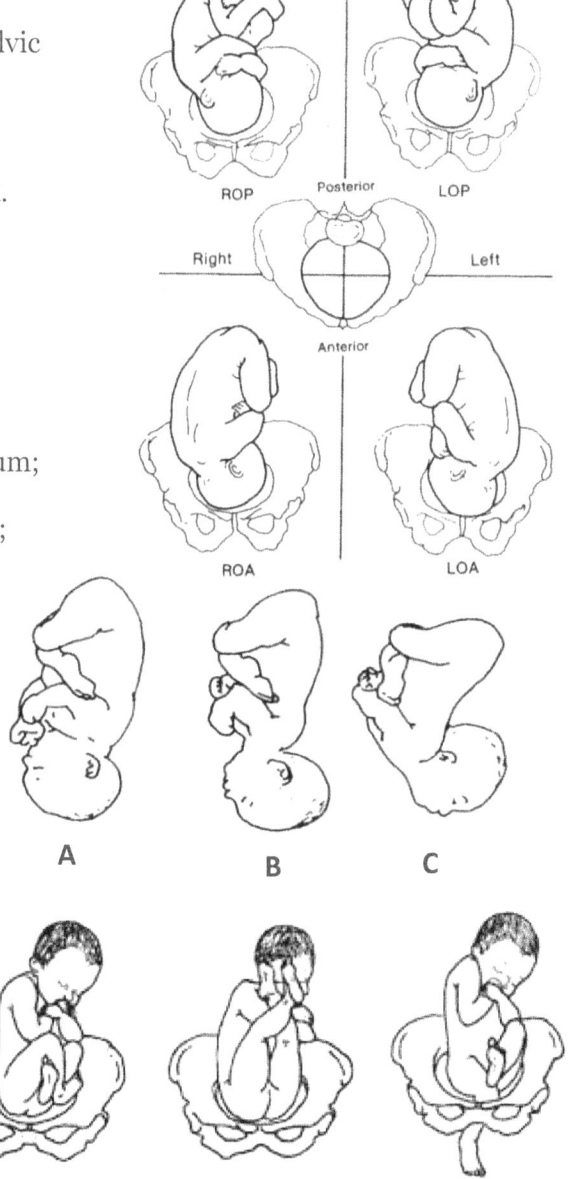

Other Cephalic Variants

A. **Military:** head neither flexed nor extended.
B. **Brow:** forehead presents; vaginal birth often not possible.
C. **Face:** head hyperextended; chin (mentum) determines position—*mentum anterior* may permit vaginal birth; *mentum posterior* usually does not.

Breech Presentations

When buttocks or feet present first (3–4% of term births).
A. **Complete breech:** hips and knees flexed, legs crossed.
B. **Frank breech:** hips flexed, knees extended, feet near head.
C. **Footling breech:** one or both feet first; more common in preterm.
There is also a very rare kneeling breech.

Positions use the **sacrum** as denominator (e.g., LSA, RSA, LSP, RSP, LST, RST).

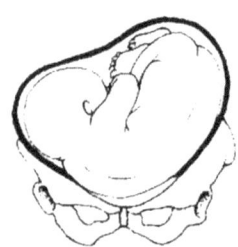

Shoulder (Transverse or Oblique) Presentation
Fetal spine lies crosswise or at an angle.
Denominator: **acromion** (shoulder tip).
Common positions: LScA, RScA, LScP, RScP.
Cannot deliver vaginally, requires correction or cesarean birth.

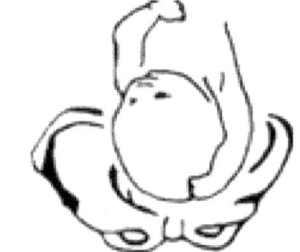

Compound Presentation
An extremity (hand/arm) descends with the presenting part. Usually transient and resolves spontaneously.

Synclitism and Asynclitism
Synclitism describes how the fetal head aligns within the maternal pelvis during descent. When the **biparietal diameter** of the fetal head is **parallel to the plane of the pelvic inlet**, both parietal eminences enter the pelvis evenly, and the sagittal suture is centered between the symphysis and sacrum. This position—**synclitic**—usually occurs when the pelvis is roomy and contractions are effective.

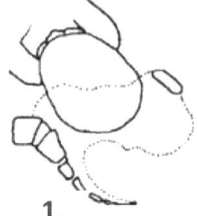

1. ASYNCLITISM occurs when the head enters the pelvis at a tilt, the parietal bones are not level, and the sagittal suture is displaced toward the front or back of the pelvis.

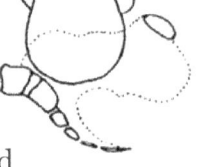

2. ANTERIOR ASYNCLITISM when the anterior parietal bone leads and the sagittal suture lies closer to the sacrum.

3. POSTERIOR ASYNCLITISM when the posterior parietal bone leads and the sagittal suture lies closer to the symphysis.

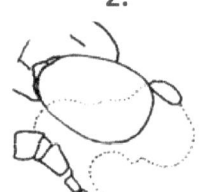

Mild asynclitism is common and can help the head engage more easily by presenting a slightly smaller diameter to the pelvic inlet. Marked asynclitism, however, may slow descent or cause uneven cervical dilation. Midwives can sometimes identify asynclitism by palpating the sagittal suture and fontanelles during a vaginal examination or by noting asymmetric molding.

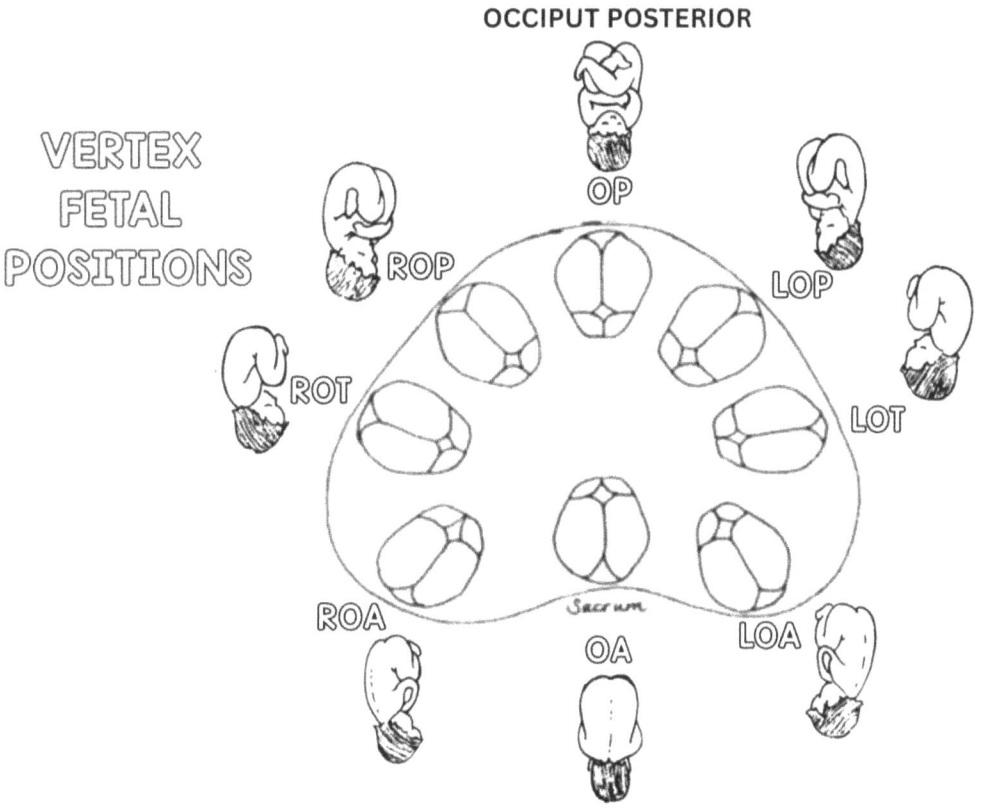

Fetal Station

Exercise 11.1: Fetal Position and Presentation
Match each term:

1. _____ LOA   A. Head flexed, occiput toward maternal sacrum; may cause longer labor or back pressure.
2. _____ ROA
3. _____ OP   B. Buttocks or feet present first; may be complete, frank, or footling.
4. _____ OT
5. _____ Breech   C. Head flexed, occiput toward maternal left front; most common and favorable.
6. _____ Face presentation
7. _____ Brow presentation   D. Head neither flexed nor extended; forehead presents.
    E. Occiput toward maternal right front; generally favorable.
    F. Head hyperextended; chin is presenting part.
    G. Occiput directed toward maternal hip; often rotates spontaneously to anterior.

Engagement

Station describes the relationship of the presenting part to the ischial spines of the maternal pelvis.
- When the presenting part is at the **level of the spines,** it is **0 station**.
- **Above the spines**: negative numbers (−1 to −5).
- **Below the spines**: positive numbers (+1 to +5).

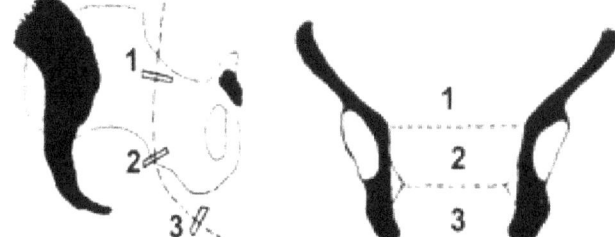

Engagement occurs when the widest diameter of the presenting part passes through the pelvic inlet.
- In a cephalic presentation, this is the **biparietal diameter**.
- In a breech, it is the **intertrochanteric diameter**.
- Engagement is sometimes called *lightening*, as the woman may feel the baby "drop," making breathing easier but increasing pelvic pressure.

A high head (−2 or above) at term may suggest disproportion or other factors affecting descent, especially in primiparas.

A. FLOATING indicates the head is not yet entering the pelvis.

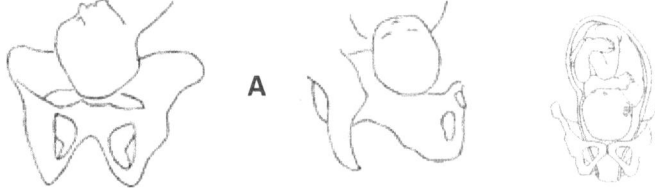

B. DIPPING means partial descent.

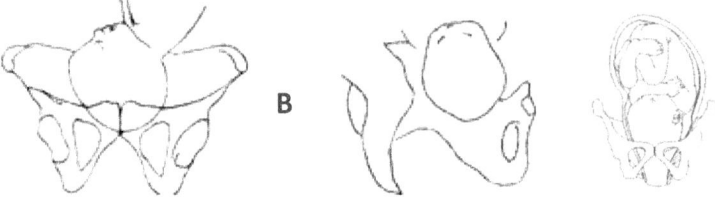

C. Fully ENGAGED means the head has reached 0 station.

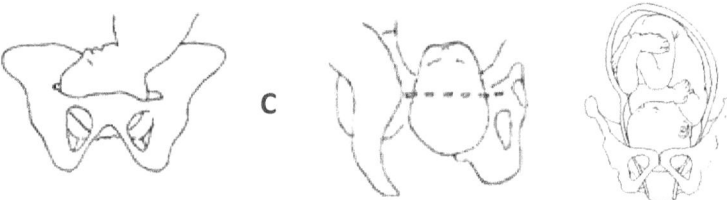

Fetal Physiologic Response to Labor

The fetus participates actively in the process of labor through a complex hormonal and circulatory response. The fetal hypothalamus and pituitary stimulate the adrenal glands to release cortisol and other hormones that prepare for birth and transition to life outside the uterus. Fetal cortisol promotes lung maturation, regulates fluid balance, and supports the production of prostaglandins and oxytocin that help coordinate uterine activity.

During contractions, temporary reductions in uterine blood flow occur as the muscle tightens and compresses the uterine vessels. This transient constriction, along with thickening of the upper uterine segment, momentarily decreases placental circulation and oxygenation. These brief reductions are well tolerated by a healthy fetus and are an expected part of normal labor physiology. Between contractions, uterine relaxation restores placental perfusion. This rhythmic alternation strengthens the fetal cardiovascular system and prepares it for independent circulation after birth.

Key fetal responses to labor include:
- Hormonal activation that promotes lung maturity and readiness for breathing after birth
- Mild, temporary shifts in oxygen and pH that stimulate adaptive cardiovascular responses
- Intermittent early decelerations of the fetal heart rate that mirror contractions and are considered normal
- Redistribution of blood flow to vital organs, ensuring protection during brief reductions in oxygenation

Mild changes in acid–base balance are expected as contractions intensify. Fetal pH may decline slightly during first stage and more rapidly in second stage but typically remains at or above 7.25. Early decelerations in fetal heart rate are usually gradual **decreases of up to about 20–30 beats per minute below baseline during contraction**, and they are typically benign and caused by increased intracranial pressure as the fetal head is compressed during descent. Decelerations in excess of 30–40 beats per minute are less characteristic of classic early decelerations and may warrant additional evaluation for other causes.

The presence of intact membranes and adequate amniotic fluid cushions the cord and distributes pressure evenly. After membrane rupture, decreased fluid volume may increase cord or head compression, making position changes or hydration support useful to optimize circulation. Together, these adaptive responses reflect the fetus's resilience and readiness for extrauterine life.

Exercise 11.2: Label the Passenger	
Label the following structures on the fetal skull diagrams:	
1. One occipital bone 2. Two parietal bones 3. Two frontal bones	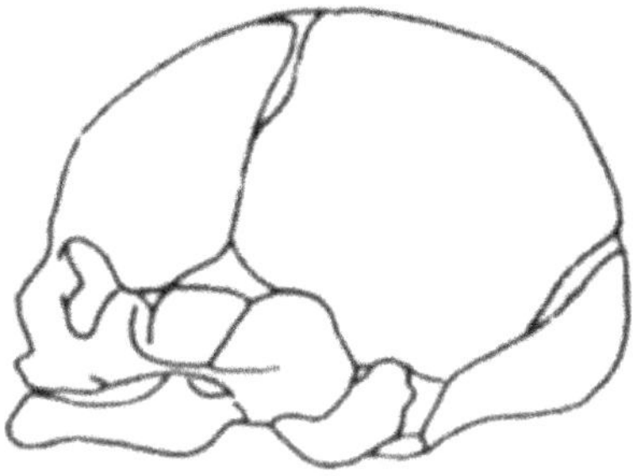
1. Frontal suture 2. Coronal suture 3. Lambdoid suture 4. Sagittal suture 5. Anterior fontanelle 6. Posterior fontanelle	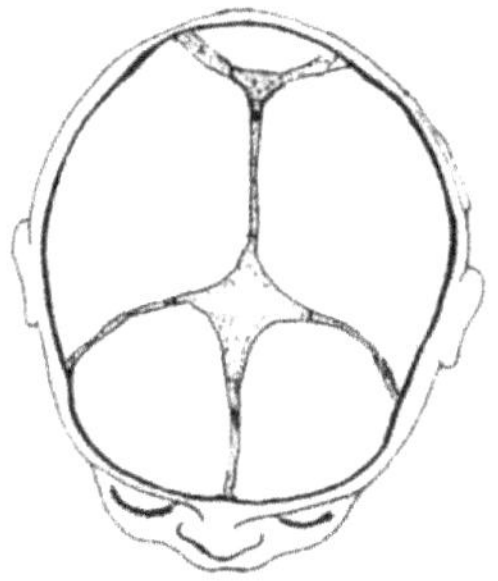

Passage: The Pelvis and Soft Tissues

The passage is formed by the bony pelvis and the surrounding soft tissues. Together, these structures create the pathway through which the fetus must navigate during birth. The pelvis provides the framework and shape, while the cervix, vagina, pelvic floor, and perineum stretch and adapt to guide fetal descent.

During labor, the maternal pelvis is not fixed but moves subtly in response to contractions and positioning. The fetal head follows a curved path through the pelvic planes, adjusting to the contours of the inlet, midpelvis, and outlet. The way these maternal and fetal structures interact determines how smoothly labor progresses. Understanding this relationship allows the midwife to support physiologic birth through positioning, movement, and reassurance.

Pelvic Types and Their Relevance

The bony pelvis forms the framework of the birth canal and is broadly classified into four types—**gynecoid, anthropoid, android,** and **platypelloid.** Each type has distinct characteristics that affect the shape and dimensions of the pelvic inlet and outlet, influencing the ease of rotation and descent during labor.

While the **gynecoid pelvis** is generally considered most favorable for vaginal birth because of its rounded, symmetric inlet, the other types may present unique challenges. In reality, few women have a "pure" type; most pelvises show mixed features. Recognizing these variations helps midwives interpret labor progress and anticipate potential complications such as cephalopelvic disproportion (CPD).

There are four primary shapes of the pelvis:

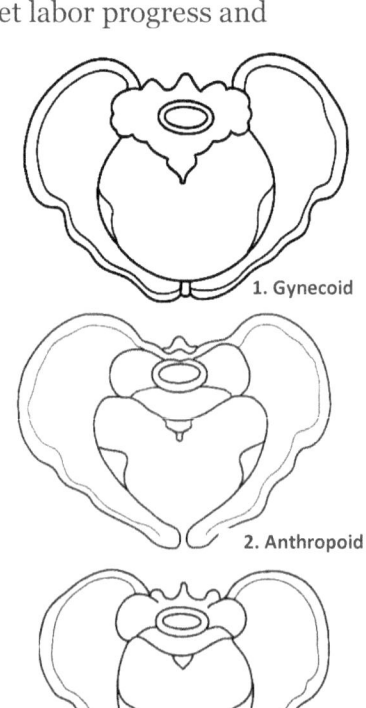

1. **GYNECOID** The most common type in women. It has a rounded, oval pelvic inlet, generous pelvic cavity, and wide pubic arch. Its balanced proportions typically allow for smooth rotation and descent of the fetal head, making it the most favorable type for childbirth.

2. **ANTHROPOID** Long and narrow, with an anteroposterior (AP) diameter greater than the transverse. This shape often encourages occiput anterior or occiput posterior positions. Though descent may take longer, the increased AP diameter provides adequate space for vaginal birth in most cases.

3. **ANDROID** Heart-shaped or triangular, resembling a typical male pelvis. It has a narrower inlet and reduced midpelvic dimensions it is associated with a higher likelihood of labor dystocia, persistent occiput posterior or transverse positions, and operative delivery.

4. **PLATYPELLOID** The least common type, characterized by a flat, wide pelvic inlet with a short AP diameter and broad transverse dimension. Engagement may be delayed until the head descends deeply and flexes well. Upright or forward-leaning positions can help optimize the inlet angle and encourage descent.

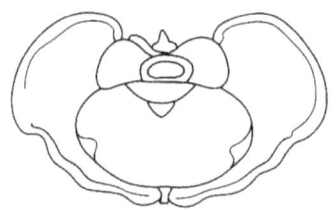

Although pelvic shape influences labor mechanics, **functional mobility and maternal positioning often compensate for anatomic variation.** Upright and asymmetrical positions can help open different pelvic diameters and create space for fetal rotation and descent.

Pelvic types rarely exist in pure form—many people have mixed characteristics. This is clinically relevant when interpreting labor progress or cephalopelvic disproportion (CPD).

Pelvic Inlet

The pelvic inlet marks the entry to the true pelvis. It is widest in the transverse diameter and slightly oval in shape. At engagement, the fetal head usually enters the inlet in a transverse or oblique orientation, with the occiput directed toward the left or right anterior quadrant of the pelvis (LOA or ROA).

Successful engagement depends on:
- The relationship between fetal head size and the pelvic inlet
- Adequate fetal flexion, which reduces the presenting diameter
- Alignment between the uterine axis and the pelvic inlet, aided by upright or forward-leaning positions

Upright positions in labor allow the maternal sacrum to move backward, widening the pelvic inlet angle and improving engagement. Supine or reclining positions tend to narrow the inlet and may hinder fetal descent.

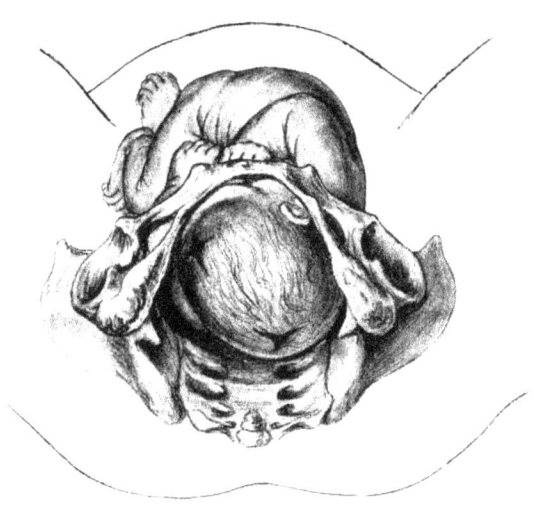

LOP Presentation

Midpelvis

The midpelvis lies between the inlet and the outlet and is the narrowest portion of the bony canal. Its boundaries include the ischial spines, lower pubic symphysis, and sacrum. Rotation of the fetal head typically occurs here, guided by the shape of the pelvis and the resistance of the pelvic floor.

- The fetal head must rotate from its transverse position at the inlet toward an anterior position to align with the outlet.
- As descent continues, fetal flexion deepens, allowing smaller diameters to present.
- The pelvic floor muscles act like a sling, directing the occiput anteriorly when tone and positioning are optimal.

Maternal mobility and asymmetrical postures, such as lunges or side-lying, can enhance these relationships and help correct delayed rotation.

Pelvic Outlet

The outlet is widest in the anteroposterior diameter, bounded by the pubic arch, ischial tuberosities, and tip of the coccyx. As the fetus descends, the fetal head extends beneath the pubic arch while the maternal sacrum moves backward to increase space by up to 2 cm.

The pelvic outlet becomes largest when:
- Upright, kneeling, or hands-and-knees positions are used
- The sacrum and coccyx are free to move, avoiding pressure against a firm surface
- The thighs are slightly apart, creating a wide pubic arch

During crowning, controlled extension of the fetal head allows gradual stretching of the perineum, reducing trauma and optimizing tissue perfusion.

Functional Mobility of the Pelvis

Although bony structures appear rigid, the maternal pelvis moves continuously during labor. Subtle adjustments occur through:
- **Nutation and counternutation:** rocking movements of the sacrum that widen either the inlet (counternutation) or the outlet (nutation)
- **Pelvic tilt and rotation:** movements that shift the uterine axis and create more room for the fetal head
- **Ligament flexibility:** the sacroiliac and pubic joints expand slightly under hormonal influence, especially in late pregnancy

Gentle asymmetry of the pelvis created through frequent movement—rocking, swaying, lunging, or alternating side-lying—helps open different pelvic diameters. These natural shifts promote balance, provide mechanical assistance to descent, and often encourage rotation when progress slows. Even when resting or using passive positions, the body should be repositioned every 3 to 5 contractions to alter pelvic mechanics and maintain flexibility in the joints and soft tissues. Regular position changes help ensure that the fetus continues to navigate through the most favorable spaces within the pelvis.

Exercise 11.3: The Dynamic Pelvis
Read each scenario and answer briefly.

A first-time mother has slow descent during active labor. The baby's head remains high at −2 station, despite good contractions. Which pelvic or positional factors might be contributing?

1. During a vaginal exam, you note the sagittal suture is closer to the sacrum and the anterior parietal bone is leading. What does this finding indicate, and how might you encourage rotation?

2. A client with a flat (platypelloid) pelvis is in early labor. What positions might help engagement and descent?

3. How could upright, asymmetrical postures improve progress in a woman with an android pelvis?

4. Why is the concept of the "living, moving pelvis" important for midwives supporting physiologic birth?

Exercise 11.4: Pelvis Types
Name and Label the Pelvic Types

_____

_____

_____

_____

POWERS: UTERINE CONTRACTIONS AND MATERNAL EFFORT

Maternal Physiologic Responses to Labor

The powers of labor are the physiologic forces that move the fetus through the pelvis and bring about birth. These forces include the involuntary contractions of the uterus—called the **primary powers**—and the voluntary bearing-down efforts of the mother—called the **secondary powers.** When these elements work in harmony, the cervix effaces and dilates, the fetus descends and rotates, and the rhythm of labor unfolds with efficiency and grace.

Labor involves whole-body adaptations that support uterine work and fetal oxygenation.

- **Cardiovascular system:** cardiac output rises by about 30 percent in first stage and up to 40 percent in second stage with pushing. Each contraction shifts 300–500 mL of blood from the uteroplacental circulation into the systemic circulation, briefly increasing blood pressure and pulse pressure.
- **Respiratory system:** oxygen consumption increases up to 40 percent in early labor and may double in second stage. Calm, paced breathing prevents hyperventilation and supports oxygen delivery.
- **Gastrointestinal system:** motility slows during labor; food eaten early may be vomited later in transition. Light nourishment and clear fluids help prevent dehydration, hypoglycemia, and ketosis.
- **Renal system:** sensation to void may diminish; a full bladder can obstruct descent or weaken contractions. Regular voiding maintains space and comfort. Trace proteinuria (+1 to +2) can occur as a normal result of muscle exertion.
- **Musculoskeletal system:** large muscle groups work continuously. Movement, hydration, and stretching reduce cramping and fatigue.
- **Endocrine and metabolic systems:** placental corticotropin-releasing hormone (CRH) triggers estrogen and prostaglandin production, enhancing myometrial contractility as progesterone declines. Cortisol and catecholamines modulate stress and energy balance; excessive stress hormones may inhibit contractions, underscoring the importance of a calm environment.

These adaptations demonstrate the mother's physiologic resilience and highlight the need for rest, hydration, and emotional safety during labor.

Hormones of Labor and the Biochemical Axis

Labor is sustained by a coordinated neuroendocrine and inflammatory cascade that activates the uterus, ripens the cervix, and synchronizes contractions. Several systems work together: the maternal brain, the fetal–placental unit, the myometrium, and local immune signaling in the decidua and cervix.

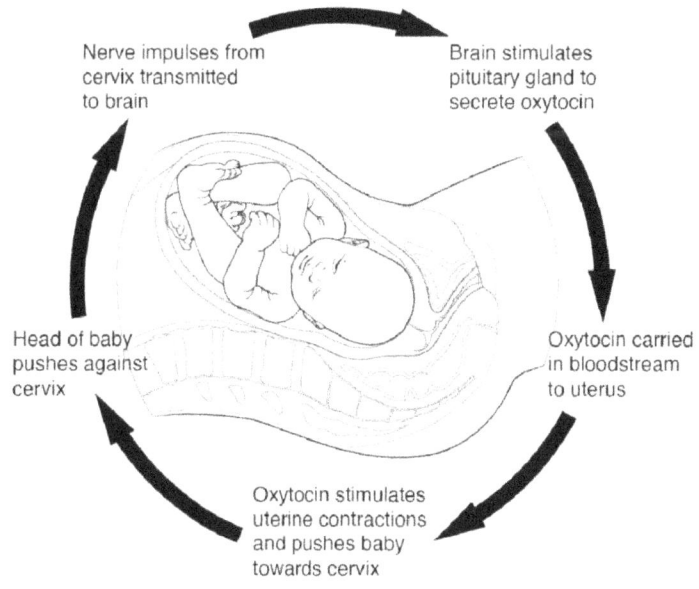

Uterine Activation in Late Pregnancy

- **Estrogen–progesterone balance:** as term approaches, functional progesterone "withdrawal" and rising estrogen activity shift the uterus from quiescence to responsiveness. Estrogen upregulates **oxytocin receptors** and **gap junctions** (notably **connexin-43**) in the myometrium, enabling coordinated, fundal-to-cervical contraction waves.
- **Placental CRH–fetal HPA axis:** placental **CRH** rises near term. The fetal hypothalamic–pituitary–adrenal axis responds with increased **cortisol**, which supports lung maturation and amplifies prostaglandin production in the membranes and decidua, promoting both contractions and cervical change.
- **Prostaglandins: PGE2** and **PGF2α** increase via COX-2 pathways in the decidua, membranes, and cervix. They enhance myometrial contractility and drive **cervical ripening** through collagen remodeling, increased water content, and leukocyte infiltration

Contraction Physiology
- **Oxytocin:** pulsatile **oxytocin** from the posterior pituitary binds upregulated uterine receptors, increasing intracellular **calcium** through membrane channels and sarcoplasmic release. Calcium binds **calmodulin** to activate **myosin light-chain kinase**, producing actin–myosin cross-bridging and contraction.
- **Synchronization:** estrogen-induced **gap junctions** electrically couple myocytes so that depolarization and calcium waves sweep from fundus to lower segment, thickening the upper uterus and thinning the lower.
- **Resting tone:** between contractions, calcium is resequestered, the uterus relaxes, and placental perfusion is restored. Adequate rest intervals protect fetal oxygenation.

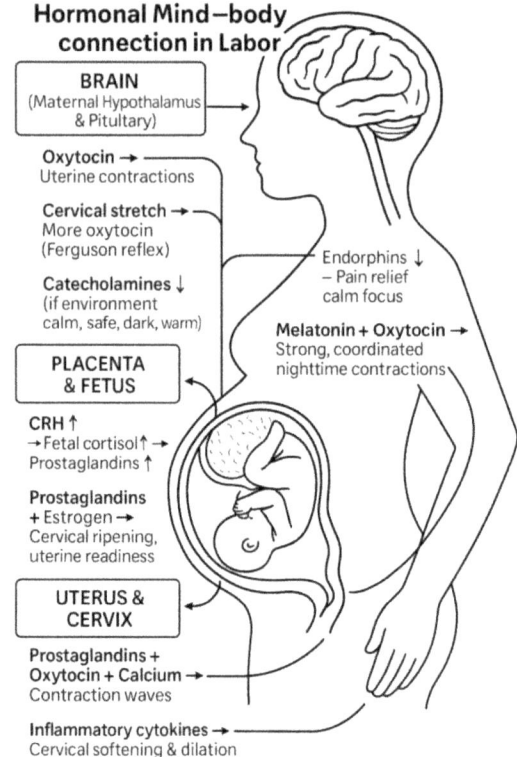

Cervical Ripening and Local Inflammation
- **Inflammatory mediators:** IL-1, IL-6, TNF-α and related cytokines upregulate COX-2 and matrix-modifying enzymes in the cervix. Collagen fibrils loosen; glycosaminoglycans and water content increase.
- **Nitric oxide and relaxin:** local **NO** and **relaxin** contribute to softening and increased compliance, complementing prostaglandin effects.

Neuroendocrine Feedback Loops
- **Ferguson reflex:** cervical and vaginal stretch receptors send signals to the hypothalamus; oxytocin release increases; stronger contractions create more stretch, reinforcing the loop. Continuous support, touch, and privacy enhance this cycle.
- **Endorphins:** rising **endorphins** modulate pain perception and support focused, rhythmic coping.
- **Catecholamines: epinephrine/norepinephrine** rise with fear, cold, bright lights, or perceived threat. Beta-adrenergic effects can relax the myometrium; peripheral vasoconstriction can reduce uterine perfusion. A calm, warm, private environment lowers catecholamines and protects uterine efficiency.
- **Circadian modulation: melatonin** can synergize with oxytocin; nighttime conditions often support more organized contraction patterns.

Fetal Contributions
- **Fetal cortisol surge:** enhances surfactant, fluid clearance, and prostaglandin synthesis.
- **Adaptive circulation:** with each contraction, transient reductions in uterine blood flow are buffered by fetal redistribution of blood to vital organs. **Early decelerations** that mirror contractions reflect normal intracranial pressure changes during descent.
- **Membranes and fluid:** intact membranes and adequate fluid reduce cord compression; after rupture, hydration and position changes help maintain placental flow.

Modulators That Stall or Support Labor
- **Supportive:** warmth, dim light, privacy, continuous presence, hydration, light nourishment, upright/forward-leaning positions, and empty bladder/rectum.
- **Disruptive:** fear, cold, bright lights/noise, unfamiliar observers, dehydration, exhaustion, supine positioning with sacral pressure, and sustained Valsalva outside the urge to push.

> **Exercise 11.5: Sequence of the Hormonal Cascade**
> *Number the following steps 1-6 in the correct order from late pregnancy to active labor.*
> _____Oxytocin from the posterior pituitary stimulates rhythmic contractions.
> _____Fetal cortisol increases, promoting prostaglandin synthesis.
> _____Estrogen rises relative to progesterone, sensitizing the uterus.
> _____Prostaglandins ripen the cervix and trigger myometrial activity.
> _____Cervical stretch activates the Ferguson reflex and additional oxytocin release.
> _____Endorphins rise to modulate pain and maintain focus.

Clinical Implications for Midwives

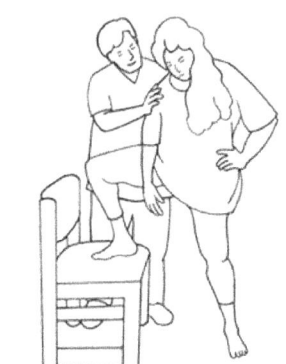

- Encourage **upright, asymmetrical movement** to align the uterine axis with the inlet, deepen flexion, and aid rotation; this may improve oxytocin efficiency and prostaglandin effect.
- Protect the **environment** to minimize catecholamine interference with oxytocin and prostaglandins.
- Monitor the **pattern**: progressive lengthening, strengthening, and shortening intervals with preserved resting tone suggests efficient hormonal coupling; loss of rest, tachysystole, or rising maternal distress may signal the need to adjust hydration, position, or environment.
- Recognize that the **living pelvis** and **responsive myometrium** are part of one system: hormonal readiness, mechanical alignment, and emotional safety work together.

Primary Power: Uterine Contractions

Uterine contractions are involuntary, rhythmic tightening of the myometrium that bring about effacement and dilation of the cervix and guide fetal descent. Each contraction has a beginning, a peak, and a gradual release, known as the **increment**, **acme**, and **decrement**. Between contractions, the uterus rests, restoring oxygen to the placenta before the next wave begins.

Healthy contractions are coordinated and progressive. They begin at the uterine fundus and move downward in a wave that thickens the upper segment while thinning the lower segment. This polarity directs pressure downward, encourages cervical change, and supports descent. Over time, contractions become longer, stronger, and closer together—signaling that labor is advancing.

Rest between contractions is essential. It allows the uterus to recover, prevents fatigue, and ensures adequate oxygen exchange for the fetus.

Secondary Power: Maternal Effort

When the cervix is fully dilated, voluntary bearing-down efforts join the uterine forces to complete birth. The **Ferguson reflex**, triggered by pressure from the fetal head on the pelvic floor, increases oxytocin release and strengthens the urge to push.

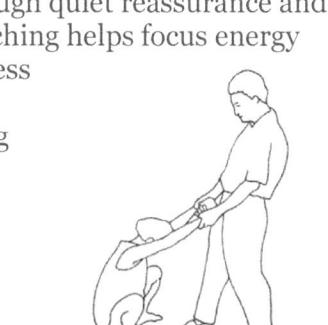

Most mothers push spontaneously with an open-glottis technique that coordinates breath and muscle effort naturally. The midwife supports this instinctive rhythm through quiet reassurance and observation. Sometimes, especially in first births, gentle coaching helps focus energy when the baby needs to move under the pubic bone or progress has slowed. Directed pushing should be brief, timed with contractions, and always balanced by rest and deep breathing between efforts. The goal is never to override instinct but to channel power effectively when anatomy, energy, or position require support.

Exercise 11.6: Matching — Contraction and Pushing Concepts		
Match each term with its correct description.		
1. ___Primary powers	A. Coordinated waves of involuntary uterine contractions
2. ___Secondary powers	B. Hormone that stimulates uterine contractions and bonding
3. ___Resting tone	C. Voluntary maternal bearing-down effort
4. ___Ferguson reflex	D. Pressure from fetal head triggers oxytocin release
5. ___Oxytocin	E. Period of uterine relaxation that restores oxygen exchange
6. ___Increment	F. Beginning of a contraction as intensity rises
7. ___Acme	G. Peak of contraction strength
8. ___Decrement	H. Gradual easing of contraction intensity

PSYCHE: EMOTIONAL AND ENVIRONMENTAL FACTORS IN LABOR

The psyche of the laboring individual profoundly influences the course of labor. Emotional state, sense of safety, past experiences, and the surrounding environment all interact with the hormonal systems that regulate uterine activity. Labor unfolds most efficiently when the person giving birth feels safe, supported, and respected. Anxiety, fear, or unresolved trauma can inhibit oxytocin release, increase stress hormones, and disrupt the rhythm of labor.

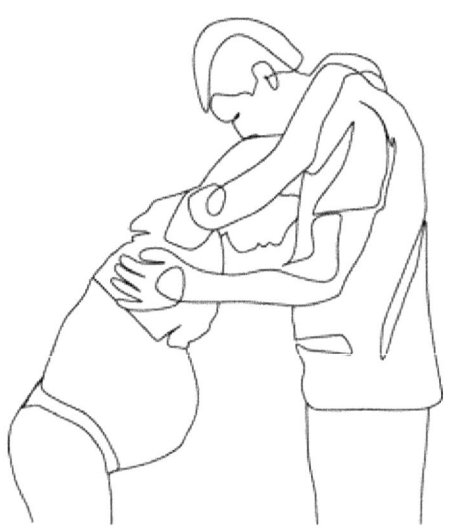

The mind and body are inseparable in the birth process. The same hormones that cause contractions also govern trust, connection, and relaxation. Understanding this interplay helps the midwife create conditions in which the physiologic process of birth can progress smoothly and with minimal intervention.

Midwives understand that labor is a dynamic interaction among the passenger, passage, powers, and psyche. Each birth reflects a unique combination of anatomy, physiology, and emotion. The role of the midwife is not to control this process but to protect the physical, emotional, and environmental conditions that allow it to unfold safely and with respect for the body's innate intelligence. Through presence, patience, and trust, the midwife supports the hormonal balance that guides labor and helps each individual find strength, focus, and resilience on the path to birth.

> **Neuroscience of Trust in Birth**
> Recent research in perinatal neuroscience shows that oxytocin not only drives uterine contractions but also promotes trust and reduces fear responses in the brain. This dual action links emotional safety directly to labor efficiency. When midwives foster connection and reassurance, they activate the same neurobiological pathways that make contractions strong and coordinated.

The Hormonal Landscape of Labor

Oxytocin strengthens contractions while also fostering calm, bonding, and focus. Its release depends on a sense of safety and emotional connection. Endorphins rise alongside oxytocin, creating a trance-like state that helps the individual cope with pain and enter the instinctive rhythm of birth.

As labor deepens, many experience an altered state of consciousness. Brain activity shifts from predominantly beta-wave patterns, associated with alert and analytical thinking, to slower alpha and theta waves linked to intuition, rhythm, and inward focus. This neurologic shift allows the laboring brain to move into an instinctive state where time perception fades and attention centers on bodily sensation and breath.

This altered state is normal and should be protected. French physician Michel Odent described how all mammals share a need for privacy, safety, and protection from observation during birth. When mammals—including humans—are disturbed by bright light, cold, noise, or the sense of being watched, the neocortex becomes stimulated, catecholamine levels rise, and labor can slow or stop. Conversely, a warm, dim, private, and quiet environment suppresses neocortical activity and allows the primitive brain to guide the process through oxytocin release and parasympathetic dominance.

Odent's research reminds midwives that effective labor is not achieved through control but through protection of the physiologic conditions that allow the body and brain to work together. Adrenaline and noradrenaline, the catecholamines of stress, can interfere with this process. When fear or overstimulation triggers a fight-or-flight response, blood flow is redirected away from the uterus, contractions may slow, and dilation can stall. This response once protected birthing mammals by pausing labor in unsafe settings. In modern contexts, bright lights, loud voices, and frequent interruptions can cause the same physiologic reaction.

A calm, private, and emotionally safe environment allows oxytocin, endorphins, and parasympathetic balance to work harmoniously. When these systems are in equilibrium, labor typically progresses with efficiency, focus, and resilience. These conditions are not always achievable in low-resource or high-volume birth settings. Importantly, safe and effective labor can still occur without ideal environmental control when respectful care, emotional support, and basic comfort measures are provided.

The Role of Safety and Trust

Safety is both physical and emotional. The presence of familiar, trusted attendants reduces anxiety and supports hormonal flow. Clear communication and respectful consent build trust and empower the individual to participate fully in decisions about their body and care.

Midwives who move quietly, speak softly, and maintain presence without intrusion help sustain the calm and rhythm of labor. This approach is especially important for individuals with a history of trauma, who may experience heightened sensitivity to touch, tone, or environment. Trauma-informed midwifery care acknowledges the potential for emotional triggers during labor and prioritizes safety, consent, and control at every step.

Fear and tension can slow or even stop labor. Education, counseling, and preparation are tools the midwife uses to help women overcome fear and enter labor with confidence. Prenatal education, childbirth classes, reading, and peer discussions can all help parents develop realistic expectations and a sense of readiness. When parents are informed and supported, they can make choices aligned with their values, leading to a more satisfying and empowering birth experience.

The Birth Environment

The setting of labor has a measurable effect on its progress. Environments that protect privacy and minimize unnecessary stimulation support physiologic labor. Odent's research on mammalian birth behavior emphasizes that undisturbed, dark, and warm spaces are essential for the release of oxytocin and endorphins. Privacy, quiet, and a sense of being unobserved allow the neocortex to rest and the primitive brain to lead.

Dim lighting, warmth, limited staff changes, and continuous familiar support enhance feelings of safety and hormonal flow. Midwives can advocate for small but meaningful environmental adjustments such as lowering voices, softening light, or reducing unnecessary conversation during contractions. Each of these actions helps maintain the delicate hormonal equilibrium required for efficient labor.

When labor occurs in a clinical or high-stimulus environment, the midwife's role is to buffer external stressors and preserve a sense of privacy and calm. Reassurance, gentle touch, and steady presence can offset overstimulation and help maintain the natural physiology of birth.

When the environment feels safe and the individual in labor feels seen, heard, and respected, oxytocin and endorphins flow freely. Labor becomes not only a physical process but an emotional and spiritual journey toward birth and new life. The steady, grounded presence of the midwife supports this transformation and protects the innate physiology of birth.

> **Protecting the Space for Birth**
>
> Birth unfolds best in spaces that honor safety, rhythm, and privacy. Soft voices, dim light, steady presence, and gentle touch help the laboring person remain in an instinctive state, guided by the body's natural wisdom.
>
> Each act of protection—closing a door, lowering a light, or offering reassurance—strengthens the hormonal feedback loops that sustain labor. When the space feels safe, the body feels free to open.

Mechanism of Labor

The mechanism of labor, also known as the **cardinal movements of labor** describes the series of movements and positional adjustments the baby makes to navigate through the birth canal. These movements allow the presenting part, usually the head, to adapt to the shape of the maternal pelvis. The process begins with engagement and continues through the birth of the body. Although each baby's path is unique, the sequence is remarkably consistent in a vertex presentation. They occur most predictably when the baby is in a left occiput anterior (LOA) position, which is the most common and favorable orientation for vaginal birth.

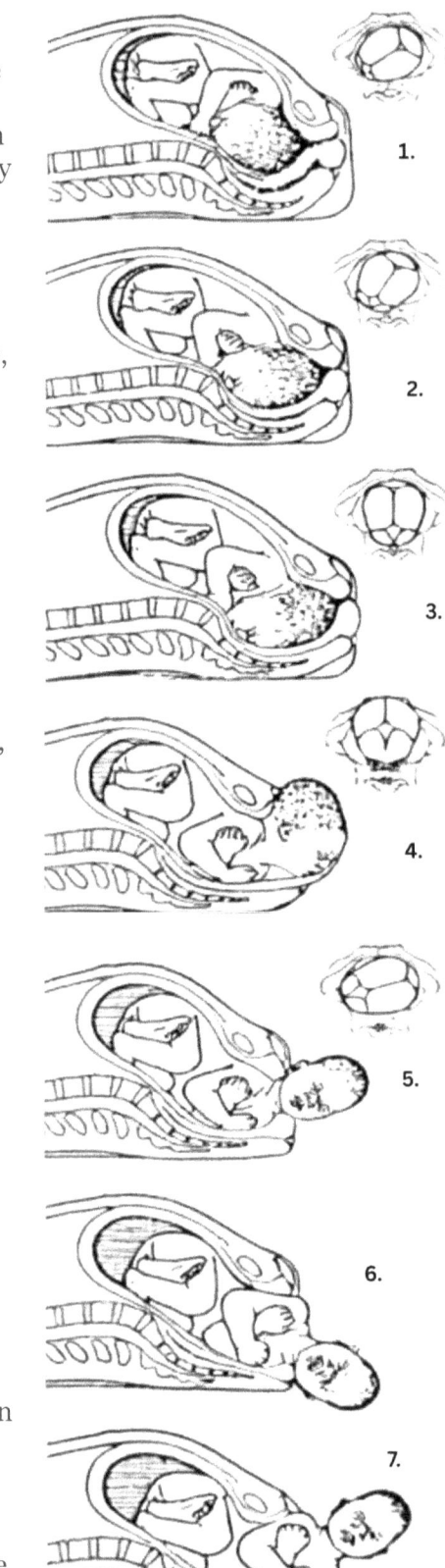

1. ENGAGEMENT occurs when the widest part of the fetal head, the **biparietal iameter**, passes through the pelvic inlet and settles into the true pelvis. In primiparas, this often happens before labor begins; in multiparas, it may occur later or even during labor.

2. DESCENT continues throughout labor as the baby moves deeper into the pelvis. *It results from:*
- Downward pressure from uterine contractions
- Maternal bearing-down efforts during second stage
- The influence of gravity and upright positioning

Progressive descent occurs in coordination with cervical dilation and thinning of the lower uterine segment.

3. FLEXION occurs as the fetal head meets resistance from the cervix, pelvic walls, and pelvic floor. The chin tucks toward the chest, reducing the presenting diameter.
- Proper flexion decreases the head's diameter by about one centimeter.
- Complete flexion usually develops at the pelvic inlet but may occur earlier or later.

A well-flexed head presents the smallest possible dimension—the **suboccipitobregmatic diameter**—for passage through the pelvis.

4. INTERNAL ROTATION: As the head descends, it typically enters the pelvis in a transverse or slightly oblique position. When it meets the pelvic floor, resistance guides the occiput to rotate anteriorly.
- In an LOA position, the occiput rotates toward the symphysis pubis.
- In posterior positions (ROP or LOP), rotation may take longer or remain incomplete.

This movement aligns the long axis of the fetal head with the anteroposterior diameter of the pelvic outlet.

5. EXTENSION: After the occiput clears the pubic arch, the head extends so the face and chin sweep over the perineum. The occiput, brow, face, and chin appear in sequence, a process known as **crowning**. Extension allows the head to be born gradually and in control.

6. EXTERNAL ROTATION: (Restitution) Once the head is born, it briefly turns to one side to realign with the shoulders—this is restitution. At the same time, the shoulders rotate internally into the oblique diameter of the pelvis.
- In an LOA presentation, the head typically turns to the left.
- The anterior shoulder emerges first, followed by the posterior shoulder and body.

7. EXPULSION: After the shoulders are delivered, the rest of the body follows smoothly as the curve of the sacrum guides the baby outward.

Physiology of Labor

Labor is a coordinated physiologic process that unfolds uniquely for each mother. It begins when maternal, fetal, hormonal, and emotional factors align to activate uterine contractions and cervical change. Signals from the baby—such as lung maturity and hormonal messengers in the amniotic fluid—help initiate labor, while shifts in maternal hormone balance increase uterine sensitivity to oxytocin and prostaglandins. Understanding the integrated function of the uterus, cervix, pelvis, and fetal head allows midwives to support labor with patience and precision.

Stages of Labor

Labor is divided into three main stages, each with a distinct physiologic focus:

1. **FIRST STAGE (Dilation Stage):** Begins with the onset of regular contractions and ends with full cervical dilation at 10 cm.
   It includes three phases:
   - *Latent Phase:* mild, irregular contractions efface the cervix but cause slow dilation.
   - *Active Phase:* the cervix dilates from approximately 5-6 cm, with stronger contractions and steady fetal descent.
   - *Transition:* the final phase (8–10 cm), marked by powerful, closely spaced contractions and intense focus.

2. **SECOND STAGE (Expulsive Stage):** begins with full dilation and ends with the birth of the baby. It includes both passive descent and active pushing.

3. **THIRD STAGE (Placental Stage):** begins with the birth of the baby and ends with delivery of the placenta.
   A Fourth Stage (Immediate Postpartum) is also identified: covers the first one to four hours after birth, when maternal and neonatal stabilization and bonding occur.

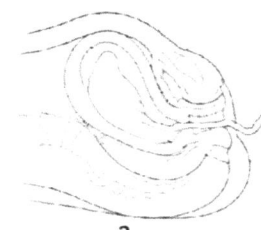

1.

2.

3.

4th Stage Immediate Postpartum

Before Labor Begins

In the days or weeks before labor, the body begins preparing through physical and hormonal changes that may occur gradually or suddenly. Recognizing these signs helps distinguish normal pre-labor adaptations from active labor.

Common experiences include:
1. **Engagement or "lightening"**—often two to three weeks before term in primiparas, though anytime for multiparas.
2. **Increased vaginal discharge** due to rising estrogen; burning or itching should be evaluated.
3. **Cervical softening and effacement**, with early dilation possible in multiparas.
4. **Persistent backache** or pelvic pressure.
5. **More noticeable Braxton Hicks contractions** as labor approaches.
6. **Loss of the mucus plug or "bloody show"**, which may appear days or weeks beforehand.

Exercise 11.7: Stages and Phases of Labor
Fill in the Blank:
1. The _____ stage begins with regular contractions and ends with full cervical dilation.
2. The _____ stage begins with full dilation and ends with the birth of the baby.
3. The _____ stage involves delivery of the placenta.
4. The _____ phase is marked by strong, regular contractions and steady dilation.
5. The _____ phase is the most intense, lasting from about 8 to 10 cm dilation.
6. The _____ phase of the first stage includes mild, irregular contractions and cervical effacement.

Biochemistry of Labor Onset

Labor begins when maternal and fetal signals align.
- **Fetal signals:** maturing fetal lungs release proteins into the amniotic fluid that increase uterine readiness and inflammatory signaling. Rising fetal cortisol and placental corticotropin-releasing hormone contribute to timing.
- **Maternal hormones:** estrogen rises relative to progesterone, increasing uterine sensitivity. Oxytocin receptor density and gap junctions in the myometrium increase, allowing contractions to synchronize.
- **Prostaglandins and cytokines:** produced by the decidua, membranes, and cervix, these promote uterine contractions and cervical ripening.
- **Emotional and environmental factors:** a sense of safety, privacy, and continuous support allows oxytocin and endorphins to flow. High stress or fear elevates catecholamines, which can slow progress.

Triggers and Onset of Labor

The exact mechanism initiating labor is not fully understood, though several factors contribute:

1. **Uterine distention**: stretching may trigger uterine nerve endings.
2. **Hormonal shifts**: progesterone withdrawal, estrogen and prostaglandin rise, and fetal cortisol changes.
3. **Fetal pressure**: stimulation of cervical nerves by the presenting part.
4. **Sexual activity**: oxytocin from orgasm and prostaglandins in semen may aid cervical ripening.
5. **Physical stress**: illness or emotional stress can trigger labor.
6. **Gastrointestinal stimulation**: bowel activity or laxatives may increase uterine tone.

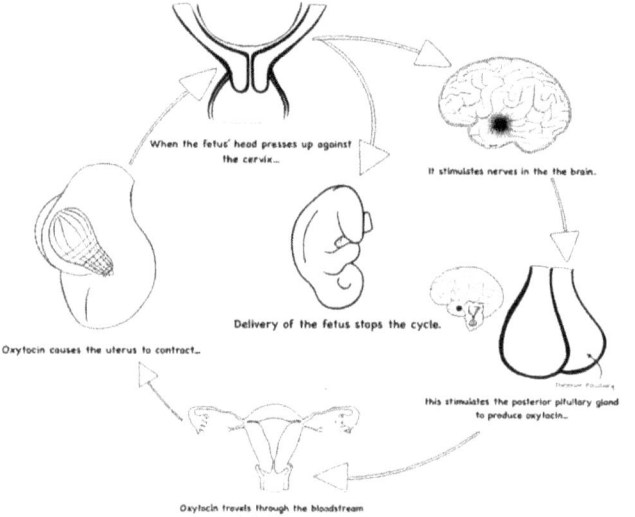

Together, these influences increase uterine responsiveness and promote the first coordinated contractions that define labor onset.

Prodromal Labor

Prodromal labor refers to contractions and other signs of labor that are present but not yet causing regular cervical change. This stage may last hours or days, helping position the baby and soften the cervix. It can also be tiring or discouraging. Supportive care includes rest, hydration, warm baths, massage, and reassurance. Reassure clients that all pre-labor contractions are productive, helping the cervix ripen and the baby descend.

Differentiating Prodromal and Active Labor

It can be difficult to tell when prodromal labor becomes true latent labor or when the latent phase turns active. Prodromal labor, sometimes called false labor, can go on and off for weeks, causing frustration and uncertainty to the mother and family.

Prodromal Labor	Active Labor
Contractions are irregular.	Contractions are regular.
Contractions remain the same intensity.	Contractions grow stronger and longer.
Walking slows or stops contractions.	Walking or movement increases intensity.
Contractions remain spaced apart.	Contractions get closer together.
Pain begins in the front and may radiate to the back.	Pain begins in the back and moves to the front.
Head is ballotable between contractions.	Fetal head remains fixed between contractions.
Contractions stop with rest or sleep.	Sleep or sedation does not stop contractions.
Cervix shows no change.	Cervix effaces and dilates.
No change in station.	Descent occurs or station changes.

Supporting the Onset of Labor

As pregnancy reaches term, many mothers look for gentle ways to encourage labor to begin naturally. Midwives can help clients distinguish between supportive traditions and riskier or ineffective methods. The goal is to encourage the body's physiologic readiness—not to force labor before it is time. These methods should not be used prior to forty weeks.

When to Consider Induction

Although most pregnancies continue safely until labor begins on their own, post-dates pregnancies (beyond forty-two weeks) carry increased risks of complications such as placental insufficiency, meconium aspiration, and decreased amniotic fluid. Babies who remain significantly post-dates are at higher risk for stillbirth and distress during labor.

For this reason, significantly post-dates pregnancies are at risk for out-of-hospital delivery. When the pregnancy extends beyond forty-one weeks, careful monitoring, including fetal movement, non-stress testing, or biophysical profiles may be recommended. If concerns arise, induction or hospital-based care should be discussed.

Castor Oil

Castor oil has long been used to stimulate contractions by increasing bowel activity, which may in turn activate uterine response. Research findings are mixed: some studies show a greater likelihood of labor onset within twenty-four hours, while others report nausea, cramping, or dehydration. Many midwives take a cautious approach, using it only when the cervix is ripe, the pregnancy is full term, and the client provides informed consent.

Herbs

Some midwives recommend herbs such as blue or black cohosh or motherwort, used either in the final week or just before labor. While there is little scientific evidence confirming their effectiveness, generations of traditional midwives have relied on these herbs.

Sexual Activity

Sex is one of the most natural ways to encourage labor. **Semen contains prostaglandins**, which can help soften the cervix, and orgasm releases oxytocin, the same hormone that drives contractions. Both partners should be comfortable, and intercourse is contraindicated if membranes have ruptured or there are concerns such as placenta previa or preterm labor. Midwives may explain that prostaglandins in semen work whether absorbed vaginally or orally, in a way that is respectful with cultural and personal sensitivity. Comfort, consent, and emotional readiness are always paramount.

Food as Medicine: Dates in Late Pregnancy

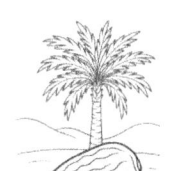

Recent research confirms that eating dates (*Phoenix dactylifera*) during the final weeks of pregnancy may promote cervical ripening, spontaneous labor, and shorter first-stage duration.
- Women who ate about six dates daily from thirty-six weeks onward were more likely to go into spontaneous labor and had more favorable cervical ripening.
- Those who ate dates tended to have a shorter first stage of labor and fewer medical interventions.
- Dates provide natural sugars, fiber, and potassium—offering sustained energy and nutrients that may support endurance during labor.

Suggested Use: Eat approximately six dates per day starting around thirty-six to thirty-seven weeks of pregnancy, continuing until labor begins. Dates can be eaten plain, chopped into oatmeal, or blended into smoothies.

Clinical Tip for Midwives

When clients ask about "natural induction," gentle options such as dates, rest, hydration, and intimacy can be discussed as part of physiologic readiness. Avoid harsh or extreme methods unless clearly indicated and supervised.

LENGTH OF LABOR

The length of labor varies greatly from one individual to another. Many factors influence its duration, including parity, fetal size and position, pelvic dimensions, cervical readiness, and the emotional and physical condition of the mother. Supportive environment, hydration, and freedom of movement can also affect the pace and comfort of labor.

Average labor times serve as general guidelines rather than strict limits. Current evidence suggests that the active phase of labor typically begins around five to six centimeters of dilation, rather than four as previously thought. Latent phase can vary widely; prolonged latent labor is not necessarily abnormal.

Typical ranges include:
- **Latent phase:** 6–20 hours for first labors; 4–14 hours for subsequent labors
- **Active phase:** starting at five to six cm, progresses at approximately 1 cm per hour in nulliparas and somewhat faster in multiparas
- **Second stage:** 1–2 hours for nulliparas; about 1 hour for multiparas, can be longer if mother and fetus is stable
- **Third stage:** Usually completed within 30 minutes

Multiparas who experience longer latent phases may progress quickly through the active phase, while nulliparas may take longer without indication of abnormality. Both slower and faster labors can still fall within the normal physiologic range.

A labor lasting less than three hours for nulliparas or two hours for multiparas may be considered **precipitous**. **Prolonged** or protracted labor refers to minimal cervical or fetal descent progress despite adequate contractions. When this occurs, midwives assess contributing factors such as fetal position, hydration, fatigue, or emotional stress before considering medical intervention.

Modern midwifery emphasizes physiologic variation, nourishment, and emotional safety as essential to supporting effective, healthy labor progress.

Progress and Patterns

Progress in labor involves more than cervical dilation. It reflects the dynamic interplay of uterine strength, fetal position, emotional state, and maternal adaptation. Midwives look for *patterns of change*, not fixed intervals or arbitrary time limits.

Signs of progress may include:
- Increasing contraction strength, duration, or frequency
- Bloody show or release of the mucus plug
- A shift in behavior, vocal tone, or focus
- Sensations of pelvic pressure or an urge to bear down
- Fetal descent or rotation by palpation or vaginal examination

Each labor follows its own rhythm. Modern understanding recognizes a wide range of normal variation, and effective midwifery care means supporting physiologic progress without pathologizing natural differences.

Exercise 11.8: Hormonal Cascade of Labor	
Match each hormone with its primary action during labor	
1. Oxytocin	**A.** Softens cervix and stimulates contractions
2. Prostaglandins	**B.** Increases pain tolerance and promotes calm focus
3. Estrogen	**C.** Signals readiness for birth; enhances prostaglandin production
4. Progesterone	**D.** Increases uterine receptor sensitivity to oxytocin
5. Cortisol	**E.** Relaxes uterus during pregnancy; decreases toward labor
6. Catecholamines	**F.** Inhibits contractions when stress or fear is high
7. Endorphins	**G.** Stimulates contractions; released in a feedback loop with cervical pressure

FIRST STAGE PHYSIOLOGY

The first stage of labor represents a complex and beautifully coordinated series of physiologic changes within the uterus, cervix, and fetal environment. These changes work together to open the cervix, thin the lower uterine segment, and gradually move the baby downward. Although the process unfolds differently for each individual, several mechanisms occur in every normal labor.

Contraction and Retraction of the Uterine Muscle

Uterine contractions are coordinated by the nervous system and influenced by hormonal signals such as oxytocin, prostaglandins, and estrogen. Contractions generally begin about every 15 to 20 minutes and gradually increase in frequency, strength, and duration as labor progresses.

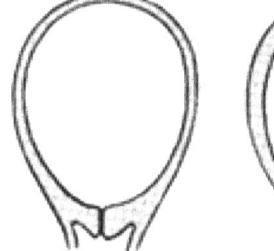
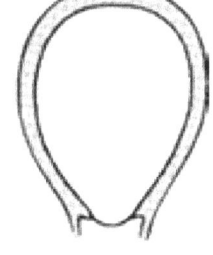

Each contraction follows a three-part rhythm:
- **Increment**—the buildup of intensity
- **Acme**—the peak of the contraction
- **Decrement**—the gradual relaxation phase

Between contractions, the uterus never fully relaxes. Some muscle fibers remain slightly shortened—a process called **retraction**. Over time, retraction causes the **upper uterine segment** to become shorter and thicker, while the **lower segment** becomes thinner and more pliable. This structural change helps draw the cervix upward and provides the force needed for fetal descent.

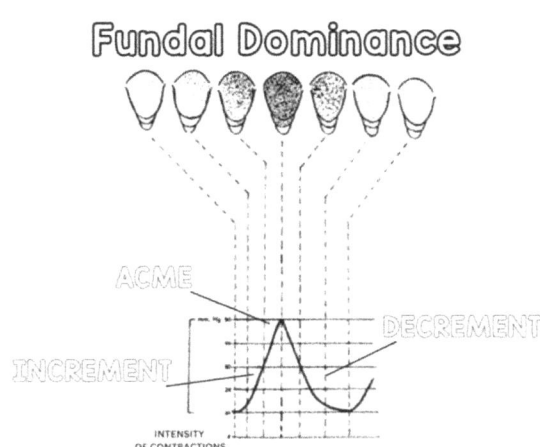

Fundal Dominance

Contractions begin at the top of the uterus and spread downward, a pattern known as **fundal dominance**. The upper segment generates the greatest power, while the lower segment accommodates the descending baby. Fundal dominance peaks at the **acme** of each contraction and ensures smooth, downward pressure that advances labor and assists cervical dilation. When fundal dominance is disrupted, as can occur with uterine overdistention or abnormal fetal position, contractions may become less effective.

Formation of the Upper and Lower Uterine Segments

As the uterus works, it divides into two functional parts:
- The **upper segment**, composed of retracted muscle fibers, becomes thick and contractile.
- The **lower segment**, composed of stretched fibers, becomes thin and passive.

Together, these create a piston-like action that directs the baby toward the cervix.

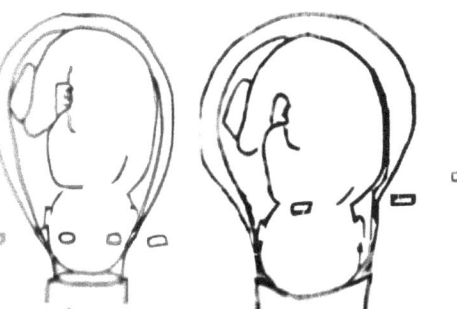
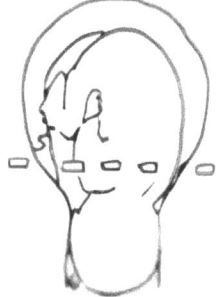
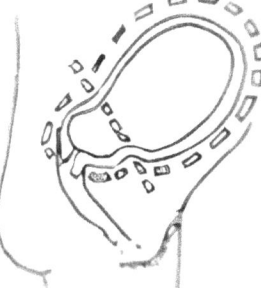

In early labor the retraction ring is barely visible | Force of the contraction is in the upper segment | Thinning of the lower segment | Formation of the retraction ring

The dividing ridge between these two areas is called the **physiologic retraction ring** (or **Bandl's ring**). It is normally present in all labors and typically lies below the level of the symphysis pubis. If the ring rises abnormally high or becomes prominent, it may indicate obstruction and requires evaluation.

Effacement and Dilation of the Cervix

The cervix undergoes two major changes during the first stage: **effacement** (thinning) and **dilation** (opening).

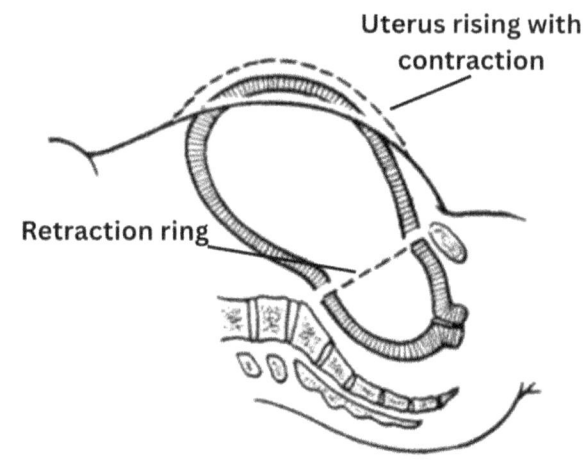

Effacement often begins before labor, especially in first pregnancies. As contractions continue, the circular muscle fibers of the cervix are drawn upward, becoming part of the lower uterine segment.

1. **0% effaced:** cervix is long and firm, approximately 1 cm dilated
2. **30% effaced:** cervix is beginning to shorten and soften, about 2 cm dilated
3. **50% effaced:** cervix is halfway thinned, about 3 cm dilated
4. **80% effaced:** cervix is nearly fully thinned, about 7 cm dilated
5. **100% effaced:** cervix is paper-thin and completely taken up, about 10 cm dilated

Dilation follows effacement and progresses more slowly in early labor, accelerating once active labor begins. A well-flexed fetal head applies even pressure to the cervix, aiding dilation. The mucus plug is often released during this process, sometimes streaked with blood—commonly known as **bloody show**.

Effacement

1.	2.	3.	4.	5.
1 cm	2 cm	3 cm	7 cm	10 cm
0%	30%	40%	80%	100%

Dilation of the Cervix

Dilation is the gradual opening of the cervix from a closed os to approximately 10 cm. Normal variation is wide; progress should be assessed in context with contraction pattern, fetal position, and the individual's overall adaptation.

- Dilation may begin before labor, typically not more than 1–2 cm.
- As labor progresses—especially after effacement—dilation accelerates with effective, rhythmic contractions.
- A well-flexed presenting part applies uniform pressure to the cervix and facilitates dilation.
- Release of the mucus plug, often streaked with blood ("bloody show"), commonly accompanies dilation.

Dilation

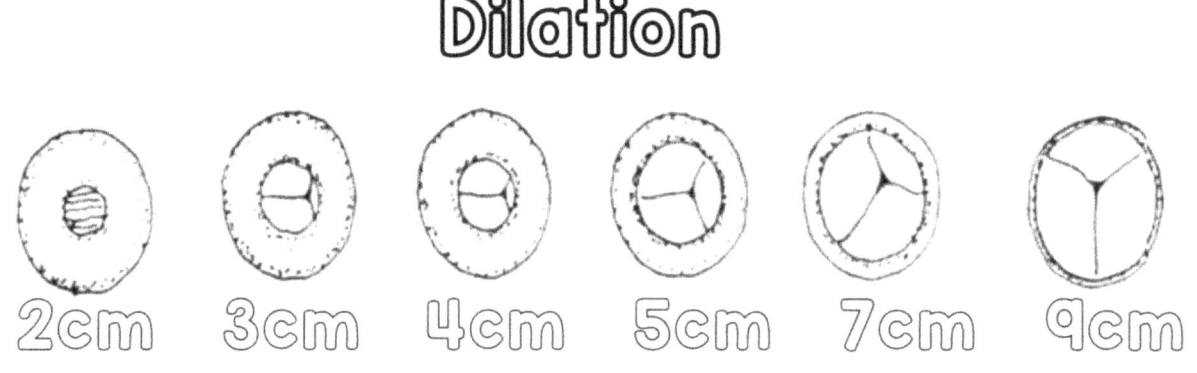

2cm   3cm   4cm   5cm   7cm   9cm

Checking cervical dilation

> **Activity: Estimating Cervical Dilation**
> Draw and cut ten circles from heavy paper, ranging from 1 to 10 centimeters in diameter. Practice estimating the diameter of each circle to develop visual and tactile awareness of cervical dilation.

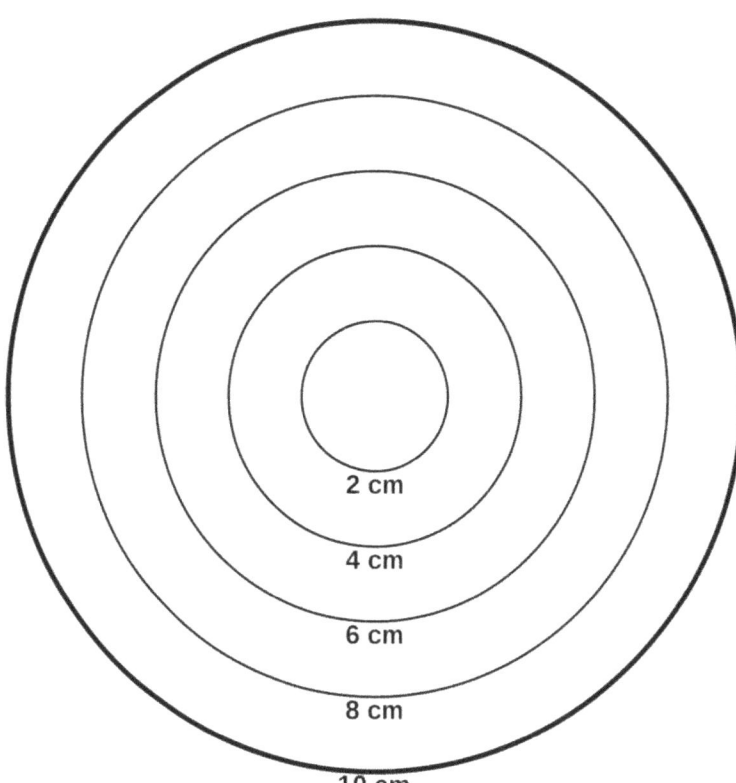

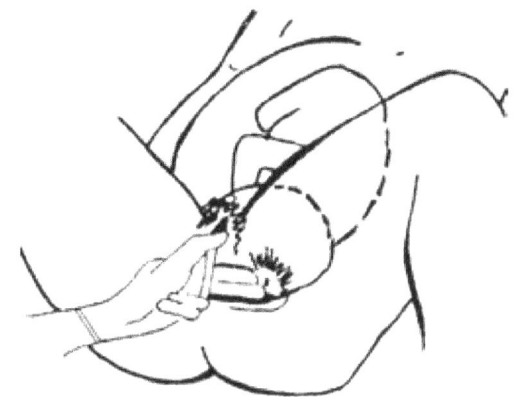

Formation of the Bag of Waters

As the lower uterine segment stretches, the **chorion** may loosen slightly, allowing part of the amniotic sac to bulge into the cervical opening. The fetal head fits snugly within the cervix, forming two distinct fluid compartments:

A. FOREWATERS—fluid in front of the head

B. HINDWATERS—fluid behind the head

The intact membranes maintain **general fluid pressure**, evenly distributing uterine force and protecting the placenta, cord, and fetus from excessive compression. This cushioning effect helps prevent fetal hypoxia and promotes steady progress.

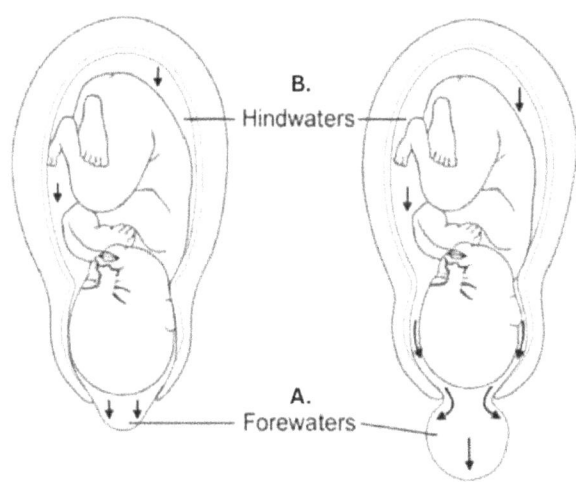

Rupture of the Membranes

The amniotic sac may rupture at any point during labor, or occasionally before contractions begin. Spontaneous rupture of membranes (SROM) is normal and may occur with a gush or a slow, steady leak of clear fluid. When the "waters break," amniotic fluid is released, reducing the cushioning effect but allowing the fetal head to engage more deeply.

Artificial rupture of membranes (AROM) should only be performed when clinically indicated, as it can increase infection risk and alter labor dynamics. After rupture, the midwife notes the **time**, **color**, and **odor** of the fluid—normal amniotic fluid is clear or pale straw-colored, with a mild, earthy scent. Green or brown discoloration suggests meconium, while cloudy or foul-smelling fluid may indicate infection. Once membranes are ruptured, temperature and fetal heart rate are monitored more frequently, and birth is generally expected within 24 hours unless otherwise determined safe by the midwife's assessment. The membranes should not be artificially ruptured to hasten labor without clear medical indication, such as evidence of fetal or maternal distress. The intact sac provides protection, maintains hydration, and supports normal physiologic birth.

> **Exercise 11.9: Sequence of the First Stage of Labor**
> *Place the following events in the correct order (1–6) to show how the progress through the first stage of labor.*
>
> ___Effacement and dilation of the cervix
> ___Formation of the upper and lower uterine segments
> ___Contraction and retraction of the uterine muscle
> ___Formation of the bag of waters
> ___Rupture of the membranes
> ___Fundal dominance directs the force of contractions downward

Maternal Response to Labor

Labor initiates widespread physiologic changes throughout the mother's body. These adaptations ensure adequate oxygenation, energy supply, and blood flow for both mother and baby. Most of these responses are temporary and return to baseline within hours or days after birth. Understanding these systemic shifts helps midwives support comfort, endurance, and safety throughout the labor process.

It begins when maternal, fetal, hormonal, emotional, and environmental factors align. Signals from the baby—such as lung maturity and chemical messengers in the amniotic fluid—help initiate labor. The birthing body contributes through changes in hormone levels, increased sensitivity to oxytocin, and a gradual shift away from progesterone dominance. Emotional readiness, stress, and a sense of safety also influence timing and rhythm.

Temperature Regulation and Fluid Balance

Mild increases in temperature and sweating are expected from muscular work and hormonal activity. Hydration, cool compresses, or warm baths help regulate temperature naturally.
- Slight rise in temperature is physiologic.
- Sweating and fluid loss increase in second stage.

Hydration and environmental comfort aid regulation.

Cardiovascular System

With each contraction, uterine blood flow briefly decreases as the muscle tightens, forcing blood from the placental bed into circulation. Cardiac output increases by 30–50 percent during labor, peaking in second stage. Blood pressure and pulse rise during contractions, returning to normal between them.

Supine positioning can compress the inferior vena cava, reducing venous return and causing dizziness, hypotension, or fetal heart rate changes. Upright, side-lying, or forward-leaning positions prevent this compression and support uteroplacental flow.
- Cardiac output rises progressively throughout labor.
- Blood pressure and pulse increase during contractions.
- Avoid supine positions to reduce vena cava compression.
- Slightly elevated pulse may persist until after birth.

Respiratory System

Oxygen consumption doubles during labor as breathing becomes deeper and faster to meet increased metabolic demand. Hyperventilation may lead to mild respiratory alkalosis, causing dizziness or tingling in the lips and fingers.

> **Whole-Body Adaptation**
>
> Every system in the mother's body contributes to the work of birth. The heart pumps harder, the lungs breathe faster, and the muscles endure waves of effort. These changes are not signs of strain but of strength—proof of the body's intricate design to sustain life, adapt to intensity, and recover swiftly once the work is done.

Encouraging rhythmic breathing, gentle exhalation, and relaxation between contractions helps maintain oxygen and carbon dioxide balance. Sips of water, cool cloths, or moist air relieve dryness.
- Oxygen demand and ventilation increase substantially.
- Mild respiratory alkalosis may occur with rapid breathing.
- Focused breathing techniques stabilize gas exchange.

Hematologic System

Labor activates clotting mechanisms to minimize bleeding after birth. Fibrinogen and clotting factors rise, and leukocyte counts increase as part of the normal stress and inflammatory response. Slight hemoconcentration occurs from plasma shifts into uterine muscle.

Average blood loss at vaginal birth is 250–500 mL—well tolerated because of pregnancy's expanded blood volume.
- Clotting factors and WBC count are elevated.
- Moderate blood loss is physiologic.
- Increased blood volume protects against hemorrhage.

Gastrointestinal System

Gastrointestinal motility slows as blood flow shifts to the uterus and skeletal muscles. Nonetheless, maintaining hydration and energy is vital for endurance. Restricting oral intake during uncomplicated labor is no longer supported by evidence.

Light foods—fruit, broth, yogurt, honey, or toast—and small sips of fluids maintain strength and prevent ketosis. Nausea or vomiting may occur during transition due to hormonal shifts and pressure on the stomach.
- GI motility slows, but oral intake should not be routinely restricted.
- Light foods and clear fluids sustain energy and comfort.

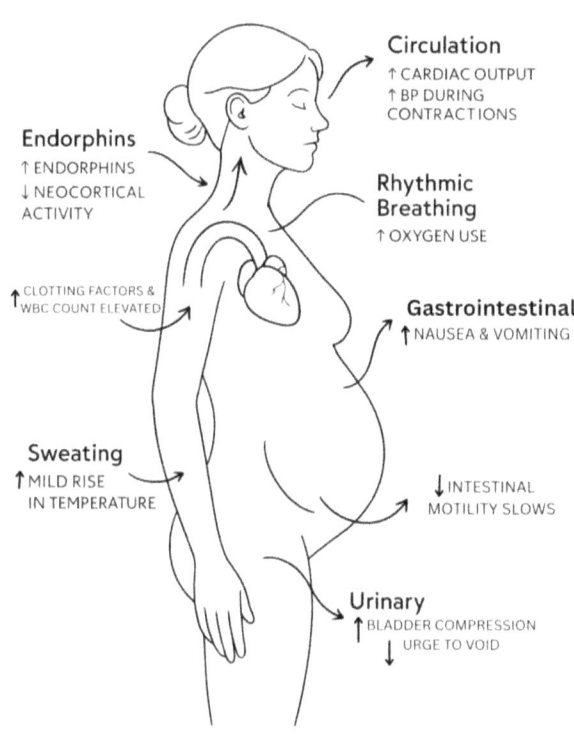

Urinary System

Descending fetal parts compress the bladder and reduce capacity. The urge to void may diminish, but a full bladder can obstruct descent or cause pain. Encourage voiding every one to two hours during labor.

After birth, temporary bladder hypotonia is common due to pressure on the urethra and pelvic nerves. Monitoring postpartum voiding helps prevent retention.
- Bladder compression is normal but may impede descent.
- Encourage voiding every 1–2 hours.
- Observe for postpartum urinary retention.

Musculoskeletal System

Sustained contractions and exertion increase muscle tone and metabolic demand. Tremors or shaking—especially during transition—reflect fatigue or hormonal surges, not pathology.

Position changes, massage, warmth, and hydration help reduce strain, while upright postures enhance pelvic mobility and circulation.
- Tremors and muscle fatigue are common.
- Movement relieves strain and improves circulation.
- Comfort measures support endurance.

Neurologic and Emotional Response

Labor activates both the autonomic nervous system and emotional centers of the brain. Early labor often brings excitement and alertness; active labor encourages inward focus and rhythmic coping behaviors.

Endorphins rise steadily, promoting pain relief and a trance-like concentration. In late labor, adrenaline and noradrenaline increase energy and alertness for birth. After delivery, oxytocin surges, fostering calm, bonding, and strong uterine contractions.
- Endorphins promote focus and pain relief.
- Catecholamines energize the body for birth.

- A calm, private environment supports hormonal balance.

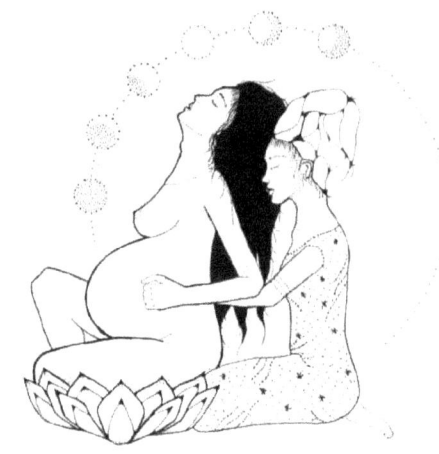

Exercise 11.10: Maternal Responses During Labor	
Match each term with its correct description.	
1. May cause dizziness or tingling if breathing is too rapid	A. Cardiovascular
2. Slows as blood flow shifts toward the uterus	B. Respiratory
3. Encourages energy and alertness in second stage	C. Gastrointestinal
4. Increases cardiac output and blood pressure during contractions	D. Neurologic
5. Causes tremors or shaking due to exertion and hormonal change	E. Musculoskeletal

Exercise 11.11: Hormonal Flow of Labor
Fill in the Blank.

1. Rising _____ and functional withdrawal of _____ prepare the uterus for contractions.
2. The fetal–placental unit releases _____, which stimulates fetal cortisol and maternal prostaglandin production.
3. _____ increases uterine sensitivity to oxytocin and promotes formation of gap junctions between uterine muscle cells.
4. _____, released from the posterior pituitary, binds to uterine receptors and triggers rhythmic contractions.
5. _____ and _____ work together to soften and ripen the cervix.
6. The _____ reflex reinforces oxytocin release through cervical stretch feedback.
7. _____ reduce uterine efficiency when fear or stress is high, while _____ promote calm and pain relief.

Exercise 11.12: Four "P's" Fill in the Blank
Fill in the blank:

1. The pelvic inlet is widest in the _____ diameter.
2. The urge to push is caused by pressure on the pelvic floor, triggering the _____ reflex.
3. _____ and _____ work together to create strong, efficient contractions and pain relief.
4. Frequent movement and position changes every ___ contractions help optimize pelvic mechanics
5. The pelvic floor acts as a _____, guiding the fetal head to rotate anteriorly.
6. The fetal head presents the smallest diameter when it is _____.
7. When adrenaline levels rise due to fear, contractions may _____ or _____.
8. The four essential factors that influence labor are _____, _____, _____, and _____.

The Midwife's Role in Labor and Delivery

Every labor unfolds in its own rhythm. The midwife's role is to witness, support, and safeguard that process with patience, skill, and adaptability. Midwives bring both clinical expertise and intuitive understanding to birth. Although clinical frameworks define stages and phases, labor does not always follow a predictable pattern. Some individuals move quickly through early labor, while others progress gradually. Midwives balance assessment with patience, supporting the natural process while remaining ready to intervene when needed.

Foundations of Effective Intrapartum Care
- **Maintain safety:** through skill and vigilance.
- **Observation:** maintain ongoing awareness of the labor pattern, ensuring progress remains within a normal range.
- **Monitoring:** track maternal vitals, fetal heart tones, contractions, and overall well-being.
- **Documentation:** accurate, detailed and complete charting is important to good care. This is especially important if the woman is transferred to another provider.
- **Support:** offer physical, emotional, and informational care while protecting privacy and calm.
- **Clinical Judgment:** recognize the difference between physiologic variation and early signs of complication.
- **Confidence in Normal Birth:** trust the process while remaining ready to respond if needs change.
- **Preparedness:** having equipment, protocols, and a plan in case of complications.

The Partner in Labor and Birth

While midwives and doulas bring a wealth of knowledge, experience, and skill to support birthing families, it is equally important not to overshadow or exclude the partner. The midwife's role includes showing the partner how to provide comfort, such as demonstrating a back massage rather than doing it herself, and finding ways to include them meaningfully in the birth process.

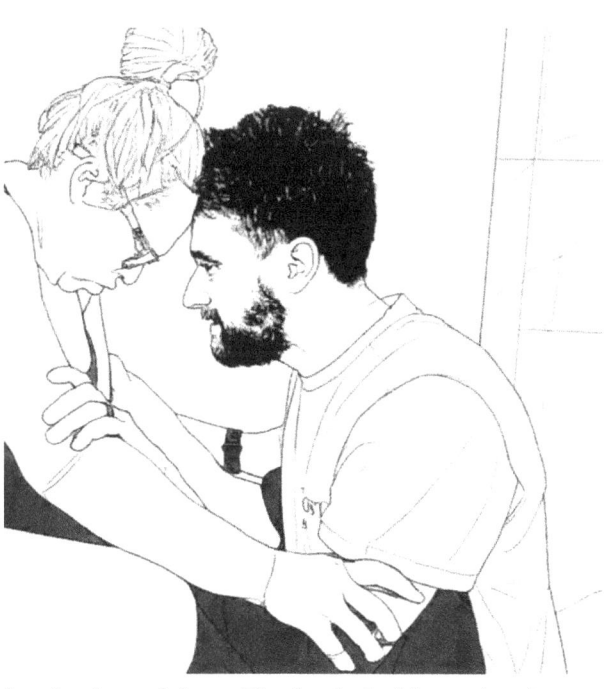

Six weeks after the baby is born, the midwife will move on, but the partner remains. The connection a couple builds during labor forms a lifelong bond. When a woman looks back on her birth, her first thought should not be "My midwife or doula was so wonderful; she helped me so much," but rather "My partner was really there for me. He (or she) supported me in every way." Midwives and doulas serve best when they protect that sacred partnership, guiding without taking over.

The Power of Natural Birth

Childbirth without drugs connects women to the ancient rhythm of the way mothers have given birth since the beginning of time. The body holds an intricate design of hormones, microbiome interactions, and neurologic responses that we are only beginning to understand. During natural labor, surges of oxytocin and endorphins guide both body and mind, creating a perfect sequence of physiologic balance. These natural processes shape early bonding, brain chemistry, and lifelong health in ways that science continues to uncover.

Choosing to labor without medication is an act of strength and trust. It allows the mother to experience the full power of her body and to meet birth with awareness and resilience. Midwives play a vital role in this process, offering the tools, presence, and encouragement that help mothers access their innate coping mechanisms. Through movement, touch, breath, and support, midwives help sustain the body's natural endorphins—honoring birth as a transformative and empowering journey that benefits both mother and child.

First Stage Intrapartum Care

Latent Phase

In early labor, contractions soften and thin the cervix and help position the baby. They may be mild or irregular, with long pauses between them. The goal of care is reassurance, rest, and energy conservation.

Midwifery care includes confirming that labor is established, encouraging nourishment and hydration, and offering comfort measures such as warm baths or gentle movement. Early labor may last for hours or even days; patience and reassurance support progress.

Midwifery care includes:
- Confirming that labor is established and normal in character
- Encouraging rest, nourishment, and gentle movement as desired
- Promoting hydration with water, broths, or electrolyte drinks
- Suggesting warm baths or showers to encourage relaxation
- Monitoring fetal heart tones and maternal vitals periodically
- Offering reassurance that early labor may take time and does not require haste

Nutrition

Digestion slows down during labor, and some women become nauseated or vomit, especially during transition. However, energy is needed to sustain strength and prevent ketosis. Hospitals often discourage eating in labor because of the possibility of surgery; in such cases, they may provide glucose intravenously.

The mother should eat frequently. Familiar, light, high-protein foods that are comforting and easy to digest—such as yogurt, soup, fruit, snacks, and date energy bars—are ideal.

Hydration

Keeping hydrated during labor is essential. In addition to water or mild herbal tea, fruit juice, coconut water, and electrolyte drinks—which can be made in advance into ice cubes—are useful.

A classic "labor aid" drink recipe is:
- 2 cups coconut water
- 1 cup water or cold raspberry leaf tea
- Juice from 1 lemon
- Juice from 1 lime
- 2 tbsp unpasteurized honey or maple syrup
- ¼ tsp unrefined Himalayan or sea salt

Rest and Conservation

Encourage the mother to sleep or rest whenever possible. Labor is a marathon, not a sprint—rest whenever possible; but when not sleeping, being upright and moving is important as well. Dim lighting, minimal noise, and a sense of privacy help maintain calm and hormonal balance.

Active Phase

Active labor is the time when the midwife's clinical awareness becomes most important. Subtle changes in tone, movement, or response may signal either steady progress or an emerging need for reassessment. Ongoing observation and risk evaluation guide decisions about hydration, rest, position, and when additional support or consultation may be needed.

As labor deepens, contractions become longer, stronger, and closer together. The mother turns inward, focusing on the rhythm of contractions and the work of labor. The midwife monitors fetal and maternal well-being while encouraging movement, hydration, and position changes. Ongoing assessment ensures progress remains physiologic and helps identify any emerging signs that require attention or consultation.

Midwifery responsibilities:
- Monitor fetal heart tones every 15–30 minutes, based on risk and stage.
- Assess maternal vitals, contraction strength and frequency, and overall coping.
- Reassess risk status throughout labor, noting any new findings such as fever, prolonged rupture of membranes, slow progress, meconium-stained fluid, or concerning fetal heart patterns.
- Observe for changes in emotional state, fatigue, and hydration—signs that can influence the course of labor.
- Support frequent position changes to promote descent and rotation.
- Encourage rhythmic breathing, grounding techniques, and relaxation.
- Maintain hydration and a comfortably empty bladder.
- Document findings clearly, noting both physiologic variation and any emerging risk factors that may require escalation or consultation.
- Maintain infection-prevention protocols and sterile technique as needed.

Movement and Comfort

Upright positions, walking, leaning forward, and water immersion all support comfort and progress. Resting positions such as side-lying or semi-upright help conserve energy without slowing labor unduly. The midwife's quiet presence and continual assessment create both reassurance and clinical safety—anchoring the birth process in confidence and attentive care.

Movement and Positioning
- **Walk and rock:** encourage gentle walking, slow dancing, or rocking in a chair to support fetal descent and rhythm.
- **Use a birthing ball:** sitting, kneeling, or leaning on a birthing ball promotes pelvic mobility.
- **Vary positions:** encourage frequent position changes—hands-and-knees, lunging, or side-lying—to reduce strain and aid rotation.

Hydrotherapy
- **Warm shower:** direct warm water onto the shoulders or back to relieve muscle tension.
- **Warm bath or birth pool:** immersion supports relaxation, reduces perception of pain, and promotes buoyancy and mobility.

Touch and Pressure

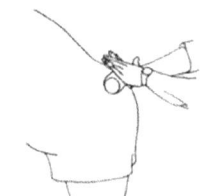

- **Massage:** gentle, rhythmic touch or massage enhances relaxation.
- **Counterpressure:** firm, steady pressure on the lower back can ease discomfort from posterior positions or back labor.
- **Heat or cold:** use warm compresses for back or abdominal discomfort, or cool cloths for the face and neck.

Mind-Body Techniques
- **Breathing:** guide slow, rhythmic breathing to promote calm focus.
- **Focal point:** use a visual or tactile cue to help the mother channel concentration during contractions.
- **Guided imagery and meditation:** support relaxation through visualization, mindfulness, or affirmations.
- **Intentional relaxation:** encourage conscious release of muscle tension between contractions.

> **Quiet Protects Progress**
>
> The hormones of birth thrive in privacy and peace. When the room grows still, endorphins rise, fear recedes, and the body's rhythm returns. Silence is not emptiness—it is medicine.

Environmental and Sensory Support
- **Adjust the environment:** keep lighting soft, voices quiet, and the temperature comfortable.
- **Soothing sensory input:** incorporate music, aromatherapy, or familiar items from home to increase emotional ease.

POSITIONS FOR LABOR

Freedom of movement during labor allows the body and baby to work together efficiently. Upright, forward-leaning, and side-lying positions optimize the relationship between the uterus, pelvis, and gravity. Evidence shows the use of upright and alternative maternal positions during labor as beneficial for physiological childbirth and maternal outcomes. Encouraging regular position changes helps prevent fatigue, improve circulation, and maintain optimal pelvic space for descent and rotation. Even small shifts—changing sides, rocking, or adjusting posture—can make a meaningful difference in comfort and progress.

Midwives understand that movement, touch, and environment profoundly influence the hormones of labor. When the mother feels safe and supported, oxytocin and endorphins flow freely, strengthening contractions and easing pain. The midwife's calm presence, reassurance, and encouragement of movement embody the art and science of physiologic birth.

Each stage of labor benefits from a variety of positions that promote comfort, mobility, and progress. No single position is best for everyone; the goal is to respond to the body's cues and use gravity and alignment to advantage.

WALKING or swaying to encourage descent and rotation

LEANING forward on a birth ball, bed, or partner to ease back pressure

HANDS-AND-KNEES to relieve back pain and assist with posterior rotation

SQUATTING increases the pelvic outlet by up to 30%, aiding descent.

PELVIC TILTS help align the baby's head with the cervix and relieve lower back discomfort.

LUNGES encourage fetal rotation in cases of malposition.

ASYMMETRICAL (one knee up, one down) opens different pelvic diameters to help babies navigate the pelvis.

Sitting upright or TAILOR SITTING to open the pelvic inlet

SIDE-LYING for rest while maintaining pelvic alignment

KNEELING and leaning forward during transition for pelvic relaxation

Monitoring Fetal Well-Being

Monitoring fetal well-being is one of the midwife's most essential responsibilities. During labor, fetal heart assessment confirms that the baby is tolerating contractions and maintaining good oxygen exchange. In community birth settings, midwives rely on intermittent auscultation (IA)—a safe, evidence-based method that preserves mobility and supports family-centered care.

Fetal monitoring is both a science and an art. Through attentive listening, midwives interpret what they hear within the broader context of labor progress, maternal condition, and emotional tone. Experience refines their ability to recognize subtle changes in rhythm and tempo that reveal how the baby is adapting to labor. Balancing technology with touch, the midwife turns listening into connection, communication, and trust between mother, baby, and caregiver.

Listening Tools

Midwives use several instruments to assess the fetal heart rate, including manual fetoscopes and Dopplers. While fetoscopes work well for prenatal care, they can be difficult to use during contractions. Many birth centers now use small electronic fetal monitoring (EFM) machines for external use only, providing brief tracings during labor or nonstress tests when needed. These portable units offer reassurance without limiting mobility or requiring continuous monitoring.

Methods of Assessment

Two main methods are used to monitor fetal well-being:

- **Intermittent auscultation (IA)** – Listening before, during, and after contractions at regular intervals (about every 15–30 minutes in active labor and every 5–15 minutes in second stage). The midwife notes baseline rate, rhythm, and any accelerations or decelerations, along with maternal pulse and fetal movement.
- **Electronic fetal monitoring (EFM)** – Provides continuous tracings of fetal heart rate and uterine activity, typically in hospital settings or when specific interventions (such as oxytocin use) are in place.
    EFM may be external or internal:
    - *External monitoring* uses two transducers on the abdomen—one for contractions and one for fetal heart rate via Doppler ultrasound.
    - *Internal monitoring*, requiring ruptured membranes, attaches a small spiral electrode to the fetal scalp and may use an intrauterine pressure catheter to measure contraction strength.

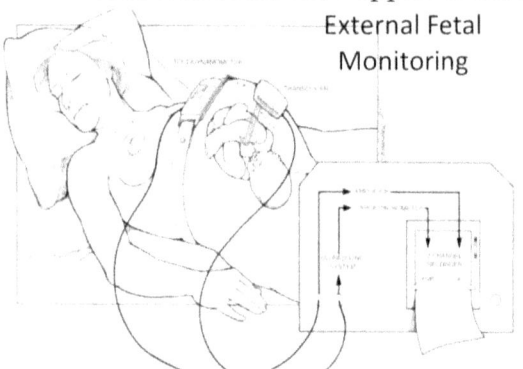

External Fetal Monitoring

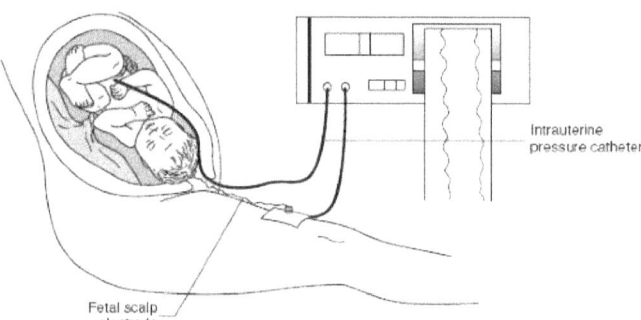

While EFM can identify some acute events, research shows no improvement in outcomes for low-risk births and an association with higher operative delivery rates. Internal monitoring also carries small risks, such as scalp injury or infection, and should be avoided when maternal infections (HIV, hepatitis, or active herpes) are present.

Supporting Fetal Oxygenation

When changes occur, midwives respond with physiologic interventions that enhance circulation and oxygen delivery:
- Change maternal position (side-lying, hands-and-knees, upright)
- Offer hydration or nourishment
- Encourage rest between contractions

- Reduce uterine stimulation if contractions are too frequent
- Evaluate for fever, dehydration, or hypotension
- Consult or transfer if abnormalities persist

Interpreting Fetal Heart Rate Patterns

Fetal heart monitoring gives insight into how the baby is adapting to contractions and maintaining oxygenation. Four key features—**baseline rate**, **variability**, **accelerations**, and **decelerations**—are assessed together for a complete picture of well-being. Full competency requires ongoing study of current guidelines and supervised clinical practice.

Baseline Rate
The baseline is the average heart rate between contractions over about ten minutes, normally 110–160 bpm.
- **Tachycardia (>160 bpm):** may reflect maternal fever, infection, dehydration, anxiety, or early hypoxia.
- **Bradycardia (<110 bpm):** may occur with cord compression or maternal hypotension. Brief changes are common, but persistent alterations warrant evaluation.

Variability
The small, irregular fluctuations in heart rate that indicate oxygenation and nervous system integrity.
- **Absent:** none visible—concerning; may reflect hypoxia or medication effects.
- **Minimal (≤5 bpm):** possible fetal sleep or medication influence.
- **Moderate (6–25 bpm):** reassuring, reflects healthy autonomic activity.
- **Marked (>25 bpm):** usually temporary, may occur with fetal stimulation or stress.

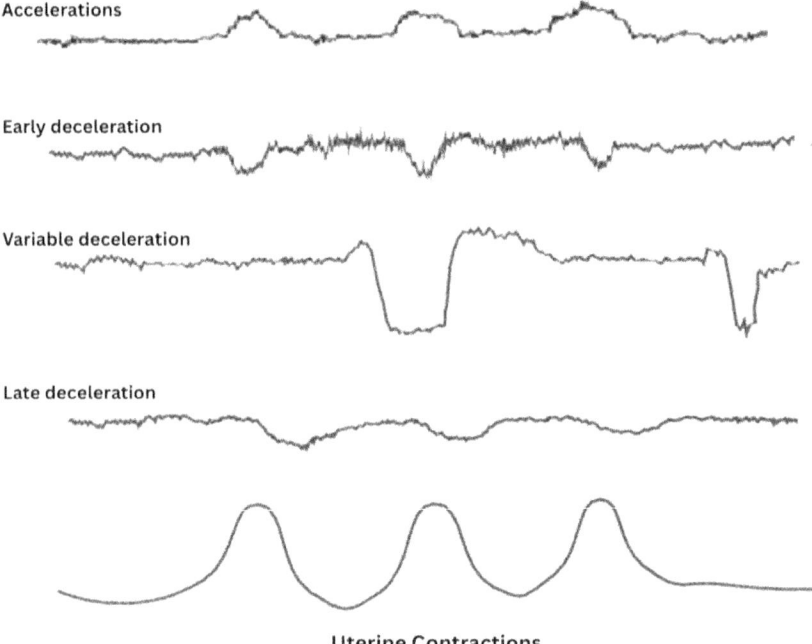

Accelerations
The brief rises in heart rate that demonstrate good oxygenation and nervous system responsiveness.
- **Term fetus:** ≥15 bpm above baseline for at least 15 seconds.
- **Preterm fetus:** ≥10 bpm for at least 10 seconds.
They often occur with movement, vaginal exams, or contractions and are almost always reassuring.

Decelerations
Temporary decreases in fetal heart rate during contractions or movement.
- **Early decelerations:** gradual decreases that mirror contractions, caused by head compression and vagal stimulation—normal and benign.
- **Variable decelerations:** abrupt "V" or "W"-shaped drops; usually due to temporary cord compression. Brief variables are common and well tolerated, but repetitive or prolonged ones may need attention.
- **Late decelerations:** begin after the contraction starts and recover after it ends; associated with uteroplacental insufficiency (reduced oxygen transfer). Evaluate for causes such as hypotension, dehydration, or excessive uterine activity.
- **Prolonged decelerations:** drops of ≥15 bpm lasting **2–10 minutes**; may occur with sustained cord compression, maternal hypotension, or rapid descent. If the rate stays low beyond 10 minutes, it becomes a new baseline.

Patterns showing moderate variability and accelerations are reassuring. Their timing and shape help identify the cause and how well the baby is compensating. Absent variability with recurrent late or variable decelerations suggests possible compromise and warrants immediate evaluation or transfer.

Exercise 11.13: Evaluating Fetal Heart Rate Patterns		
Check the box that best describes each fetal heart rate pattern.		
Pattern	Reassuring	Concerning
Baseline 120–150 bpm with moderate variability	☐	☐
Baseline 170 bpm with maternal fever	☐	☐
Early decelerations that mirror contractions	☐	☐
Variable decelerations lasting less than 30 seconds with quick recovery	☐	☐
Late decelerations that begin after the contraction starts	☐	☐
Prolonged deceleration lasting 3 minutes before returning to baseline	☐	☐
Accelerations of 15 bpm for 15 seconds during movement	☐	☐
Absent variability with recurrent late decelerations	☐	☐

Transition

As the first stage of labor draws to a close, the body's work becomes fully visible. The cervix has softened, thinned, and opened; the baby has settled deeper into the pelvis. The rhythm of contractions builds to its peak, guiding the transition toward birth. When full dilation is reached, care shifts naturally toward the second stage—supporting descent, pushing, and the safe, gentle emergence of the baby.

The transition between first and second stages marks a shift in intensity and focus as the body prepares for birth. Contractions are often strong and close together, with little rest between them. Emotional expression may peak, sometimes marked by self-doubt, irritability, or exhaustion.

During this phase, emotional reassurance and simple direction are most effective. Encourage rest between contractions, fluid intake, and an empty bladder. The midwife quietly prepares the birth space, maintaining an atmosphere of calm and confidence.

Common observations:
- Strong, frequent contractions with increasing pelvic pressure
- Shaking, chills, or sweating
- Feelings of doubt, overwhelm, or surrender
- Behavioral shift, loss of control, vocalization, or withdrawal
- Nausea or vomiting

Midwifery care:
- Remain close and calm; speak sparingly and clearly
- Encourage sips of fluid and emptying of the bladder as needed
- Monitor fetal and maternal well-being closely
- Prepare the birth space and supplies while maintaining calm surroundings
- Encourage low-pitched vocalizations, singing, or chanting.
- Use focused, patterned breathing such as "pant-pant-blow" breathing, taking several shallow breaths followed by a longer exhale.
- Encourage visualization and affirmations, like, "You're so close to holding your baby, or your cervix is opening like a flower.

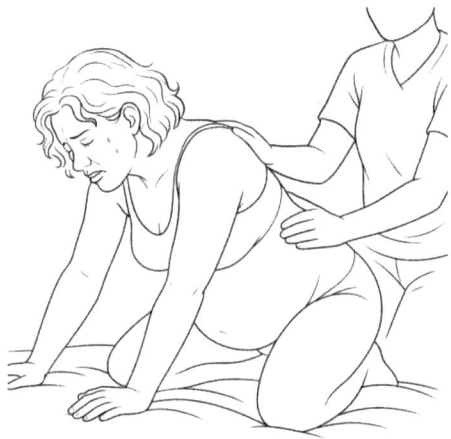

Transition
Strength and surrender in motion.

SECOND STAGE CARE

The second stage of labor begins with full cervical dilation and ends with the birth of the baby. In community birth, it is a time of focused observation, calm reassurance, and skilled support. The midwife's role is to balance patience with vigilance, recognizing what is normal, what may need guidance, and when consultation or transfer is indicated.

Through steady observation, the midwife reads the language of labor: the rhythm of breathing, the change in tone as the urge to push emerges, the gradual stretch and color shift of the perineum, the descent of the fetal head, and the reassuring beat of the baby's heart. Each cue informs care without unnecessary interference.

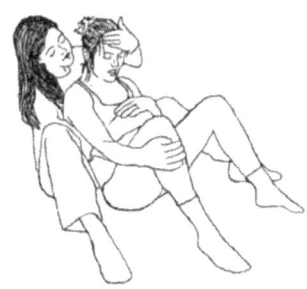

Physiologic pushing, upright positions, and freedom of movement are encouraged to enhance descent and oxygenation. Communication remains calm and grounded through short phrases, a steady tone, and quiet confidence that reinforces safety and trust. Ultimately, the midwife's presence and skill protect both flow of birth and the health and safety of the mother and baby.

Clinical Assessment in Second Stage

Second stage care requires continuous awareness rather than continuous intervention. The midwife monitors progress through behavioral, physical, and clinical cues.

Maternal Cues
- Urge to push or change in vocalization
- Involuntary bearing-down efforts
- Changes in breathing, focus, or tone
- Signs of fatigue, frustration, or renewed energy

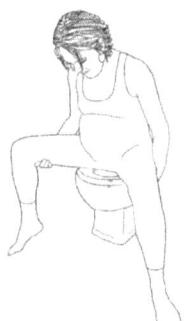

Physical Signs
- A full bladder can impede the baby's descent, so check and empty if necessary.
- Increasing perineal pressure or bulging
- Visible descent and rotation of the fetal head
- Crowning, when the head remains visible between contractions
- Thinning, stretching, or color change in vulvar and rectal tissues

Fetal Assessment
- Intermittent auscultation of heart tones before, during, and after contractions
- Recognition of reassuring versus nonreassuring patterns
- Position changes or hydration if variables appear
- Consultation or transfer if abnormalities persist

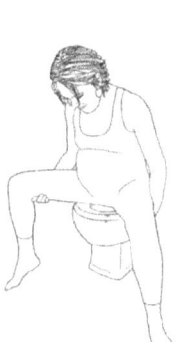

Pacing and Support

The second stage unfolds best when allowed to follow its natural rhythm. Some mothers rest briefly before pushing; others feel an immediate urge. The midwife reassures that both patterns are normal and supports physiologic pushing, which involves bearing down in response to the body's own reflex.

Encourage open-throated breathing, open glottis low moans, and exhalations to maintain oxygenation and release tension. Common positions include upright, squatting, side-lying, kneeling, and hands-and-knees. When available, warm water immersion offers comfort and buoyancy.

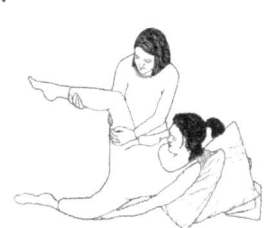

Let the woman follow her body's natural urge to push, rather than forcing her to push with every contraction, which can help save energy and prevent uterine hyperstimulation.

Communication and Emotional Grounding

The second stage can be emotionally intense and deeply transformative. Midwives use communication as a clinical tool—offering clear, calm, and concise guidance when needed, and a quiet presence when not.

Effective communication includes:
- Using low, steady tones to help the laboring person stay centered
- Giving short, actionable directions only when necessary
- Reinforcing progress with specific observations ("Your baby is moving down beautifully")
- Maintaining privacy, calm, and continuity of care

The goal is to protect the hormonal and emotional environment that supports spontaneous birth while keeping everyone informed and safe.

Safety Markers and Decision Points

In out-of-hospital birth, second stage assessment focuses on ongoing progress, stable vital signs, and reassuring fetal tones.

Midwives continually assess:
- Descent and rotation (steady or stalled)
- Maternal fatigue, hydration, and coping
- Fetal heart rate patterns (normal, variable, or prolonged decelerations)
- Condition of the perineum and any swelling or bruising
- Evidence of edema, bleeding, or cord prolapse

When second stage becomes prolonged, descent stalls, or fetal tones become concerning, the midwife reassesses with the team and may initiate consultation or transfer. Safety depends on both skillful observation and timely escalation when indicated.

Birth Positions

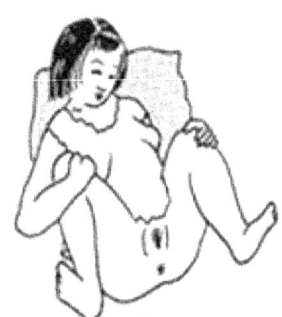

Just as every labor follows its own rhythm, every birth unfolds in its own position. The best position for giving birth is the one that allows the mother to feel grounded, supported, and free to follow her instincts. Midwives observe and adapt, helping the mother find what works best for her body and her baby. Upright positions often use gravity to assist descent and rotation, while side-lying or kneeling positions can help slow a rapid birth and protect the perineum.

Ultimately, the right position is the one that honors both physiology and intuition. When mothers feel free to move, shift, and choose, birth tends to unfold more smoothly and with greater confidence.

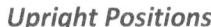

Upright Positions

Standing, squatting, or supported kneeling positions make use of gravity, open the pelvis, and can increase the efficiency of contractions. Squatting widens the pelvic outlet and often feels powerful and instinctive. Some mothers prefer to stand and lean forward on a partner or birth ball between contractions, using movement to help the baby descend.

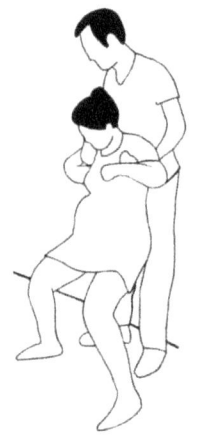

Kneeling and Forward-Leaning Positions

Kneeling on hands and knees or leaning forward over a birth ball, chair, or the side of a tub can relieve pressure on the lower back and sacrum, especially if the baby is in a posterior position. These positions also allow the pelvis to move freely and help rotation during descent.

Side-Lying Positions

Side-lying offers rest and control, particularly during crowning. It helps slow a fast birth and reduces perineal strain while allowing the midwife easy access for support and observation. This position can also be ideal for clients with elevated blood pressure, fatigue, or epidural anesthesia.

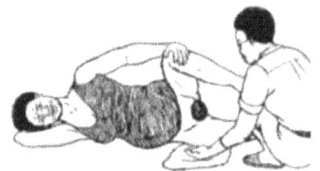

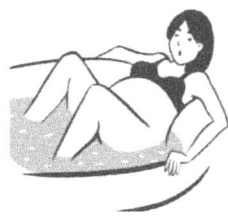
Water Birth
Warm water supports the body, reduces pain, and allows buoyant movement as the baby emerges.

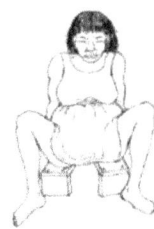
Birth Stools
A birthing stool or chair offers upright support while keeping the perineum visible and accessible.

Normal Delivery Steps

Preventing Perineal Trauma
Most tears occur when the fetal head delivers too quickly or when tissues are tense and poorly supported.

The midwife minimizes trauma by:
- Encouraging the mother to breathe or pant instead of pushing during crowning
- Using warm compresses to increase circulation and elasticity
- Applying gentle counterpressure to the head only if it begins to extend rapidly
- Supporting the perineum and labia to guide gradual stretching
- Encouraging upright or lateral positions, which allow better pelvic mobility and natural perineal expansion

If the perineum appears pale, white, or blanched, stretching may be excessive. Slowing or pausing the birth allows blood flow to return and tissues to recover.

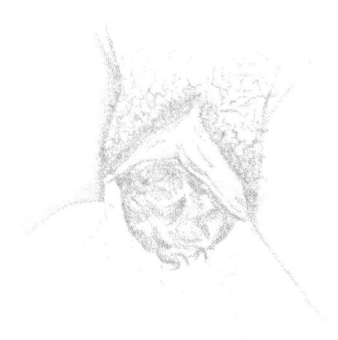

Routine episiotomy is **not indicated.** Evidence consistently shows that spontaneous tears are often less severe and heal more effectively than surgical incisions. Episiotomy should be reserved only for rare, urgent circumstances such as severe fetal distress requiring immediate birth or unavoidable tissue rigidity.

Hand Positions and Perineal Support
The midwife's hands guide the speed and direction of the baby's emergence, never forcing or pulling. The goal is to slow the delivery of the head, allowing gradual stretching and time for the tissues to adapt.

Common hand techniques include:
- One hand on the fetal head, applying gentle counterpressure to prevent rapid extension as the head crowns
- One hand supporting the perineum, providing light upward pressure to support the perineal body and control the rate of expulsion
- Hands-poised approach: the midwife keeps her hands ready to assist but avoids direct pressure until necessary, allowing spontaneous stretching and descent

The chosen technique depends on the situation, maternal position, and perineal elasticity. Warm compresses, perineal oil, or immersion in warm water can all increase comfort and circulation.

- Use the least amount of pressure needed to slow the birth.
- Avoid pushing the head back into the perineum.
- Maintain a calm, steady voice to help the mother release tension.

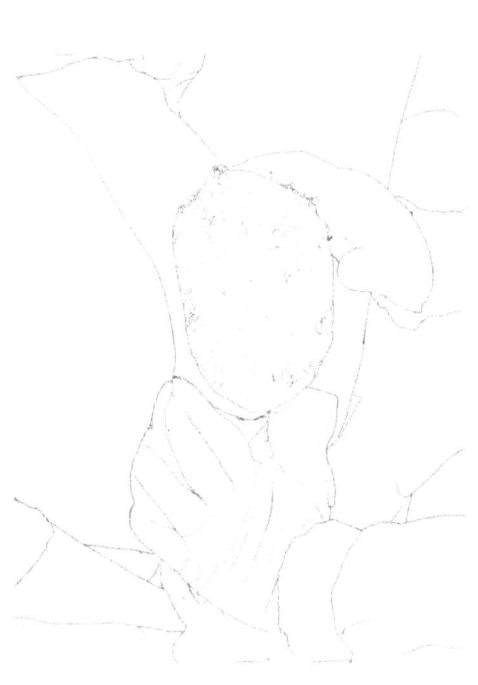

Normal Vaginal Birth: Step-by-Step

1. **Support crowning:** encourage slow, open-mouthed breathing as the head crowns ("ring of fire"). Continue perineal support with a warm compress or gauze-covered hand over the perineum, loosening the tissues and preventing tearing. If fetal heart tones remain strong and the scalp color is pink, the slow, controlled delivery of the head can proceed safely.
2. **Guide controlled extension:** with the next gentle effort, support the occiput as it slips under the pubic bone. Allow the forehead, nose, mouth, and chin to emerge slowly. Avoid pulling; let the tissues stretch gradually.
3. **Check for a nuchal cord:** as the head is born, run a finger along the neck to determine if a cord is present and assess whether it is loose or tight.
   - If the cord is loose, lift it over the head.
   - If snug, try to create space for the shoulders to pass.
   - If very tight, manage with the Somersault Maneuver

   Somersault Maneuver for a Tight Nuchal Cord
   The goal is to keep the baby's head close to the perineum during birth so the body can deliver without traction on the cord, maintaining placental circulation.

   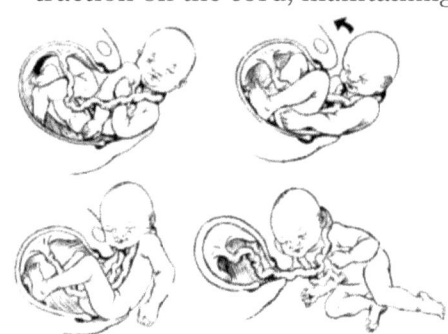

   A. Identify the nuchal cord as the head is born.
   B. Do not pull on the cord or the baby's head; keep the head close to the perineum.
   C. Flex the baby's head gently toward the mother's thigh so the face stays near the perineum as the shoulders deliver.
   D. Allow the baby to perform a small "somersault," bringing feet toward the mother's knees as the body is born.
   E. Once the body is fully delivered, unwrap the cord from the neck.

4. **Pause and wait.**
   Support the head near the perineum and wait for the next contraction. During this interval, observe for spontaneous restitution (the head turning to align with the shoulders) and ensure good color and tone. The body often delivers spontaneously; if not, gentle guidance may be needed to assist delivery.
5. **Deliver the anterior shoulder.**
   With the next contraction, guide the head gently downward so the anterior shoulder slips under the pubic bone. If the mother is upright, gravity often completes this motion without assistance. Use both hands to support the head as the body is born.
6. **Deliver the posterior shoulder.**
   Lift slightly to free the posterior shoulder, then allow the rest of the body to follow in a smooth motion.
7. **Receive and support the baby.**
   Support the baby with both hands as the body is born. If the mother is upright, be ready for a quick release into her hands or yours.
8. **The mother may be invited** to reach down and lift the baby onto the abdomen if desired.
9. **Place baby skin-to-skin.**
   Keep the cord intact. Dry the baby, observe color and respirations, and encourage bonding and breastfeeding as desired.
10. **Observe mother and prepare for third stage.**
    Monitor bleeding, uterine tone, and signs of placental separation. Maintain calm and warmth as you transition into care of the third stage.

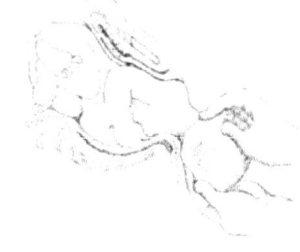
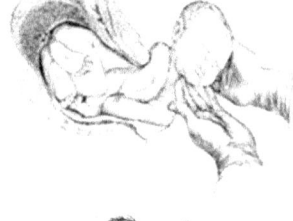
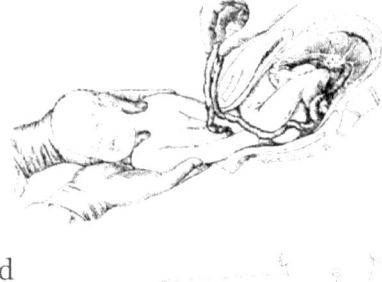

Immediate Newborn Care

Immediately assess the baby's color, tone, and breathing. If the newborn is vigorous, dry and place skin-to-skin on the mother's abdomen or chest, with the head turned slightly downward for drainage. Suction with a bulb syringe if indicated. Cover with a warm blanket or hat to prevent heat loss. Continue to observe respirations, color, and tone while allowing uninterrupted bonding.

Umbilical Cord Clamping

Keeping the umbilical cord intact by **delaying cord clamping** for at least three minutes, or until the cord has stopped pulsating, allows for placental transfusion. During this brief delay, about one quarter to one third of the baby's blood volume transfers from the placenta. This additional blood increases red blood cells, hemoglobin, and iron stores, supporting healthy growth and brain development during infancy. It also improves blood pressure stability, oxygenation, and temperature regulation, helping the newborn adapt smoothly to life outside the womb. When the third stage is well managed, delayed clamping does not increase the mother's risk of bleeding.

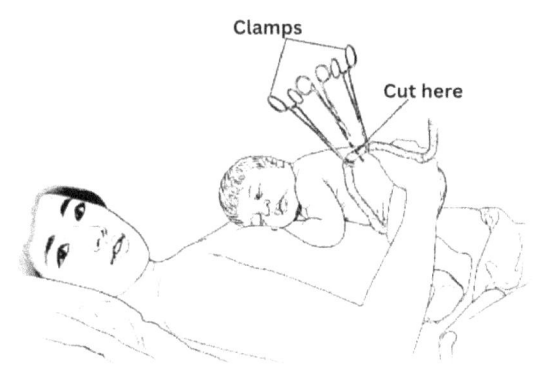

Once pulsation has ceased, the cord is clamped with two hemostats, or with one hemostat and a plastic cord clamp, and cut using sterile scissors between the two clamps. The midwife then continues to observe both mother and baby quietly, documenting findings while honoring the sacred first moments of bonding.

Benefits of Skin-to-Skin Contact

Immediately after birth, the midwife's role is to support uninterrupted skin-to-skin contact whenever possible. Holding the baby directly against the mother's bare chest helps stabilize vital functions, fosters bonding, and promotes physiologic adaptation.

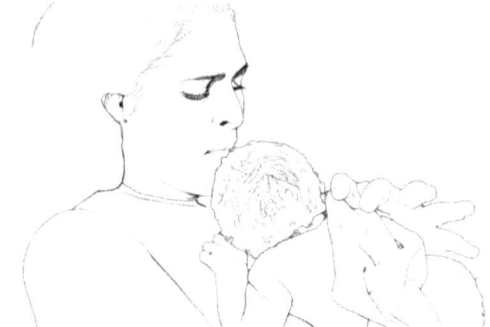

Regulating Temperature, Breathing, and Heart Rate

Skin-to-skin is one of the most effective ways to help a newborn transition smoothly from womb to world. The mother's body acts as a natural warmer or cooler, adjusting temperature to meet the baby's needs. Close contact also synchronizes the newborn's breathing and heart rate, promoting calm and stability during the first hours of life.

Supporting Breastfeeding and Hormonal Flow

Skin-to-skin contact triggers the release of oxytocin in both mother and baby, enhancing the "let-down" reflex and stimulating milk flow. The baby's proximity allows them to smell, feel, and instinctively locate the breast, which supports early feeding success and helps establish long-term breastfeeding patterns.

Promoting Neurologic and Emotional Development

When midwives encourage sustained skin-to-skin contact, they are helping lay the foundation for secure attachment and emotional regulation. Oxytocin released during this contact fosters relaxation, connection, and trust. For families who experience separation or difficulty bonding, skin-to-skin remains one of the most effective ways to reconnect and restore that sense of closeness.

Building the Newborn Microbiome

During the early hours after birth, the baby's microbiome begins to form. Direct contact with the mother's skin helps transfer her protective microbes, supporting immune function and long-term well-being.

Encouraging Healing and Recovery

Even if immediate skin-to-skin contact is delayed due to medical needs, its benefits continue long afterward. Midwives can teach families to use **kangaroo care**, holding the baby skin-to-skin for extended periods in the days or weeks that follow. This practice improves outcomes for preterm and unwell infants and enhances recovery for both mother and baby. Skin-to-skin can also be shared with partners, strengthening family bonds and promoting confidence in early caregiving.

Third Stage Management

An important responsibility of the midwife lies in the immediate postpartum, third stage, delivery of the placenta and fourth stage until the mother has stabilized. This includes monitoring bleeding and uterine tone, watching for placental separation, delivery of the placenta and making sure it is intact. This will be covered in detail in Chapter Twelve: Placenta & Postpartum.

LABOR & BIRTH ESSENTIAL TAKEAWAYS

Labor is a dynamic, whole-body process that unites physiology, emotion, and environment in the work of birth. The *Four P's*—passenger, passage, powers, and psyche—frame the midwife's understanding of how the mother, baby, and birth space interact. Each contraction, position change, and breath reflects a living dialogue between structure and spirit. When midwives observe these subtle relationships, they can respond with skill and patience, helping birth unfold in its own rhythm.

The pelvis is not fixed but a flexible, responsive structure that adapts with movement, gravity, and position. The baby's descent and rotation depend on this mobility as much as on uterine strength. Midwives use touch, observation, and positioning to facilitate this balance, encouraging upright, forward-leaning, or asymmetrical postures that open space and enhance alignment. Supporting hydration, nourishment, and rest preserves endurance and helps contractions remain efficient.

Labor also depends on hormonal and emotional harmony. Oxytocin, prostaglandins, and endorphins create the rhythm and flow of birth, but they are deeply influenced by safety and trust. When the environment is warm, private, and undisturbed, these hormones rise naturally; when fear or intrusion occurs, stress hormones can slow or halt progress. The midwife's calm presence, quiet reassurance, and respect for privacy protect this delicate hormonal balance and strengthen confidence.

Every birth teaches the midwife to balance vigilance with trust. Observation, gentle guidance, and the willingness to wait allow the physiologic process to lead. By protecting the conditions in which labor thrives—movement, calm, hydration, and emotional safety—the midwife becomes both guardian and witness to the power of the body and the intelligence of birth. Labor, when supported in this way, affirms the deep connection between mother and baby, and between human strength and the natural order that sustains life.

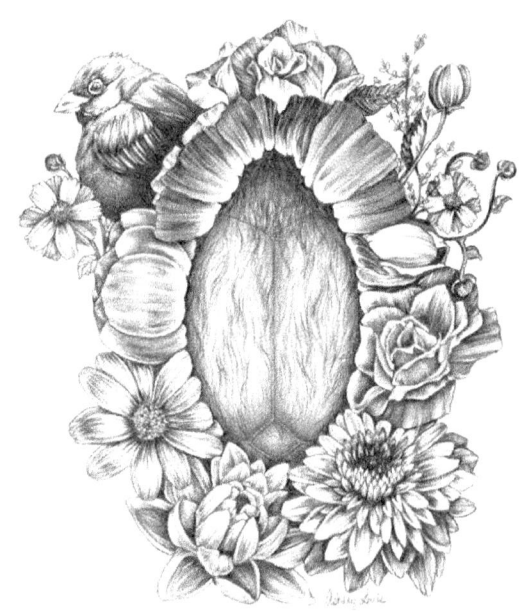

Chapter Eleven Self-Assessment

Multiple Choice
1. Which physiologic change contributes most to uterine efficiency in labor?
   a) Uterine retraction and fundal dominance
   b) Equal contraction strength throughout the uterus
   c) Relaxation of the upper uterine segment
   d) Decreased oxytocin sensitivity

2. Which physiologic change supports normal postpartum hemostasis?
   a) Increased fibrinogen and clotting factors
   b) Decreased blood volume
   c) Reduced cardiac output
   d) Lowered blood pressure

3. Which of the following best describes the mechanism of labor in a typical vertex presentation?
   a) Descent, internal rotation, flexion, extension, restitution, expulsion
   b) Engagement, flexion, internal rotation, extension, restitution, expulsion
   c) Engagement, extension, internal rotation, restitution, expulsion
   d) Descent, flexion, external rotation, restitution, expulsion

4. Which comfort measure most effectively relieves back labor associated with a posterior fetal position?
   a) Semi-reclined positioning
   b) Counterpressure or hands-and-knees
   c) Supine rest
   d) Quiet environment

5. Which maternal adaptation supports normal blood flow during contractions?
   a) Elevated fibrinogen levels
   b) Uterine retraction
   c) Increased cardiac output
   d) Decreased heart rate

6. Which hormone primarily promotes relaxation and bonding after birth?
   a) Estrogen
   b) Cortisol
   c) Oxytocin
   d) Progesterone

7. The most reassuring indicator of progress in second stage is:
   a) Maternal fatigue
   b) Consistent descent and rotation
   c) Contraction frequency alone
   d) Time elapsed since full dilation

8. During second stage, the best indicator of fetal well-being is:
   a) Contraction strength
   b) Fetal heart rate pattern
   c) Maternal urge to push
   d) Amniotic fluid color

9. The most effective position for fetal rotation with back pressure is:
   a) Supine
   b) Side-lying
   c) Hands-and-knees

d) Semi-reclined

10. Which of the following describes a normal contraction pattern in active labor?
    a) Irregular, mild contractions every ten minutes
    b) Strong contractions every two to three minutes lasting about sixty seconds
    c) Continuous uterine tone without relaxation
    d) Random short contractions every twenty minutes

11. The primary powers of labor are:
    a) Voluntary bearing-down efforts
    b) Involuntary uterine contractions
    c) Hormonal regulation of oxytocin
    d) Emotional support from the care team

12. During which pelvic plane does rotation of the fetal head usually occur?
    a) Inlet
    b) Midpelvis
    c) Outlet
    d) Perineum

13. Which maternal position best increases the pelvic outlet diameter?
    a) Supine with legs extended
    b) Semi-reclined
    c) Hands-and-knees or squatting
    d) Sitting with knees together

14. The hormone most responsible for the rhythmic contractions of labor is:
    a) Estrogen
    b) Oxytocin
    c) Relaxin
    d) Progesterone

Fill in the Blank

15. The second stage begins with full cervical _____ and ends with the birth of the _____.
16. The Ferguson reflex stimulates the _____ to push.
17. Crowning occurs when the fetal _____ remains visible between contractions.
18. The best indicator of ongoing fetal health is a reassuring _____ pattern.
19. The uterus contracts most strongly at the _____, a pattern known as fundal dominance.
20. The partial shortening of muscle fibers that thickens the upper uterine segment is called _____.
21. The ridge between the upper and lower uterine segments is known as the _____ ring.
22. Effacement refers to the _____ of the cervix.

Matching

23. Match each term with its correct description. Write the letter in the blank.
    1. ___Gynecoid pelvis   **A.** Emotional and hormonal balance influencing labor
    2. ___Asynclitism   **B.** The uterus as the involuntary force of labor
    3. ___Passenger   **C.** Pelvic type most favorable for vaginal birth
    4. ___Powers   **D.** Fetal head enters pelvis tilted to one side
    5. ___Psyche   **E.** Fetus, membranes, and placenta

24. Match each observation to its clinical meaning.
    1. ___Crowning   **A.** Indicates fetal head is distending tissues and nearing birth
    2. ___Guttural/bearing-down sounds   **B.** Reflects involuntary bearing-down efforts

3. ____ Lengthening perineum   **C.** Suggests perineum is stretching and descent is progressing
4. ____ Slow, controlled breathing   **D.** Helps protect perineal integrity and regulate oxygen flow

True or False
25. _____ Supine positioning improves oxygen flow during second stage.
26. _____ Continuous electronic monitoring is standard for community birth.
27. _____ Nuchal cords always require immediate clamping and cutting.
28. _____ Blood pressure typically decreases during contractions.
29. _____ A slight elevation in temperature can be a normal finding in active labor.
30. _____ The bladder should be emptied at least every two hours during labor.
31. _____ The uterus contracts and fully relaxes between contractions during active labor.
32. _____ Fundal dominance refers to contractions that begin at the lower segment and spread upward.
33. _____ Supine positioning can reduce blood flow to the uterus and cause maternal hypotension.
34. _____ The bag of waters forms during early labor.
35. _____ Mild hyperventilation during labor can cause temporary lightheadedness.
36. _____ Light nourishment and fluids should be encouraged during normal labor.
37. _____ Endorphins help reduce pain perception and promote emotional focus.
38. _____ Internal rotation aligns the occiput with the pelvic outlet.
39. _____ Movement and gravity assist in shortening the duration of labor.
40. _____ Artificial rupture of membranes should be performed routinely to speed labor progress.
41. _____ The Four P's of labor are Passenger, Passage, Powers, and Position.
42. _____ The fetal head usually enters the pelvis in a transverse or oblique orientation.
43. _____ The pelvic outlet is widest in the transverse diameter.
44. _____ Rest between contractions allows for placental reperfusion and fetal oxygenation.
45. _____ Emotional safety and privacy enhance oxytocin release and support effective contractions.
46. _____ Catecholamines released during fear or stress can slow or stall labor progress.
47. _____ The bony pelvis is a fixed structure that cannot change during labor.
48. _____ The Ferguson reflex is triggered when the fetal head presses on the pelvic floor.

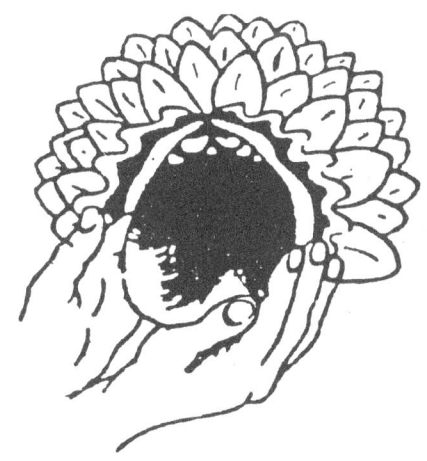

Chapter Eleven Reading & References

Recommended Reading for Labor & Birth

- Buckley, S. ***Gentle Birth, Gentle Mothering*** (2nd ed.). Explores the hormonal physiology of birth, emphasizing calm, privacy, and trust to support safe, satisfying experiences.
- Chapman, V., & Charles, C. ***The Midwife's Labour and Birth Handbook*** (4th ed.). Offers guidance on labor progress, complications, emergencies, and best practices in intrapartum care.
- Coad, J., & Dunstall, M. ***Anatomy and Physiology for Midwives*** (5th ed.). Comprehensive foundation text linking biological systems to the physiology of labor and birth.
- Frye, A. ***Holistic Midwifery, Volume II: Labor and Birth.*** In-depth exploration of physiologic and practical aspects of labor emphasizing individualized, woman-centered care.
- Gaskin, I. M. ***Ina May's Guide to Childbirth*** (Updated ed.). A classic work combining physiology, empowerment, and first-person stories illustrating normal, healthy birth.
- Johnson, R., & Taylor, W. ***Skills for Midwifery Practice*** (5th ed.). Practical guide covering the technical, observational, and communication skills required for intrapartum care.
- Oxnard, C., & Foote, W. ***Anatomy and Mechanics of the Human Birth Process.*** Classic text on the biomechanics of labor, fetal positioning, and maternal structural adaptation.
- Simkin, P., Ancheta, R., & Durham, J. ***The Labor Progress Handbook*** (4th ed.). Practical manual of early interventions to support physiologic progress and prevent dystocia.
- Varney, H., Kriebs, J. M., & Gegor, C. L. ***Varney's Midwifery*** (7th ed.). Comprehensive professional reference covering the full scope of midwifery practice with detailed labor management guidance.
- Walsh, D., & Downe, S. ***Essential Midwifery Practice: Intrapartum Care.*** Evidence-based clinical text promoting normal birth and minimizing unnecessary intervention.

References

Buckley, S. J. (2015). *Gentle birth, gentle mothering: A doctor's guide to natural childbirth and gentle early parenting choices* (2nd ed.). Celestial Arts.

Chapman, V., & Charles, C. (2020). *The midwife's labour and birth handbook* (4th ed.). Wiley-Blackwell.

Coad, J., & Dunstall, M. (2020). *Anatomy and physiology for midwives* (5th ed.). Elsevier.

Davis, E. A. (2019). *Heart and hands: A midwife's guide to pregnancy and birth* (6th ed.). Ten Speed Press.

Frye, A. (2013). *Holistic midwifery: Labor and birth* (Vol. 2). Labrys Press.

Gaskin, I. M. (2003). *Ina May's guide to childbirth*. Bantam Dell.

Johnson, R., & Taylor, W. (2016). *Skills for midwifery practice* (5th ed.). Elsevier.

Lawrence A, Lewis L, Hofmeyr GJ, Styles C. Maternal positions and mobility during first stage labour. *Cochrane Database of Systematic Reviews.* https://pubmed.ncbi.nlm.nih.gov/19370591

Musie MR, Peu MD, Bhana-Pema V. Factors hindering midwives' utilisation of alternative birth positions during labour in a selected public hospital. *African Journal of Primary Health Care & Family Medicine.* 2019. https://phcfm.org/index.php/phcfm/article/view/2071/3338

Odent, M. (2003). *The nature of birth and breastfeeding: Rediscovering the needs of women during pregnancy and childbirth*. Pinter & Martin.

Oxnard, C., & Foote, W. (1975). *Anatomy and mechanics of the human birth process*. Charles C Thomas Publisher.

Queyam, A., Pahuja, S., & Dahiya, D. (2017). Non-invasive feto-maternal well-being monitoring: A review of methods. *Journal of Engineering Science and Technology Review, 10*(1), 177–190. https://doi.org/10.25103/jestr.101.25

Simkin, P., Ancheta, R., & Durham, J. (2018). *The labor progress handbook: Early interventions to prevent and treat dystocia* (4th ed.). Wiley-Blackwell.

Uvnäs-Moberg, K. (2019). *The oxytocin factor: Tapping the hormone of calm, love, and healing* (3rd ed.). Pinter & Martin.

Varney, H., Kriebs, J. M., & Gegor, C. L. (2023). *Varney's midwifery* (7th ed.). Jones & Bartlett Learning.

Walsh, D., & Downe, S. (2010). *Essential midwifery practice: Intrapartum care*. Wiley-Blackwell.

World Health Organization. (2018). *WHO recommendations: Intrapartum care for a positive childbirth experience*. https://www.who.int/reproductivehealth/publications/intrapartum-care-guidelines/en/

Chapter Twelve
Placenta & Postpartum

Objectives
After completing this chapter, the student should be able to:

1. **Describe** the structure, circulation, and membranes of the placenta, including the maternal and fetal surfaces and their interrelationship.

2. **Explain** the major functions of the placenta, including respiratory, nutritional, endocrine, protective, and excretory roles, and their importance in maintaining fetal and maternal physiology.

3. **Identify** the clinical signs of placental separation and describe normal mechanisms of placental expulsion during the third stage of labor.

4. **Discuss** evidence-based management of the third stage of labor, comparing physiologic and active management approaches, and describe methods for assessing and estimating blood loss.

5. **Describe** the normal process and timeline of uterine involution and the progression of lochia as indicators of healing.

6. **Summarize** the physiologic changes of major body systems during the postpartum period, including reproductive, cardiovascular, endocrine, musculoskeletal, urinary, gastrointestinal, and integumentary adaptations.

7. **Identify** common postpartum discomforts, such as perineal pain, uterine cramping, hemorrhoids, and breast tenderness, and describe appropriate comfort and self-care measures.

8. **Describe** essential components and timing of postpartum follow-up care, including vital signs, fundal assessment, lochia, perineal healing, elimination, rest, nutrition, and emotional wellbeing.

9. **Explain** the purpose and key components of the comprehensive six-week postpartum exam, including physical assessment, emotional screening, and family planning discussion.

10. **Identify** and classify perineal and genital tract lacerations by degree and location, including labial, urethral, and vaginal sidewall trauma, and recognize signs of hematoma or infection.

11. **Discuss** the physiologic and emotional significance of the early postpartum or golden hour, including maternal-neonatal bonding, hormonal influences, and uninterrupted skin-to-skin contact.

12. **Describe** the stages of maternal role adaptation and the factors that influence adjustment to parenthood, including support, rest, cultural expectations, and emotional health.

13. **Recognize** the spectrum of postpartum mood and anxiety disorders and outline the midwife's role in screening, support, and referral, including the use of validated screening tools and appropriate follow-up intervals.

Chapter Twelve: Placenta & Postpartum

The placenta and membranes sustain fetal life throughout pregnancy and play a vital role in the safe completion of birth. Together, they form the bridge between mother and child, supporting growth, nourishment, and protection until birth is complete.

During the third and fourth stages of labor, the midwife's role expands from attending the birth of the baby to guiding the physiologic completion of the birth process. Careful observation of placental separation, uterine tone, and maternal adaptation protects against hemorrhage and supports a smooth transition into the postpartum period.

The postpartum phase continues this continuum of care. As the uterus involutes and hormone levels shift, the mother's body restores balance and the family learns new rhythms. Midwives safeguard recovery through presence, teaching, and attentive follow-up, ensuring that healing, bonding, and confidence unfold naturally within the circle of support.

STRUCTURE AND FUNCTION OF THE PLACENTA

The placenta is the primary organ of fetal life support and serves as the interface between the mother and the developing fetus. It maintains pregnancy, provides nutrition and oxygen, removes waste, and produces hormones vital for fetal growth and maternal adaptation. Understanding its structure and function allows midwives to assess normal physiology and recognize early signs of dysfunction.

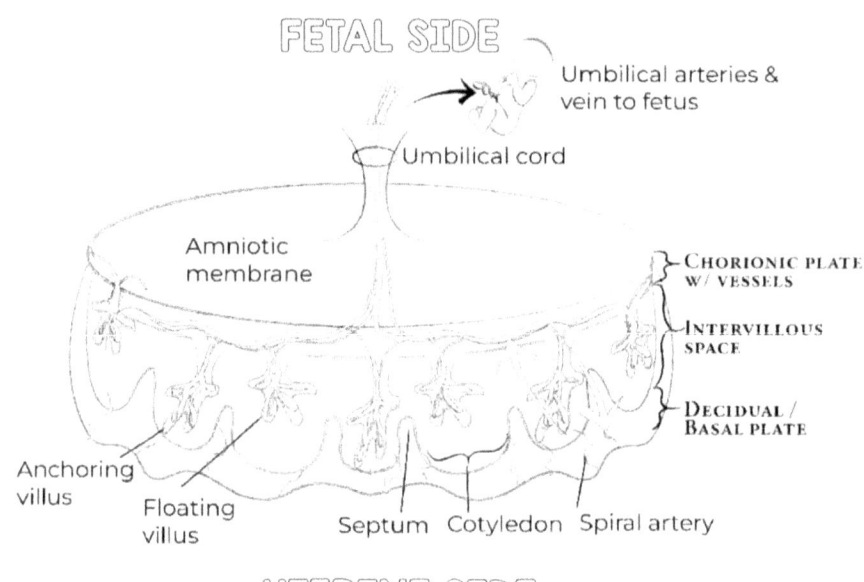

The placenta begins forming soon after implantation, when trophoblastic cells from the fertilized ovum invade the uterine lining to create chorionic villi. These villi burrow into the decidua basalis, establishing intervillous spaces filled with maternal blood. Within the villi, fetal blood circulates through a dense capillary network. Although maternal and fetal blood never mix directly, diffusion and selective transport across thin cellular membranes enable vital exchange.

By the end of the first trimester, the placenta is fully functional. At term it is typically discoid, about 15–20 cm in diameter, 2–3 cm thick, and weighs roughly one-sixth of the newborn's weight.

The **fetal surface** is smooth and glistening, covered by the fused chorion and amnion membranes. Umbilical vessels branch outward from the cord insertion site across this surface.
The **maternal surface** is dark red, lobulated, and divided into 15–20 **cotyledons**, which correspond to attachment areas of the uterine wall. Shallow grooves between them are called sulci, and small calcareous deposits sometimes appear as whitish specks with no clinical significance.

Chapter twelve: Placenta & Postpartum

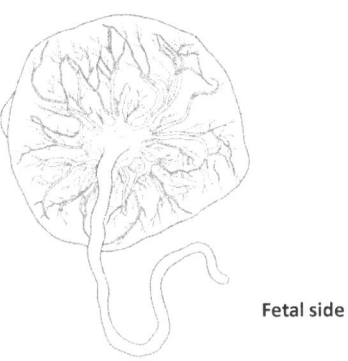
Fetal side

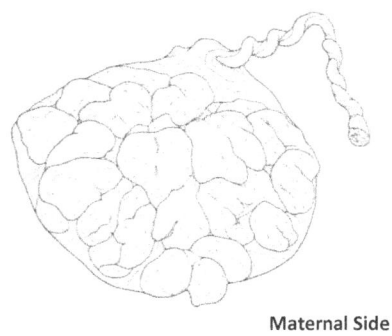
Maternal Side

Placental Variations

While the typical placenta is a single, round organ, variations may occur:

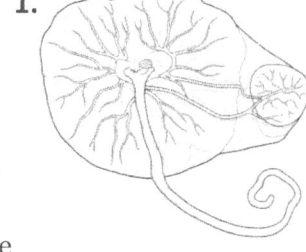

1. **SUCCENTURIATE LOBE** One or more smaller accessory lobes of placental tissue develop separately from the main disc and connect by vessels running through the membranes. These vessels may tear or an accessory lobe may be retained after birth, increasing the risk of postpartum hemorrhage.

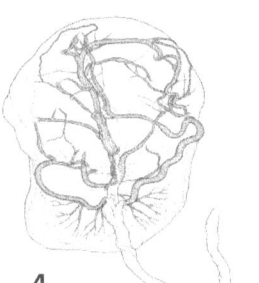

2. **BILOBED PLACENTA** The placental tissue develops as two nearly equal lobes connected by membranes and vessels. This configuration is usually benign but may increase the risk of retained membranes or vasa previa if connecting vessels lie near the cervical os.

3. **CIRCUMVALLATE PLACENTA** The membranes fold back over the placental edge, creating a thickened, raised ring that makes the fetal surface smaller than the maternal surface. This configuration is sometimes linked to antepartum bleeding, placental abruption, or preterm labor.

4. **VELAMENTOUS CORD INSERTION** The umbilical cord inserts into the membranes instead of the placental disc, leaving vessels to travel unprotected before entering the placenta. If these vessels cross the cervix (vasa previa), they can be compressed or rupture during labor, endangering the fetus.

5. **BATTLEDORE INSERTION** The cord attaches at the placental margin rather than near the center, giving a "paddle" or "tennis-racket" appearance. Usually benign, it may occasionally be associated with growth restriction or preterm birth.

MAJOR FUNCTIONS OF THE PLACENTA

1. Respiratory Exchange: Oxygen diffuses from maternal arterial blood (carried as oxyhemoglobin) into fetal blood, while carbon dioxide diffuses in the opposite direction. This gas exchange occurs entirely through diffusion; no direct mixing of maternal and fetal blood occurs.

2. Nutritional Transfer The placenta facilitates nutrient passage from the mother to the fetus. Complex foods are broken down into simpler compounds for easier assimilation. Glucose, amino acids, fatty acids, and electrolytes cross by active or facilitated transport. Fat-soluble vitamins A, D, E, and K pass more slowly and may be stored temporarily within placental tissue.

3. Endocrine Production The placenta functions as a hormone-producing organ, synthesizing progesterone, estrogens, human chorionic gonadotropin (hCG), human placental lactogen (hPL)—also known as human chorionic somatomammotrophic hormone—and several lesser-known peptides that regulate metabolism, fetal growth, and breast preparation for lactation.

4. Protective and Storage Functions: The placenta provides partial immune protection by transferring maternal IgG antibodies to the fetus. It also stores glycogen, iron, and fat-soluble vitamins for short-term use. However, the placental barrier is imperfect—many viruses, medications, alcohol, and other harmful substances cross easily.

5. Excretory Function: The placenta aids in removing carbon dioxide, urea, and other waste products from fetal blood, returning them to the maternal circulation for elimination.

THE THIRD STAGE OF LABOR: BIRTH OF THE PLACENTA

The third stage of labor begins after the birth of the baby and ends with the birth of the placenta and membranes. During this stage, the uterus contracts and retracts to separate and expel the placenta, while the midwife observes closely, supports normal physiology, and remains prepared to respond if separation or bleeding does not proceed as expected.

During this stage, the umbilical cord and fetal membranes play key roles in completing the birth process. As the placenta separates from the uterine wall, the membranes help contain it and guide its expulsion. The umbilical cord provides an external indicator of progress and assists in determining when the placenta has fully separated.

The membranes form the amniotic sac, which attaches around the margins of the placenta. As the uterus contracts, these membranes peel away from the uterine wall and follow the placenta during expulsion. The cord remains attached to the placenta and serves as a visual guide to its descent. Changes in cord tension and length are among the most reliable signs that the placenta has separated and is descending into the lower uterine segment.

As the uterus continues to contract, it becomes smaller and firmer, reducing the surface area at the placental site and helping the placenta detach from the uterine wall. A small amount of blood, usually about 30–60 mL, collects behind the placenta as separation occurs. Once detachment is complete, the uterus contracts strongly to close maternal vessels and minimize bleeding.

If the placenta is delivered before full separation, hemorrhage or retained tissue may result. The midwife's primary tools during this stage are patience, observation, and a calm presence to support the body's natural process.

The third stage of labor begins after the birth of the baby and ends with the birth of the placenta and membranes. During this stage, the uterus continues to contract and retract, separating and expelling the placenta. The midwife's primary tools are patience, observation, and readiness to respond if separation or bleeding does not proceed as expected.

Signs of Placental Separation

Recognizing the signs of placental separation helps determine when it is safe to assist in delivery:

1. **Cord lengthening:** the cord visibly lengthens as the placenta descends. A clamp or hemostat placed near the vulva helps gauge movement.
2. **Gush of blood:** a small gush (about 30–60 mL) may occur as the placenta separates. Not all bleeding indicates completion, so confirm with other signs.
3. **Change in uterine shape and position:** the uterus becomes firm, globular, and rises in the abdomen as the placenta moves into the lower segment.
4. **Maternal awareness:** the mother may feel renewed cramping or an urge to bear down as the placenta is ready to deliver.

Do not massage the uterus or apply fundal pressure before the placenta is expelled. These actions can interfere with natural separation or cause partial detachment.

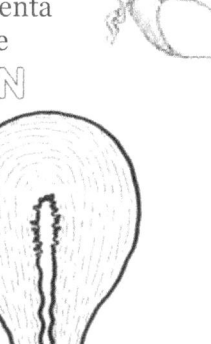

Uterus changing shape

PLACENTA SEPARATION

Mechanisms of Placental Delivery

Two main patterns of placental delivery are recognized:
- **Schultze mechanism:** the placenta separates from the center outward and delivers fetal (shiny) side first. This is the most common pattern and is usually accompanied by minimal bleeding.
- **Matthew-Duncan mechanism:** the placenta separates from the edges first and delivers maternal (rough) side first. Slightly more bleeding may occur before expulsion.

The mechanism cannot be chosen or controlled, but understanding these patterns helps the midwife interpret the timing and amount of bleeding during the third stage.

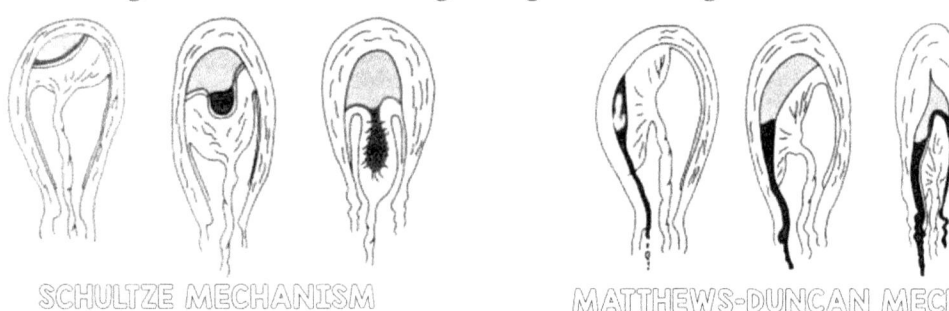

Steps in Third Stage Care

The safest third stage is one that progresses naturally with minimal interference and attentive observation. Calm presence, respect for physiology, and timely action when needed form the foundation of effective midwifery care.

1. **Observe and measure blood loss.**
   Normal blood loss averages 250–500 mL (one to two cups). Chart the estimated amount and monitor pulse, blood pressure, and uterine tone frequently. A rising pulse is often the earliest sign of excessive loss.
2. **Encourage uterine contractions.**
   Support early breastfeeding or gentle nipple stimulation to increase natural oxytocin release. Ensure the bladder is empty, since a full bladder can inhibit placental descent.
3. **Wait for placental separation.**
   Most placentas deliver spontaneously within 5–30 minutes. Encourage gentle pushing only when signs of separation are present.
4. **Assist with controlled cord traction.**
   Once separation is confirmed and the uterus is firm, apply steady downward traction on the cord while supporting the uterus above the pubic bone.
5. Allow the **placenta** to slide out slowly, **twisting it gently** to help the membranes follow intact. Do not pull forcefully or prematurely.
6. **Perform fundal massage after delivery.**
   Massage the uterus firmly while "guarding" it with the other hand just above the symphysis pubis to prevent inversion. This helps expel clots and promotes contraction to minimize blood loss.
7. **Administer a uterotonic.**
   Depending on birth setting and protocol, oxytocin is usually given after the birth of the baby or placenta to support uterine tone and prevent hemorrhage.

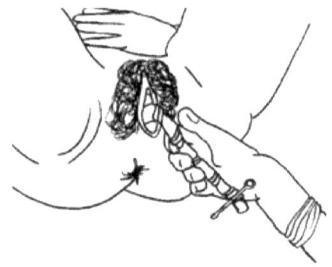
Controlled Cord Traction

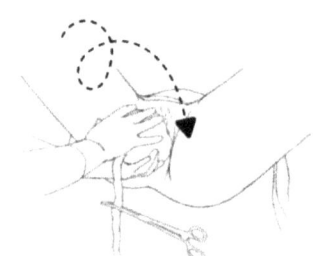
Twisting as placenta slides out

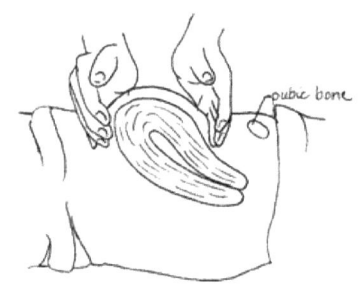
Guarding the uterus

Chapter twelve: Placenta & Postpartum

Exercise 12.1: Structure and Function of the Placenta
Match each placental structure or function with its correct description.

1. ____Chorionic villi
2. ____Decidua basalis
3. ____Intervillous spaces
4. ____Amnion and chorion
5. ____Umbilical cord
6. ____Fetal surface
7. ____Maternal surface
8. ____Endocrine function
9. ____Nutritional function
10. ____Respiratory function

A. Outer fetal membrane that contributes to the placenta's formation
B. Network of finger-like projections that allow exchange between maternal and fetal blood
C. Stores nutrients and provides a partial immune barrier between mother and fetus
D. Maternal tissue layer where the placenta implants
E. Contains two arteries and one vein that transport blood between fetus and placenta
F. Smooth, glistening membrane covered by amnion where umbilical vessels branch outward
G. Rough, lobulated surface divided into cotyledons
H. Produces hormones like progesterone, estrogen, hCG, and hPL
I. Transfers glucose, amino acids, and other nutrients to the fetus
J. Facilitates diffusion of oxygen to the fetus and removal of carbon dioxide

Cord Blood Collection and Banking:

Cord blood may be collected for two main purposes: **newborn blood typing** and **cord blood banking** (including donation or storage for future medical use).

1. Newborn blood typing: when the mother's blood type is O or Rh negative, a small cord blood sample is collected after birth to determine the newborn's ABO and Rh type. This helps identify possible incompatibility and determines whether Rh immune globulin (Rhogam) is needed to prevent sensitization in future pregnancies. This sample is taken while the cord remains intact and pulsating and does **not** interfere with delayed cord clamping.

2. Donation, research, or family banking: families may choose to donate or store cord blood for potential future medical use. These collections are usually performed while the cord is still intact and pulsating. Although they do not require early clamping, removing larger volumes for banking may slightly reduce the amount of blood transferred to the newborn during placental transfusion. Midwives should provide accurate information about cord blood options, obtain informed consent before birth, and document any collection. Families planning donation or banking should make arrangements early with their care team to ensure proper timing and safety.

Exercise 12.2: Management of the Third Stage of Labor
Write the number 1–7 in the correct order to reflect physiologic third-stage management.

____Support early breastfeeding or nipple stimulation to enhance natural oxytocin release.

____Observe for signs of placental separation such as cord lengthening, gush of blood, and change in uterine shape.

____Wait for spontaneous separation while monitoring maternal vitals and estimated blood loss.

____Collect cord blood sample for newborn typing or cord blood banking, if indicated, while the cord remains intact and pulsating.

____Once separation is confirmed, assist with gentle, controlled cord traction while supporting the uterus.

____Deliver the placenta slowly, twisting it slightly to help membranes follow intact.

____Perform firm fundal massage while guarding the uterus to expel clots and ensure contraction.

Assessment of Blood Loss

Evaluating blood loss accurately during the third stage of labor is one of the midwife's most important responsibilities. Even small errors in estimation can delay recognition of hemorrhage. Combining visual and quantitative methods provides the best protection for maternal safety.

Qualitative Assessment (Visual Estimation)

Visual estimation, or *estimated blood loss* (EBL), involves judging the color, amount, and spread of blood on pads, chux, and linens. While convenient, this approach alone often underestimates actual loss by 30 to 50 percent. Regular practice and comparison with measured results improve accuracy.

Quantitative Blood Loss (QBL)

Quantitative blood loss is a measured method that provides a more accurate picture of total loss and is now standard in many birth centers and hospitals.

Steps in QBL:
1. Use graduated containers to collect and measure blood from under-buttocks drapes or suction canisters.
2. Weigh blood-soaked items with a digital scale (zero out first). One gram equals one milliliter of blood. *Example:* A chux pad weighing 200 g dry and 450 g wet contains 250 mL of blood.
3. Add all sources, including blood from pads, gauze, and any clots expelled after delivery, to obtain a total QBL.
4. Record findings promptly and reassess if bleeding continues.

> **Helpful Visual Guides**
> - A 50 mL spot on most chux or underpads is about 4–5 inches across, roughly the width of an adult palm.
> - A 100 mL pool fills the center of a chux pad and begins to spread outward.
> - A 250 mL loss saturates half of a standard pad.
> - A 500 mL loss soaks through the entire pad or forms a visible puddle beneath the mother.
> - When blood mixes with amniotic fluid, reassess carefully because dilution can disguise true volume.

When to Be Concerned

- **Normal blood loss:** up to 500 mL after vaginal birth
- **Early warning:** 500–1000 mL or any quantitative blood loss with clinical signs of maternal compromise such as tachycardia, hypotension, pallor, or dizziness
- **Hemorrhage:** more than 1000 mL or any amount accompanied by tachycardia, pallor, dizziness, or delayed uterine contraction

Frequent pulse and blood-pressure checks during the third stage help identify early signs of hypovolemia before visible symptoms appear. Developing an "eye for blood loss" by comparing visual estimates with weighed measurements builds clinical accuracy over time.

Maternal Comfort and the Golden Hour

The first hour after birth, often called the *golden hour*, marks a powerful physiologic shift in the mother's body. As the uterus empties and contracts, blood from the uterine sinuses returns to circulation, briefly increasing cardiac output and stabilizing vital signs.

At the same time, catecholamines that surged during pushing begin to fall, allowing the parasympathetic nervous system to create a sense of calm, warmth, and relaxation. Oxytocin remains elevated, stimulating uterine contraction to prevent bleeding while promoting feelings of connection and safety. Rising prolactin levels prepare the breasts for lactation and reinforce nurturing behavior.

Environmental factors strongly influence this balance. A quiet, dimly lit space and uninterrupted skin-to-skin contact help maintain oxytocin flow and parasympathetic dominance, supporting uterine tone and early lactation. Bright light, noise, or unnecessary procedures raise stress hormones such as cortisol, which can slow uterine involution and delay milk let-down.

Midwives can enhance the golden hour by maintaining warmth and privacy, encouraging rest, offering fluids, and supporting early breastfeeding and comfortable positioning. When the environment supports this transition, the body's natural hormones complete their work—closing vessels, initiating milk production, and grounding the early bond between mother and baby.

Inspection of the Placenta and Cord

After the placenta and membranes are delivered, they should always be examined for completeness and normal appearance. This inspection confirms that no fragments remain in the uterus—which could lead to bleeding or infection—and provides important information about fetal health and placental function. Midwives routinely perform and document this examination at every birth.

Placenta

Place the placenta on a flat surface with the **maternal side facing up**. Ensure all cotyledons are present and none are missing or torn. Missing sections may indicate retained tissue.

- Check for **hematomas**, which appear as dark, raised areas of clotted blood under the surface and may indicate partial abruption or vascular compromise during pregnancy.
- Small white or gritty areas known as **calcareous deposits** are often seen, especially in post-term placentas, and are usually benign.

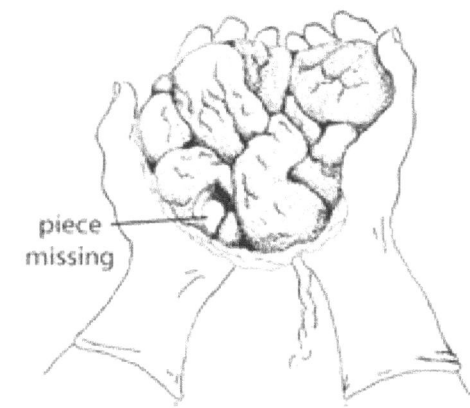

Next, turn the placenta over to view the **fetal surface**, which should appear smooth and glistening with a gray-blue tint. Confirm that the membranes are intact and note the point and type of **cord insertion** (central, marginal, or velamentous).

- A healthy placenta is typically about 20 cm in diameter, 2–3 cm thick, and weighs 400–600 g
- Minor findings such as small infarcts, calcifications, or marginal insertions are common and generally not concerning.

Membranes

Spread the membranes out gently to confirm they form a complete circle around the placental edge.

- Identify both layers: the **amnion** (thin and shiny) and the **chorion** (thicker and opaque).
- Torn or missing membranes suggest that part may remain inside the uterus.
- Check for a **succenturiate lobe**, a small accessory lobe connected by membranes, which increases the risk of retained tissue and postpartum hemorrhage.

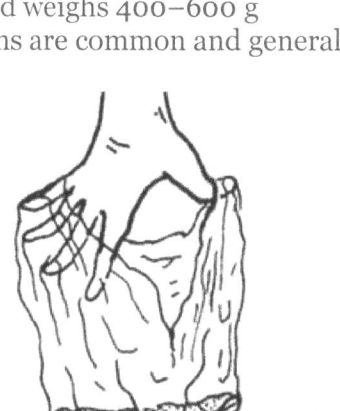

Umbilical Cord

Inspect the umbilical cord for its characteristics and integrity.

- Note **length, coiling, and color.** A normal cord is about 50–60 cm long.
- A **short cord** (under 30 cm) may be associated with delayed descent or traction during birth, while a **long cord** increases the likelihood of loops or knots.
- **True knots** form before birth and are usually harmless if loose; **false knots** are simply folds in the vessels within Wharton's jelly.
- Confirm the presence of **three vessels**—two arteries and one vein. A **two-vessel cord** should be documented, as it may occasionally be associated with congenital anomalies.
- Note the **cord insertion type** (central, marginal, or velamentous) and record any abnormalities, such as hematomas, thrombosis, or color changes.

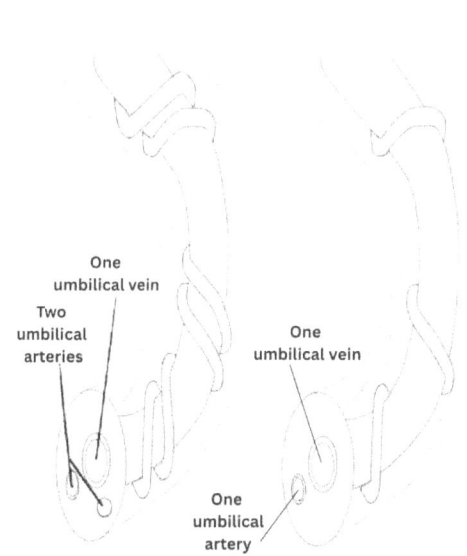

Documentation

After inspection, record findings promptly and completely, including:
- Time and mechanism of placental delivery (**Schultze** or **Matthews–Duncan**)
- Appearance of maternal and fetal surfaces
- Cord length, insertion type, and number of vessels
- Completeness of membranes and presence of accessory lobes
- Estimated or measured blood loss
- Any abnormalities (hematoma, infarct, calcification, or others)
- Whether a specimen was sent for pathology

Cultural and Traditional Practices

Across many cultures, the placenta is viewed as sacred, a companion to the newborn and a symbol of the bond between mother, child, and the earth. Rituals surrounding its handling reflect beliefs about health, protection, and the cycle of life. Respecting each family's tradition, whether ceremonial, artistic, or spiritual, honors the deep meaning that surrounds the placenta in every culture. In many Indigenous and traditional societies, the placenta is buried as an act of honoring and reconnection.

- **Navajo (Diné)** families may bury the placenta near their home so the child will always have a spiritual tie to family and homeland.
- Among the **Māori** of Aotearoa (New Zealand), *whenua* means both "placenta" and "land." Burying the *whenua* returns the child's life essence to the earth, linking them to their ancestors and place of birth.
- **Hawaiian** families often bury the *iewe* (placenta) with a tree, symbolizing growth and life.
- In **Malaysia**, families may bury the placenta beneath the home with objects such as pencils or books to encourage wisdom and learning.
- In **Turkey**, it may be buried near a mosque so the child will grow to be devout.
  In many regions, the placenta is ritually washed, wrapped in cloth, and buried in a special vessel, sometimes with herbs or offerings, before planting a tree above it to symbolize continued life.
- Some European traditions, such as those once practiced in **Hungary**, involved burning the placenta to prevent future pregnancies.
- In parts of East Africa, including Tanzanian groups such as the **Chaga**, the dried placenta may be kept before burial as a symbol of family continuity. Among several West and East African societies, the placenta is buried under trees, near the home, or in a family compound to connect the child to the land, protect against harm, and honor ancestral ties. In some **Nigerian** and **Ghanaian** communities, the placenta is viewed as the baby's deceased twin or spiritual companion and is buried with rituals to safeguard the child's destiny. In **Zambian** and **Kenyan** cultures, burial beneath a fertility tree or at specific locations reflects beliefs about fertility, future well-being, and familial belonging. **Ethiopian** traditions also include placenta burial customs that vary by region and gender of the newborn, where the placenta's burial site conveys cultural beliefs about lineage, home, and child-parent connection. In several belief systems, the placenta is regarded as the baby's twin, guardian, or spiritual double, a being deserving of gratitude and respect.

Placentophagy

Some families choose to consume the placenta as part of cultural or personal belief. It may be eaten raw, cooked, or prepared through dehydration and encapsulation. A few small studies have explored possible benefits such as improved mood or increased milk supply, but no strong evidence supports these claims. Midwives should provide balanced information and support safe handling if families choose this practice.

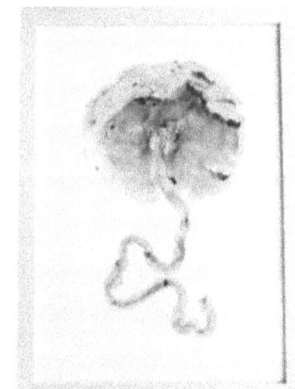

Placenta Prints and Keepsakes

Many families today create placenta prints, artistic impressions made by pressing the placenta onto paper to reveal its branching vessels that resemble a "tree of life." Some use the placenta's natural color, while others apply natural pigments to create keepsake art. Umbilical cords may also be dried into spiral or heart shapes, symbolizing continuity and love.

Exercise 12.3: Placenta and Cord Inspection
Match each term with its correct description.

1. ____Cotyledon
2. ____Hematoma
3. ____Calcareous deposit
4. ____True knot
5. ____False knot
6. ____Amnion
7. ____Chorion
8. ____Two-vessel cord
9. ____Velamentous insertion
10. ____Succenturiate lobe

A. Raised, dark area of clotted blood beneath the maternal surface.
B. Folded area of vessel within Wharton's jelly that resembles a knot.
C. Finger-like lobule on the maternal surface that forms part of the placental structure.
D. Dense, gritty white spot often found in post-term placentas; usually benign.
E. Actual loop formed in the cord before birth; usually harmless if loose.
F. Inner, thin, transparent fetal membrane that covers the placenta.
G. Outer, thicker fetal membrane lying beneath the decidua.
H. Umbilical cord variation with one artery and one vein; may require follow-up.
I. Cord attaches to membranes before reaching the placental disc.
J. Small accessory placental lobe connected by membranes.

POSTPARTUM PHYSIOLOGY

The postpartum period, or puerperium, encompasses the six weeks following birth. During this time, every organ system gradually returns toward its pre-pregnant state while adapting to lactation, emotional change, and the work of caring for a newborn. The midwife's role is to observe normal recovery, recognize early signs of imbalance, and support the body's natural restoration process.

Integumentary System

Stretch marks and the linea nigra fade as hormone levels stabilize. Temporary hair loss is common between two and four months postpartum as hair follicles shift back to their normal growth pattern. Profuse sweating, especially at night, occurs as the body eliminates excess plasma and regulates temperature. Persistent dryness or slow wound healing can signal dehydration or nutritional depletion, so hydration and meals rich in protein, zinc, and vitamin C are encouraged to promote tissue repair.

Musculoskeletal System

The hormone relaxin may remain in circulation for several weeks, keeping joints and ligaments looser than normal and increasing the risk of strain. Pelvic stability improves as muscles regain tone. Gentle movement, walking, and pelvic floor exercises are helpful, while heavy lifting and strenuous workouts should be postponed until stability returns. Coccyx soreness or pelvic discomfort from birth positioning usually resolves within a few weeks but may need attention if persistent. Observing how a mother moves, stands, or walks offers useful clues to her comfort and recovery.

Respiratory System

With the uterus no longer pressing on the diaphragm, lung expansion improves, and breathing feels easier. Most women experience an immediate sense of relief and deeper respiration. Shortness of breath that continues beyond the first few days may suggest anemia, fluid overload, or, rarely, cardiomyopathy and should be evaluated promptly.

Urinary System

Increased urination during the first few days helps remove up to two liters of excess fluid. Swelling or bruising near the urethra can make urination difficult, and pain from small tears may cause hesitancy. A distended bladder can push the uterus upward and increase bleeding, so midwives monitor bladder fullness and encourage frequent voiding. If no urination occurs within six hours of birth, gentle assessment and possible intervention are warranted. Stress incontinence is common during early recovery but generally improves with pelvic floor strengthening.

Gastrointestinal System

Bowel movements often resume within two to three days. Mild constipation, hemorrhoids, or fear of pain can delay the first movement. Warm fluids, fiber, gentle walking, and relaxation help restore normal function. The gut microbiome also plays a role in postpartum mood and immunity, and foods containing probiotics or fermented ingredients may support both digestion and emotional balance.

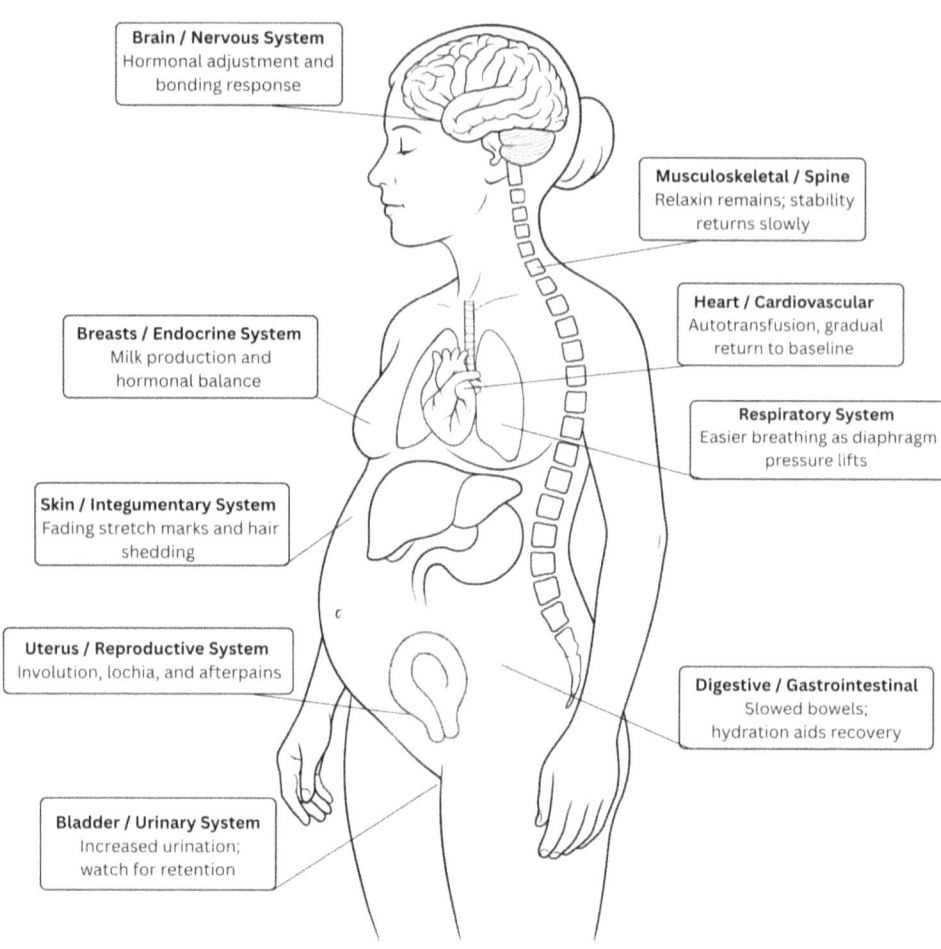

Postpartum Physiological Changes

Nervous System

Tremors or chills are common in the minutes following birth and typically last 10–20 minutes. They result from hormone shifts and temperature regulation rather than infection. Quiet reassurance and physical warmth usually bring comfort. Heightened sensitivity—such as sharper hearing, a keener sense of smell, or emotional intensity—is also normal, as the nervous system integrates hormonal and sensory changes. Any tremors accompanied by fever or confusion should be assessed for infection or blood loss.

Cardiovascular System

When the uterus contracts after birth, blood from the placental site returns to circulation, temporarily increasing cardiac output. This rise helps maintain blood pressure and oxygen delivery despite normal blood loss. Over the next several days, diuresis and sweating reduce plasma volume, and heart rate gradually stabilizes. A slower pulse is common for a few days as the heart adjusts to increased stroke volume. The body remains slightly hypercoagulable for several weeks, which aids healing but increases the risk of blood clots. Early ambulation, leg movement, and hydration are simple, effective ways to prevent thrombosis.

Endocrine System

After the placenta is delivered, estrogen and progesterone levels drop sharply, while prolactin rises to initiate milk production. Oxytocin released during breastfeeding strengthens uterine contraction and fosters emotional bonding. Temporary thyroid suppression may cause fatigue or low mood. Hormonal shifts often produce mood swings or "baby blues," which typically resolve within two weeks. Persistent sadness, anxiety, or detachment signals the need for further evaluation and support.

Uterine and Reproductive Recovery

Immediately after birth, the uterus begins **involution**, the process of contracting and shrinking to close blood vessels at the placental site and return to its pre-pregnant size. At birth, it weighs about **1000 grams** and can be felt at or just below the umbilicus. The fundus descends approximately **one centimeter (one fingerbreadth) per day** and is usually no longer palpable by the tenth day. By one week, it weighs around **500 grams**, by two weeks about **350 grams**, and by six weeks it returns to **60–90 grams**.

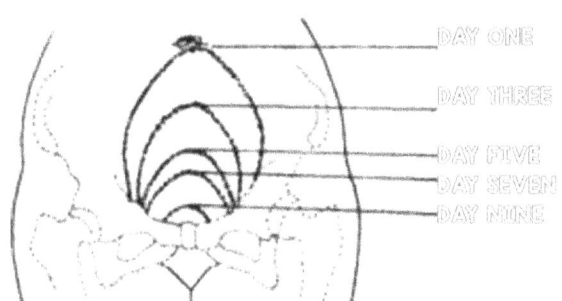

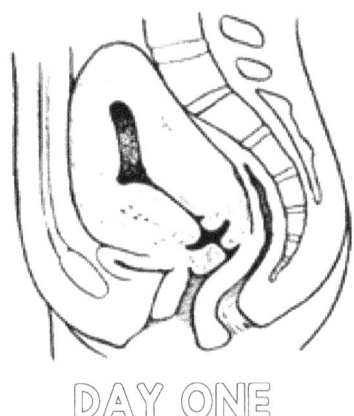
DAY ONE

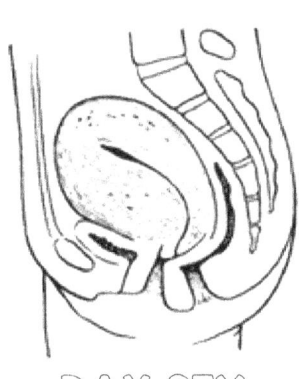
DAY SIX

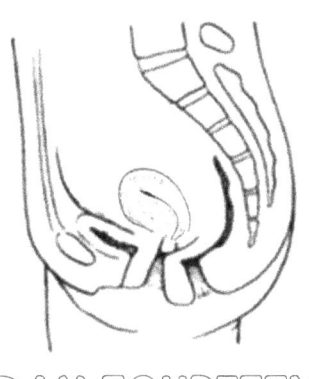
DAY FOURTEEN

Contractions known as **afterpains** assist this process and may cause discomfort, especially in multiparous women. These cramps often intensify during breastfeeding due to oxytocin release and typically subside by the fifth day. Breastfeeding, adequate hydration, and gentle rest support uterine recovery. Persistent or severe pain, however, may indicate infection or retained fragments and should be evaluated.

As involution progresses, the superficial layer of the decidua undergoes **autolysis**, breaking down and shedding through the vaginal flow known as **lochia**. Lochia is composed of blood, exfoliated decidua, epithelial cells, and leukocytes.

- **Lochia rubra:** dark red discharge, moderate flow for the first 3–4 days.
- **Lochia serosa:** pink or brownish discharge from about day 4–10.
- **Lochia alba:** pale yellow or white discharge lasting 2–6 weeks.

An increase in bright red bleeding after it has lightened, especially if accompanied by clots, odor, or uterine tenderness, requires assessment for infection or retained tissue. A firm, midline fundus indicates good tone, while a boggy or displaced uterus suggests bladder distention or uterine atony.

Perineum and Vaginal Tissue

The perineum heals quickly due to its rich blood supply. Minor lacerations or skin splits usually heal within a week, while deeper tears or episiotomy repairs may take longer. Swelling peaks within 24 hours and then gradually subsides. Applying ice in the first day and using warm sitz baths after the initial 24 hours help reduce swelling and increase circulation.

A drop in estrogen levels, especially in breastfeeding mothers, can cause temporary dryness and reduced elasticity of vaginal tissue. This may make early intercourse uncomfortable. Reassure mothers that these changes are normal and will resolve as hormone balance returns. Lubrication, gentle communication, and adequate rest support comfort and confidence during recovery.

Breasts

Colostrum production begins during pregnancy and continues immediately after birth. By day three to five, transitional milk replaces colostrum, and the breasts may feel full or tender as milk volume increases. Frequent nursing or expression relieves engorgement and helps establish supply. Warm compresses before feeding promote milk flow, while cool compresses afterward reduce swelling.

Firm, localized tenderness may indicate a blocked duct, which can usually be relieved by massage, continued feeding, and ensuring complete drainage. Persistent pain, fever, or redness suggests mastitis and requires evaluation. Breast changes reflect both endocrine adaptation and infant feeding patterns, so midwives monitor for comfort, temperature, and symmetry.

Menstrual Cycle and Sexual Health

Ovulation and menstruation remain suppressed in most breastfeeding mothers due to high prolactin levels. This **lactational amenorrhea** may last up to a year with frequent, around-the-clock nursing. As prolactin levels fall with reduced feeding, ovarian function gradually resumes.

Low estrogen levels during this time can cause decreased libido and vaginal dryness, contributing to discomfort during intercourse. Open discussion about these temporary changes helps normalize the experience. Reassure that sexual interest and comfort typically improve with rest, hormonal recovery, and adequate lubrication.

SUMMARY OF PHYSIOLOGIC RECOVERY BY TIMEFRAME

Time Period	Primary Changes	Midwifery Focus
First 24 hours	Autotransfusion, diuresis, uterine contraction	Monitor bleeding, fundal tone, and vital signs
Days 1–3	Afterpains, lochia rubra, perineal swelling	Encourage rest, hydration, and early mobility
Days 3–10	Lochia serosa, milk onset, joint tightening	Support lactation and monitor emotional well-being
10 days–6 weeks	Involution complete, lochia alba, hormonal balance	Guide gradual return to activity and assess overall health

---

Exercise 12.4: Postpartum System Changes
Match each body system with its primary postpartum adaptation.

1. _____ Integumentary
2. _____ Musculoskeletal
3. _____ Respiratory
4. _____ Urinary
5. _____ Gastrointestinal
6. _____ Nervous
7. _____ Cardiovascular
8. _____ Endocrine
9. _____ Reproductive
10. _____ Breasts

A. Involution and lochia progression
B. Autotransfusion and mild bradycardia
C. Fading linea nigra, sweating, and hair shedding
D. Drop in estrogen and progesterone; prolactin rise
E. Diuresis and temporary incontinence
F. Easier breathing as diaphragm pressure resolves
G. Tremors, chills, and emotional sensitivity
H. Relaxin persists; gradual return of tone
I. Constipation and sluggish peristalsis
J. Milk production, engorgement, and tenderness

Postpartum Discomforts and Comfort Measures

Mild to moderate discomfort is normal in the postpartum period. Healing, hormonal shifts, and fluid changes create predictable patterns of soreness and fatigue. The midwife's role is to distinguish between normal recovery and early signs of complication, offering comfort measures that support physiology. Observation, reassurance, and simple practical care often provide as much benefit as medical intervention. Most discomforts resolve within the first two weeks, but awareness of their timing, location, and intensity helps identify concerns early.

Uterine Cramping (Afterpains)

Afterpains result from uterine involution and the release of oxytocin during breastfeeding or nipple stimulation. They are stronger in multiparous mothers and usually last three to five days postpartum. Intermittent cramps that coincide with nursing are expected, but continuous or severe pain may suggest retained tissue, infection, or clot formation.

Comfort measures include frequent voiding to prevent bladder distention, relaxed breathing, and gentle movement. Ibuprofen can be used when pain interferes with rest. Once bleeding and uterine tone are stable, a warm compress on the lower abdomen may ease discomfort. Normal cramping with a firm fundus indicates effective uterine contraction and protection from hemorrhage.

Perineal and Vaginal Discomfort

Perineal soreness is common after birth due to stretching, small tears, or surgical repair. Swelling peaks within the first 24 hours and gradually subsides. Mild bruising and tenderness are expected, but increasing pain, hematoma formation, or separation of sutures requires evaluation.

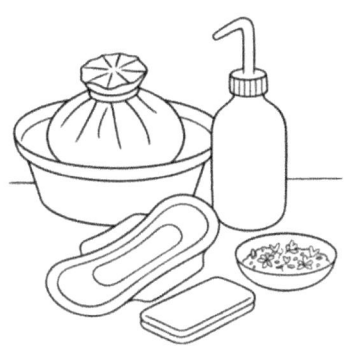

Ice packs or cold compresses during the first day reduce swelling, followed by warm sitz baths to promote circulation and healing. However, in many traditional care systems, exposure to cold, wind, or drafts is believed to slow healing and disturb body balance. Midwives should honor cultural preferences whenever possible. Gentle compression with cloths at room temperature can also provide relief without cold exposure.

Resting in a side-lying position, using peri-bottle rinses with warm water, and keeping the area clean all help prevent irritation. If pain persists with a firm uterus and normal bleeding, inspect for a possible hematoma rather than assuming normal discomfort.

Perineal Comfort Care Checklist
☐ Use peri bottle with warm water or sage/uva ursi tea after voiding.
☐ Keep area clean and dry; change pads frequently.
☐ Apply ice packs in first 24 hours; use warm sitz baths afterward.
☐ Avoid powdered herbs or salves directly on tears.
☐ Rest in side-lying position; avoid prolonged sitting or squatting.
☐ Use witch hazel pads for itching or swelling.
☐ Report increasing pain, foul odor, or difficulty urinating promptly.

Hemorrhoids and Rectal Pressure

Hemorrhoids are common after birth, caused by venous pressure during pushing and increased intra-abdominal strain. They often worsen temporarily in the first week. Relief measures include cool compresses or witch hazel, hydration, high-fiber foods, and stool softeners to ease passage. Gentle walking improves circulation and prevents congestion.

Mothers should be reassured that most hemorrhoids regress within a few weeks. If bright red bleeding is observed, confirm the source is rectal rather than vaginal before documenting blood loss.

Breast and Nipple Discomfort

Breast tenderness and fullness occur as milk transitions from colostrum to mature milk between days three and five. Engorgement results from increased blood flow and milk volume. Both breasts should feel full and soften after feeding; one-sided pain, redness, or fever may indicate a blocked duct or mastitis.

Comfort measures include frequent breastfeeding or gentle expression, warm compresses before feeding, and cool compresses afterward to reduce swelling. Supportive but nonrestrictive bras help prevent congestion. A few drops of expressed milk can soothe sore nipples and should be air-dried after feeding. Regular, complete emptying maintains comfort and supply while preventing overfilling.

Fatigue and General Muscle Soreness

Postpartum fatigue is universal. Labor depletes muscle glycogen and electrolytes, and hormonal changes may disrupt normal sleep cycles. Diaphoresis and fluid shifts further contribute to exhaustion. Encourage frequent rest, hydration, and balanced meals rich in protein and iron. Gentle stretching and light activity help restore circulation and energy. Fatigue usually peaks around day three and gradually improves. Persistent exhaustion, pallor, or mood changes should prompt assessment for anemia, thyroid imbalance, or infection.

When Discomfort Becomes a Warning Sign

Pain or fatigue that increases rather than improves may indicate developing complications.
Warning signs include:
- Bleeding that becomes heavier or includes large clots
- Fever over 100.4°F (38°C)
- Unilateral breast pain or redness with chills
- Calf pain, swelling, or warmth
- Persistent dizziness, pallor, or malaise: midwives should recheck vital signs, uterine tone, and bladder function, and seek consultation if infection, deep vein thrombosis, or hemorrhage is suspected. Many serious conditions begin with discomfort that feels "different" or disproportionate to the exam findings. Listening carefully to a mother's report of pain or fatigue is often the first step in early recognition.

Exercise 12.5: Postpartum Comfort Measures
Match each postpartum discomfort with the most appropriate comfort measure or herbal support.

1. _____ Uterine cramping (afterpains)
2. _____ Perineal soreness or swelling
3. _____ Breast engorgement
4. _____ Hemorrhoids or rectal pressure
5. _____ Fatigue and night sweats
6. _____ Constipation
7. _____ Perineal healing (episiotomy or tears)
8. _____ Emotional sensitivity or "baby blues"
9. _____ General muscle soreness

A. Sitz baths with calendula or comfrey infusion to promote healing
B. Nipple care with expressed milk or lanolin; frequent nursing
C. Gentle heat or red raspberry leaf tea to ease cramping and support tone
D. Warm fluids, fiber, and dandelion tea to aid bowel movement
E. Nettles or oatstraw tea to rebuild strength and replace minerals
F. Witch hazel compresses and avoiding prolonged sitting
G. Ice in first 24 hours, then warm soaks and rest
H. Gentle exercise, hydration, and magnesium-rich foods
I. Lemon balm or motherwort tea for calming and hormonal support

Genital and Perineal Assessment and Care

The tissues of the vulva, vagina, and perineum stretch extensively during birth. While the perineum often bears the most visible strain, tears and bruising can also occur in the labia, clitoral hood, urethral area, and vaginal walls. These structures are richly supplied with blood vessels, so even minor trauma may appear dramatic or bleed heavily. Postpartum assessment of the entire genital area is an essential midwifery skill. Careful visualization allows early recognition of injuries that might otherwise be missed, preventing excessive bleeding, infection, or long-term discomfort. The goal of care is to identify trauma accurately, support healing, and ensure that the client can rest and recover comfortably. Suturing techniques and repair methods are taught separately in the clinical skills sequence.

Laceration Classification
Perineal tears are classified by the structures involved:
- **First degree:** involves only the skin and mucosa.
- **Second degree:** extends into the perineal muscles.
- **Third degree:** involves the anal sphincter.
- **Fourth degree:** extends into the rectal mucosa.

Small first-degree or periurethral tears often heal without suturing if bleeding is minimal and edges are well aligned. Second-degree or deeper tears generally require repair. At each postpartum visit, inspect for redness, separation, or discharge, and explain that absorbable sutures dissolve gradually, sometimes causing mild itching or pulling.

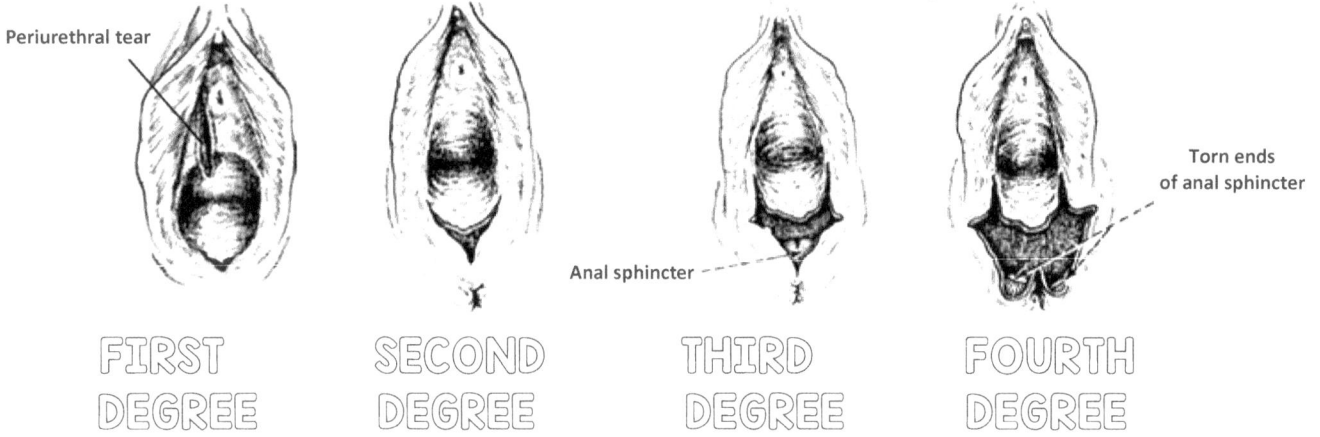

Recognition of Hematoma and Excessive Bleeding

Hematomas develop when a blood vessel is injured beneath intact tissue, allowing blood to collect and form a firm swelling. They most often appear within the first few hours after birth, typically unilaterally in the labia or perineum. Persistent pain with minimal bleeding often signals hematoma.

Early signs include deep pelvic or rectal pressure, localized pain out of proportion to visible trauma, or one-sided swelling that feels tense and warm. Because bleeding is concealed, the external flow may appear normal while the client shows restlessness, pallor, or rising pulse. Bleeding from tears, in contrast, is usually brisk and visible. Bright red flow from the vaginal opening despite a firm fundus suggests a genital tract source rather than uterine atony. Inspection with good lighting is essential to locate and control the site.

Exercise 12.6: Perineal Laceration Classification	
Match each degree of tear with the structures involved.	
1. _____ First degree	A. Involves only the skin and vaginal mucosa
2. _____ Second degree	B. Extends into the perineal muscles
3. _____ Third degree	C. Includes the anal sphincter
4. _____ Fourth degree	D. Extends through the rectal mucosa

Assessment Technique

Examine the genital area after placental delivery when bleeding is stable. Explain the procedure, ensure privacy, and use warm lighting and clean technique.

Inspect systematically from the urethra toward the anus:
1. **Urethral and clitoral region:** check for small splits or abrasions that may sting during urination or bleed freely.
2. **Labia and vaginal walls:** separate the labia gently to visualize both sides. Note any linear or deeper tears and document their location, size, and depth.
3. **Perineum:** observe color, swelling, bruising, and tissue integrity. Palpate gently if tolerated to assess firmness and symmetry.

Even small periurethral or labial lacerations should be recorded since they may swell later or interfere with urination. Persistent pain with minimal bleeding often indicates a hematoma rather than normal bruising and warrants further assessment.

Normal Tissue Response and Healing

After birth, it is common to see generalized swelling, mild bruising, and tenderness in the vulvar and perineal tissues. This is a normal inflammatory response that protects against infection and initiates repair.

Healing occurs in three overlapping stages:
- **Inflammatory phase (first 24–48 hours):** small vessels constrict, white blood cells clear debris, and swelling peaks.
- **Proliferative phase (days 2–10):** granulation tissue and new epithelial cells form to close small breaks in the skin.
- **Remodeling phase (weeks 2–6):** collagen fibers strengthen and tenderness gradually subsides.

A small amount of serosanguinous drainage is expected in the first day. Pain and swelling should steadily decrease by the end of the first week. Any increase in pain, swelling, or bleeding after initial improvement warrants re-evaluation.

Regardless of temperature preference, hygiene is essential. The vulvar area should be rinsed with warm water after urination or stooling and gently dried. Loose clothing and breathable fabrics prevent irritation. Over-the-counter analgesics such as ibuprofen can be used when appropriate and within the midwife's prescribing parameters.

Indicators of Infection or Delayed Healing

Signs of infection include redness spreading beyond wound margins, increasing swelling, pain, or foul-smelling discharge. Fever or malaise reinforce this concern. A wound that reopens or begins bleeding again (dehiscence) requires prompt evaluation. Both infection and separation may need antibiotics or re-closure.

Exercise 12.7: Postpartum Genital Assessment Checklist
Identify findings that require further evaluation or follow-up.

☐ Mild swelling and bruising that improve daily
☐ Increasing pain or swelling after initial improvement
☐ Bright red bleeding with a firm uterus
☐ Pink drainage with steady healing
☐ Foul odor, new drainage, or visible wound separation
☐ Localized pressure or swelling that feels tense or warm
☐ Itching or mild pulling sensation as sutures dissolve
☐ Fever, malaise, or generalized discomfort
☐ Temporary stinging during urination that improves with rinsing
☐ Light spotting with firm fundus and normal tone

Postpartum Emotional Health and Adjustment

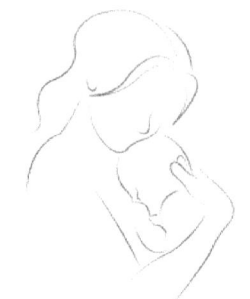

Emotional well-being is a vital part of postpartum recovery. The time after birth brings rapid hormonal change, physical healing, sleep disruption, and major shifts in identity and relationships. These changes affect bonding, lactation, body image, and the overall sense of safety and capability. The midwife's role is to understand what is normal, recognize when something needs attention, and respond with reassurance, education, screening, and referral when needed.

By listening closely, observing emotional tone, and validating the mother's experience, the midwife can promote healing and resilience in the early weeks after birth.

Normal Emotional Adjustment

Emotional sensitivity in the first days after birth is common and expected. The sudden drop in estrogen and progesterone after placental delivery, combined with rising levels of prolactin and oxytocin, creates a period of hormonal readjustment. Many new mothers describe emotions that shift quickly from joy and relief to tears, irritability, worry, or feeling overwhelmed.

This temporary state, often called the "baby blues," affects approximately seventy to eighty percent of postpartum individuals. It usually begins around the third to fifth day after birth and resolves within about two weeks. Typical symptoms include tearfulness, restlessness, mood swings, feeling easily upset, trouble sleeping even when tired, or feeling overstimulated by noise, touch, and responsibility. The condition generally improves with reassurance, warmth, food, and sleep.

It is important to normalize this experience and encourage open conversation. Validation, loving presence, and practical support help prevent isolation and shame.

When these feelings begin in the first week and improve by two weeks, they are considered part of normal recovery. When they worsen or persist beyond two weeks, they are not "just hormones" and require evaluation.

POSTPARTUM EMOTIONAL HEALTH: NORMAL ADJUSTMENT AND WHEN TO SEEK HELP

Emotional Pattern	Typical Timing and Duration	Common Symptoms	When to Seek Help
Baby Blues (Normal Adjustment)	Begins around day 3–5; resolves within 2 weeks	Tearfulness, irritability, mood swings, fatigue, temporary anxiety; improves with sleep and support	If symptoms persist beyond 2 weeks or worsen
Postpartum Depression	Onset anytime in first year; often within 3 months	Persistent sadness, hopelessness, guilt, lack of pleasure, detachment from baby	If sadness or disinterest interferes with self-care or bonding
Postpartum Anxiety	First days to months postpartum	Excessive worry, racing thoughts, restlessness, heart palpitations, trouble sleeping	When anxiety feels constant or exhausting
Postpartum OCD	Within weeks to months postpartum	Intrusive thoughts or mental images of harm, compulsive checking, avoidance	If intrusive thoughts are distressing or interfere with daily life
Postpartum Psychosis	First 2 weeks postpartum	Confusion, hallucinations, delusions, rapid mood shifts, agitation	**Medical emergency**—seek immediate evaluation and ensure safety for mother and infant

Risk Factors for Postpartum Emotional Distress

No single factor causes emotional illness after birth. Most serious postpartum mood and anxiety disorders arise from an interaction between biology (hormonal shifts, neurologic sensitivity), lived experience (trauma, disrespect in care), and environmental stress (lack of rest, isolation, or unsafe conditions). Understanding risk helps the midwife anticipate who may need more support and closer follow-up.

Before Pregnancy
- Personal or family history of depression, anxiety, bipolar disorder, or other mental health conditions
- History of trauma, including childhood trauma, sexual assault, or intimate partner violence
- Chronic stress, unresolved grief, or ongoing crisis
- Limited social support or unstable family relationships
- Ongoing financial or housing insecurity even before conception

During Pregnancy
- High-risk or medically complicated pregnancy
- Unplanned or unwanted pregnancy
- Ongoing financial strain or unstable housing
- Anxiety about the baby's health or survival
- Relationship conflict, including emotional or physical abuse
- Feeling judged, unheard, or unsafe in clinical encounters

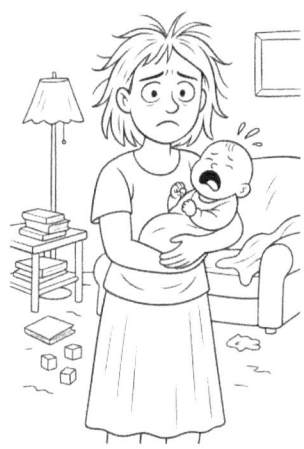

During Birth and Immediate Postpartum
- Traumatic or prolonged labor
- Emergency transport or surgical delivery
- Feeling powerless, disrespected, or physically violated during care
- Severe pain, hemorrhage, or fear for the baby's survival
- Neonatal separation or NICU stay
- Sleep deprivation and exhaustion
- Lack of in-home support after discharge

Clients with a prior history of depression or anxiety are at high risk for recurrence. Those with bipolar disorder are particularly vulnerable to postpartum psychosis and should be co-managed with behavioral health providers beginning in pregnancy.

Perinatal Mood and Anxiety Disorders (PMADs)

When emotional distress lasts longer than two weeks, intensifies instead of easing, or interferes with daily functioning, a mood or anxiety disorder may be developing. These are collectively known as Perinatal Mood and Anxiety Disorders (PMADs). PMADs affect approximately fifteen to twenty percent of postpartum individuals, and rates are higher for those with prior trauma, low support, racism, and discrimination in care, or financial instability.

PMADs include depression, anxiety, obsessive-compulsive symptoms, trauma responses, and, rarely, psychosis. They can appear anytime in the first year after birth.

Postpartum Depression

Postpartum depression occurs in about one in seven births. It is more than sadness. It may include hopelessness, persistent guilt, low self-worth, irritability, difficulty concentrating, or a sense of numbness. Mothers may feel emotionally flat, disconnected from the baby, or convinced they are "not a good mother." They may describe going through the motions but feeling no joy.

Onset is most common within the first three months postpartum, but it can appear later in the first year. Without support, postpartum depression can strain bonding, feeding, sleep, and safety. With support, most people recover.

Postpartum Anxiety

Postpartum anxiety affects about ten percent of postpartum individuals and often coexists with depression. It is marked by constant worry, racing thoughts, restlessness, feeling "wired and tired," irritability, and physical symptoms such as a pounding heart, chest tightness, or shortness of breath.

Unlike typical new-parent vigilance ("Is the baby breathing?"), postpartum anxiety feels relentless, intrusive, and exhausting. Mothers may have difficulty resting because they believe something terrible will happen if they are not actively watching.

Postpartum Obsessive-Compulsive Disorder (OCD)

Postpartum obsessive-compulsive disorder occurs in approximately three to five percent of postpartum individuals. It is characterized by intrusive, unwanted thoughts or mental images of harm coming to the baby, along with compulsive checking, avoiding certain objects (for example, knives), or refusing to let others hold the baby.

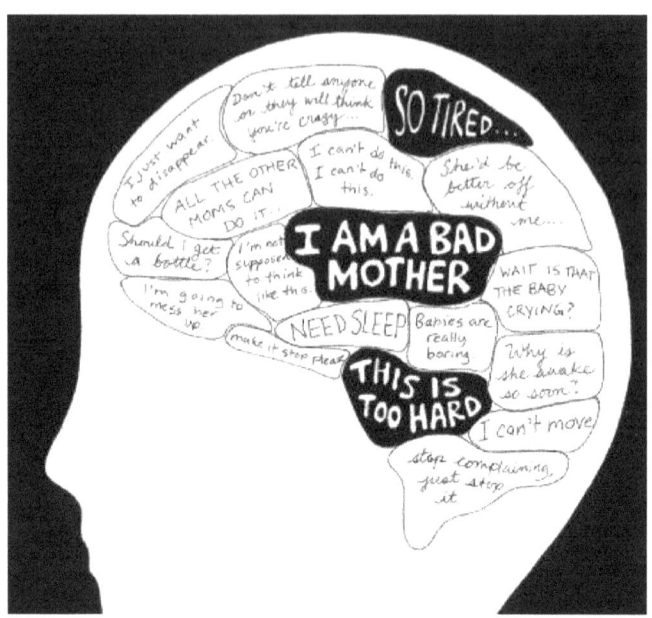

Key point: these thoughts are ego-dystonic. The mother knows the thoughts are frightening and not who she is. She is horrified by them, not driven by them. Intrusive thoughts alone do not mean she is a danger to her baby. They are, however, extremely distressing and deserve calm, nonjudgmental assessment and possible referral.

Birth Trauma and Postpartum PTSD

Postpartum post-traumatic stress disorder (PTSD) can develop even when the baby is physically healthy. It is more likely when the mother felt powerless, unheard, or in danger during labor or medical procedures. PTSD may follow perceived threat, actual emergency, or violation of bodily autonomy. Prior trauma increases risk.

Symptoms may include:
- Nightmares
- Flashbacks or unwanted replay of moments from the birth
- Avoidance of reminders (for example, refusing follow-up care because the clinic itself is triggering)
- Hypervigilance, jumpiness, and constant scanning for danger
- Emotional numbing or a sense of disconnection from the body or from the baby

Rates are estimated at three to six percent of all births, and higher after obstetric emergencies, hemorrhage, unplanned surgery, forced procedures, or neonatal separation.

It is essential to recognize that PTSD after birth is not "overreacting." It is a nervous system response to trauma. Recovery improves when the experience is acknowledged and processed rather than minimized or dismissed. Midwives support healing by listening to the birth story without interruption, reflecting the parent's feelings back to them, and making clear that what happened matters.

Postpartum Psychosis

Postpartum psychosis is rare but life-threatening. It affects approximately one to two per one thousand births and usually begins suddenly in the first two weeks postpartum.

Symptoms include confusion, disorganized thinking, hallucinations (hearing or seeing things that are not there), delusions (fixed false beliefs, such as believing the baby is cursed or unsafe in ordinary situations), agitation, or extreme and rapidly shifting mood.

Postpartum psychosis is a medical emergency. The client should never be left alone. Immediate psychiatric evaluation and safety planning for both mother and baby are required.

Resilience and Protective Factors

Not all stress becomes illness. Many women navigate intense physical and emotional change without developing a disorder. Protective factors lower risk and also support recovery for those who are already struggling.

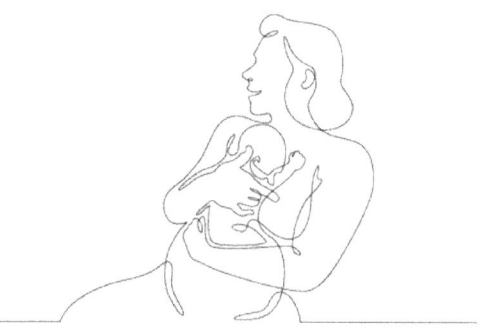

These include:
- Strong social and family support
- Positive partner involvement
- Access to home visits, peer support, or community-based postpartum care
- Stable housing and financial security
- Adequate sleep, food, fluids, and skilled breastfeeding help
- A sense of being respected during birth, even if it was medically complex
- Cultural or traditional postpartum practices that emphasize rest, ceremony, warmth, and protection

Midwives can strengthen resilience by normalizing emotional fluctuation, supporting rest and nourishment, encouraging culturally meaningful practices, and reminding mothers that needing help is expected, not a failure.

Screening and Assessment

Screening for emotional well-being is routine postpartum care. The purpose of screening is not to label someone. The purpose is to identify who may need more support, and to open a door to honest conversation. All screening should be done with privacy, compassion, and clear reassurance that mental health changes are common and treatable.

Commonly Used Screening Tools in Midwifery Practice

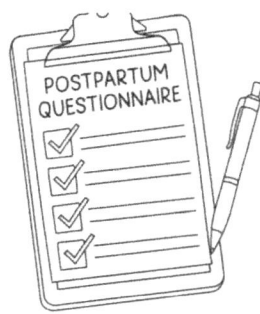

- *Edinburgh Postnatal Depression Scale (EPDS):* A ten-item questionnaire used worldwide. A score of ten or higher suggests possible depression and the need for further assessment.
- *Patient Health Questionnaire (PHQ-9):* Screens for depressive symptoms and can also be used to monitor response to treatment over time.
- *Generalized Anxiety Disorder Scale (GAD-7):* Screens for anxiety by measuring worry, tension, and somatic symptoms.
- *Mood Disorder Questionnaire (MDQ):* Used when there is concern for bipolar spectrum disorder. This is important because untreated bipolar disorder increases the risk of postpartum psychosis.

Recommended Screening Intervals (per ACOG, ACNM, and AWHONN):
- At least once during pregnancy, and in each trimester for clients with elevated risk
- At the first postpartum contact, ideally within seventy-two hours after birth
- At every subsequent postpartum visit (for example, two weeks and six weeks), and any time a concern arises
- Whenever a client, partner, or other family member voices worry about mood, anxiety, or behavior

Screening works best when it is paired with open-ended questions such as, "How have you been coping?" "What has felt hardest?" and "How are you sleeping emotionally, not just physically?" Quiet space and nonjudgmental listening invite honest answers.

The midwife should document scores, observations, and statements in clear, objective language and have a plan for referral before screening begins.

Midwifery Role in Assessment, Referral, and Ongoing Support

Screening is the first step, not the last step. When a client's responses suggest concern, the midwife's responsibilities include:
- Listening without minimizing or rushing
- Assessing immediate safety for both mother and baby
- Distinguishing urgent situations (such as suicidal thoughts, psychosis, or inability to safely care for the baby) from situations that need follow-up but are not emergent
- Referring to appropriate resources such as counseling, support groups, lactation support, primary care, psychiatry, or crisis services
- Following up, not assuming that "they will call if they need something"

Most clients improve with early counseling, peer support, and rest. Some benefit from medication. Normalizing help-seeking protects both mother and infant.

Midwifery Support and Community Resources

Holistic postpartum care is not limited to physical assessment. It also includes the living situation, family dynamics, access to food, and the emotional climate of the home. The midwife should know who is helping, who is staying in the house, how feeding is going, and how the mother is resting. Asking, "Who is taking care of you while you take care of the baby?" is as important as checking the fundus.

The midwife can:
- Assess bonding and attachment
- Support breastfeeding and infant care skills without judgment
- Connect families to postpartum doulas, parenting circles, breastfeeding support groups, peer lactation counselors, crisis lines, and community programs
- Encourage practical help such as meal trains, housework support, and safe sleep planning

Follow-up visits are a chance to notice early strain: a flat affect, guarded answers, tension with a partner, anxiety about finances, or signs of exhaustion. Sometimes the most helpful act in that moment is reassurance, quiet presence, or even folding a load of laundry while continuing the conversation.

When a mother feels seen, supported, and not alone, she is more likely to bond positively with her baby, recover her strength, and grow in confidence.

PREPARING FOR THE POSTPARTUM PERIOD

Thoughtful preparation for the postpartum period can make the difference between exhaustion and balance, between feeling isolated and feeling supported. Many challenges that arise after birth are not medical; they are practical, social, and emotional. When the midwife helps families plan ahead for rest, nourishment, and community support, recovery and adaptation occur more smoothly.

Postpartum education begins during pregnancy. Discussing what to expect, what is normal, and when to ask for help gives families the tools they need to adjust with confidence. The midwife's guidance can prevent unnecessary stress, promote bonding, and strengthen resilience in the first weeks after birth.

Families who plan for postpartum care as intentionally as they plan for birth often experience smoother recoveries and greater satisfaction. Creating a written postpartum plan helps organize meals, rest, and support before the baby arrives. Warm, nourishing foods such as soups, stews, and broths provide comfort and hydration while honoring cultural traditions that emphasize keeping the mother warm during recovery. These foods support digestion, healing, and milk production and can be easily adapted to each family's preferences.

Core Elements of Postpartum Preparation

During the third trimester, families should begin developing a flexible plan for the early postpartum period. This plan includes practical arrangements for food, rest, emotional support, and newborn care. Each family's needs are unique, and cultural values surrounding warmth, recovery, and family involvement should guide the discussion.

Rest and Recovery

Adequate rest is central to healing. The birthing parent's body undergoes dramatic changes as it returns to a nonpregnant state, and rest supports uterine involution, lactation, and mental health.
- Plan for at least two weeks with minimal household responsibilities.
- Arrange childcare or household help when possible.
- Encourage naps and early bedtimes to reduce fatigue and irritability.

Nourishment and Hydration

Simple, easy-to-digest meals made from whole foods provide steady energy and promote tissue repair.
- Prepare and freeze meals before birth or organize a meal train with friends and family.
- Keep snacks and water near the feeding area to support hydration.
- Warm, brothy soups and stews are especially beneficial. They provide comfort, hydration, and align with traditional practices that emphasize keeping the mother warm after birth. These foods support digestion, circulation, and milk production.

Community and Social Support

Social connection is one of the strongest protective factors in the postpartum period.
- Identify at least two people who can offer practical or emotional support.
- Encourage partners and family to learn the signs of postpartum complications.
- Connect families with local postpartum groups, lactation support, or home visiting programs when available.

Feeding and Infant Care

Feeding on cue strengthens bonding and milk supply while helping regulate parental hormones.
- Encourage unrestricted access to the newborn for frequent feeding.
- Avoid strict feeding schedules unless medically indicated (e.g., prematurity, low birth weight, or poor weight gain).
- When schedules are necessary, ensure close supervision and frequent reassessment.

Emotional and Mental Well-Being

Preparation should include emotional awareness and early support planning.
- Normalize emotional changes and provide education on postpartum mood variations.
- Encourage open communication among family members and care providers.
- Provide written information for mental health and community resources before birth.

Exercise 12.8: Postpartum Planning Checklist

Check off the plans you have already made for your clients postpartum recovery.
Add one example of your own under each category.

☐ **Rest and Recovery:** Have arranged help for chores, meals, or childcare.
Your example: _____

☐ **Nourishment and Hydration:** Have prepared or planned for easy meals and snacks.
Your example: _____

☐ **Community and Social Support:** Have identified at least two people who can offer emotional or practical help.
Your example: _____

☐ **Feeding and Infant Care:** Have discussed feeding goals and support options.
Your example: _____

☐ **Emotional and Mental Well-Being:** Have information on postpartum mood changes and support resources.
Your example: _____

Postpartum Assessment

Postpartum assessment allows the midwife to observe the physical, hormonal, and emotional recovery that occurs after birth. Regular follow-up visits support comfort, early detection of problems, and confidence in the transition to parenthood.

In community midwifery, the typical schedule includes a home visit within twenty-four hours, another at three days, a follow-up at about two weeks, and a final comprehensive visit at five to six weeks. Additional visits may be arranged for clients who need extra support or closer monitoring.

BUBBLE-HE: A Framework for Postpartum Assessment

The acronym BUBBLE-HE provides a simple and systematic guide for postpartum assessment. It helps midwives remember the key areas to evaluate after birth and ensures that no major aspect of recovery is overlooked. The letters stand for Breasts, Uterus, Bladder, Bowels, Lochia, Episiotomy or perineum, Homan's sign, and Emotional status. The BUBBLE-HE framework can be applied during every postpartum visit to maintain a complete picture of maternal health. It helps organize assessment, documentation, and communication among care providers.

Midwives often use it as a quick mental checklist during home visits, ensuring that both physical and emotional aspects of recovery are addressed. This systematic approach builds confidence in comprehensive postpartum care and supports early recognition of complications.

Each element represents a vital part of maternal recovery:

B–Breasts: assess breast fullness, softness, and symmetry. Observe the nipples for cracking or soreness and evaluate the latch if breastfeeding. Discuss comfort measures, feeding frequency, and any signs of blocked ducts or mastitis.

U–Uterus: palpate the fundus to determine firmness and position. A firm, midline uterus indicates good tone and reduced bleeding. A boggy or displaced uterus may suggest atony or bladder distention.

B–Bladder: ask about frequency and comfort with urination. A full bladder can push the uterus upward and increase bleeding. Encourage voiding every few hours and observe for burning, retention, or difficulty starting the stream.

B–Bowels: discuss the return of bowel movements, stool consistency, and comfort. Mild constipation is common. Encourage hydration, fiber, and gentle mobility. Check for hemorrhoids and discuss relief options.

L–Lochia: observe color, amount, and odor of vaginal flow. Normal progression is from lochia rubra (red) to serosa (pink-brown) to alba (pale yellow). Bright red bleeding, clots, or foul odor require evaluation.

E–Episiotomy or Perineum: inspect for swelling, bruising, separation, or hematoma formation. Healing should progress steadily, with discomfort decreasing over time. Reinforce perineal hygiene and use of sitz baths or ice packs as indicated.

H–Homan's Sign: screen for signs of deep vein thrombosis when indicated.

E–Emotional Status: observe affect, tone, and bonding. Ask open-ended questions about sleep, support, and adjustment to parenting. Normalize emotional fluctuations while screening for signs of depression, anxiety, or overwhelm.

Postpartum Maternal Assessment

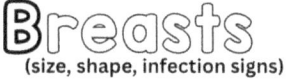
Breasts (size, shape, infection signs)

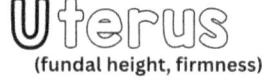
Uterus (fundal height, firmness)

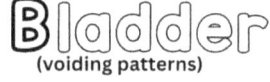
Bladder (voiding patterns)

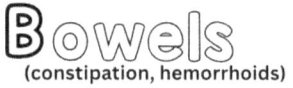
Bowels (constipation, hemorrhoids)

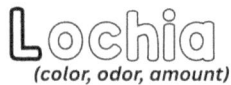
Lochia (color, odor, amount)

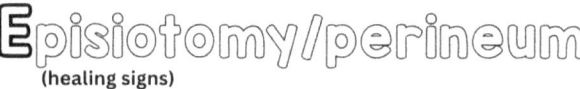
Episiotomy/perineum (healing signs)

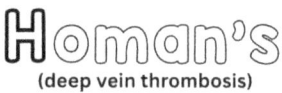
Homan's (deep vein thrombosis)

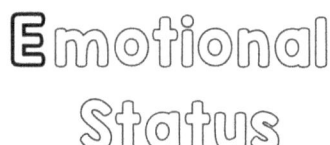
Emotional Status

The 24-hour Visit

The first visit focuses on physical stability, bleeding control, and reassurance. Families are often in a heightened emotional state, and calm midwifery presence helps normalize early adjustment to life with a newborn.

Assessment should include:
- **Breasts:** feeding should be underway, although milk may not yet be in. Observe latch, nipple comfort, and suckling behavior.
- **Uterus:** the fundus should be firm and just below the umbilicus. Mild cramping is normal when palpated.
- **Bleeding:** lochia should be moderate, not excessive. Passing small clots is common.
- **Perineum:** inspect for swelling, bruising, or hematoma. Review hygiene and comfort care.
- **Vital signs:** temperature, pulse, and blood pressure should be within normal limits.
- **Rest and activity:** the client should be mobile without dizziness and encouraged to rest.
- **Elimination:** urination should be spontaneous and not painful. Bowel movement may not yet have occurred.
- **Hydration and nutrition:** appetite should be good; encourage warm fluids and small, frequent meals.
- **Bonding and emotions:** observe interactions with the baby and offer space to discuss the birth experience.
- **Documentation:** record all findings, education, and any early referrals.

The Three-day Visit

By the third day, milk production increases and hormonal shifts often cause emotional sensitivity. This visit focuses on early healing, lactation comfort, and family adjustment.

Assessment should include:
- **Breasts:** milk is in; mild engorgement may occur. Review comfort and feeding frequency.
- **Uterus:** fundus should be midway between the umbilicus and pubic bone.
- **Bleeding:** lochia is lighter, similar to a menstrual period.
- **Perineum:** healing tissue may itch slightly. No swelling, redness, or discharge should be present.
- **Vital signs:** continue to monitor for fever or tachycardia.
- **Elimination:** bowel function should have resumed. Urination should be comfortable.
- **Rest and activity:** encourage naps and limited household work.
- **Emotional well-being:** normalize tearfulness and reassure that mood swings are common.

The Two-week Visit

This midpoint visit assesses uterine involution, perineal healing, and emotional wellbeing while reinforcing rest, nutrition, and support. It often uncovers early signs of fatigue or delayed healing, allowing timely intervention before problems escalate.

Assessment should include:
- **Uterus:** should have involuted into the pelvis and no longer be easily palpable.
- **Lochia:** should be lighter, pink or brown, and steadily decreasing.
- **Perineum and vulva:** healing should be well progressed, with no separation or infection.
- **Breasts:** softening after feeds indicates good milk transfer. Address any discomfort or fullness.
- **Vital signs:** continue monitoring for fever or fatigue.
- **Elimination:** bladder and bowel function should be normal. Hemorrhoids or mild stinging may persist.
- **Emotional and social well-being:** ask open questions about mood, sleep, and support. Screen for early symptoms of postpartum depression or anxiety.
- **Family adjustment:** discuss partner involvement, older children's adaptation, and division of responsibilities.
- **Activity:** gentle walking or stretching may begin; avoid heavy lifting or strenuous exercise.
- **Education:** reinforce contraceptive counseling, normal menstrual suppression during lactation, and the need for continued nutrient-dense foods and hydration.

The Six-week Postpartum Exam

By six weeks, most clients have completed early physical recovery. This visit provides a comprehensive review of physical healing, emotional health, and readiness to resume normal activities.

Assessment should include:

- **General health:** review any illnesses or complications since birth. Record weight, temperature, pulse, and blood pressure.
- **Laboratory tests:** check hemoglobin or hematocrit if indicated; perform a Pap test if due.
- **Emotional health:** discuss mood, stress, and satisfaction with birth and parenting. Screen for persistent depression or anxiety.
- **Bonding:** observe parent-infant interaction and confidence.
- **Sleep and rest:** review infant sleep patterns and coping strategies for fatigue.
- **Nutrition:** encourage balanced meals, fluids, and continuation of supplements.
- **Breasts:** should be soft and non-tender. Nipples intact without cracking.
- **Abdomen:** check for **diastasis recti**, a separation of the rectus muscles that may occur during pregnancy, especially in clients with decreased muscle tone or multiple pregnancies.

    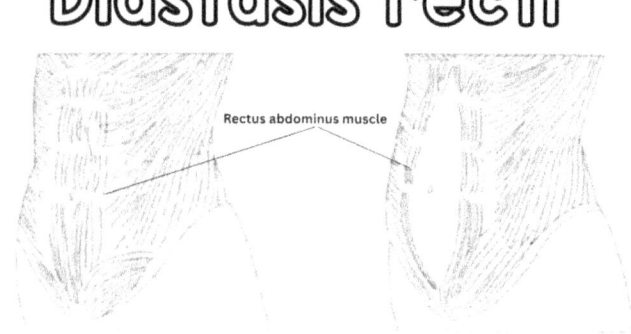

    - *Technique:* have the client lie flat and lift her head and shoulders slightly. Palpate the midline above and below the umbilicus to assess for a gap or ridge.
    - *Documentation:* record the width and length of the separation (for example, "diastasis 4 cm × 1 cm").
    - *Care:* provide reassurance and review gentle strengthening exercises once cleared for activity.

- **Uterus:** should not be palpable.
- **Lochia:** usually resolved; a slight pink discharge with exertion can be normal.
- **Perineum and vagina:** tissues should be healed and comfortable. Evaluate tone and check for cystocele or rectocele.
- **Cervix:** closed with a lateral slit.
- **Lower extremities:** assess for **Homan's sign** to screen for deep vein thrombosis if indicated.

    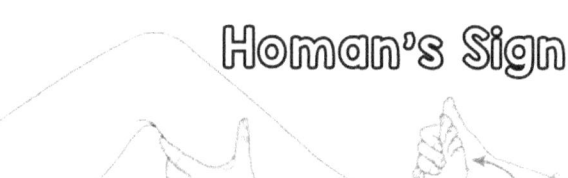

    - *Technique:* with the client's leg extended, gently dorsiflex the foot and note any calf pain or tenderness.
    - *Findings:* a positive Homan's sign (pain with dorsiflexion) may indicate thrombophlebitis.
    - *Care:* Do not repeat the test if pain is present; refer for medical evaluation.

- **Sexuality and contraception:** discuss comfort, desire, and family planning preferences.
- **Urinary and bowel function:** should be normal and pain-free.
- **Education and reflection:** encourage reflection on the transition to parenthood. Provide information about pelvic floor health, emotional balance, and long-term well-being.

> **Exercise 12.9: Postpartum Assessment Checklist**
> *Mark each item that should be evaluated during postpartum visits.*
> *Leave unchecked any that are not typically part of the midwife's maternal assessment.*

☐ Breastfeeding latch and nipple comfort
☐ Uterine firmness and location
☐ Vaginal pH testing
☐ Lochia color and amount
☐ Perineal healing or swelling
☐ Temperature, pulse, and blood pressure
☐ Bowel and bladder function
☐ Sleep patterns and emotional tone
☐ Glucose and protein in urine
☐ Partner involvement and family support
☐ Pelvic floor tone and comfort
☐ Amniotic fluid color and odor
☐ Education on nutrition, rest, and contraception
☐ Cervical dilation progress
☐ Umbilical cord condition and clamp placement

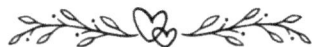

PLACENTA AND POSTPARTUM ESSENTIAL TAKEAWAYS

The placenta sustains life throughout pregnancy, performing respiratory, nutritional, endocrine, and excretory functions that maintain fetal growth. Safe completion of the third stage of labor depends on recognizing signs of separation, supporting uterine contraction, and avoiding unnecessary intervention. Inspection of the placenta and membranes confirms completeness and provides valuable information about pregnancy health. Thorough documentation of findings, blood loss, and cord characteristics ensures both safety and continuity of care.

Following birth, the midwife's focus shifts toward the mother's recovery. The postpartum period is one of profound physical, hormonal, and emotional change as every body system gradually returns toward a pre-pregnant state. Regular assessment, guided by the BUBBLE-HE framework, helps identify normal healing and early signs of imbalance. Evaluating uterine involution, lochia, perineal integrity, breast comfort, urinary and bowel function, and emotional tone supports early detection of complications and promotes confident adjustment.

Emotional health is central to postpartum wellbeing. Hormonal changes, sleep disruption, and new responsibilities can create vulnerability to mood disorders. Distinguishing normal "baby blues" from conditions such as postpartum depression, anxiety, or trauma response allows timely support and referral. Compassionate screening, education, and conversation normalize the emotional spectrum of recovery and strengthen resilience.

Preparation during pregnancy sets the foundation for a smooth postpartum transition. Families who plan ahead for nourishment, rest, and community support experience less stress and faster recovery. Cultural traditions such as warm foods, shared care, and placenta rituals reflect universal needs for protection and connection during this sensitive time. Midwives honor these practices while offering evidence-based guidance that supports healing, bonding, and long-term wellbeing.

Chapter Twelve Self-Assessment

Multiple Choice

1. Which physiologic process defines uterine involution after birth?
   a) Uterine enlargement through fluid retention
   b) Gradual shrinking and firming of uterine muscle
   c) Loss of uterine tone with retained fragments
   d) Increased uterine elasticity

2. Which finding at the two-week postpartum visit indicates normal recovery?
   a) Fundus palpable at the umbilicus
   b) Firm uterus below the symphysis pubis
   c) Uterus no longer palpable abdominally
   d) Soft uterus with lateral displacement

3. Which visit most often reveals emerging physical or emotional concerns?
   a) Twenty-four-hour visit
   b) Three-day visit
   c) Two-week visit
   d) Six-week visit

4. Which sign confirms placental separation?
   a) Decrease in uterine tone
   b) Cord lengthening and gush of blood
   c) Absent lochia
   d) Maternal shivering

5. What is the safest time to apply controlled cord traction?
   a) Before uterine contraction
   b) After signs of separation and a firm fundus
   c) While the uterus is relaxed
   d) During fundal massage

6. The main newborn benefit of delayed cord clamping is:
   a) Reduced third-stage bleeding
   b) Increased iron stores
   c) Earlier milk production
   d) Shorter recovery time for the mother

7. Which structure cushions umbilical vessels?
   a) Vernix caseosa
   b) Wharton's jelly
   c) Chorionic plate
   d) Amniotic fluid

8. Torn or jagged membranes after delivery may indicate:
   a) Normal variation
   b) Retained placental tissue
   c) Short cord
   d) Two-vessel cord

9. Which lochia description is normal at one week postpartum?
   a) Bright red with clots
   b) Pink or brown moderate flow
   c) Yellow-white discharge with odor
   d) Heavy red bleeding

10. Which comfort measure best reduces perineal swelling in the first 24 hours?
    a) Warm compress
    b) Ice or cold pack
    c) Sitz bath
    d) Massage

11. Which finding requires immediate evaluation?
    a) Mild perineal tenderness
    b) Intermittent afterpains
    c) Firm one-sided swelling with pressure
    d) Light pink lochia

12. The most common site for postpartum hematoma formation is the:
    a) Cervical region
    b) Vulvar or perineal region
    c) Abdominal wall
    d) Upper thigh

13. Which hormone primarily promotes uterine contraction and bonding?
    a) Estrogen
    b) Cortisol
    c) Oxytocin
    d) Progesterone

14. Which emotional response is considered a normal adjustment?
    a) Persistent sadness and detachment
    b) Mood swings resolving within two weeks
    c) Paranoia or hallucinations
    d) Extreme anxiety lasting several months

15. Which condition is a psychiatric emergency?
    a) Postpartum depression
    b) Postpartum psychosis
    c) Postpartum anxiety
    d) Postpartum obsessive-compulsive disorder

16. Which screening tool identifies risk for postpartum depression?
    a) PHQ-9
    b) GAD-7
    c) Edinburgh Postnatal Depression Scale
    d) Mood Disorder Questionnaire

17. Which physiologic change supports normal postpartum hemostasis?
    a) Decreased clotting factors
    b) Increased fibrinogen and platelet activity
    c) Reduced blood viscosity
    d) Lowered blood pressure

18. Which maternal adaptation supports venous return and prevents thrombosis?
    a) Early ambulation
    b) Prolonged bed rest
    c) Supine positioning
    d) Fluid restriction

19. What best supports milk flow and emotional stability during the golden hour?
    a) Bright light and conversation
    b) Quiet, warm, dimly lit environment
    c) Routine procedures and stimulation
    d) Immediate relocation to postpartum room

20. Which protective factor lowers risk for postpartum depression?
    a) Sleep deprivation
    b) Limited support
    c) Positive partner involvement and community help
    d) Returning to work right away

True or False

21. _____ By two weeks postpartum the uterus is usually no longer palpable abdominally.
22. _____ Bright red bleeding with a firm uterus suggests a genital tract laceration rather than uterine atony.
23. _____ Delayed cord clamping increases the risk of postpartum hemorrhage.
24. _____ Postpartum chills are a normal response to hormone and fluid shifts.
25. _____ The umbilical cord normally contains one vein and two arteries.
26. _____ Breastfeeding mothers ovulate sooner than non-breastfeeding mothers.
27. _____ The "baby blues" typically resolve within two weeks.
28. _____ Postpartum psychosis occurs in about one to two per thousand births.
29. _____ A temperature of 101 °F or higher on day three is considered normal when the milk comes in.
30. _____ Clients with prior depression are at higher risk for perinatal mood disorders.

Fill in the Blank

31. The process by which the uterus returns to its pre-pregnant size is called _____.
32. Lochia should gradually change from red to pink or brown by about _____ week(s) postpartum.
33. The most common site for postpartum hematoma formation is the _____ region.
34. Each gram of soaked material equals approximately _____ milliliter(s) of blood loss.
35. The Edinburgh Postnatal Depression Scale is used to screen for _____.

Matching

36. Match each Postpartum visit with its primary purpose.
    1. ____ Twenty-four-hour   A. Stability and immediate recovery
    2. ____ Three-day   B. Milk production and early healing
    3. ____ Two-week   C. Midpoint assessment of recovery and mood
    4. ____ Six-week   D. Comprehensive review of physical/emotional health

37. Match each type of Lochia with its color and timing.
    1. ____ Lochia rubra   A. Pink or brown, days 4–10
    2. ____ Lochia serosa   B. Bright red, days 1–4
    3. ____ Lochia alba   C. Yellow or white, up to six weeks

38. Match the Mood Disorders condition with its key feature.
    1. ____ Postpartum depression   A. Persistent sadness and loss of interest
    2. ____ Postpartum anxiety   B. Excessive worry and restlessness
    3. ____ Postpartum OCD   C. Intrusive thoughts and compulsive checking
    4. ____ Postpartum psychosis   D. Hallucinations or delusions

Chapter Twelve Recommended Reading & References

Recommended Reading for Placenta and Postpartum

- Beck, C. T. ***Postpartum Mood and Anxiety Disorders: A Guide for Nurses and Midwives*** (2nd ed.). Evidence-based overview of perinatal mood disorders, screening tools, and trauma-informed approaches for care.
- Buckley, S. ***Gentle Birth, Gentle Mothering*** (2nd ed.). Explores the hormonal physiology of labor, birth, and early postpartum, emphasizing calm and connection.
- Cleveland, L. M., & Gill, S. L. ***Mood and Anxiety Disorders in the Perinatal Period: A Guide for Health Professionals***. Practical manual integrating research with therapeutic and community-based support strategies.
- Coad, J., & Dunstall, M. ***Anatomy and Physiology for Midwives*** (5th ed.). Comprehensive foundation text linking physiologic systems to perinatal and postpartum adaptation.
- Cohen, L. S., & Nonacs, R. ***Mood and Anxiety Disorders During Pregnancy and Postpartum*** (2nd ed.). Medical and psychological perspectives on perinatal mental health and treatment safety in breastfeeding.
- Johnson, R., & Taylor, W. ***Skills for Midwifery Practice*** (5th ed.). Covers assessment, communication, and practical postpartum care techniques for community midwifery.
- Kendall-Tackett, K. A. ***Depression in New Mothers: Causes, Consequences, and Treatment Alternatives*** (3rd ed.). Comprehensive text exploring biological, cultural, and social contributors to postpartum depression.
- Stern, D. N., & Bruschweiler-Stern, N. ***The Birth of a Mother: How the Motherhood Experience Changes You Forever***. Insightful exploration of psychological and emotional transitions into motherhood.
- Walsh, D., & Downe, S. ***Essential Midwifery Practice: Intrapartum Care***. Evidence-based guide promoting normal birth and minimizing unnecessary intervention, with sections on early postpartum physiology.

References

Beck, C. T., & Gable, R. K. (2001). Postpartum depression screening scale: Development and psychometric testing. *Nursing Research, 50*(5), 275–282. https://doi.org/10.1097/00006199-200109000-00004

Cleveland, L. M., & Gill, S. L. (2019). *Mood and anxiety disorders in the perinatal period: A guide for health professionals*. Routledge.

Cohen, L. S., & Nonacs, R. (2019). *Mood and anxiety disorders during pregnancy and postpartum* (2nd ed.). American Psychiatric Publishing.

Dennis, C.-L., & Dowswell, T. (2013). Psychosocial and psychological interventions for preventing postpartum depression. *Cochrane Database of Systematic Reviews, 2013*(2), CD001134. https://doi.org/10.1002/14651858.CD001134.pub3

Johnson, R., & Taylor, W. (2016). *Skills for midwifery practice* (5th ed.). Elsevier.

Kendall-Tackett, K. A. (2017). *Depression in new mothers: Causes, consequences, and treatment alternatives* (3rd ed.). Routledge.

O'Hara, M. W., & McCabe, J. E. (2013). Postpartum depression: Current status and future directions. *Annual Review of Clinical Psychology, 9*, 379–407. https://doi.org/10.1146/annurev-clinpsy-050212-185612

Stern, D. N., & Bruschweiler-Stern, N. (1998). *The birth of a mother: How the motherhood experience changes you forever*. Basic Books.

Walsh, D., & Downe, S. (2010). *Essential midwifery practice: Intrapartum care*. Wiley-Blackwell.

Yim, I. S., Tanner Stapleton, L. R., Guardino, C. M., Hahn-Holbrook, J., & Dunkel Schetter, C. (2015). Biological and psychosocial predictors of postpartum depression: Systematic review and call for integration. *Annual Review of Clinical Psychology, 11*, 99–137. https://doi.org/10.1146/annurev-clinpsy-101414-020426

Chapter Thirteen
Midwifery Care of the Newborn

Objectives
After completing this chapter, the student should be able to:
1. **Explain** the midwife's role and responsibilities in the care and ongoing assessment of the newborn.
2. **Describe** the physiologic and environmental factors that stimulate the newborn's first breath and extrauterine adaptation.
3. **Outline** the immediate steps of newborn care, including:
    a. Preventing heat loss and recognizing cold stress;
    b. Clearing the airway appropriately and understanding when suctioning is indicated;
    c. Performing and interpreting the APGAR assessment;
    d. Safely clamping and cutting the umbilical cord.
4. **Assess** neonatal respirations, heart rate, temperature, and color, and identify normal parameters for each.
5. **Describe** the physiologic basis and emotional importance of bonding and the "golden hour."
6. **Conduct** a complete head-to-toe newborn examination, identifying normal findings and common variations.
7. **Estimate** gestational age using the Dubowitz/Ballard assessment.
8. **Explain** the indications, methods, and parental options for common newborn procedures, including:
    a. Vitamin K administration;
    b. Eye prophylaxis;
    c. Metabolic and genetic screening (PKU);
    d. Hearing screening and CCHD pulse oximetry;
    e. Glucose testing in at-risk infants;
    f. Circumcision and informed parental decision-making.
9. **Recognize** the types, causes, and management of neonatal jaundice, distinguishing physiologic from pathologic findings.
10. **Describe** appropriate cord care and expected healing patterns.
11. **Explain** expected weight changes, feeding frequency, and elimination patterns in the first weeks of life.
12. **Demonstrate** how to prepare families for newborn care through effective parent education, including safe sleep, car seat safety, and home readiness.
13. **Identify** key criteria for newborn discharge and early follow-up visits.
14. **Discuss** the midwife's role in continuity of care, pediatric collaboration, and community support for new families.

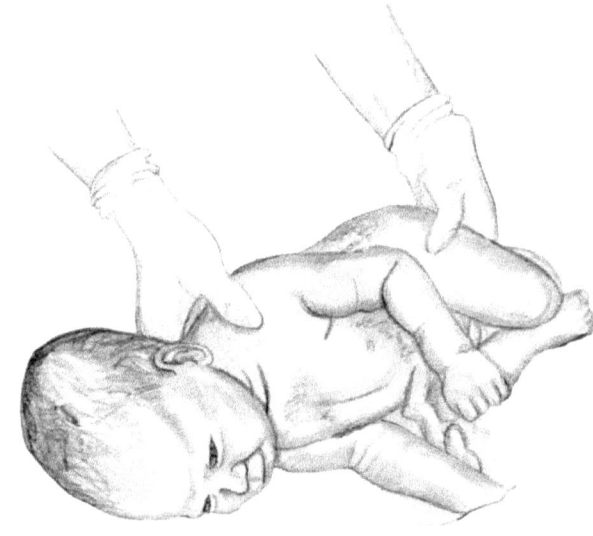

Midwifery Care of the Newborn

The midwife's care of the newborn begins well before birth. During pregnancy, she becomes familiar with the mother's health history, nutritional status, and any prenatal conditions that may influence newborn adaptation. By observing fetal well-being and the course of labor, she anticipates how factors such as maternal exhaustion, meconium-stained fluid, or prolonged labor might affect the baby's transition. This awareness allows her to prepare with focused awareness, attentive, observant, and grounded in readiness for all possibilities.

Before every delivery, the midwife reviews the pregnancy record, noting any maternal or fetal risk factors that could influence the newborn's condition. Equipment for warmth, lighting, suction, and oxygen, if available, should be organized and checked before each birth. This intentional preparation ensures that she can respond quickly and effectively if the baby requires assistance.

When risk factors are present, the midwife's demeanor becomes a steadying presence in the room. A composed, focused environment supports both physiologic transition and parental confidence. Communication with parents and birth attendants remains clear, concise, and free of unnecessary alarm. By modeling grounded professionalism and quiet confidence, the midwife helps preserve the peaceful energy of the birth space while ensuring safety.

> **Key Vocabulary**
>
> - **Neonate:** A baby from birth to 28 days of life.
> - **Newborn:** Often used interchangeably with *neonate*; generally refers to the baby during the early postpartum period under midwifery care.
> - **Infant:** A child from one month to one year of age.
> - **Transition:** The newborn's physiologic adjustment from intrauterine to extrauterine life.
> - **Golden hour:** The first hour after birth, marked by heightened alertness, hormonal synchrony, and physiologic regulation.
> - **Thermoregulation:** The ability of the newborn to maintain normal body temperature through heat production and conservation.

As the baby is born, the midwife maintains a centered and protective atmosphere, honoring the sacred first moments of family connection. The newborn is placed directly in the mother's arms or on her chest, where skin-to-skin contact promotes warmth, regulation, and bonding. The midwife begins her assessment gently and unobtrusively, observing color, tone, and breathing while respecting the intimacy of these first minutes, often called the *golden hour*, a time of powerful physiologic and emotional adjustment for both mother and baby. Witnessing the moment parents first meet their child is one of midwifery's greatest privileges.

Within the first few hours after birth, the midwife performs a complete newborn assessment to confirm normal transition and identify any concerns that may require follow-up or referral. This exam is done in the presence of the family whenever possible, encouraging transparency and shared learning. The midwife provides guidance about newborn screenings, vitamin K, eye prophylaxis, and any procedures that may be recommended based on community standards or family preference.

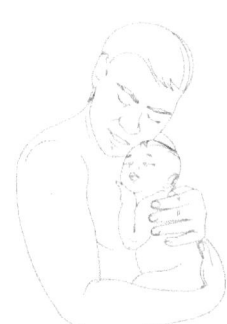

Midwifery care of the newborn continues through the early weeks of life. The midwife monitors feeding, elimination, weight, and temperature stability, while also observing the developing mother–infant bond. Education about newborn cues, feeding patterns, and normal behaviors helps families feel confident in their care. Support for breastfeeding is especially vital, as early and exclusive feeding contributes to both immediate and long-term health.

Cultural and family traditions surrounding newborn care vary widely, and when safe, they should be respected and supported. The midwife's role includes helping families integrate traditional or cultural practices into newborn care in ways that promote safety, attachment, and well-being.

Because the midwife is deeply involved with the family, she is often the first to recognize early concerns such as feeding difficulties, delayed bonding, or signs of neglect or abuse. Midwives are legally and ethically obligated to report any suspected abuse or neglect and to collaborate with community partners to ensure the baby's safety. Early home visits, parent support programs, and public health services may play an important role in meeting emerging needs.

Community collaboration is a vital part of midwifery practice. The midwife connects families with pediatric or public health providers, lactation consultants, and parenting resources. Most midwives recommend that every newborn be evaluated by a physician or nurse practitioner trained in newborn care within the first week or two of life. This visit helps identify any medical issues that may develop after birth and establishes continuity of care with the child's long-term healthcare provider.

Midwifery care of the newborn gradually transitions to another provider over the first six weeks after birth. During this time, the midwife helps the family build confidence and healthy patterns that will support the child's growth and development for years to come.

ANTENATAL AND INTRAPARTUM RISK ASSESSMENT FOR THE NEWBORN

Newborn assessment begins before birth. By monitoring maternal health, fetal development, and the course of labor, the midwife anticipates how the baby may respond to life outside the womb. This proactive approach allows for thoughtful preparation, timely intervention, and a smoother transition after delivery. Understanding antenatal and intrapartum risk factors supports individualized care planning and safe observation of the newborn in the first hours of life.

Antenatal Risk Factors

Antenatal risk factors may influence newborn adaptation and should be reviewed at every prenatal visit.
Examples include:
- Maternal anemia, hypertension, diabetes, thyroid disease, or infection
- Substance use, poor nutrition, or limited prenatal care
- Fetal growth restriction, multiple gestation, or abnormal ultrasound findings
- Environmental or social concerns that may affect newborn safety or care

Intrapartum Risk Factors

Intrapartum factors observed during labor help guide immediate newborn management.
These may include:
- Prolonged or precipitous labor, shoulder dystocia, or assisted delivery
- Abnormal fetal heart rate patterns or other signs of fetal stress
- Meconium-stained amniotic fluid or evidence of chorioamnionitis
- Maternal fever, dehydration, or excessive blood loss

Observation and Preparedness
- Anticipate the need for assistance when multiple risk factors are present.
- Prepare equipment in advance, including warmth, lighting, suction, and oxygen if available.
- Establish a clear plan for consultation or transfer if the newborn requires additional care.

Documentation and Communication
- Record all known antenatal and intrapartum factors in the newborn chart at birth.
- Communicate findings clearly to the receiving provider to ensure continuity of care.

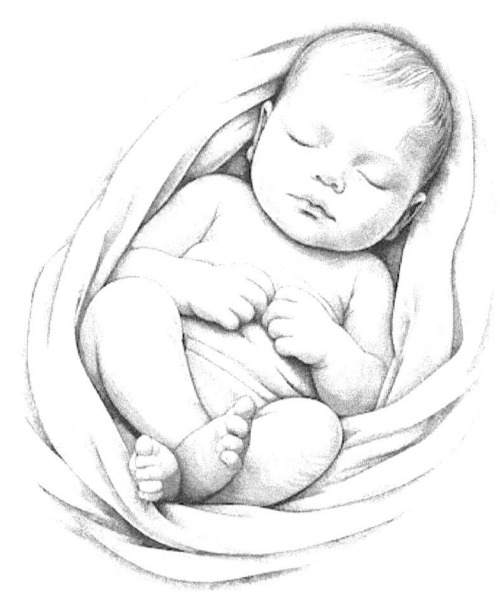

CLINICAL EQUIPMENT CHECKLIST: NEWBORN RESUSCITATION

Every midwife attending births outside of a hospital must be prepared to assist a newborn who does not begin breathing spontaneously. Equipment should be organized, checked before each birth, and ready for immediate use. This checklist reflects current Neonatal Resuscitation Program (NRP) standards and out-of-hospital best practices.

Airway and Ventilation
- ☐ Self-inflating bag (240–500 mL, newborn size)
- ☐ Clear newborn face masks (sizes 0 and 1) with airtight seal
- ☐ Bulb syringe for gentle suctioning
- ☐ Portable or hand-powered suction device with adjustable pressure
- ☐ Suction catheters (sizes 6F, 8F, 10F)
- ☐ Oxygen source with flowmeter and tubing
- ☐ Oxygen mask for blow-by administration

Airway Adjuncts (Advanced Use)
- ☐ Laryngoscope with straight blades (sizes 0 and 1) and spare batteries
- ☐ Endotracheal tubes (sizes 2.5, 3.0, 3.5 mm) with stylet
- ☐ Meconium aspirator (if trained and indicated for non-vigorous infants)

Monitoring and Assessment
- ☐ Newborn stethoscope
- ☐ Pulse oximeter with neonatal sensor
- ☐ Timer or stopwatch
- ☐ Thermometer
- ☐ Portable light source (headlamp or flashlight)
- ☐ Neonatal scale

Thermal Support
- ☐ Warm, dry towels and blankets (multiple sets)
- ☐ Pre-warmed receiving blanket
- ☐ Radiant heat source or heating pad (covered, temperature-checked)
- ☐ Newborn hat to prevent heat loss
- ☐ Plastic wrap or food-grade bag for very small or premature babies

Medications (Per Local Regulation)
- ☐ Epinephrine 1:10,000 (0.1 mg/mL)
- ☐ Normal saline for volume expansion
- ☐ Glucose gel or D10W for hypoglycemia
- ☐ Water-soluble airway lubricant

Circulation and Access
- ☐ Umbilical clamps and sterile scissors
- ☐ Umbilical catheter kit (3.5F and 5F catheters, saline, syringes)
- ☐ Normal saline (0.9%) for flushes
- ☐ Syringes (1 mL, 3 mL, 10 mL) and assorted needles

Infection Control and General Supplies
- ☐ Sterile and clean gloves
- ☐ Hand sanitizer and disinfectant wipes
- ☐ Sharps container
- ☐ Waste disposal bags
- ☐ Towels, drapes, and chux pads

Recommended Additions
- ☐ Oxygen-saturation reference chart (by minute of life)
- ☐ Laminated NRP algorithm for quick reference
- ☐ Spare batteries for all powered devices
- ☐ Backup face masks and tubing in sealed storage

Immediate Care of the Newborn

The newborn should be placed skin-to-skin on the parent's abdomen or chest immediately after birth. This position supports warmth, bonding, and physiologic stability. The baby is gently dried with a warm blanket while remaining in contact. Wet linens are replaced promptly. Hats are not used routinely but may be applied if the environment is cool or if the newborn has thermoregulation concerns.

Observation begins the moment the baby is born. The midwife assesses color, tone, breathing, and activity while the baby remains skin-to-skin. Most newborns begin breathing or crying within the first 30 seconds. Gentle stimulation, such as drying or rubbing the back, is usually sufficient to encourage respirations. Routine suctioning is not indicated. If secretions obstruct airflow, the mouth and nose may be cleared with gauze or a bulb syringe.

Step-by-Step Observation and Assessment

1. Place the newborn skin-to-skin on the parent's chest; dry thoroughly and replace any wet linens.
2. Observe immediately for color, tone, breathing, and activity while maintaining skin-to-skin contact.
3. Within the first 30 seconds, look for a spontaneous cry or effective respirations.
4. If breathing is present and the baby is vigorous, continue quiet observation; do not suction routinely.
5. If breathing is not established, provide gentle stimulation: complete drying, rub the back, or give a brief flick to the soles if needed.
6. If secretions obstruct airflow, position the head neutrally or slightly to the side and clear the mouth and nose with gauze. Use gentle bulb suction only if needed, mouth first, then nose. Avoid deep or mechanical suction unless specifically indicated.
7. Reassess work of breathing and chest movement. Auscultate respirations and heart rate. Target 30 to 60 breaths per minute and 120 to 160 beats per minute.
8. If breathing remains poor, color does not improve, or heart rate is below 100, initiate newborn resuscitation steps per protocol and call for assistance.
9. Maintain warmth and contact. Keep the room warm, replace damp linens promptly, and use a hat only if there are thermoregulation concerns.
10. Perform and record Apgar scores at one and five minutes without separating the newborn from the parent.
11. Document observations, timing, and any interventions.

> **Practice Tips**
>
> Prepare towels, clamps, and equipment before every birth, but use only what is needed. Maintain a warm, quiet environment to support newborn transition. Perform assessments gently and without separating the baby from the parent. Speak softly and describe what you are observing to reassure parents and involve them in their baby's care. A confident, centered presence and clear communication create safety and trust during this sensitive time.

Auscultation of the heart and lungs can be done while the baby remains in skin-to-skin contact. Normal respirations range from 30 to 60 per minute, and the heart rate from 120 to 160 beats per minute. The Apgar score, recorded at one and five minutes, evaluates appearance, pulse, grimace, activity, and respirations.

Umbilical cord clamping is delayed until pulsations have stopped unless immediate intervention is required. The cord may be cut by the midwife or a family member using sterile scissors and a secure tie or clamp about one inch from the abdomen.

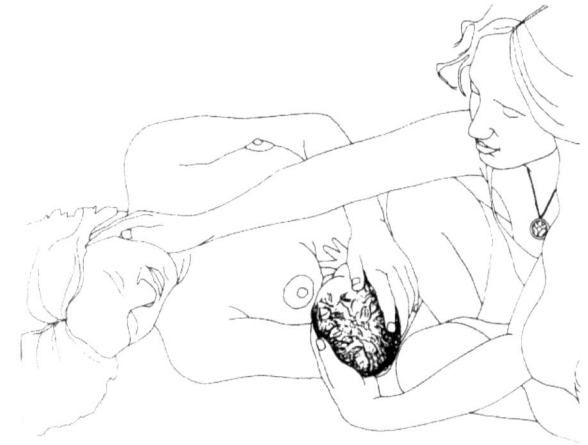

The Newborn's First Breath

The first breath marks one of the most dramatic transitions in human physiology. Within seconds of birth, the baby's lungs shift from fluid-filled organs of potential to functioning centers of oxygen exchange. Several factors work together to stimulate this vital first breath and the beginning of independent respiration.

Mechanical Events

As the baby's chest is compressed during birth, amniotic fluid is expelled from the lungs. When the chest is released, air rushes in, helping the lungs expand for the first time. This physical change creates negative pressure, drawing oxygen into the alveoli and establishing the first rhythm of breathing.

Chemical Stimuli

A brief decrease in oxygen and increase in carbon dioxide levels during birth stimulate the respiratory center in the brain. This change, along with the sudden cutting off of placental gas exchange, triggers the baby's first spontaneous inhalation.

Thermal Stimuli

The sudden change from the warm uterine environment to the cooler temperature of the outside world activates sensory receptors in the skin. This thermal shift acts as a natural signal that initiates breathing.

Sensory Stimuli

Touch, sound, and light in the birth environment awaken the newborn's senses and encourage respiratory effort. The tactile stimulation of being touched, dried, and held supports the start of effective breathing.

Physical Stimuli

Handling, drying, and gentle stimulation—such as rubbing the back or flicking the soles of the feet—help the baby sustain regular respirations. These actions, combined with skin-to-skin contact and parental voices, reinforce physiologic adaptation and emotional security.

Underwater Birth Considerations

In water births, the newborn's first breath is influenced by several protective mechanisms, including oxygenation through the umbilical cord and the natural *dive reflex*, which prevents breathing until the baby's face meets air. The midwife ensures a safe transition by lifting the baby gently to the surface only after the head and shoulders are fully born. The water should remain warm, calm, and clean to support this smooth adaptation.

Clearing the Airway

As the baby passes through the birth canal, the chest is compressed, pushing amniotic fluid and mucus from the lungs and airways. When the chest expands again, air fills the lungs for the first time. A small amount of fluid may remain in the nose and mouth. Clearing these secretions helps ease the baby's breathing and prevents aspiration.

Using a **bulb syringe** or **gauze** is a gentle and effective way to clear the airway. Suctioning should be minimal and performed only when needed. If the baby has spontaneous respirations and is vigorous, wiping the mouth and nose is usually sufficient. Position the baby's head slightly to the side to allow secretions to drain naturally.

For many years, routine suctioning was recommended, especially when meconium-stained fluid was present. Traditional practice included suctioning the mouth and nose before the shoulders were delivered, or intubating the newborn after birth to remove meconium from the trachea. Research, has shown that these procedures may not prevent **meconium aspiration syndrome** and can sometimes cause harm. Current evidence supports avoiding routine deep suctioning or intubation unless clearly indicated by poor tone, depressed respirations, or persistent airway obstruction.

Suction mouth first than nose, only if needed

CUTTING AND CARE OF THE UMBILICAL CORD

The umbilical cord serves as the newborn's lifeline throughout pregnancy, carrying oxygen and nutrients from the placenta. After birth, its work is complete, but the transition from fetal to newborn circulation continues as the remaining cord blood finishes its flow. The midwife's role is to manage the cord safely, support delayed clamping whenever possible, and provide clear guidance for cord care in the days after birth.

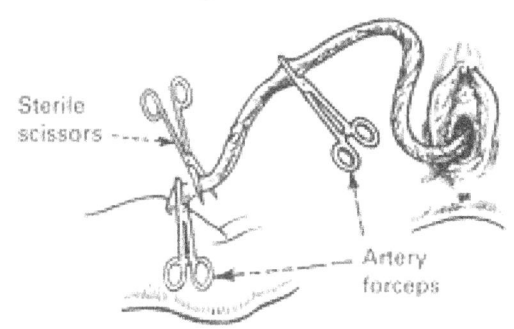

Families should be encouraged to discuss cord clamping preferences during prenatal care so decisions are made ahead of time. Before the birth, the midwife prepares sterile instruments, ensuring clamps and ties are within easy reach. Delayed clamping is supported whenever the newborn is vigorous and stable. Parents or family members may participate in cutting the cord if they wish, using sterile scissors and under supervision. The cord may be cut while the baby remains on the mother's abdomen or chest, preserving warmth and bonding. Two hemostats are applied—one near the baby and one quite few inches farther along the cord—and the cut is made between them using sterile scissors. The longer hemostat remains attached to the baby's side until it is time for newborn examination.

At that time, the cord can be shortened, and a plastic cord clamp applied about one inch above the baby's abdomen. If plastic cord clamps are not available or desired, sterile cord tape or sterile, sturdy string may be used instead. The tie should be placed securely using a **square knot**, ensuring firm closure without excessive tension. After cutting, check carefully for bleeding and confirm that the clamp or tie is secure before completing documentation. If the cord continues to ooze, apply a second tie or clamp closer to the base. A later trimming may be done once bleeding has stopped and the newborn is stable.

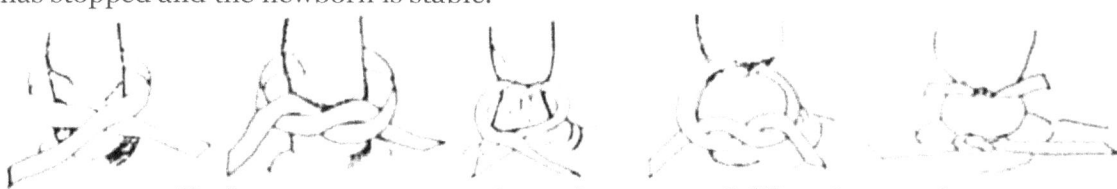

Cord Care After Birth

The remaining cord stump requires only simple, gentle care.

- Keep the area clean and dry.
- Fold the diaper below the cord to allow air circulation.
- Do not apply alcohol, ointments, or powders unless specifically indicated.
- Observe daily for redness, swelling, or odor that may signal infection.
- The clamp or tie can be removed once the cord is dry and there is no bleeding, typically within 24 to 48 hours. Some parents wish to keep clamp on until it falls off with the dried cord to save.
- The stump will darken, shrink, and separate naturally within one to two weeks.

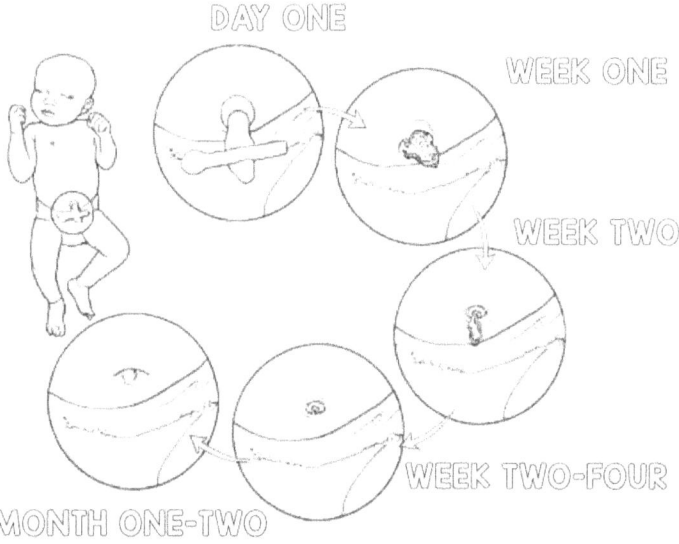

Educating parents about normal cord healing helps prevent unnecessary interventions and reassures them during this brief transition period. The midwife's calm explanation and guidance reinforce confidence in the baby's natural adaptation and the family's growing caregiving skills.

APGAR ASSESSMENT

The **Apgar score** is a simple, standardized tool used to quickly evaluate a newborn's physical condition and response to extrauterine life. Developed by Dr. Virginia Apgar in 1952, the scoring system helps the birth attendant recognize which babies may need additional support during transition. The Apgar score is not designed to predict long-term outcomes but provides valuable information about the baby's adaptation in the first few minutes after birth.

Purpose and Timing

The Apgar score evaluates **five criteria**—appearance, pulse, grimace, activity, and respiration. Each category is scored from 0 to 2 for a maximum total of 10 points.

- The **one-minute score** reflects how well the newborn tolerated birth.
- The **five-minute score** indicates how effectively the newborn is adapting to life outside the uterus.

If the five-minute score is below seven, the assessment should be repeated every five minutes until the score reaches seven or higher, or until twenty minutes of life.

APGAR Scoring System

Appearance (Color)
0 = Pale or blue all over
1 = Pink body with blue extremities (acrocyanosis)
2 = Completely pink

Pulse (Heart Rate)
0 = Absent
1 = Below 100 beats per minute
2 = 100 or higher

Grimace (Reflex Irritability)
0 = No response to stimulation
1 = Grimace or weak cry with stimulation
2 = Strong cry, cough, or sneeze with stimulation

Activity (Muscle Tone)
0 = Limp or flaccid
1 = Some flexion of extremities
2 = Active movement with good flexion

Respiration (Breathing Effort)
0 = Absent
1 = Weak, irregular, or gasping respirations
2 = Strong cry with regular respirations

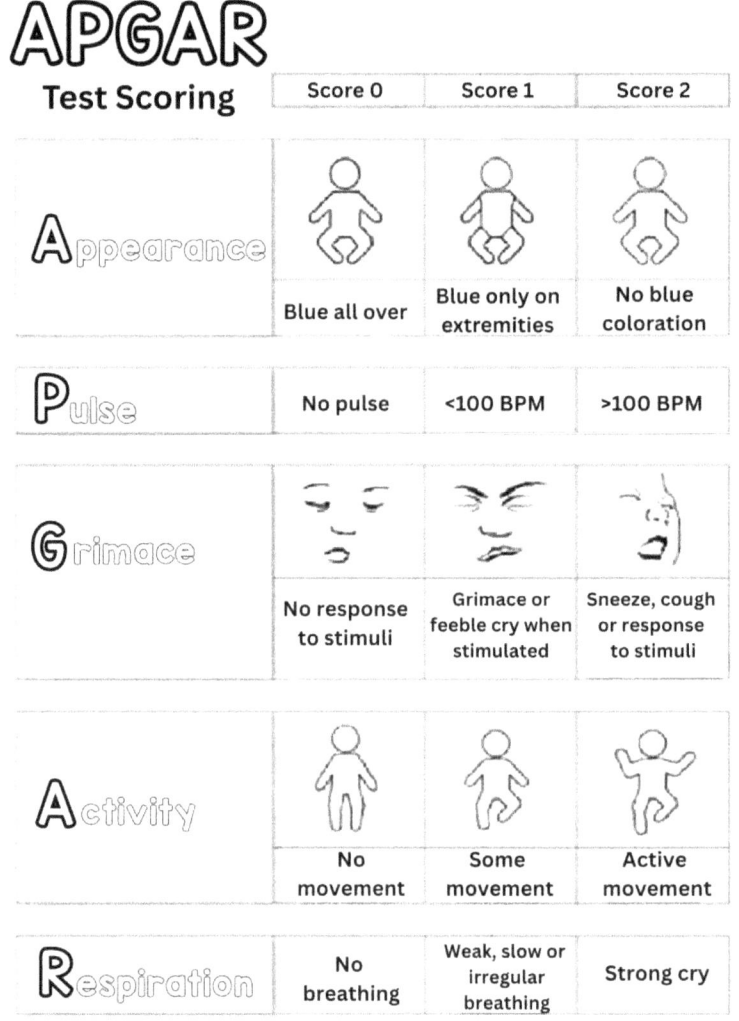

Interpreting the Score

- **7–10:** Normal adaptation. Continue observation and skin-to-skin care.
- **4–6:** Moderate difficulty. Provide stimulation, clear the airway, or assist with ventilation as indicated.
- **0–3:** Severe distress. Begin immediate resuscitation and evaluation.

A low one-minute Apgar score that improves by five minutes usually indicates effective transition. Persistent low scores require further assessment for respiratory, cardiac, or neurologic concerns. The Apgar score should always be interpreted alongside clinical observations and never used as a stand-alone measure of newborn well-being.

Exercise 13.1: APGAR Score
Match the APGAR category with the finding being evaluated.

1. Reflex response to stimulation	A. Appearance
2. Heart rate by auscultation or palpation	B. Pulse
3. Color of the newborn's skin	C. Grimace
4. Muscle tone and movement	D. Activity
5. Breathing effort and cry	E. Respiration

THERMOREGULATION AND COLD STRESS

Maintaining normal body temperature is one of the newborn's most important physiologic tasks after birth. The change from the warm intrauterine environment to cooler external air can quickly lead to heat loss. Because the newborn's thermoregulation system is immature, the midwife plays a vital role in prevention, recognition, and management of cold stress. Supporting temperature stability also conserves oxygen and glucose—two key components of the newborn's energy triangle.

The newborn's temperature can drop rapidly if heat is lost faster than it is produced. Full-term infants can generate heat through metabolism of brown fat, but preterm and growth-restricted infants are at higher risk because they have less brown fat and thinner skin. When the newborn becomes cold, oxygen consumption and glucose use increase, placing stress on the respiratory and metabolic systems.

Mechanisms of Heat Loss
- **Evaporation:** When amniotic fluid or other moisture on the baby's skin turns to vapor; the most common cause of heat loss immediately after birth.
- **Conduction:** When the baby is placed on a cold surface such as a scale or examination table.
- **Convection:** When cool air currents pass over the baby's body, often from open windows or fans.
- **Radiation:** When heat transfers from the baby's body toward nearby cooler objects, even without direct contact.

Key Vocabulary
- **Thermoregulation:** The process by which the newborn maintains normal body temperature through heat production and conservation.
- **Neutral thermal environment:** The environmental temperature at which the newborn uses the least energy to maintain normal temperature.
- **Brown adipose tissue:** Specialized fat used for nonshivering heat production in the newborn.
- **Cold stress:** A condition in which heat loss exceeds the baby's ability to produce heat, resulting in metabolic and respiratory instability.
- **Nonshivering thermogenesis:** Heat production through the metabolism of brown fat rather than muscle activity.
- **Hypothermia:** An abnormally low body temperature, defined in the newborn as below 36.5°C (97.7°F).

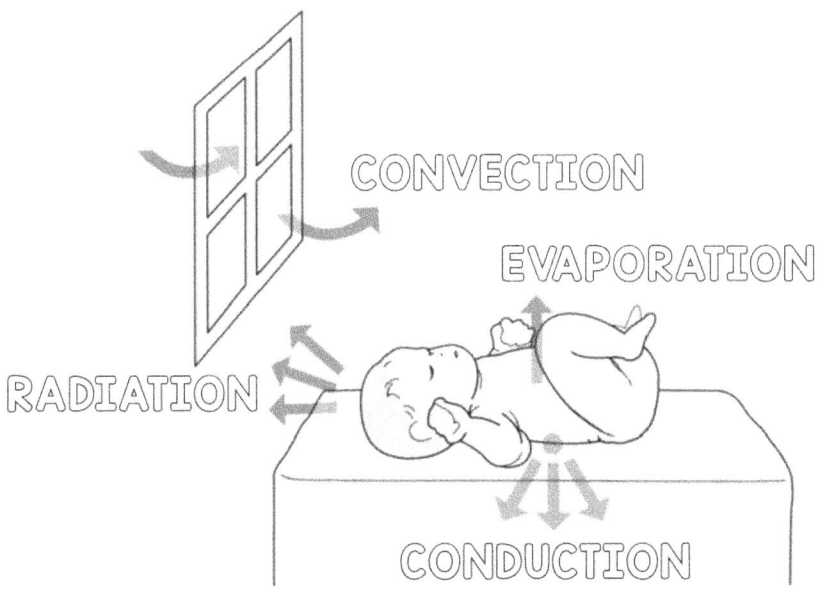

Prevention of Heat Loss
- Keep the room comfortably warm and free of drafts.
- Place the newborn skin-to-skin on the parent's chest as soon as possible after birth.
- Dry the baby thoroughly with a warm blanket and replace wet linens promptly.
- Cover both parent and baby with a dry blanket or shawl to retain warmth.
- Delay bathing until the temperature is stable for several hours.
- Use warmed equipment and blankets for any procedures requiring temporary separation.
- Apply a hat only when the environment is cool or if the newborn shows temperature instability.

Recognition of Cold Stress

Early signs of cold stress include cool or mottled skin, lethargy, weak cry, poor feeding, and acrocyanosis that persists beyond the first ten minutes of life. If cold stress continues, respirations may become shallow and glucose levels may fall. The midwife should rewarm the baby gradually through skin-to-skin contact, warm blankets, or a prewarmed radiant heat source if needed.

Monitoring Temperature

Axillary temperature is the preferred method for healthy newborns. Normal temperature ranges from 36.5°C to 37.4°C (97.7°F to 99.3°F). Temperatures below 36.5°C indicate the need for rewarming and assessment for contributing factors such as prematurity, wet linens, or a cool environment.

Relationship to the Energy Triangle

Thermoregulation, oxygenation, and glucose metabolism form the newborn's energy triangle. When temperature drops, energy is diverted from breathing and glucose regulation to heat production, increasing the risk of hypoxia and hypoglycemia. Maintaining warmth therefore protects the baby's overall physiologic stability.

Exercise 13.2: Newborn Heat Loss

Match the method of heat loss with its example.

1. Air blowing over the baby's body from a fan	A. Conduction
2. Placing the baby on a cold surface	B. Convection
3. Heat transfer to cooler objects nearby	C. Radiation
4. Moisture on the skin turning to vapor	D. Evaporation

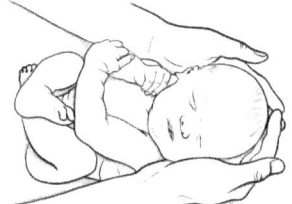

Exercise 13.3: Immediate Care of the Newborn

Number each step in the correct order to show the sequence of care during the first minutes after birth.

_____ Apply a cord tie or clamp about one inch above the baby's abdomen.
_____ Dry the baby thoroughly with a warm blanket and replace any wet linens.
_____ Encourage parents to remain close and speak softly to their newborn.
_____ Allow delayed cord clamping until pulsations stop or the cord appears white and flaccid.
_____ Cut the cord between two clamps using sterile scissors.
_____ Avoid routine suction unless secretions obstruct airflow; use gentle bulb suction if needed.
_____ Continue observing for effective respirations and normal color.
_____ Document timing, observations, and any interventions
_____ Observe color, tone, and respirations while maintaining skin-to-skin contact.

The Newborn's Experience of Birth and the Golden Hour

Birth is both a physiologic and emotional transformation for the newborn. Within minutes, the baby moves from the dark, fluid-filled security of the uterus into a world of air, light, and sound. This first hour of life, known as the **golden hour**, is a sensitive period when both newborn and family are biologically primed for connection. Protecting this time supports physiologic stability, emotional security, and the foundation for lifelong attachment. These first moments are sacred; when the newborn's life begins in peace and is surrounded with love and joy, the roots of lifelong well-being are nurtured.

The Newborn's Experience of Birth

From the baby's perspective, birth is a profound sensory awakening. After months of gentle motion, muffled sounds, and constant warmth, the baby encounters light, cool air, and gravity for the first time. The sudden expansion of the lungs replaces fluid with air. Oxygen flows through the bloodstream, and circulation redirects from the placenta to the lungs.

- The baby's eyes open in dim light, drawn instinctively to faces and voices.
- The familiar heartbeat and scent of the mother provide reassurance in the new environment.
- The sound of a partner's familiar voice is soothing and grounding.
- Gentle touch and the sound of calm voices signal safety, helping the newborn integrate sensory input.
- Within the first minutes, the baby's alert state supports recognition, rooting, and the first attempt to feed.

This quiet, alert awareness is the newborn's way of learning the world. Physiologic stability and emotional security are intertwined in this moment.

> **Cultural Traditions in the First Hour**
>
> *Across cultures, early contact and gentle welcome are seen as essential to the baby's well-being.*
>
> - In many Indigenous traditions, newborns are greeted with song or prayer before being touched by anyone else.
> - Scandinavian and Dutch midwives refer to the first hour as *the sacred hour*, emphasizing quiet, warmth, and family togetherness.
> - In parts of Latin America, early wrapping and skin contact are accompanied by whispered blessings to honor the baby's spirit.
> - Some Asian cultures place importance on covering the baby's ears and head immediately to protect from wind and spirits, balancing spiritual safety with warmth.
>
> *These traditions, though diverse, share a universal truth: the way a baby is welcomed matters.*

The Science of Imprinting

Research shows that newborns recognize the parent's voice and smell within hours after birth. Familiar sounds heard in utero—such as speech and heartbeat rhythms—help orient the baby to their family after delivery. The baby's brain releases oxytocin and endorphins that enhance calmness and receptivity, strengthening early memory pathways. Visual recognition develops quickly; newborns prefer to focus on human faces at the distance typical of breastfeeding.

Hormones of Connection

During the golden hour, both baby and parent experience a cascade of hormones that deepen emotional and physical connection.

- **Oxytocin** encourages uterine contraction, reduces bleeding, and enhances feelings of affection.
- **Prolactin** stimulates milk production and supports nurturing behavior.
- **Endorphins** provide pain relief, euphoria, and relaxation for both baby and parent.
- **Catecholamines** heighten alertness and energy during the immediate transition, gradually subsiding as bonding and rest begin.

Together, these hormones create a physiologic state of calm and attachment that supports both healing and emotional connection.

The Golden Hour in Practice

The golden hour is a period of natural synchrony between the newborn and the family.

- Skin-to-skin contact stabilizes heart rate, temperature, and breathing.
- Early breastfeeding stimulates milk production and uterine contraction.
- The parent's voice and scent help regulate the baby's heart rate and cortisol levels.
- Minimal lighting and noise preserve the baby's ability to focus and bond.
- Delaying routine procedures such as weighing or bathing protects uninterrupted contact.

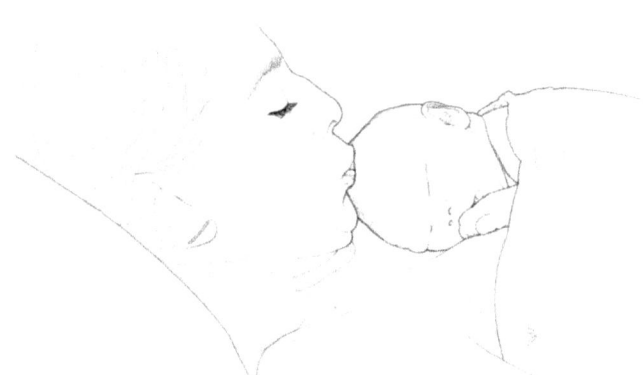

Neuroprotective Benefits of the Golden Hour

Modern research supports what midwives and families have known for generations. Early skin-to-skin contact and breastfeeding lower stress hormones, stabilize blood sugar, and improve oxygenation. Close contact reduces crying, enhances sleep organization, and supports brain development through regulated cortisol patterns. The combination of warmth, touch, and calm presence acts as neuroprotection, buffering the newborn's brain from the physiologic stress of transition.

Bonding and Attachment

Bonding is the beginning of attachment\—a lifelong pattern of connection. Parents who experience uninterrupted early bonding often show greater confidence and responsiveness in caring for their baby. Partners, siblings, and extended family can also participate through gentle touch, eye contact, and quiet interaction. Protecting bonding time contributes to healthier relationships and emotional well-being for both parents and children.

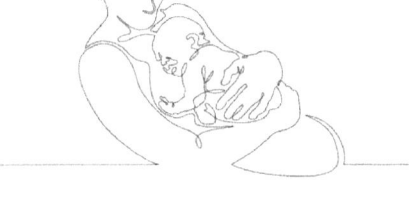

Exercise 13.4: Golden Hour
Match the term with its description.

1. _____ Hormone promoting uterine contraction and emotional connection
2. _____ The first hour after birth marked by alertness and readiness to bond
3. _____ Early recognition of familiar sensory cues
4. _____ Hormone supporting milk production and nurturing response
5. _____ The newborn's quiet alert state
6. _____ Natural pain relief and relaxation during birth and bonding
7. _____ Skin-to-skin contact

A. Golden hour
B. Oxytocin
C. Regulates temperature, heart rate, and stress hormones
D. Imprinting
E. Prolactin
F. A period of focused awareness that supports bonding and early feeding
G. Endorphins

The Newborn Examination

The newborn examination is a complete, head-to-toe assessment designed to confirm the infant's overall health, identify findings that may require follow-up, and reassure the family about normal adaptation. For many midwives, especially in home or low-resource settings, it may be the only full exam performed before discharge. A systematic, gentle, and well-documented assessment establishes trust with the family and ensures early detection of conditions that need further care.

Preparation and Environment

Perform the exam in a warm, draft-free space, ideally while the baby remains close to the parent. Use clean or gloved hands, a warm blanket, and a firm surface. Before touching the baby, quietly observe color, tone, posture, and breathing. Wash hands thoroughly. Use clean gloves when handling the cord, umbilicus, or genitalia. Replace linens if soiled.

If the baby appears cyanotic, limp, or apneic, stabilize first—warmth, airway, breathing—then proceed once stable.

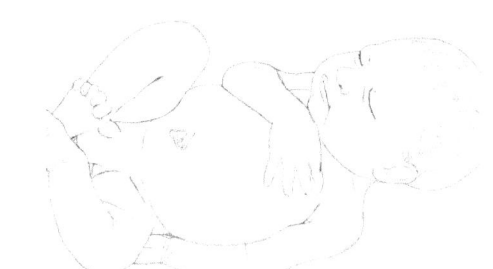

Have ready:
- Clean tape measure and scale
- Stethoscope and thermometer
- Penlight
- Cord and hip assessment supplies
- Documentation form

Initial Observation and Vital Signs

Observe the infant's general appearance: alertness, cry, color, posture, and movement symmetry. Then measure and record vital signs:

Parameter	Normal Range	Notes
Temperature	36.5–37.4°C (97.7–99.3°F)	Axillary preferred; rewarm if <36.5°C
Heart Rate	120–160 bpm	Up to 180 when crying, 100 when asleep
Respirations	30–60 per minute	Irregular pauses <10 seconds are normal
Weight	2.5–4.0 kg typical	Up to 10% loss in first week
Length	48–53 cm typical	Measure crown to heel
Head Circumference	32–38 cm	Head usually 1–2 cm > chest circumference

General Appearance and Color

A healthy newborn is pink to red, with flexed limbs, spontaneous movement, and a strong cry.

Note:
- **Central cyanosis** (blue lips/tongue) = oxygenation problem
- **Pallor or gray tone** = anemia or shock
- **Mottling** = may indicate cold stress or sepsis

Skin
- Should be warm and smooth with good turgor and capillary refill under 3 seconds.
- **Normal findings:** acrocyanosis, vernix residue, milia, erythema toxicum, Mongolian spots, lanugo, transient peeling.
- **Abnormal findings:** generalized cyanosis, jaundice <24 hours, pallor, petechiae, or large bruises.
- **Document:** birthmarks, hemangiomas, and rashes for future comparison.

Head and Scalp
- Measure head circumference.
- Inspect sutures and fontanelles; they should be soft and flat.
- **Anterior fontanelle:** diamond-shaped, 2–3 cm; **posterior:** smaller and triangular.
- **Bulging** may indicate increased intracranial pressure; **sunken** suggests dehydration.
- **Molding** is normal after vaginal birth and resolves in days.

Caput Succedaneum
A diffuse swelling of serum and blood into scalp tissue, caused by pressure from a tight cervix or prolonged labor.
- Present at birth
- May cross suture lines
- Pits on pressure
- Disappears in a few days
- Benign, no treatment needed

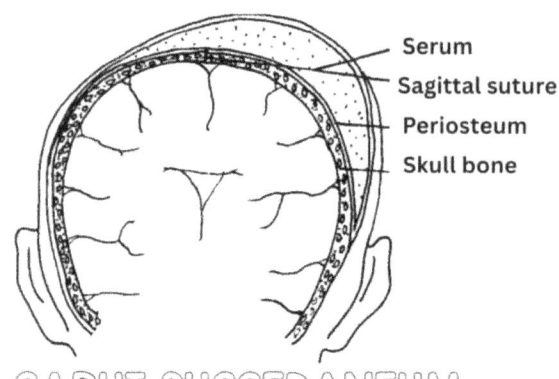

Cephalohematoma
A collection of blood beneath the periosteum, usually from cephalopelvic disproportion or long pressure on the skull.
- Appears several hours after birth (not immediately)
- Does not cross suture lines
- May enlarge for 1–2 days, then resolve over weeks
- Does not pit on pressure
- Usually benign; observe for jaundice as it resolves

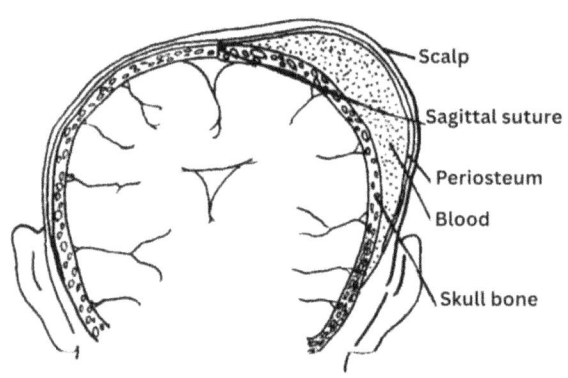

Eyes, Nose, and Mouth
- **Eyes:** open spontaneously; sclerae may show tiny hemorrhages. Red reflex should be present; absence may indicate cataract or retinoblastoma.
- **Nose:** may appear flattened or bruised; sneezing is normal. Confirm both nostrils open by occluding one side at a time.
- **Mouth:** inspect lips, gums, and palate for clefts. Palpate the roof of the mouth with a gloved finger. Observe sucking reflex and tongue symmetry.
- **Normal variants:** Epstein pearls, small natal teeth.
- **Abnormal findings:** thrush (white plaques), cleft lip or palate, persistent drooling (possible esophageal atresia).

Ears and Neck
- Ears should align with outer canthi of eyes. Low-set or malformed ears may suggest renal anomalies; note for referral.
- Confirm patent ear canals and response to sound.
- Neck should be supple without webbing or masses. Palpate for cysts or goiter.

Chest, Lungs, and Heart
- Observe for symmetry and equal chest rise.
- Count respirations for one full minute; look for retractions, nasal flaring, or grunting.
- Auscultate lungs bilaterally; breath sounds should be clear and equal.
- Clavicles should be straight and smooth—crepitus may indicate fracture.
- Auscultate heart at the apex for rate and rhythm.
- Normal heart rate: 120–160 bpm.
- Soft murmurs may be transient; loud or persistent murmurs need follow-up.
- Check femoral pulses for strength and equality. Weak or absent pulses suggest coarctation of the aorta.
- Note capillary refill and perfusion.

Abdomen and Umbilicus
- Abdomen soft, round, non-distended.
- Palpate liver and spleen edges gently; they should not be enlarged.
- Auscultate for bowel sounds—should be active within one hour.
- Check umbilical cord for **two arteries and one vein**.
- Observe stump for redness, odor, or bleeding.
- Confirm urination and passage of meconium within 24 hours.

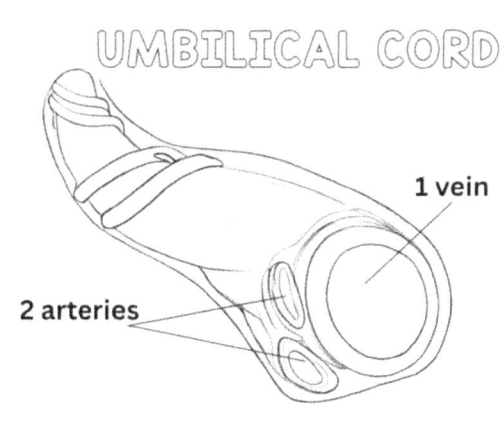

Common Findings:
- **Umbilical hernia:** small, soft bulge, usually resolves in months.
- **Granuloma:** moist tissue at cord base; may need silver nitrate if persistent.
- **Omphalitis:** spreading redness or discharge—refer immediately.

Genitalia
- **Males:**
  - Scrotum enlarged with rugae; testes should be descended.
  - Urethral meatus at tip; note **hypospadias** or **epispadias.**
  - Hydroceles are common and self-limiting.
- **Females:**
  - Labia majora may be edematous; vaginal discharge or small blood-tinged fluid (**pseudomenstruation**) normal from hormone withdrawal.
  - Observe for ambiguous genitalia and refer if uncertain.
- Palpate femoral pulses; inspect for inguinal hernia.

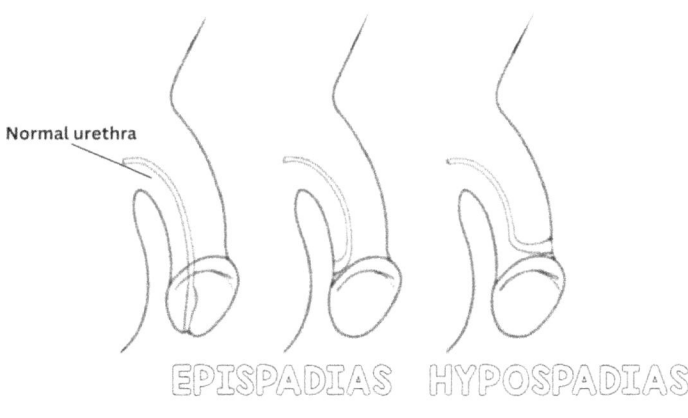

Extremities and Musculoskeletal
- Count fingers and toes; check for **syndactyly**, **polydactyly**, or clubfoot.
- Observe tone, spontaneous movement, and symmetry.
- Assess for fractures, particularly clavicle or humerus.
- Note **simian crease** or abnormal limb proportions.
- Inspect spine for straight alignment, sacral dimples, or tufts of hair; a deep pit may suggest **spina bifida occulta**.

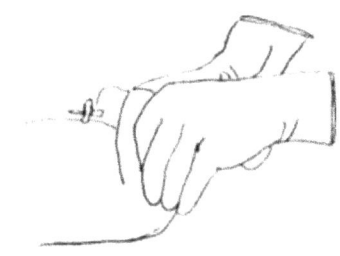

Hip Assessment
Congenital hip dislocation occurs in 0.1–0.2% of newborns, more in breech births and girls. Positive findings require prompt referral for orthopedic evaluation.

- Observe thigh-fold symmetry; one leg may appear shorter.

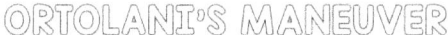

Congenital Hip Screening (Ortolani's Maneuver):
1. Place the baby supine with hips and knees flexed to 90°.
2. Hold thighs with thumbs on inner thighs and fingers on femoral heads.
3. Gently abduct hips while lifting the femur anteriorly.
4. A palpable or audible *clunk* indicates dislocation.

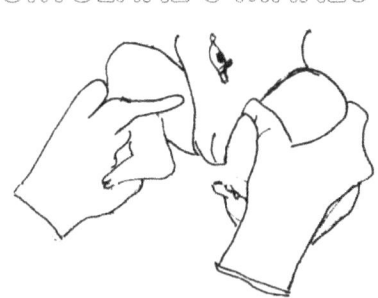

Neurologic Reflexes

Healthy term infants display the following primitive reflexes:

Reflex	Response	Appears / Disappears
Rooting	Turns head toward touch on cheek	Birth–4 mo
Sucking	Rhythmic sucking when lips touched	Birth–4 mo
Palmar grasp	Fingers close around object	Birth–6 mo
Moro	Arms extend then flex when startled	Birth–4 mo
Babinski	Toes fan when sole stroked	Birth–1 yr
Tonic neck	"Fencing" posture	2 wk–6 mo
Stepping	Alternating leg motion	Birth–2 mo
Gallant	Trunk curves to side of spinal touch	Birth–2 mo

Absence, asymmetry, or persistence beyond expected ages may indicate neurologic or muscular issues.

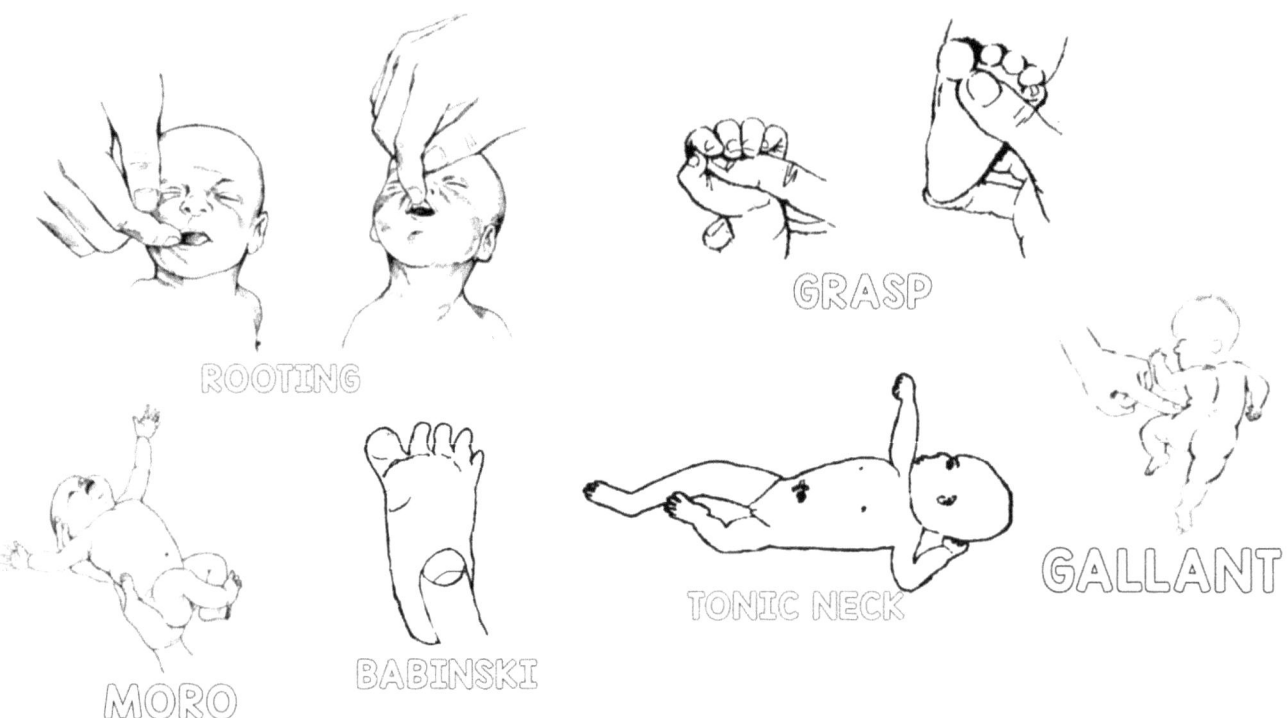

Measurements and Growth

Record:
- Weight, length, and head circumference
- Chest circumference (normally 1–2 cm smaller than head)
- Note proportions and symmetry
- Calculate percentage of weight loss in early days and observe for dehydration.

Documentation and Education
- Chart all findings clearly and review them with the parents.
- Demonstrate normal reflexes and show how to observe warmth, color, and feeding cues.
- Explain when to call for help: fever, poor feeding, lethargy, jaundice, breathing difficulty, or umbilical infection.
- Arrange follow-up within 48 hours if any uncertainty remains.

Common Benign Findings

Finding	Description	Care / Teaching
Vernix caseosa	White, creamy coating on skin	Leave to absorb; protects and moisturizes.
Milia	Small white papules on nose / cheeks	No treatment; resolve spontaneously.
Erythema toxicum	Red blotches with pale centers	Common rash; fades in 3–5 days.
Mongolian spots	Bluish patches over sacrum / shoulders	Document to distinguish from bruises.
Acrocyanosis	Blue hands and feet	Normal first 24 hr; rewarm if persistent.
Transient peeling	Dry skin on hands / feet	Apply gentle oil; normal exfoliation.
Breast engorgement/ "Witch's milk"	Maternal-hormone effect	Do not squeeze; resolves in 1–2 weeks.
Pseudomenstruation	Blood-tinged vaginal mucus	Normal; reassure parents.

Danger Signs Requiring Immediate Referral or Transport

Category	Warning Signs
Respiratory	Grunting, persistent nasal flaring, retractions, apnea > 20 sec, central cyanosis
Cardiac / Perfusion	HR < 100 or > 180 bpm, cap refill > 3 sec, weak femoral pulses
Temperature	< 36.5 °C (97.7 °F) or > 37.5 °C (99.5 °F) despite warming
Neurologic	Lethargy, poor feeding, seizures, jitteriness, persistent high-pitched cry
Gastrointestinal / Umbilical	Abdominal distention, bilious vomiting, no meconium / urine > 24 hr, omphalitis
Skin / Jaundice	Generalized pallor, gray color, jaundice in first 24 hr, petechiae
Other	Bleeding from cord / sites, significant weight loss > 10 %, refusal to feed

Parental Teaching Points

Topic	Key Guidance
Thermal care	Keep baby warm and dry; delay bathing; cover head if cool.
Cord care	Keep stump clean and dry; fold diaper below; seek help for redness or odor.
Feeding	Feed on demand; at least 8–12 times / 24 hr.; monitor wet diapers.
Elimination	Expect urine / stool within 24 hr.; 6+ wet diapers by day 4.
Sleep	Place on back, firm surface, no loose bedding.
When to call for help	Trouble breathing, poor feeding, fever, jaundice, lethargy, umbilical redness.

Exercise 13.5: Newborn Exam

Match each condition or term with its description.

1. Soft scalp swelling that crosses sutures	A. Cephalohematoma
2. Blood collection under periosteum that does not cross sutures	B. Caput succedaneum
3. Screening for hip dislocation	C. Ortolani maneuver
4. Bluish hands and feet from immature circulation	D. Acrocyanosis
5. Fluid-filled swelling in the scrotum	

	E. Hydrocele

Gestational Age Assessment

Determining gestational age helps identify whether a newborn is preterm, term, or postterm and guides care planning for temperature regulation, feeding, and observation. When the due date is uncertain or ultrasound data are unavailable, physical and neurologic assessment offers valuable information. The **Dubowitz/Ballard Assessment** is the most widely used method. It assigns maturity scores to specific physical and neuromuscular characteristics observed within the first day of life. Each item is scored from −1 to 5, and the total corresponds to an estimated gestational age in weeks. Scores are lower in premature infants and highest in postmature babies.

Perform the physical portion of the exam within the first two hours after birth, before skin changes progress, while maintaining warmth and observing the baby in a quiet, alert state. Review findings with parents to support understanding of their baby's development, document all scores clearly, and communicate any concerns to the newborn's health care provider.

> **Clinical Note**
>
> In low-resource settings, where ultrasound or electronic records may be unavailable, the Dubowitz/Ballard exam is a vital tool for estimating gestational age and identifying at-risk newborns. Accurate scoring helps midwives recognize prematurity-related concerns early and provide timely care or referral.

Physical Maturity Assessment

Completed within the first two hours after birth, the physical maturity exam evaluates features that change predictably with gestational age:

- **Skin:** Ranges from thin, sticky, and translucent in very preterm infants to smooth and then cracking or peeling in postmaturity.
- **Lanugo:** Fine, downy hair that is absent in very premature babies, appears with mid-maturity, and disappears again with postmaturity.
- **Plantar Creases:** Soles are smooth in immature infants; creases gradually extend to cover the entire foot as maturity advances.
- **Breast Tissue:** The areola and breast bud enlarge and thicken with gestational age; larger tissue indicates greater maturity.
- **Eyes and Ears:** Fused eyelids and soft, pliable ears suggest immaturity; open eyes and firm ear cartilage that recoils indicate term maturity.
- **Genitalia (Male):** Testes descend and scrotal rugae deepen with increasing maturity.
- **Genitalia (Female):** With maturity, the labia majora enlarge and cover the labia minora and clitoris.

Neuromuscular Maturity Assessment

Performed within the first 24 hours of life, this part of the exam evaluates posture, tone, and reflex responses that reflect neurologic development:

- **Posture:** Preterm infants lie with extended limbs; term infants flex arms and legs tightly toward the trunk.
- **Square Window:** The angle between the hand and forearm decreases with advancing maturity.
- **Arm Recoil**: When extended and released, the arm of a mature infant quickly recoils to flexion.
- **Popliteal Angle:** Resistance to leg extension increases with maturity.
- **Scarf Sign**: Preterm infants can draw one arm easily across the chest; term infants resist crossing the arm beyond the midline.
- **Heel-to-Ear**: The greater the resistance when bringing the heel toward the ear, the more mature the infant.

Clinical Interpretation

- Compare the **estimated gestational age** to **birth weight** to classify the infant as **appropriate (AGA), small (SGA),** or **large for gestational age (LGA)**.
- Significant discrepancies between gestational age and weight may indicate **intrauterine growth restriction (IUGR), maternal diabetes,** or **placental insufficiency**.
- Findings help guide **feeding support, temperature management,** and **follow-up** for potential complications of prematurity or postmaturity.
- When gestational age assessment is uncertain, repeat the exam within 12–24 hours and combine findings with maternal history and prenatal data.

Neuromuscular Maturity

Score	-1	0	1	2	3	4	5
Posture							
Square window (wrist)	>90°	90°	60°	45°	30°	0°	
Arm recoil		180°	140°–180°	110°–140°	90°–110°	<90°	
Popliteal angle	180°	160°	140°	120°	100°	90°	<90°
Scarf sign							
Heel to ear							

Physical Maturity

Skin	Sticky, friable, transparent	Gelatinous, red, translucent	Smooth, pink; visible veins	Superficial peeling and/or rash; few veins	Cracking, pale areas; rare veins	Parchment, deep cracking; no vessels	Leathery, cracked wrinkled
Lanugo	None	Sparse	Abundant	Thinning	Bald areas	Mostly bald	
Plantar surface	Heel-toe 40-50 mm: −1 <40 mm: −2	>50 mm, no crease	Faint red marks	Anterior transverse crease only	Creases anterior 2/3	Creases over entire sole	
Breast	Imperceptible	Barely perceptible	Flat areola, no bud	Stippled areola, 1–2 mm bud	Raised areola, 3–4 mm bud	Full areola, 5–10 mm bud	
Eye/Ear	Lids fused loosely: −1 tightly: −2	Lids open; pinna flat; stays folded	Slightly curved pinna; soft; slow recoil	Well curved pinna; soft but ready recoil	Formed and firm, instant recoil	Thick cartilage, ear stiff	
Genitals (male)	Scrotum flat, smooth	Scrotum empty, faint rugae	Testes in upper canal, rare rugae	Testes descending, few rugae	Testes down, good rugae	Testes pendulous, deep rugae	
Genitals (female)	Clitoris prominent, labia flat	Clitoris prominent, small labia minora	Clitoris prominent, enlarging minora	Majora and minora equally prominent	Majora large, minora small	Majora cover clitoris and minora	

Maturity Rating

Score	Weeks
-10	20
-5	22
0	24
5	26
10	28
15	30
20	32
25	34
30	36
35	38
40	40
45	42
50	44

Exercise 13.6: Gestational Age Assessment Practice

Read the case scenario below and use the Dubowitz/Ballard criteria to estimate gestational age. Record your scores in the chart, calculate the total, and determine the baby's maturity level.

Case Scenario: A newborn is delivered at home following a healthy pregnancy with uncertain dates. The baby is vigorous, weighs 2.6 kg (5 lb 12 oz), and shows the following characteristics:
- Skin smooth with a few areas of superficial peeling
- Sparse lanugo on shoulders and upper back
- Plantar creases covering the anterior two-thirds of each sole
- Firm ear cartilage with quick recoil
- Breast tissue with raised areola and palpable buds
- Labia majora nearly covering the labia minora
- Limbs flexed with strong tone
- Arm recoils promptly after extension
- Square window angle about 30 degrees
- Heel-to-ear maneuver shows resistance halfway to the ear

Scoring Table

Category	Observed Finding	Score (−1 to 5)
Skin	Smooth with light peeling	_____
Lanugo	Sparse on shoulders	_____
Plantar Creases	Anterior ⅔ of sole covered	_____
Breast Tissue	Raised areola, palpable bud	_____
Eyes/Ears	Firm cartilage, quick recoil	_____
Genitalia (Female)	Labia majora nearly cover minora	_____
Posture	Flexed arms and legs	_____
Square Window	30° angle	_____
Arm Recoil	Quick recoil	_____
Heel-to-Ear	Moderate resistance	_____

Total Score: _____   **Estimated Gestational Age:** _____ weeks

Questions for Reflection

1. Based on your findings, is this infant **preterm**, **term**, or **postterm**? _____

2. How would the baby's gestational age influence your priorities for warmth, feeding, and observation?

3. What follow-up care or referrals would you recommend?

4. How might cultural or resource differences affect how gestational age is assessed in various birth settings?

Newborn Screenings and Procedures

Newborn screenings and preventive procedures identify early health concerns and support a safe transition to life outside the womb. Midwives play a vital role in educating parents, performing procedures within their scope, and coordinating follow-up with pediatric providers. In community birth settings, screenings are usually completed through a combination of home visits, in-office care, and referrals to local programs.

Discuss all procedures with families before birth to support informed decision-making. Maintain sterile technique and gentle handling, document findings and parental consent clearly, and encourage families to keep a copy of all results and vaccine records.

Vitamin K

Newborns have limited vitamin K stores because placental transfer is minimal and intestinal bacteria that synthesize vitamin K are not yet established. Without supplementation, **vitamin K deficiency bleeding (VKDB)** can occur and may cause life-threatening hemorrhage, including intracranial bleeding. Studies show that a single intramuscular dose shortly after birth reduces the risk of late VKDB by about 98 percent.

Purpose: Prevent hemorrhage, especially intracranial bleeding, caused by vitamin K deficiency.

Standard Dose and Timing: 0.5–1 mg phytonadione intramuscularly (IM) in the lateral thigh within the first hours after birth

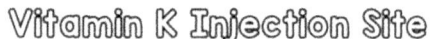

Technique
- Wash hands and don clean gloves.
- Identify the **vastus lateralis** (outer thigh).
- Clean the site with alcohol and allow to dry.
- Use a 5/8-inch, 25- or 27-gauge needle.
- Insert at a 90-degree angle into the muscle.
- Inject the dose slowly, then withdraw the needle and apply gentle pressure with sterile gauze.
- Observe for any immediate reaction.
- Document the dose, route, site, manufacturer, and lot number in the newborn record.

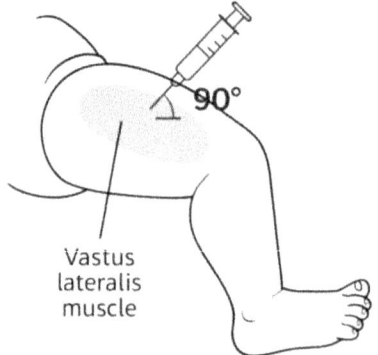

Effectiveness and Route Comparison

Intramuscular vitamin K provides the most reliable protection against both early and late VKDB. Prenatal herbal approaches have been suggested, but there is no clear evidence supporting their effectiveness. Mild discomfort or swelling may occur at the injection site; serious reactions are rare. Oral regimens have been offered as an alternative when parents decline injection. Oral dosing requires multiple carefully timed doses and provides less reliable protection, particularly against late VKDB.

Vaccinations

The **hepatitis B vaccine** is the only immunization recommended at birth in the United States. All other routine infant vaccines begin at or after the two-month visit. Midwives should encourage families to schedule timely pediatric follow-up to ensure continuity of preventive care and adherence to local immunization schedules.

In many community birth settings, midwives do not administer vaccines directly but discuss vaccine benefits and potential risks during prenatal and postpartum visits. They should provide evidence-based written materials and encourage families to establish follow-up with their pediatric provider or local health department for vaccination scheduling.

It is important for midwives to recognize the influence they have on the decisions their clients make. Many families who choose out-of-hospital birth do so because they prefer to limit medical interventions and may be hesitant about some or all vaccines. A midwife's role is to present clear, evidence-based information about immunizations and the potential consequences of declining them, offering guidance without judgment or personal bias.

Eye Prophylaxis

Purpose: Prevent ophthalmia neonatorum—conjunctivitis caused by exposure to maternal organisms such as *Neisseria gonorrhoeae* or *Chlamydia trachomatis*—which can lead to blindness if untreated. Erythromycin remains effective against *N. gonorrhoeae* but offers limited protection for chlamydial infection. Some midwives delay application until after initial bonding and breastfeeding, provided it is administered within the legally required timeframe. Families with negative STI results may decline prophylaxis in jurisdictions where this is permitted.

Medication and Timing: Erythromycin 0.5 percent ophthalmic ointment, both eyes, within two hours after birth (per most state laws).

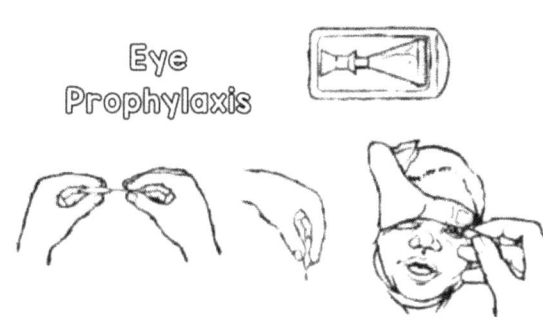

Technique:
1. Wash hands and wear gloves.
2. Gently pull down the lower eyelid.
3. Apply a thin ribbon of ointment along the conjunctiva from inner to outer canthus.
4. Avoid contact between the tube tip and the eye.
5. Allow the ointment to remain for one minute, then gently wipe away excess.
6. Document time, medication, and parental consent or declination.

Newborn Metabolic Screening (PKU)

Newborn metabolic screening identifies inherited metabolic, endocrine, and hematologic disorders that may not be evident at birth but can cause severe disability or death if untreated. Early detection allows for timely intervention and improved outcomes.

Timing: Collected between 24 and 72 hours after birth, with a repeat specimen as required by state protocol.

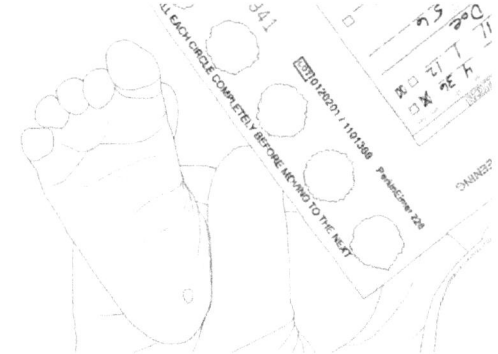

Technique:
- Warm the infant's heel and clean with alcohol.
- Puncture the lateral or medial heel with a sterile lancet.
- Allow free-flowing blood to saturate each circle on the filter paper card.
- Air-dry the sample thoroughly before mailing to the state laboratory.
- Complete all documentation and verify submission.

Follow-up: Each state determines which conditions are screened, typically ranging from 30 to 50 disorders. Results requiring confirmation are reported promptly for medical evaluation. Midwives should confirm that families understand the purpose of screening and know how to obtain follow-up results.

Critical Congenital Heart Disease (CCHD) Screening

Pulse oximetry screening detects serious heart defects that may not be apparent on physical exam. Early identification prevents delayed diagnosis and complications.

Purpose: Detect critical heart defects that cause low blood oxygen before symptoms develop.

Timing: Between 24 and 48 hours after birth.

Technique:
- Place pulse oximeter sensors on the **right hand** and **one foot.**
- Record both readings.
- A result below 95 percent in either extremity or a difference greater than 4 percent between them requires medical referral.

- Document results and explain results clearly to the family, and provide written documentation for the pediatric provider or local public health office.

Hearing Screening

Hearing loss affects approximately 2 to 4 newborns per 1,000 births. Early identification allows for prompt language, social, and developmental support. Inform families that the test is painless and noninvasive, usually performed while the baby is calm or feeding. For home or birth center clients, coordinate referral to an approved newborn hearing program.

Purpose: Detect congenital hearing loss by one month of age.

Methods:
- **Otoacoustic emissions (OAE)** – Measures inner-ear response to sound.
- **Automated auditory brainstem response (AABR)** – Measures brainwave response to sound.

Technique:
- Place a small probe or earphone in the ear canal while the infant rests quietly.
- The device records auditory responses and displays results as "pass" or "refer."
- Refer to a certified hearing center within one week if not performed on-site or if the result is "refer."

Glucose Testing

Neonatal hypoglycemia refers to abnormally low blood glucose levels in the first days of life. Transient drops are common during adaptation to extrauterine life, but persistent or symptomatic hypoglycemia may lead to neurologic injury if untreated. Routine glucose testing is not recommended for all newborns. Midwives should assess risk factors, feeding effectiveness, and temperature stability during early postpartum visits. Early skin-to-skin contact and prompt initiation of breastfeeding are typically sufficient for maintaining normal glucose levels in healthy term infants.

Purpose: Identify infants with low blood glucose who require feeding support or medical evaluation.

At-Risk Infants:
- Preterm or late-preterm infants
- Small for gestational age (SGA) or large for gestational age (LGA) infants
- Infants of diabetic parents
- Infants who experienced birth stress, asphyxia, or hypothermia

Normal and Abnormal Values:
- Within the first 24 hours: less than 40 mg/dL is considered low.
- After 24 hours: less than 45–50 mg/dL is considered low.
- Normal range for term newborns: approximately 60–90 mg/dL.

Symptoms: Jitteriness, tremors, weak cry, lethargy, poor feeding, apnea, cyanosis, seizures, or temperature instability.

Technique:
- Warm the heel to increase blood flow.
- Clean with alcohol and allow to dry.
- Use a sterile lancet on the lateral or medial heel.
- Collect a drop of blood on a glucose test strip or glucometer.
- Record and interpret results with attention to symptoms and feeding history.

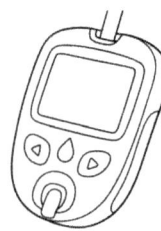

Management:
- Encourage early and frequent breastfeeding.
- If the infant cannot latch or feed effectively, express breast milk and feed with a syringe or cup.
- Repeat glucose testing after feeding to confirm response.
- Persistent or symptomatic hypoglycemia requires medical evaluation and possible intravenous glucose therapy.

CIRCUMCISION AND CULTURAL PRACTICES IN NEWBORN CARE

Midwives often support families in making informed, evidence-based decisions about newborn procedures, including circumcision. These decisions are influenced by culture, religion, family tradition, and personal values. The midwife's role is to provide accurate information, ensure consent is fully informed, and advocate for the newborn's comfort and safety in all cases.

Male Circumcision

Male circumcision is the surgical removal of the foreskin (prepuce) that covers the glans of the penis. In the United States, it remains a common procedure, although the American Academy of Pediatrics (AAP) does not recommend it routinely for all newborns. The AAP recognizes potential health benefits—such as reduced urinary tract infection rates and lower transmission of certain infections—but emphasizes that these benefits are not sufficient to justify universal circumcision.

> **Circumcision Trends**
> Routine newborn circumcision is declining worldwide. In the U.S., rates fell below 50% in 2025, while most European countries report rates under 10%, primarily for religious or medical reasons. The global trend reflects a growing emphasis on bodily autonomy and non-intervention.

Risks: Circumcision is a painful surgical procedure that may cause bleeding, infection, or, in rare cases, injury to the penis. Local anesthesia is used but does not fully eliminate pain. Improper technique or poor aftercare can result in complications.

Cultural and Parental Considerations: Some parents choose circumcision for religious or cultural reasons, while others decline it for ethical or personal reasons. Many parents assume it is standard practice or believe their child should "match" a circumcised father or peers. Midwives should provide balanced information that includes the procedure's risks, potential benefits, and available alternatives.

Midwifery Care:
- Provide education about the normal anatomy and natural retraction process of the foreskin.
- Emphasize that the intact penis is not unclean and requires only gentle external washing.
- Review potential complications and signs of infection or bleeding.
- Offer written materials and referrals for families seeking circumcision for religious reasons.
- Ensure informed consent is signed before any procedure.

Female Circumcision (Female Genital Mutilation)

Female genital mutilation (FGM) involves cutting or altering female genital organs for nonmedical reasons. It has no health benefits and causes significant physical and psychological harm. FGM is practiced in parts of Africa, the Middle East, and Southeast Asia, often justified by cultural or religious tradition. It is internationally condemned as a violation of human rights by the World Health Organization (WHO), the United Nations, and professional midwifery and medical associations.

FGM is illegal in the United States and most other countries. Midwives may encounter clients who have experienced FGM and must provide care with compassion and cultural sensitivity. Performing or assisting in any genital cutting is both unethical and unlawful.

Midwifery Care:
- Offer trauma-informed, nonjudgmental care.
- Recognize complications such as scarring, infection, and emotional trauma.
- Educate families about health risks and human rights issues.
- Know and follow all legal reporting requirements.

Global and Ethical Awareness: Midwives working internationally or with refugee and immigrant communities should understand FGM practices and respond with education, advocacy, and referrals for support. Ethical midwifery care balances cultural respect with the duty to protect health, safety, and autonomy.

Key Points:
- Obtain informed consent for all newborn procedures.
- Present medical facts alongside cultural understanding.
- Never condone or participate in harmful traditional practices.
- Promote education, compassion, and respect in all discussions of culture

Exercise 13.7: Newborn Screening
Match each procedure with its purpose

1. Prevents hemorrhagic disease of the newborn	A. Vitamin K injection
2. Prevents infection of the conjunctiva	B. Eye prophylaxis
3. Detects state-specific metabolic and genetic disorders	C. Metabolic screening
4. Identifies heart defects associated with low oxygen levels	D. CCHD screening
5. Detects congenital hearing loss early for timely treatment	E. Hearing screening

Follow-Up Visits and Continuing Newborn Assessment

Follow-up visits are essential for monitoring a newborn's adaptation to life outside the womb and ensuring that feeding, temperature regulation, and bonding are progressing normally. Ongoing assessments allow early recognition of complications and provide continued support for families as they adjust to their new roles. These visits also reinforce trust and strengthen the parent–midwife relationship.

Timing of follow-up visits to track adaptation, growth, and overall well-being:
- **First visit (24–48 hours):** Assess vital signs, temperature, color, feeding, weight, and elimination.
- **Three-day visit:** Evaluate weight change, feeding adequacy, and early jaundice.
- **One-week visit:** Confirm normal cord separation, milk production, and stable weight.
- **Ongoing visits:** Continue weekly or as needed until the family transitions to pediatric care.

Weight and Feeding

Newborn weight changes are among the best indicators of healthy adaptation and adequate feeding.

Normal weight changes:
- **Expected loss:** Up to 7 percent of birth weight during the first week is normal for breastfed infants.
- **Concerning loss:** Greater than 10 percent in the first week or more than 7 percent in the first 72 hours requires closer monitoring.
- **Weight gain:** Most babies regain their birth weight by two to three weeks and gain about six ounces (170 g) per week once milk supply is established.

Feeding and output expectations:
- Newborns should nurse 8–12 times in 24 hours with rhythmic suck and swallow.
- Output should increase daily: one wet diaper per day of age for the first week, then at least six wet diapers and three to four stools per day after milk is established.

A baby who is feeding well will wake on their own, be alert, and show satisfaction after nursing. If weight gain is poor, collaborate promptly with a lactation consultant or pediatric provider.

Average Newborn Feeding and Growth Pattern

Age	Feeds/24 hrs	Wet Diapers	Stools	Expected Weight Trend
Day 1–2	8–12	1–2	1–2 meconium	0–3% loss
Day 3–4	8–12	3–4	2–3 transitional	Up to 7% loss
Day 5–7	8–12	5–6	3–4 yellow	Stable or gaining
Week 2+	8–10	6–8	3–4	Regained birth weight

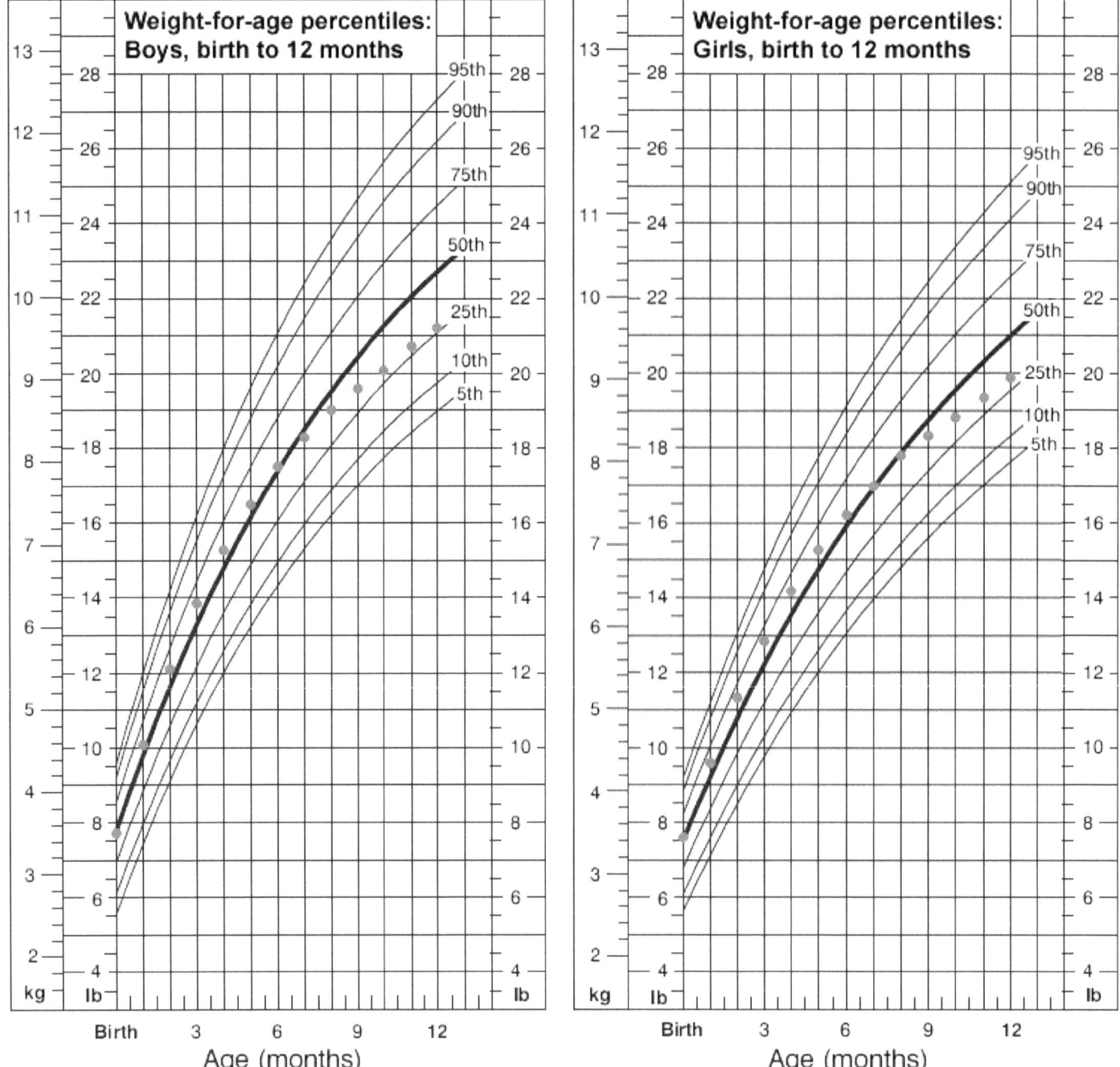

Average Growth Patterns of Breastfed Infants

The red points plotted on the CDC Growth Charts represent the average weight-for-age for a small set of infant boys and girls who were breastfed for at least 12 months (see references).

Sources:

- **Base chart** -- CDC Growth Charts: United States, Published May 30, 2000.

- **Breastfed baby data points** -- WHO Working Group on Infant Growth. An Evaluation of Infant Growth: a summary of analyses performed in preparation for the WHO Expert Committee on Physical Status: the use and interpretation of anthropometry. (WHO/NUT/94.8). Geneva. World Health Organization, 1994, p.21.

Graphic by kellymom.com, 2004

Jaundice

Jaundice is the yellow discoloration of the skin and eyes caused by elevated bilirubin in the blood. It occurs in about half of full-term infants and in most preterm infants.

Types of Jaundice

- **Physiologic jaundice:** Common in healthy newborns, appearing between days two and four, peaking by day five, and resolving within seven to ten days.
- **Breast milk (late-onset) jaundice:** Appears after the third day and may persist for several weeks but is typically benign.
- **Pathologic jaundice:** Occurs within the first 24 hours or persists beyond one week in term infants. Causes may include blood incompatibility (Rh or ABO), infection, liver disease, or significant bruising.

Causes: Bilirubin results from the breakdown of red blood cells. Before birth, the mother's liver processes bilirubin for the baby; after birth, the newborn's liver may be immature and slow to eliminate it. When bilirubin accumulates, the skin and sclera become yellow.

Risks: If levels rise excessively, bilirubin can cross the blood–brain barrier and cause kernicterus, a rare but serious form of brain injury.

Assessment

- Examine the baby in natural light for yellowing of the skin and sclera.
- Blanch the skin over the chest, nose, or thighs to observe color change.
- In darker-skinned infants, assess oral mucosa and sclera.
- Jaundice within the first 24 hours, extending to the palms or soles, or lasting beyond one week requires testing.
- Warning signs include lethargy, poor feeding, and hypotonia.

Practice Tips for Midwives

- Encourage daily checks of color, alertness, and feeding.
- Support breastfeeding and refer early if needed.
- Keep accurate logs of feeding, output, and weight.
- Give clear written guidance on when to seek help.
- Record all observations, education, and referrals.

Management and Prevention

- Encourage early and frequent breastfeeding to promote stooling and bilirubin elimination.
- Colostrum acts as a natural laxative and helps clear meconium.
- Avoid supplementing with glucose water or formula unless medically indicated.
- Filtered sunlight exposure indoors may aid mild cases.
- Phototherapy or hospital evaluation is indicated if bilirubin rises rapidly or exceeds 15 mg/dL in the first three days.

Referral and Collaborative Care

- Refer promptly for serum bilirubin testing or pediatric evaluation if:
- Jaundice appears within 24 hours of birth
- Yellowing progresses quickly or covers the entire body
- The baby shows lethargy, poor feeding, or unstable temperature
- Bilirubin levels approach treatment thresholds

Normal Bilirubin Ranges (mg/dL)
1st 24 hrs: 2–6 (term), 1–6 (preterm)
Day 2: 6–7 (term), 6–8 (preterm)
Days 3–5: 4–12 (term), 10–15 (preterm)

Parent Education and Discharge Observation

Midwives play a vital role in guiding families through the newborn period, helping them adapt to the physical, emotional, and practical changes that follow birth. While much attention is often given to pregnancy and labor, newborn education is equally important. Parent teaching begins during pregnancy, continues through the immediate postpartum period, and extends into the first weeks of life. Effective teaching empowers parents, supports bonding, and builds confidence in caring for their baby at home.

Newborn Parenting Education

New parents often feel unprepared for the realities of caring for a newborn. Even families who attend childbirth classes may miss newborn sessions due to early delivery or scheduling conflicts. The midwife's role is to offer clear, compassionate, and practical guidance before and after birth.

Teaching Topics Include:

- Normal newborn appearance, reflexes, and behavior
- Bathing, diapering, and dressing the baby
- Cord care and observing for signs of infection
- Safe sleep practices and environmental safety
- Burping, soothing, and gentle handling techniques
- Signs of feeding readiness, fullness, and effective feeding
- Managing diaper rash and skin care
- Recognizing dehydration, fever, or illness
- Car seat use, changing table safety, and choke hazards
- Medication safety and avoiding unsafe sleep surfaces such as couches or recliners

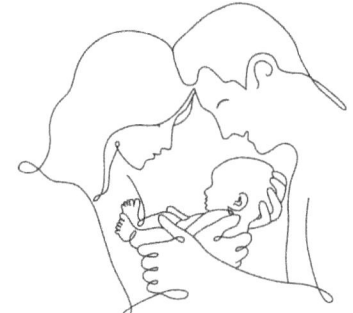

Provide written handouts and checklists to reinforce learning. Encourage parents to attend newborn-specific classes or local support groups, and consider maintaining a lending library of books and videos. Offering practical demonstrations during home visits helps parents feel capable and supported.

Safe Sleep Education

Midwives teach parents that safe sleep practices significantly reduce the risk of sudden infant death syndrome (SIDS) and suffocation. Babies should always be placed on their backs to sleep, on a firm, flat surface free of pillows, blankets, toys, or bumper pads. Keep the baby's sleep area smoke-free, cool, and uncluttered, and avoid couches or armchairs for naps. Parents should also know that breastfeeding and pacifier use (after breastfeeding is well established) are protective factors. Clear, compassionate education empowers families to create a sleep environment that's both safe and nurturing.

Emotional Adjustment and Postpartum Experience

The early postpartum weeks bring intense physical recovery and emotional change. Fatigue, self-doubt, and fluctuating moods are common, and parents may feel both joy and uncertainty as they learn to meet their baby's needs. Unrealistic expectations of being the "perfect parent," loss of personal time, and disrupted sleep can increase stress and anxiety. Midwives can normalize these experiences by reassuring families that adjustment takes time and by encouraging rest, nourishment, and open communication. Recognize signs of postpartum depression or anxiety, and refer for counseling or peer support when appropriate. Compassionate listening is often as important as clinical guidance.

Common Emotional Challenges Include

- Fatigue and sleep deprivation
- Feelings of inadequacy or guilt
- Strain in relationships or shifting roles
- Anticlimax after a difficult or unexpected birth
- Fear of harming or failing the baby

Reassure parents these emotions are temporary and support is available.

Car Seat Safety and the Midwife's Role

Safe transportation is an essential part of newborn care education. Every baby should ride in a rear-facing, federally approved car seat, installed in the back seat according to manufacturer instructions. Midwives can help families understand proper positioning—snug harness, chest clip at armpit level, and no bulky clothing that interferes with straps. For families without access to a vehicle or who cannot afford a car seat, midwives can connect them with community programs, hospitals, or fire departments that provide free or low-cost seats and installation checks. In some cases, a midwife may advise arranging alternate transportation home or delaying discharge until safe travel can be ensured. Supportive, nonjudgmental discussion about barriers to car seat use helps families find safe, realistic solutions that protect their newborn.

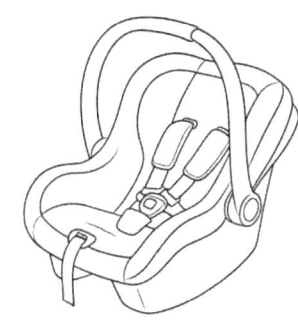

Observation Prior to Discharge

Before discharge or going home, the midwife assesses both the newborn's physical stability and the family's readiness for independent care.

The Newborn Should
- Maintain stable vital signs and temperature
- Exhibit normal color, tone, and reflexes
- Feed effectively with evidence of swallowing and rhythmic suck
- Have voided and passed meconium
- Have a clean, dry umbilical cord

The Family Should
- Demonstrate safe handling and feeding techniques
- Recognize early warning signs of illness or distress
- Verbalize understanding of follow-up plans and emergency contacts

Parent Education Prior to Discharge

Before leaving midwifery care, review essential topics to ensure confidence and safety:
- Feeding frequency, elimination patterns, and signs of adequate intake
- Umbilical cord care and infection prevention
- Jaundice awareness and when to contact the provider
- Car seat safety and travel precautions
- Written instructions for emergencies and follow-up visits

Discharge Criteria

A newborn may be discharged when:
- Vital signs and temperature are stable
- Feeding and elimination are established
- Screenings and prophylaxis are completed
- The umbilical cord is secure and clean
- Parents understand and demonstrate newborn care
- Follow-up is scheduled within 24–48 hours

Midwifery Care
- Normalize the emotional challenges of early parenthood and encourage self-compassion
- Reinforce positive caregiving and bonding behaviors
- Provide brief written summaries of key care topics
- Schedule an early postpartum visit to assess feeding, weight, and emotional health
- Offer resources for lactation, mental health, and parenting support
- Be available for questions—your reassurance and presence can make all the difference

Cultural Traditions for Newborns Around the World

- **Cradleboards** (Indigenous North America): Traditional portable infant carriers used by many Nations (e.g., Diné, Lakota, Ojibwe, Apache). The baby is swaddled and secured to a padded board, often with a hood or bow.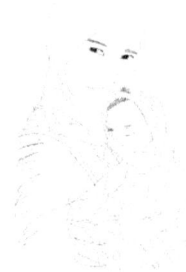
  - **Babywearing** (Global): Found in nearly every culture—African kanga cloths, Asian mei tais, and Mexican rebozos—babywearing promotes bonding, warmth, and easy feeding.
  - **Oil Massage** (India, Nepal, West Africa): Daily massage with warm oils strengthens muscles, promotes circulation, and soothes digestion.
  - **Salt and Herbal Baths** (Middle East, Latin America): Used to cleanse and protect the baby's spirit, often accompanied by blessings or prayers.
- **Naming Ceremonies** (Africa, Pacific Islands, Native Nations): The baby's name is chosen and celebrated publicly, affirming identity and community belonging.
- **Confinement Periods** (China "zuo yuezi," Latin America "la cuarentena"): Mothers and infants rest for 30–40 days, supported by family care, nourishing foods, and limited outside exposure.
  - **Swaddling** (Eastern Europe, Russia, Japan): Keeps babies calm and warm, symbolizing protection and care.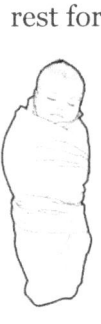
  - **Placenta Honoring** (Maori, Hawaiian, Indigenous Americas): The placenta is buried with ceremony to honor the child's connection to the land and ancestors.
  - **Evil Eye Protection** (Mediterranean, Middle East, Latin America): Amulets or red strings protect newborns from negative energy or envy.
  - **First Hair or Nail Rituals** (Islamic, Hindu, and African traditions): Hair or nails are cut ceremonially to mark growth and transition into community life.

Exercise 13.8: Continuing Care and Parent Education
Answer the following questions:

1. The first newborn follow-up visit should occur within _____ hours after birth.

2. By the end of the first week, most babies should have lost no more than _____ percent of their birth weight.

3. Healthy newborns typically regain their birth weight by _____ weeks of age.

4. The umbilical cord usually separates naturally within _____ to _____ days.

5. A baby should have at least _____ wet diapers per day after the first week.

6. Normal newborn temperature ranges from _____°C _____(°F) to _____°C _____(°F).

7. Before discharge, parents should demonstrate confidence in _____, _____, and recognizing signs of illness.

8. Safe sleep practices include placing the baby on the _____ to sleep, on a _____ surface free of loose bedding or pillows.

The Midwife's Role in Ongoing Pediatric Collaboration

Midwifery care extends beyond the first days of life, forming a vital bridge to pediatric and family practice follow-up. Continuity of care ensures that growth, development, and family adjustment remain supported after midwifery care concludes. Midwives play an essential role in maintaining communication and collaboration during this transition—providing families with clear guidance, connecting them to trusted pediatric providers, and sharing accurate records of birth and newborn findings.

Maintaining an updated list of pediatricians, lactation specialists, and family practice clinicians who are familiar with midwifery clients allows for timely referrals and seamless continuity of care. Parents should be encouraged to schedule their first pediatric visit before the birth whenever possible, ensuring follow-up care is in place at discharge. Using standardized transfer forms or SBAR (Situation, Background, Assessment, Recommendation) summaries promotes consistent, efficient communication. Collaboration should be viewed as shared care, not a transfer of authority, reinforcing a family-centered model where midwives and pediatric providers work together to safeguard newborn health.

Transition of Care

At discharge and during follow-up visits, midwives support families in establishing pediatric or family medicine care. The timing of this transition varies by setting and state regulations but typically occurs between the first week and the sixth week postpartum.

- Provide parents with the name and contact information of the pediatric provider or family physician.
- Communicate pertinent birth and newborn information, including risk factors, screenings, and any ongoing observations.
- Document the transfer of care clearly in the newborn chart, including date, provider name, and parent acknowledgment.
- Encourage families to maintain regular well-baby visits and immunization schedules as appropriate for their chosen provider.

Collaborative Communication

Effective collaboration depends on respectful communication and shared goals for the newborn's health.

- Send a concise written summary or SBAR report to the newborn's provider.
- Include information on birth details, screenings, vitamin K and eye prophylaxis, feeding status, and any follow-up needs.
- Discuss concerns about weight, jaundice, or congenital findings before transfer of care.
- Encourage direct communication between the midwife and pediatric team when complex needs arise.

Community Integration and Support

Midwives are often the first point of contact for families navigating early parenting. Building partnerships with community agencies expands support beyond the clinical setting.

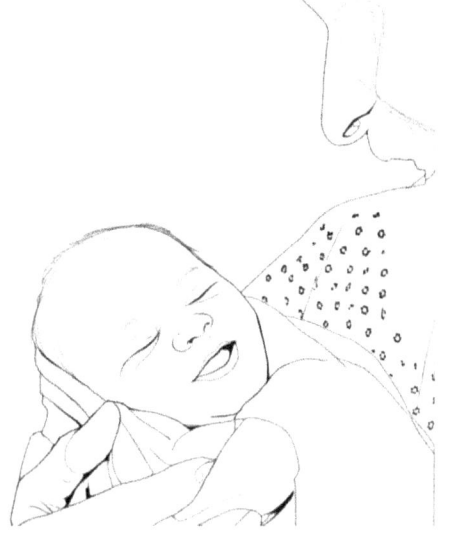

- Identify local lactation consultants, home visiting nurses, and public health programs.
- Refer families to early parenting classes or peer support groups.
- Provide educational materials about infant CPR, safe sleep, and emergency preparedness.
- Encourage use of WIC, SNAP, and other community nutrition and support services as needed.

Professional Accountability

Midwives have a professional responsibility to maintain collaborative, transparent relationships with the wider health care community.

- Stay informed about state and national newborn screening requirements.
- Maintain courtesy and professionalism through consistent communication with physicians and nurses.
- Document all consultations, referrals, and follow-ups.
- Participate in interprofessional or regional review groups when possible to strengthen standards of newborn care.

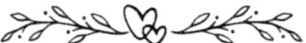

MIDWIFERY CARE OF THE NEWBORN ESSENTIAL TAKEAWAYS

Midwives are responsible for assessing and supporting the newborn's adaptation to extrauterine life from birth through the early weeks. Competence in newborn care includes recognizing normal physiologic changes, performing systematic head-to-toe assessments, and identifying deviations that require prompt evaluation or referral.

Students should understand the components of immediate newborn care, including airway management, temperature stabilization, APGAR scoring, and delayed cord clamping. Knowledge of thermoregulation, prevention of cold stress, and recognition of early feeding cues are essential to promoting stability. Accurate monitoring of weight loss and gain, feeding frequency, and elimination patterns provides the best indicators of newborn well-being.

Midwives must also be familiar with common newborn conditions such as physiologic and pathologic jaundice, appropriate timing for follow-up visits, and safe cord care. Understanding screening and prophylactic procedures—including vitamin K, eye ointment, metabolic testing, hearing assessment, glucose monitoring, and immunizations—is vital for safe practice and effective parent education.

Parent teaching is a core part of newborn care. Midwives ensure families are confident in feeding, safe sleep practices, car seat use, and recognizing signs of illness or dehydration. Ongoing collaboration with pediatric providers, lactation consultants, and community resources ensures continuity of care and early support for both baby and family.

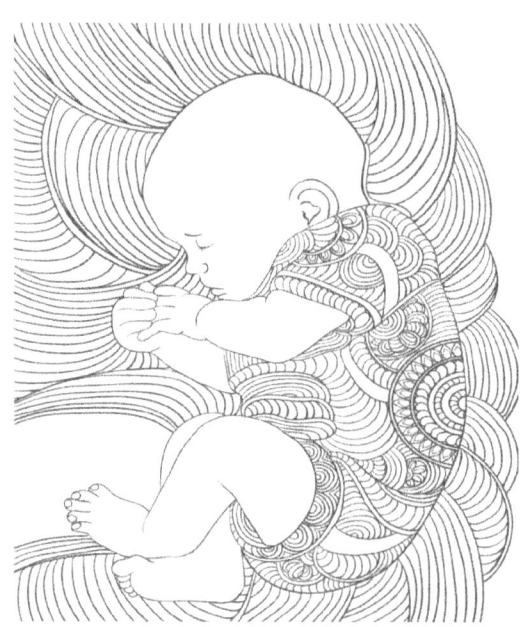

Chapter Thirteen: Self-Assessment

Multiple Choice

1. Which finding indicates a newborn is adapting normally in the first hour after birth?
   a) Persistent central cyanosis
   b) Irregular respirations with strong cry and flexed tone
   c) Heart rate below 90 bpm
   d) No movement or weak tone

2. The most accurate indicator of effective transition immediately after birth is:
   a) Loud crying alone
   b) Pink color and regular respirations
   c) Presence of meconium
   d) Rapid heart rate over 200 bpm

3. The correct intramuscular site for vitamin K administration is the:
   a) Deltoid muscle
   b) Vastus lateralis (lateral thigh)
   c) Gluteal muscle
   d) Abdomen

4. Which of the following newborn screening tests identifies metabolic disorders such as PKU or hypothyroidism?
   a) CCHD screen
   b) Hearing screen
   c) Newborn blood spot (metabolic) test
   d) Glucose heel stick

5. The recommended time for completing the first metabolic screen is:
   a) Immediately after birth
   b) Within 12 hours
   c) Between 24 and 72 hours
   d) After the cord separates

6. A pulse oximetry result of 93 percent in the right hand and 98 percent in the foot suggests:
   a) Normal findings
   b) Possible critical congenital heart disease
   c) Machine malfunction
   d) Need for vitamin K

7. Which statement about newborn glucose testing is accurate?
   a) Routine testing is recommended for all newborns
   b) Testing focuses on infants at risk for hypoglycemia
   c) All readings below 90 mg/dL are critical
   d) Water supplementation is the first treatment

8. Which baby requires closer follow-up for hypoglycemia?
   a) 8-pound term baby nursing well
   b) 6-pound preterm baby with poor feeding
   c) 7-pound term baby with strong cry
   d) 9-pound baby born after rapid labor

9. The Ballard assessment evaluates:
   a) Neonatal reflex irritability
   b) Gestational maturity
   c) Feeding reflex strength
   d) Neurologic disorders

10. A newborn with sticky skin, few plantar creases, and fused eyelids is likely:
    a) 30 weeks
    b) 36 weeks
    c) 39 weeks
    d) 42 weeks

11. Which statement about thermoregulation is correct?
    a) Newborns shiver to maintain temperature
    b) Evaporation is the most common cause of heat loss after birth
    c) Alcohol baths reduce heat loss
    d) Cold stress decreases oxygen demand

12. The normal axillary temperature for a healthy newborn is:
    a) 35.0–36.0 °C (95–96.8 °F)
    b) 36.5–37.4 °C (97.7–99.3 °F)
    c) 37.8–38.2 °C (100–100.8 °F)
    d) 34.0–35.0 °C (93–95 °F)

13. Which type of jaundice appears after the second day and resolves within 10 days?
    a) Pathologic jaundice
    b) Physiologic jaundice
    c) Hemolytic jaundice
    d) Breast-milk jaundice with infection

14. The most reliable way to promote bilirubin elimination is to:
    a) Supplement with glucose water
    b) Encourage frequent breastfeeding and stooling
    c) Delay feeds until milk is established
    d) Use sunlight outdoors

15. The newborn's cord stump should be:
    a) Clean and dry, outside the diaper
    b) Covered with alcohol daily
    c) Tightly wrapped with gauze
    d) Removed after 3 days

16. Which finding requires referral during follow-up?
    a) Cord separation at 10 days
    b) Weight loss > 10 percent by day 5
    c) Breastfeeding 10 times per day
    d) Three wet diapers per day after milk in

17. Which discharge topic should always be reviewed?
    a) Bathing frequency
    b) Cord care and infection signs
    c) Favorite sleep position
    d) Use of herbal powders

Chapter Thirteen: Midwifery Care of the Newborn

True or False
21. _____ Delayed cord clamping increases blood volume and iron stores.
22. _____ The umbilical cord usually separates between 7 and 14 days after birth.
23. _____ Routine suctioning is recommended for all newborns immediately after birth.
24. _____ Physiologic jaundice appearing after day two is a normal finding in most term infants.
25. _____ Breast-milk jaundice always requires discontinuing breastfeeding.
26. _____ Cold stress increases oxygen and glucose consumption.
27. _____ Evaporation is the most common cause of heat loss immediately after birth.
28. _____ Vitamin K deficiency bleeding can be prevented by a single intramuscular dose after birth.
29. _____ Hearing screening should ideally be completed by one month of age.
30. _____ Phototherapy converts bilirubin into compounds that can be excreted in urine and stool.
31. _____ Midwives are required to document newborn screenings and prophylaxis when transferring care.
32. _____ Co-care means shared management between qualified providers.

Fill in the Blank
33. The APGAR score is performed at _____ and _____ minutes after birth.
34. The average head circumference of a term newborn is _____ cm.
35. The newborn's normal respiratory rate is _____ to _____ breaths per minute.
36. The fine downy hair found on preterm infants is called _____.
37. The process by which the newborn maintains body temperature is _____.
38. The three elements of the newborn energy triangle are _____, _____, and _____.
39. Normal weight loss for a term breastfed infant in the first week is _____ percent.
40. The preferred site for vitamin K injection is the _____.
41. The membrane covering the bones of the skull is the _____.
42. The first pediatric or family practice visit should occur within _____ to _____ hours after community birth.

Matching
43. Match each finding with the correct description.
    1. ____ Normal rise in bilirubin after day two
    2. ____ Appears within 24 hours or persists beyond a week
    3. ____ Keep clean and dry, outside the diaper
    4. ____ > 10 percent loss requires follow-up
    5. ____ Uses light to break down bilirubin

    A. Weight loss
    B. Pathologic jaundice
    C. Phototherapy
    D. Physiologic jaundice
    E. Cord care

44. Match each provider collaboration term with its meaning.
    1. ____ Seeking advice while maintaining management
    2. ____ Transfer of specific care to another provider
    3. ____ Shared management between providers
    4. ____ Ongoing connection between birth/pediatric follow-up
    5. ____ Structured summary for safe communication

    A. Co-care
    B. Referral
    C. SBAR report
    D. Continuity of care
    E. Consultation

Chapter Thirteen: Recommended Reading & References

Recommended Reading: Midwifery Care of the Newborn
- Frye, A. (2013). ***Holistic Midwifery, Volume II: Care of the Mother and Newborn***. Labrys Press. Classic midwifery text emphasizing physiologic newborn care and mother–infant bonding in out-of-hospital settings.
- Kittredge, D., & Spencer, N. (2019). ***Community Midwifery and the Newborn: Integrating Home and Hospital Care*** (2nd ed.). Springer. Focuses on postnatal continuity, collaboration with pediatric care, and culturally responsive practice.
- Klaus, M. H., & Fanaroff, A. A. (2015). ***Care of the High-Risk Neonate*** (6th ed.). Elsevier. Comprehensive clinical text covering newborn adaptation, complications, and neonatal intensive care principles.
- Klaus, M. H., & Kennell, J. H. (2001). ***Parent–Infant Bonding*** (2nd ed.). C. V. Mosby. Seminal work exploring attachment, emotional development, and the role of early contact after birth.
- MacDonald, M. G., Ramasethu, J., & Mullett, M. (2022). ***Avery's Neonatology: Pathophysiology and Management of the Newborn*** (9th ed.). Wolters Kluwer. Offers updated guidance on newborn screening, resuscitation, and common neonatal disorders.
- Marshall, J. E., & Raynor, M. D. (2020). ***Myles Textbook for Midwives*** (17th ed.). Elsevier. Global standard midwifery reference including newborn assessment, transition, and community follow-up.
- Martin, R. J., Fanaroff, A. A., & Walsh, M. C. (2020). ***Fanaroff and Martin's Neonatal-Perinatal Medicine: Diseases of the Fetus and Infant*** (11th ed.). Elsevier. Authoritative reference integrating physiology, pathology, and evidence-based newborn management.
- World Health Organization. (2017). ***WHO Recommendations on Newborn Health: Guidelines for Essential Care***. WHO Press. Evidence-based global recommendations for safe newborn care, breastfeeding, and early follow-up.

References

American Academy of Pediatrics. (2022). Vitamin K and the newborn infant: Policy statement. *Pediatrics, 149*(3), e2021056035. https://doi.org/10.1542/peds.2021-056035

Ballard, J. L., Khoury, J. C., Wedig, K., Wang, L., Eilers-Walsman, B. L., & Lipp, R. (1991). New Ballard Score, expanded to include extremely premature infants. *The Journal of Pediatrics, 119*(3), 417–423. https://doi.org/10.1016/S0022-3476(05)82056-6

Cochrane Pregnancy and Childbirth Group. (2021). Prophylactic vitamin K for the prevention of vitamin K deficiency bleeding in newborns. *Cochrane Database of Systematic Reviews*, 2021(5), CD002776. https://doi.org/10.1002/14651858.CD002776.pub3

Greer, F. R., & McCormick, A. M. (2022). Vitamin K deficiency bleeding in infants: Updated recommendations for prevention. *Pediatrics, 149*(3), e2021056036. https://doi.org/10.1542/peds.2021-056036

Mahle, W. T., Newburger, J. W., Matherne, G. P., Smith, F. C., Hoke, T. R., Koppel, R., ... Beekman, R. H., III. (2009). Role of pulse oximetry in examining newborns for congenital heart disease: A scientific statement from the American Heart Association and American Academy of Pediatrics. *Pediatrics, 124*(2), 823–836. https://doi.org/10.1542/peds.2009-1397

Maisels, M. J., & McDonagh, A. F. (2008). Phototherapy for neonatal jaundice. *New England Journal of Medicine, 358*(9), 920–928. https://doi.org/10.1056/NEJMct0708376

Vain, N. E., Szyld, E. G., Prudent, L. M., Wiswell, T. E., Aguilar, A. M., & Vivas, N. I. M. (2004). Oropharyngeal and nasopharyngeal suctioning of meconium-stained neonates before delivery of their shoulders: Multicentre, randomised controlled trial. *The Lancet, 364*(9434), 597–602. https://doi.org/10.1016/S0140-6736(04)16854-8

Wiberg, N., Källén, K., & Olofsson, P. (2008). Delayed umbilical cord clamping at birth has effects on arterial and venous blood gases and lactate concentrations. *BJOG: An International Journal of Obstetrics & Gynaecology, 115*(6), 697–703. https://doi.org/10.1111/j.1471-0528.2008.01703.x

World Health Organization. (2017). *WHO recommendations on newborn health: Guidelines for essential care*. World Health Organization. https://www.who.int/publications/i/item/9789241550379

Chapter Fourteen
Breastfeeding Physiology & Practice

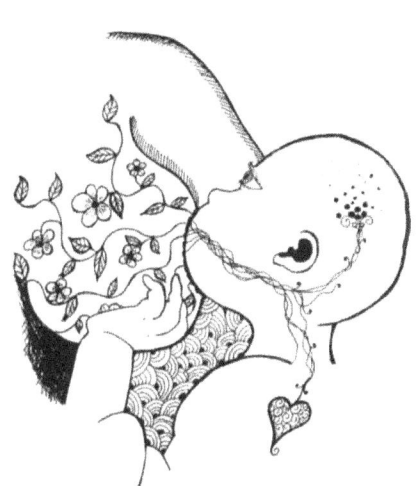

Objectives
After completing this chapter, the student should be able to:
1. **Describe** the midwife's role in promoting, supporting, and protecting breastfeeding throughout the continuum of care, including education, emotional reassurance, and culturally sensitive counseling.
2. **Identify** the anatomy of the breast, including lobes, lobules, alveoli, ducts, nipple, and areola, and explain their functions in milk production and ejection.
3. **Explain** hormonal regulation of lactation, including the roles of prolactin, oxytocin, estrogen, progesterone, and local feedback mechanisms.
4. **Describe** the stages of lactogenesis (I, II, and III) and the physiological process of milk synthesis and release.
5. **Explain** the milk ejection (let-down) reflex and how oxytocin coordinates emotional and physiologic responses during feeding.
6. **Demonstrate** understanding of preventive and supportive techniques for successful breastfeeding, including:
    - Proper positioning and latch,
    - Safe and gentle removal of the baby from the breast,
    - Management of engorgement, blocked ducts, and nipple discomfort.
7. **Describe** methods of milk expression, including hand expression, manual pumps, and electric pumps, and discuss evidence-based guidelines for milk storage and safe handling.
8. **Discuss** the midwife's role in addressing common breastfeeding challenges, such as low supply, overactive let-down, mastitis, or thrush, and identify when to refer to a lactation consultant.
9. **Explain** strategies for maintaining milk supply during separation or return to work, including realistic planning, paced bottle feeding, and emotional support for working mothers.
10. **Describe** the process of weaning, including physical, hormonal, and emotional changes, and how to support gradual, family-centered transitions.
11. **Discuss** special circumstances and maternal health considerations that may affect breastfeeding, including cesarean recovery, medication use, postpartum mood disorders, and complicated births.
12. **Recognize** the influence of culture, tradition, and trauma on lactation practices, and apply principles of cultural humility, inclusivity, and trauma-informed care.
13. **Explain** global and community perspectives on breastfeeding and lactation equity, including advocacy for policies that support breastfeeding families.

Midwifery Support of Breastfeeding

Breastfeeding is the biological norm for infant feeding and the foundation of early human health. No manufactured substitute can fully replicate the nutritional composition, immune protection, or emotional connection that breastfeeding provides. Human milk is uniquely designed for each baby, adapting over time to meet changing developmental needs.

Although nearly all lactating parents are physiologically capable of producing milk, many face barriers related to social norms, inconsistent education, lack of skilled support, or medical or psychological challenges. In Western culture, breastfeeding is widely recommended but not always fully supported in practice. Midwives play a vital role in bridging this gap through early education, practical guidance, and ongoing encouragement.

From a midwifery perspective, breastfeeding is a central component of postpartum care and family health. Colostrum provides concentrated immune protection and supports the newborn's transition to extrauterine life. Continued breastfeeding lowers the risk of sudden infant death, respiratory and gastrointestinal illness, and many chronic diseases later in life. For the lactating parent, breastfeeding promotes bonding, stimulates oxytocin release to support uterine involution, and is associated with reduced risk of postpartum hemorrhage, breast and ovarian cancer, and type 2 diabetes.

> **Key Facts**
> - Human milk is a living fluid that adapts to each baby's needs, varying by time of day and stage of lactation.
> - It contains stem cells, hormones, and bioactive compounds that shape brain development and immunity.
> - Breastfeeding supports healthy stress responses, attachment, and emotional regulation.
> - Colostrum, often called "liquid gold," provides powerful immune protection and helps establish the newborn's microbiome.

Midwives should begin lactation education early in prenatal care, normalizing breastfeeding as a natural and attainable process. Encourage parents to identify sources of support such as partners, peers, or community groups, and reinforce that early follow-up can prevent most feeding complications. Teaching should include both technical skill and emotional support, helping families understand that breastfeeding is learned through practice rather than instinct alone.

In traditional societies, breastfeeding knowledge was passed from one generation to the next. Girls grew up seeing their mothers, aunties, and sisters breastfeed, learning by observation long before they became mothers themselves. Today, many women have never seen a baby nurse until they hold their own. Restoring this visibility and sharing positive stories of breastfeeding can help rebuild confidence and normalize the experience for new mothers.

Education about breastfeeding should begin early in pregnancy, ideally during the first prenatal visits. Discussion should include the physiology of lactation, normal newborn feeding patterns, signs of effective feeding, and realistic expectations for the early days. Working parents or those planning to express milk should receive instruction on the use of breast pumps, safe storage of expressed milk, and strategies for maintaining supply.

After birth, the midwife should provide instruction on positioning, latch, milk transfer, and feeding frequency, and should directly observe a full feeding when possible. Observing a complete feeding during early postpartum visits allows correction of positioning, reinforcement of confidence, and early identification of concerns before they become problems. When challenges persist, collaboration with a lactation consultant or community-based peer support program such as La Leche League or WIC breastfeeding services can help families sustain breastfeeding. In communities where lactation consultants are not available, experienced peer counselors and midwives trained in basic lactation management are valuable resources.

With education, reassurance, and ongoing midwifery support, most families can establish and sustain a satisfying and healthy breastfeeding relationship, even when challenges arise.

Anatomy and Physiology of Lactation

Our understanding of lactation anatomy has advanced through modern imaging and physiological research. When teaching students or parents, describe the breast as a dynamic organ where milk is continually made and moved, not as a container that fills and empties. Reassure clients that breast size does not determine milk-making ability and explain that consistent stimulation and removal of milk are the true drivers of supply.

ANATOMY OF THE BREAST

The breast contains glandular, fibrous, and adipose tissue, supported by Cooper's ligaments. About fifteen to twenty lobes are arranged around the nipple, each divided into lobules containing clusters of secretory units called alveoli. The alveoli are lined with mammary epithelial cells that produce milk and are surrounded by myoepithelial cells that contract in response to oxytocin, moving milk into the ductal system.

Milk travels from the alveoli through progressively larger ducts toward the nipple. The older concept of large "lactiferous sinuses" under the areola has been revised; current imaging shows these spaces are minimal, and milk is stored mainly in the alveoli and small ducts.

The nipple contains multiple openings of terminal ducts, and the surrounding areola includes Montgomery glands that secrete a lubricating oil. These secretions protect the skin and release scent cues that help the newborn orient to the breast.

Key Vocabulary

- **Alveoli (acini):** Small sac-like structures in the mammary gland where milk is produced.
- **Cooper's ligaments:** Fibrous connective tissue that supports the structure of the breast.
- **Feedback inhibitor of lactation (FIL):** milk protein that slows production when the breast is full
- **Foremilk / Hindmilk:** Early and later portions of a feeding that differ in fat concentration.
- **Human placental lactogen (hPL):** placental hormone that prepares the breast for milk production
- **Hypotonia:** Low muscle tone that can make suckling less effective.
- **Lactiferous ducts:** Channels that carry milk from the alveoli toward the nipple.
- **Lactiferous sinus:** A slight widening of the duct beneath the areola, now known to be minimal or absent in most individuals.
- **Lactogenesis I, II, III:** phases of milk production from initiation through maintenance
- **Mammogenesis:** Growth and differentiation of mammary tissue that occurs during puberty and each pregnancy.
- **Myoepithelial cells:** Contractile cells surrounding alveoli that expel milk into the ducts during letdown.
- **Suckling reflex arc:** neural pathway connecting nipple stimulation to pituitary hormone release

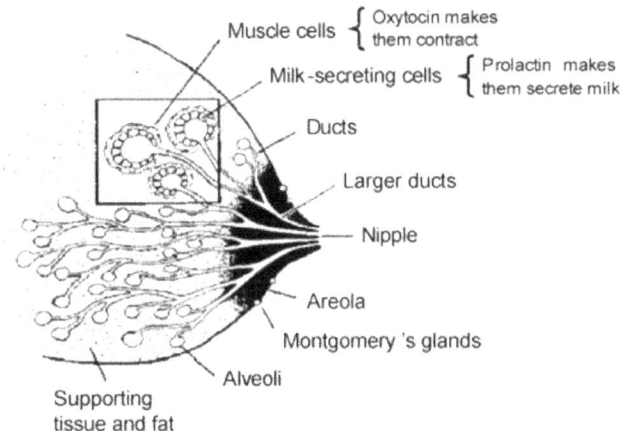

Exercise 14.1: Breast Anatomy
Match each term with its definition.

1. ____Alveoli	A.	Darker area surrounding the nipple
2. ____Myoepithelial cells	B.	Functional units where milk is produced
3. ____Montgomery glands	C.	Contract to push milk through ducts
4. ____Cooper's ligaments	D.	Sebaceous glands that lubricate and scent the areola
5. ____Areola	E.	Fibrous connective tissue supporting breast shape

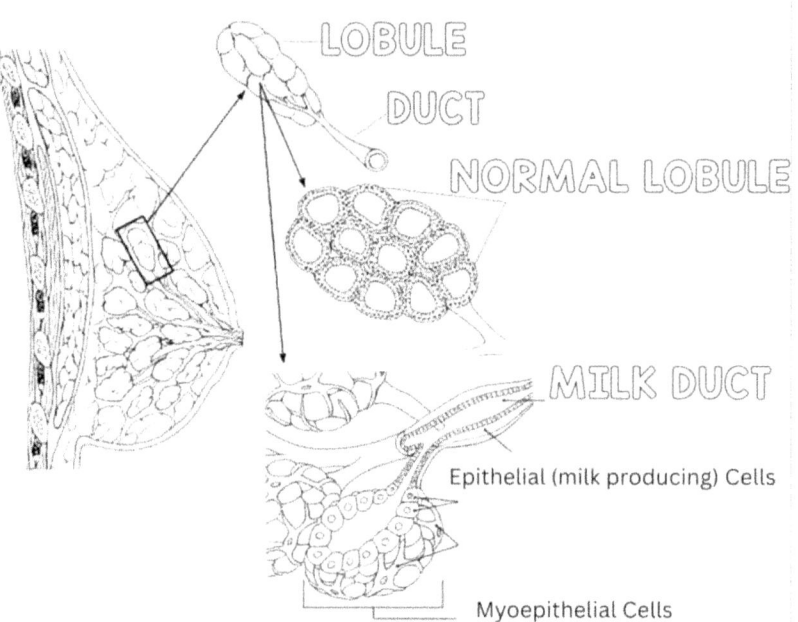

Physiology of Lactation

Lactation begins during pregnancy and continues through three overlapping stages. These changes are guided by complex hormonal and local feedback systems that ensure milk production matches the baby's needs.

Breast Growth During Pregnancy (Mammogenesis)

Each pregnancy stimulates new glandular growth under the influence of estrogen, progesterone, prolactin, and human placental lactogen. The ductal network expands, new alveoli form, and existing structures mature. By mid-pregnancy, the breasts feel fuller and more vascular, the areolae darken, and Montgomery glands enlarge. Each subsequent pregnancy builds on this development, often improving milk-making capacity over time. After weaning, glandular tissue involutes but retains the capacity to regenerate with future pregnancies.

Minimal or absent breast growth during pregnancy may suggest insufficient glandular tissue (IGT). Although breast size alone is not diagnostic, midwives should document breast changes, spacing, and symmetry during prenatal care to anticipate possible lactation challenges.

Lactogenesis: The Stages of Milk Production

Lactogenesis I (Secretory Initiation)

During pregnancy, high levels of estrogen, progesterone, prolactin, and human placental lactogen stimulate ductal and alveolar development. The breasts begin producing small amounts of colostrum, a thick, yellowish fluid rich in immune and growth factors. High progesterone levels inhibit most milk secretion during this time.

Lactogenesis II (Secretory Activation)

After birth, delivery of the placenta causes a sharp drop in progesterone, estrogen, and human placental lactogen, while prolactin remains elevated. This hormonal shift activates milk synthesis. When the nipple is stimulated, prolactin levels rise, peaking about 45 minutes after feeding and returning to baseline within about three hours. This surge triggers the alveolar cells to produce milk, and within two to four days many women feel breast fullness as milk "comes in." Frequent and effective feeding supports this transition and stabilizes supply.

> **Hormonal Control of Lactation**
>
> - **Prolactin** stimulates milk production; levels peak with suckling, especially at night.
> - **Oxytocin** triggers milk ejection and responds to touch, emotion, and relaxation.
> - **Estrogen and Progesterone** prepare the breasts but inhibit secretion until after birth.
> - **FIL** (Feedback Inhibitor of Lactation) slows milk synthesis when breasts are full and increases it with frequent emptying.
>
> *Effective latch and frequent feeding keep hormones balanced and prevent engorgement.*

Lactogenesis III (Galactopoiesis)

Once lactation is established, production becomes locally regulated through the feedback inhibitor of lactation (FIL). When the breast is full, FIL slows further synthesis; when milk is removed, production resumes. Each breast adjusts supply independently according to demand. Milk removal through suckling or pumping maintains receptor activity and ensures consistent milk supply.

The Suckling Reflex Arc

Suckling activates sensory nerves in the nipple and areola, sending signals to the hypothalamus and pituitary. The anterior pituitary releases prolactin to stimulate milk synthesis, and the posterior pituitary releases oxytocin to cause milk ejection. Oxytocin also contracts the myoepithelial cells around each alveolus, pushing milk through the ducts toward the nipple.

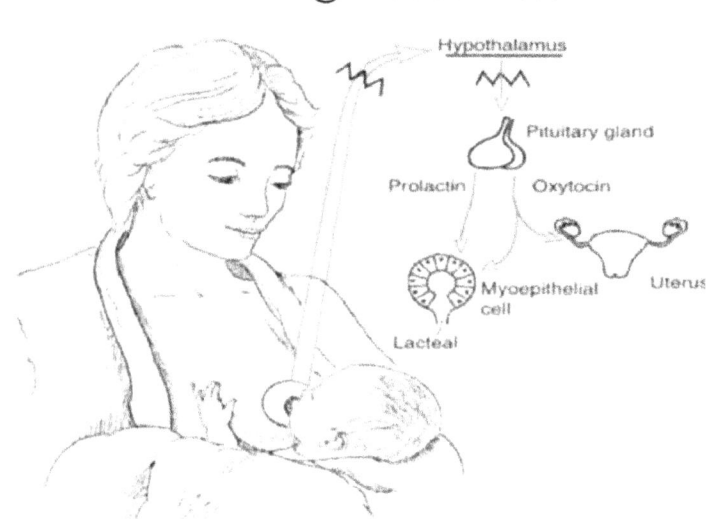

Prolactin and oxytocin release can be influenced by emotional factors such as relaxation, skin-to-skin contact, or even the sound of the baby's cry, demonstrating how emotion and physiology work together in breastfeeding.

Transition from Colostrum to Mature Milk

The composition of milk evolves in the early weeks postpartum, moving from colostrum to transitional and then mature milk.

Colostrum: Produced in late pregnancy and during the first several days after birth, colostrum is low in volume but dense in nutrition and immune factors.
- High in protein, antibodies (especially IgA), and lactoferrin
- Low in fat and lactose, easing early digestion
- Helps establish the infant's microbiome, aids meconium passage, and reduces jaundice risk

Transitional Milk: Around days three to five, milk volume increases and composition shifts as fat and lactose concentrations rise while protein decreases. The milk becomes thinner and whiter. By the end of the first week, daily output may reach 500 to 750 milliliters, depending on feeding frequency and maternal health.

Mature Milk: By about two weeks postpartum, milk stabilizes at around 20 calories per ounce (67 kcal/100 mL). It contains 3 to 5 percent fat, about 1 percent protein, and 7 percent lactose, along with antibodies, enzymes, and prebiotics that support immune and gut health.

Foremilk and Hindmilk

Milk composition changes throughout a feeding.
- **Foremilk** is produced when the breast is full and is higher in water and lactose, satisfying the infant's thirst.
- **Hindmilk** follows as the breast empties, richer in fat and calories for sustained energy.

Encourage families to allow the baby to finish the first breast before switching sides so the infant receives the natural balance of hydration and nutrition. For parents who express milk, explain that early milk may look bluish and thinner, while later milk appears creamier and more opaque.

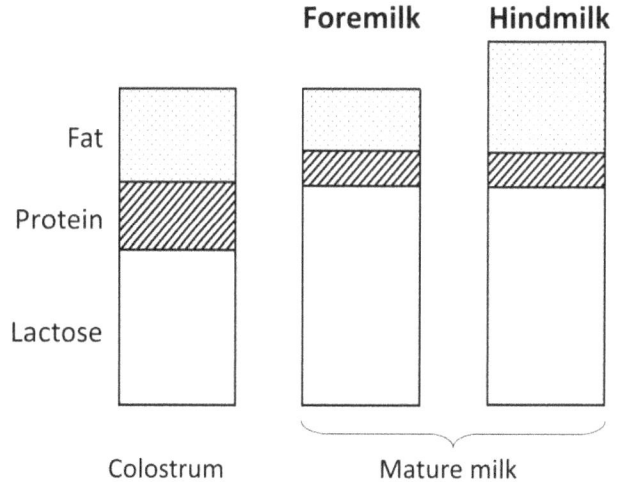

Differences between colostrum and mature milk

INFLUENCES OF STRESS, NUTRITION, HYDRATION, AND REST

Milk production depends not only on hormones and infant demand but also on the overall physiologic condition of the lactating parent. The endocrine system that supports lactation is sensitive to nutrition, hydration, rest, and emotional well-being.

Stress

Stress affects lactation through its influence on oxytocin and prolactin. When cortisol and adrenaline rise, oxytocin release can be inhibited, slowing milk ejection. Flow usually resumes once the parent feels calm or supported. Chronic psychosocial stress or unresolved trauma may delay Lactogenesis II or contribute to a perceived low supply.

Supportive care, reassurance, rhythmic breathing, and skin-to-skin contact help restore oxytocin activity and normal let-down. Midwives can normalize temporary stress-related changes and reassure parents that milk is rarely lost, only temporarily inhibited.

Nutrition

Lactation increases caloric and nutrient needs as the body transfers energy, protein, and micronutrients into milk. Most lactating parents require an additional 450 to 500 calories per day.

Macronutrients
- **Carbohydrates:** 45–65% of total calories from whole grains, fruits, and vegetables
- **Protein:** 15–25% of total calories (about 1.3 g/kg/day)
- **Fat:** 25–35% of total calories, emphasizing unsaturated fats and omega-3 sources such as nuts, avocados, and low-mercury fish

Adequate dietary fat is essential for absorbing fat-soluble vitamins A, D, E, and K, which enhance their presence in breast milk. Very low-fat diets can reduce these vitamin concentrations. Regular omega-3 intake, particularly DHA, supports infant brain and eye development and helps stabilize postpartum mood.

> **Supporting Milk Flow Under Stress**
>
> Stress and exhaustion are among the most common reasons parents believe their milk supply is low. Reassure families that milk is almost never "lost" but may be temporarily slowed.
>
> Encourage simple grounding tools such as rhythmic breathing, hydration, and skin-to-skin contact before feeding. Quiet surroundings, gentle lighting, and warm compresses can enhance oxytocin release. A calm environment and supportive reassurance often restore milk flow as effectively as any intervention.

Micronutrients

The body protects milk composition even when intake is low, but ongoing deficiencies can deplete the parent.
- **Calcium:** 1,000 mg/day
- **Iron:** 9–10 mg/day (higher if anemic)
- **Iodine:** 290 mcg/day
- **Selenium:** 70 mcg/day
- **Zinc:** 12 mg/day
- **Vitamin D:** 600 IU/day minimum
- **Vitamin B12:** 2.8 mcg/day
- **Choline:** 550 mg/day

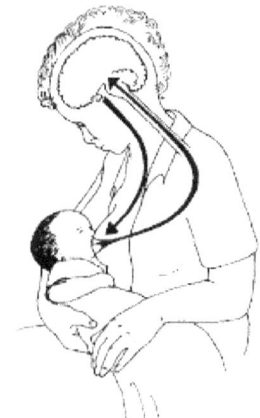

Restrictive diets or skipped meals can lead to fatigue, mood changes, or reduced energy for milk synthesis. Midwives should assess for food insecurity and connect families with WIC, food banks, or culturally familiar nutrition resources.

Weight Loss During Lactation

Gradual weight loss of about 0.5 to 1 pound per week is normal and safe. Milk production uses 400 to 600 calories daily, naturally mobilizing stored fat. Rapid dieting, fasting, or intense exercise can decrease supply and increase fatigue. Most lactating parents return to pre-pregnancy weight within 6 to 12 months, retaining mild fat reserves until weaning.

Hydration

Human milk is about 87% water. Adequate fluid intake is essential for milk synthesis, though overhydration does not increase supply. A general guideline is about 3.1 liters (13 cups) of total fluids daily, or simply drinking to thirst.

Signs of mild dehydration include dark urine, fatigue, and headache. Parents in hot climates or nursing multiples may need additional fluids. Herbal teas such as nettle or rooibos support gentle hydration, while caffeine should be limited to about 300 mg per day (roughly two cups of coffee) to avoid stimulating sensitive infants.

Rest

Rest restores hormonal balance and supports prolactin surges, which peak during nighttime sleep. Interrupted or inadequate rest elevates stress hormones and may blunt oxytocin release. Encourage parents to nap when possible, share responsibilities, and protect rest as an essential physiologic need rather than a luxury.

Milk composition also reflects circadian rhythm: daytime milk contains more cortisol, which promotes alertness, while nighttime milk has higher melatonin levels that support relaxation and help the infant regulate sleep–wake cycles. Feeding milk expressed at the same time of day it was produced may assist the newborn in establishing natural circadian balance.

INITIATION OF BREASTFEEDING

The first hours after birth are a period of powerful hormonal coordination between parent and baby. The newborn enters a quiet, alert state with regular breathing and wide, searching eyes. Elevated catecholamines from the stress of birth keep the baby awake and responsive.

Skin-to-skin contact triggers oxytocin and prolactin release, initiating the hormonal cascade that drives milk production and ejection. It stabilizes the baby's temperature and heart rate while promoting colonization with healthy skin flora. Rooting and sucking reflexes, guided by touch and scent, help the baby locate and latch onto the breast.

When left undisturbed, most newborns attach and feed within the first 30 to 60 minutes. This early feeding reinforces hormonal balance, uterine contraction, and bonding. Interrupting this process can delay the onset of full milk production and increase early feeding challenges.

> **The Instinctive Newborn**
>
> Newborns are born ready to breastfeed. In the first hour, heightened alertness, scent recognition, and coordinated reflexes guide the baby to self-attach.
>
> Allowing time for this natural sequence helps imprint feeding behaviors, regulate vital signs, and support long-term breastfeeding success.

The Breast Crawl

When placed prone on the parent's abdomen or chest immediately after birth, the newborn begins a coordinated sequence of movements known as the *breast crawl*. The baby lifts and turns the head, flexes the legs, and pushes upward in short bursts, using the feet and thighs for propulsion. These movements help the baby navigate toward the warmth and scent of the nipple.

Montgomery glands secrete an oily substance that smells similar to amniotic fluid, guiding the baby toward the areola. The baby's hands play an important role in this process—rubbing or mouthing them transfers familiar scent cues from amniotic fluid, and touching the breast stimulates rooting and oxytocin release in both parent and infant.

Covering the baby's head with a hat or the hands with mittens can interfere with these sensory cues and coordinated movements. Bare skin contact allows the baby to use smell, touch, and body movement to self-attach. A light blanket across the back helps maintain warmth without restricting motion.

The breast crawl may take up to an hour. Quiet observation and patience allow the baby to complete this instinctive sequence, building early confidence and reinforcing the bond between parent and child.

Integration

Lactation reflects the coordinated action of hormones, metabolism, and emotional stability:
- **Prolactin and oxytocin** respond to both physical and emotional cues
- **Nutrition and hydration** sustain milk synthesis and parental health
- **Rest and calm** support efficient milk ejection
- **Early skin-to-skin contact and unrestricted newborn movement** strengthen hormonal balance and bonding

Midwives can help families understand that these elements are essential components of postpartum care. Nourishment, rest, and recovery should be recognized as vital parts of the physiology of breastfeeding, not optional self-care.

Exercise 14.2: Lactation Physiology
Fill in the Blank:

1. Milk is produced in clusters called _____.
2. The hormone _____ causes milk ejection.
3. The change from foremilk to hindmilk occurs _____ during feeding.
4. The first milk produced is called _____.
5. The process by which milk volume increases after birth is known as _____.
6. The hormone responsible for milk ejection is _____.
7. The hormone that stimulates milk synthesis is _____.
8. Milk production is locally regulated by the _____.
9. Prolactin release peaks approximately _____ minutes after feeding begins.
10. Daytime milk is higher in _____, while nighttime milk is higher in _____.
11. The newborn's instinctive movement toward the breast is called the _____.
12. Milk produced early in a feeding is called _____, and milk produced later is called _____.

Positioning, Latch, and Milk Transfer Techniques

Positioning for Comfort and Effectiveness

Teaching positioning and latch is both a clinical and relational skill. The midwife's confident guidance reassures mothers that small adjustments can make a big difference. Begin each feeding by ensuring the mother is comfortable and supported, with the baby raised to breast height rather than the mother leaning forward. Use pillows or rolled blankets for support, and encourage relaxation before offering feedback. Quiet observation allows the midwife to recognize what is working and to model or gently guide hand placement only as needed.

Good positioning creates the foundation for pain-free, effective breastfeeding. The mother should feel relaxed and supported, with the baby's body turned fully toward her chest so ear, shoulder, and hip are aligned. The baby's nose should be opposite the nipple, and the chin should touch the breast first. This allows the head to tilt back slightly, enabling a wide gape and deep latch.

Normalize the learning curve and praise progress. Remind mothers that breastfeeding is a skill developed over time. The goal is not perfection but a feeding rhythm that feels natural, effective, and sustainable for both mother and baby.

Each mother–baby pair finds unique positions that work best for them. Common options include:

Cradle and Cross-Cradle Holds: in the cradle hold, the baby's head rests in the crook of the mother's arm. In the cross-cradle hold, the opposite arm supports the baby's head and neck for more control in guiding a deep latch. The cross-cradle is especially helpful for new mothers or babies still learning to coordinate suck–swallow–breathe patterns.

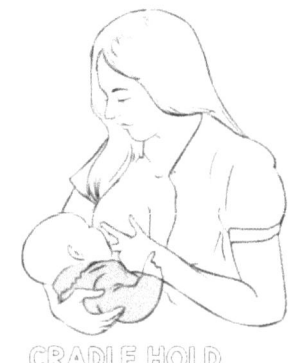
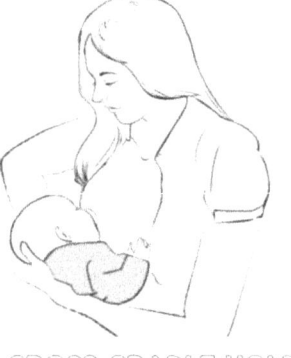

Football Hold: the baby's body lies along the mother's side, supported by the forearm with the head at the breast. This position works well for mothers recovering from cesarean birth or with larger breasts, as it avoids pressure on the abdomen.

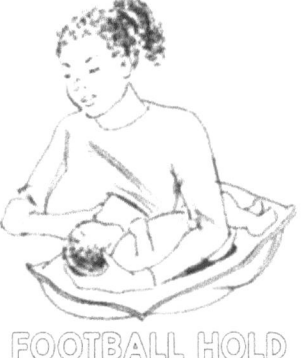

Side-Lying: this position allows rest while feeding, especially at night or during recovery. The baby's face and body should stay close, with the nose opposite the nipple and the chin touching the breast.

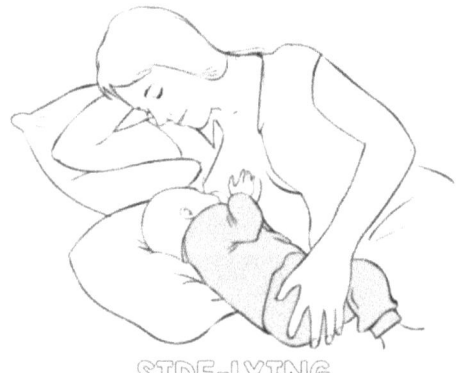

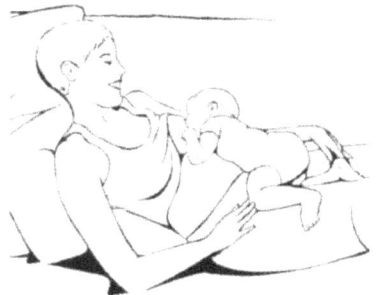

Laid-Back or Biological Nurturing Position: the mother reclines comfortably while the baby lies prone on her chest. Gravity supports deep attachment, and the baby's reflexes guide rooting and head bobbing. This position can help infants with strong gag reflexes or those who struggle with overactive let-down.

Exercise 14.3: Breastfeeding Positions
Match each term with its definition.

1. ____Cross-cradle hold
2. ____Football hold
3. ____Laid-back feeding
4. ____Deep latch
5. ____Hypotonia
6. ____Breast compression

A. Parent supports baby's neck with opposite hand for control
B. Baby's body rests alongside parent's torso
C. Reclined position using gravity and reflexes
D. Nipple reaches far back in the baby's mouth
E. Decreased muscle tone affecting suck strength
F. Gentle rhythmic squeezing to increase milk flow

Breastfeeding Challenges and Midwifery Management

Breastfeeding challenges are common and usually manageable with early, compassionate support. Midwives play a central role in identifying and addressing these issues, particularly in low-resource settings where access to specialized care may be limited.

While midwives should understand the physiology and management of lactation difficulties, collaboration with lactation consultants—when available—enhances care. Lactation consultants have additional training in complex breastfeeding management, and coordinated care between disciplines often leads to better outcomes and stronger family confidence.

When problems arise, reassurance and timely guidance are essential. Encourage mothers to seek support at the first signs of pain, swelling, or fever. Early observation, frequent feeding, and gentle adjustments in position or latch often prevent complications. Calm, consistent encouragement helps mothers stay confident through challenges, reinforcing that most difficulties are temporary and can be resolved with appropriate care.

Engorgement

Engorgement is common when milk first comes to volume, usually between days three and five postpartum. The breasts may feel heavy, warm, and firm, and the areola can become taut, making latch difficult. This fullness results from increased milk, blood, and lymphatic flow as the body adjusts to lactation.

Encourage frequent feeding, gentle breast massage, and warm compresses before nursing to soften tissue. If the baby struggles to latch due to firmness, **reverse pressure softening (RPS)** can help. RPS uses light fingertip pressure around the base of the nipple and areola to move fluid back into the deeper breast tissue. The mother presses inward toward the chest wall with fingertips evenly placed around the nipple for 30–60 seconds, rotating to soften all sides of the areola. This creates enough flexibility for the baby to grasp and latch effectively.

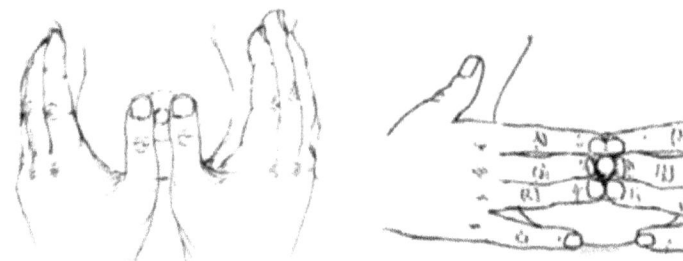

After feeding, cool compresses or chilled cabbage leaves can reduce swelling. Light hand expression may relieve residual pressure. A supportive but nonrestrictive bra prevents discomfort without compressing ducts. Persistent or painful engorgement beyond a few days may indicate incomplete drainage or blocked ducts.

Blocked Ducts

A blocked duct causes localized tenderness, swelling, and a firm, rope-like or pea-sized area without fever or systemic symptoms. Contributing factors include infrequent feeding, tight clothing, or pressure from sleeping position.

Encourage increased feeding frequency, varied positions to fully drain all areas, and gentle massage from the firm area toward the nipple during feeding. Warm compresses before and cool compresses after nursing help relieve discomfort. Adequate hydration and rest support healing.

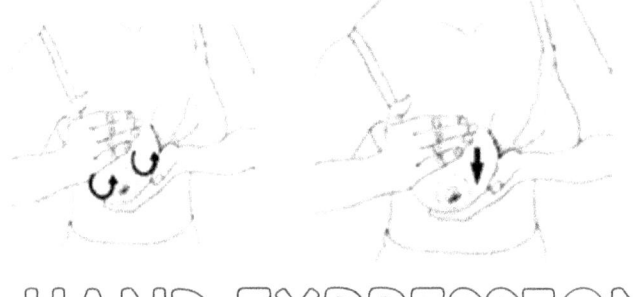

If the lump persists beyond 48 hours, evaluate for infection or abscess formation.

Thrush

Thrush presents as shiny, red, or flaky nipples with deep burning pain during or after feeding. The baby may have white patches on the tongue or inside the cheeks that do not wipe away. It often follows antibiotic use.

Treat with topical antifungals such as nystatin or miconazole for the mother and oral suspension for the baby. Sterilize pacifiers, pump parts, and bottle nipples after each use. Probiotics and air exposure to the nipples can help restore skin balance.

Nipple Pain and Trauma

Mild nipple tenderness is common at first, but persistent pain, cracks, or bleeding usually indicate a shallow latch. Early observation of a full feeding helps prevent most nipple soreness by allowing quick correction of positioning and latch.

Common causes and management strategies include:

- **Shallow latch or poor positioning:** adjust the baby's position and deepen the latch to reduce friction.
- **Incomplete attachment:** ensure the baby's mouth covers both the nipple and a large portion of the areola.
- **Improper removal from the breast:** always break suction gently before removing the baby. Insert a clean finger into the corner of the baby's mouth between the gums, turn the finger slightly to release the seal, and then remove the nipple.
- **Friction or compression:** alternate feeding positions to relieve pressure on sore areas.
- **Nipple trauma:** apply expressed breast milk to the nipples and allow them to air-dry. Hydrogel pads or lanolin may be used sparingly for comfort.

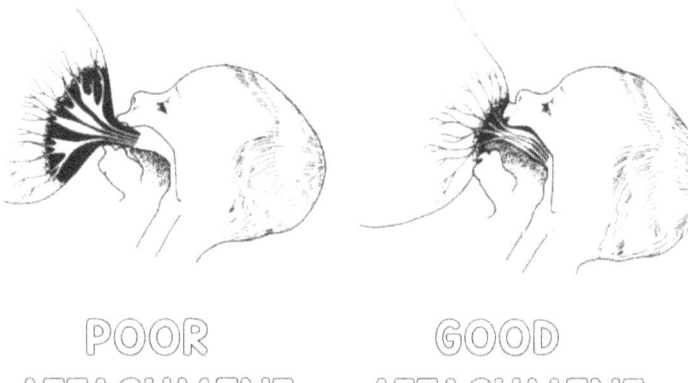

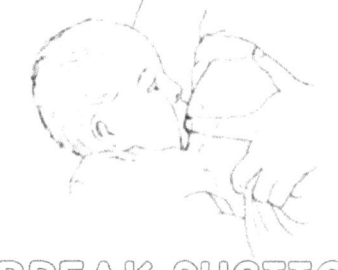

If trauma persists, assess for tongue-tie, lip-tie, or infection. For thrush, both mother and baby require treatment.

Flat or Inverted Nipples

Nipple shape varies widely and usually does not prevent breastfeeding. Some mothers have nipples that appear flat at rest or draw inward when compressed. This can make the early latch more challenging but usually improves with stimulation and frequent feeding.

Encourage early skin-to-skin contact and gentle nipple rolling or hand expression before feeding to help evert the nipple. If swelling is present, reverse pressure softening can reduce tension around the areola and improve latch. Babies learn to draw the breast tissue deeply into the mouth with practice, and most adapt well within the first week.

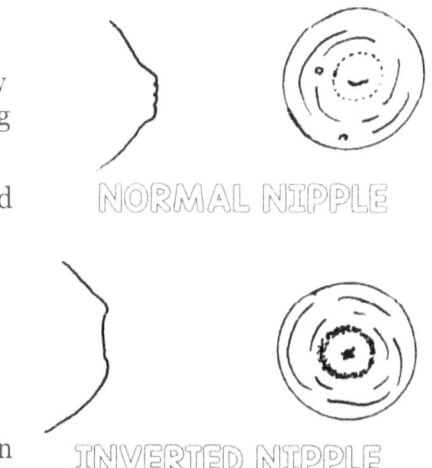

True inversion, where the nipple remains retracted despite stimulation, is uncommon. If the baby continues to struggle with attachment, temporary use of a nipple shield under midwifery or lactation consultant supervision may help establish feeding until the baby gains strength and coordination.

Mastitis

Mastitis involves inflammation of breast tissue, sometimes accompanied by infection. It presents with localized pain, warmth, redness, and systemic symptoms such as fever and body aches. It often follows unresolved engorgement or a blocked duct.

Early management includes continued breastfeeding or milk expression, rest, fluids, and anti-inflammatory medication such as ibuprofen if not contraindicated. Warm compresses and massage toward the nipple assist drainage. If symptoms do not improve within 24 hours, or if fever exceeds 101°F (38.3°C), begin antibiotics appropriate for skin flora such as dicloxacillin or cephalexin.
Reassure mothers that continued milk removal is safe and necessary; abrupt weaning increases risk of abscess formation.

Overactive Let-Down and Hyperlactation

An overactive let-down can cause coughing, sputtering, or pulling away at the breast. The baby may swallow air, leading to gassiness or irritability. Hyperlactation may result from excessive pumping, frequent switching between breasts, or hormonal variation.

Encourage nursing in a **laid-back position** so gravity slows flow, and allow the baby to finish the first breast before switching sides. Expressing a small amount of milk before feeding can ease initial pressure. If oversupply persists, **block feeding** (offering one breast for several hours at a time) can help regulate production. Monitor for plugged ducts or nipple trauma, which may result from forceful flow or shallow latch.

Low Milk Supply and Ineffective Milk Removal

Many mothers worry they are not producing enough milk, but true low milk supply is uncommon. Most cases result from ineffective milk removal rather than inadequate production. Frequent and efficient emptying of the breasts is the key to maintaining supply. When milk remains in the breast for long periods, the **feedback inhibitor of lactation (FIL)** slows further synthesis.

When milk is removed poorly or infrequently, the body receives a false signal that less milk is needed. Correcting latch, increasing feeding frequency, and supporting the baby's suck–swallow coordination usually restore normal production.

CAUSES OF APPARENT VERSUS TRUE LOW SUPPLY

Apparent or Secondary Low Supply	True Low Milk Supply
Infrequent feeding or long gaps between feeds	Insufficient glandular tissue (IGT)
Shallow latch or ineffective suck	Prior breast surgery with tissue or nerve damage
Sleepy, jaundiced, or hypotonic baby	Endocrine disorders (thyroid disease, retained placenta)
Early supplementation reducing breast stimulation	Significant postpartum hemorrhage affecting prolactin
Use of nipple shields or inefficient pumping	Structural breast hypoplasia or congenital ductal anomaly
Maternal stress, dehydration, or fatigue	Severe malnutrition or chronic illness

Assessing Milk Production and Transfer

The best indicators of adequate milk supply are the baby's growth and elimination patterns. Six or more wet diapers and three or more stools daily by the end of the first week indicate good intake. Consistent weight gain after initial loss confirms effective feeding.

Ineffective milk removal may appear as persistent breast fullness, short or weak sucking bursts, or lack of audible swallowing. The baby may gain weight slowly despite frequent feeds. The midwife should observe a full feeding to assess latch, transfer, and milk flow before concluding true low supply.

Delayed Lactogenesis II

The transition from colostrum to mature milk, known as lactogenesis II, usually occurs within 48–72 hours after birth. A delay beyond this increases risk of low production and early weaning. Contributing factors include maternal stress, obesity, diabetes, thyroid disorders, excessive blood loss, or retained placental fragments. Frequent feeding, hand expression, and skin-to-skin contact help stimulate earlier onset. When delay persists beyond five days, further evaluation is warranted.

Clinical Management

Midwifery care focuses on restoring effective milk removal and supporting the physiologic feedback system of lactation.

Assessment should include:
- Observation of latch and position
- Frequency and duration of feeds
- Infant tone and coordination of suck–swallow–breathe
- Maternal health factors affecting hormonal function

Interventions may include:
- Encouraging feeding at least 8–12 times in 24 hours
- Using hand expression or pumping after feeds to ensure drainage
- Addressing maternal endocrine or thyroid conditions
- Treating retained placental tissue if present
- Avoiding unnecessary supplementation unless clinically indicated

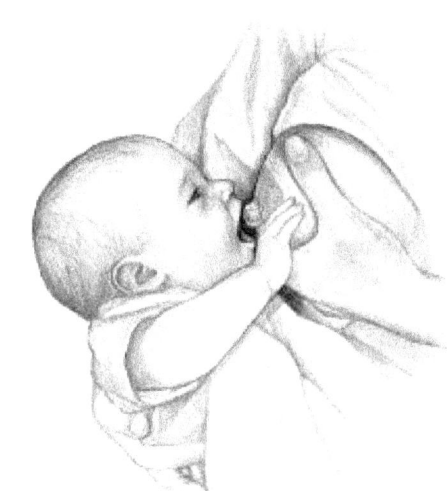

If low supply persists, consultation with a lactation specialist or physician may be needed. Galactagogues—herbal or pharmaceutical—should be used only after optimizing milk removal and correcting reversible causes.

Frequent feeding, early observation, and gentle self-care prevent most challenges. When addressed promptly, breastfeeding difficulties usually resolve quickly, and continued breastfeeding remains possible in nearly all cases. The midwife's role is not only to treat but also to teach, building the parent's confidence to manage small issues independently while knowing when to reach out for support.

Exercise 14.4: Breastfeeding Challenges
Match each term with its definition.

1. ____Engorgement	A. Temporary fullness when milk first comes to volume
2. ____Blocked duct	B. Localized lump without systemic symptoms
3. ____Mastitis	C. Painful inflammation with fever or redness
4. ____Overactive let-down	D. Rapid milk flow causing infant choking
5. ____Hyperlactation	E. Oversupply leading to engorgement or discomfort
6. ____Low milk supply	F. Inadequate production from infrequent feeding
7. ____Thrush	G. Candida infection of nipple and baby's mouth
8. ____Reverse pressure softening	H. Technique to soften areola for easier latch
9. ____Insufficient glandular tissue	I. Underdevelopment of milk-producing structures
10. ____Delayed lactogenesis II	J. Late onset of abundant milk production

PUMPING, HAND EXPRESSION, MILK STORAGE, AND RETURNING TO WORK

The Role of Expression in Lactation Support

Milk expression is an essential skill for many mothers and a valuable part of midwifery care. Expression may be needed for a variety of reasons, including early separation, return to work, or temporary feeding challenges. It also helps relieve fullness, stimulate supply, and provide milk when the baby cannot feed directly.

Midwives play a vital role in helping mothers view expression as an extension of breastfeeding, not a replacement for it. Teaching hand expression during the early postpartum period ensures that every mother has a reliable, equipment-free way to manage fullness and protect supply. Normalize the use of pumps without medicalizing the process, and tailor guidance to the mother's resources, needs, and cultural context.

When taught early, expression can prevent common issues such as engorgement, blocked ducts, or declining supply. Encourage relaxed routines and reassure mothers that output varies by time of day and emotional state. Flexibility, not perfection, supports long-term breastfeeding success.

Hand Expression

Hand expression is a simple, effective way to remove milk without equipment and is especially useful in the first days after birth when small amounts of colostrum are produced. Teaching this skill during pregnancy or the early postpartum period builds confidence and self-sufficiency.

To express milk by hand, the mother should:

1. Wash hands thoroughly and prepare a clean container.
2. Gently massage the breast in a circular motion to stimulate let-down.
3. Place the thumb and forefinger about one inch behind the nipple, forming a "C" shape.
4. Press back toward the chest wall, then compress and release rhythmically without sliding the fingers over the skin.
5. Rotate hand positions around the areola to drain different ducts.

Drops of colostrum or milk can be collected in a small sterile cup or syringe. Early expression is often easier than pumping because colostrum is thick and produced in small quantities.

Hand expression can also soften the areola for easier latch, relieve engorgement, and stimulate additional milk production after or between feedings. It is gentle, portable, and requires no equipment, making it a vital skill in all birth settings.

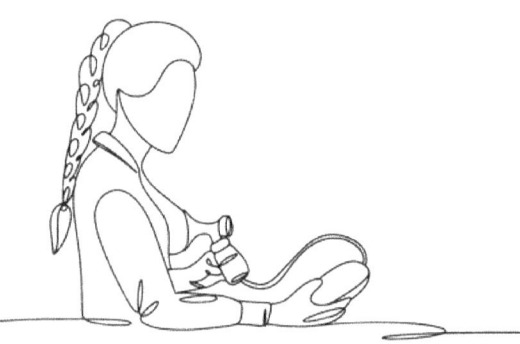

Pumping Methods

Mechanical pumps may be manual or electric, single or double. Manual pumps are inexpensive and portable, while electric pumps—especially hospital-grade models—are more efficient for maintaining supply or expressing milk for preterm or hospitalized infants.

Effective pumping depends on comfort and correct flange fit. The nipple should move freely within the tunnel without rubbing, and the areola should not be pulled excessively. Pain or blanching indicates a need for a different flange size or lower suction setting.

Pumping sessions usually last 15–20 minutes, though shorter sessions may suffice once milk is flowing easily. For mothers separated from their infants, pumping every 2–3 hours during the day and at least once at night helps maintain supply.

Relaxation enhances milk flow. Encourage mothers to use gentle breast massage, warm compresses, or visualization of their baby to stimulate let-down. Some mothers find that looking at photos or hearing their baby's voice helps trigger oxytocin release.

Milk Collection and Storage

Expressed milk should be collected in clean, food-grade containers made of glass or BPA-free plastic. Specialized storage bags designed for breast milk are convenient for freezing but should not be reused. Label each container with the date and time of expression, and if applicable, the baby's name.

Evidence-based milk storage guidelines:
- **Room temperature (up to 77°F or 25°C):** 4 hours
- **Refrigerator (up to 40°F or 4°C):** 4 days
- **Freezer (0°F or −18°C):** 6 months for optimal quality, up to 12 months if needed

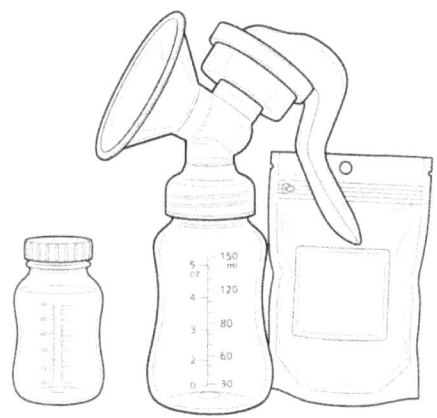

When thawing frozen milk, place it in the refrigerator overnight or warm gently in a bowl of warm water. Avoid microwaves or boiling water, as these destroy nutrients and increase the risk of scalding.

Once thawed, milk should be used within 24 hours and never refrozen. Any leftover milk from a feeding should be discarded after two hours. For preterm or hospitalized infants, use more conservative storage times due to higher infection risk.

Discuss realistic storage and transport strategies, particularly for mothers working long shifts or without easy access to refrigeration. Reinforce that small amounts of milk are valuable—every drop counts.

Maintaining Supply and Returning to Work

Returning to work or school can be a significant emotional and physical transition. Advance planning helps mothers continue lactation successfully while reducing stress.

Encourage building a small freezer supply one to two weeks before returning to work by expressing milk once daily after the first morning feeding. At work, pumping sessions should occur about every three hours in a private, clean space with access to handwashing and refrigeration. Many regions have workplace laws protecting the right to express milk; midwives can help mothers understand these rights and, when needed, provide documentation for employers.

Reuniting with the baby after work allows for direct feeding, skin-to-skin contact, and emotional reconnection. Breastfeeding in the evening and overnight helps sustain milk production and strengthen attachment. If another caregiver feeds expressed milk, recommend paced bottle feeding to mimic the flow of breastfeeding and reduce confusion.

Teaching milk expression skills is an important part of midwifery care. When mothers understand how to hand express, pump comfortably, and store milk safely, they gain flexibility and confidence to sustain breastfeeding through changing circumstances. By offering reassurance, practical guidance, and culturally sensitive support, midwives help families integrate lactation into daily life and strengthen long-term breastfeeding success.

Exercise 14.5: Breastmilk Collection
Fill in the Blank:

1. The manual technique for removing milk without equipment is called _____.
2. The hormone that triggers milk release during pumping is _____.
3. Expressed milk should be labeled with the date and _____ of expression.
4. Breast milk stored in the freezer at 0°F (-18°C) is best used within _____ months.
5. When feeding expressed milk, caregivers should use _____ bottle feeding to mimic breastfeeding rhythm.

WEANING AND EXTENDED BREASTFEEDING

Understanding Weaning

Weaning is a normal and highly individual transition that marks a new stage in the relationship between mother and child. It may occur naturally when the child gradually loses interest in nursing or be guided by the mother for personal or logistical reasons. The process often unfolds over weeks or months depending on the child's readiness and the family's needs.

Globally, the natural age of weaning varies widely, often between two and four years. In cultures where breastfeeding is socially visible and uninterrupted by early separation, extended breastfeeding is common and continues to provide immune and emotional benefits. Midwives can reassure families that breastfeeding beyond infancy remains biologically normal and beneficial, offering continued comfort, nutrition, and antibodies that support the child's health.

Midwives can help families view weaning as a natural evolution rather than a sudden event. Encourage open discussion about timing, motivation, and emotional readiness on both sides. Whether the decision is led by the child or the mother, emphasize that the process can be gradual, gentle, and respectful of their bond.

Physical and Hormonal Changes During Weaning

As feeding frequency decreases, milk production naturally declines. Falling prolactin and oxytocin levels may cause temporary breast fullness, emotional sensitivity, or fatigue. These sensations usually resolve within days to weeks as the body adapts. Gradual weaning minimizes discomfort and helps prevent engorgement or blocked ducts.

When fullness occurs, gentle expression or partial emptying provides relief. Ice packs, supportive bras, and anti-inflammatory medication can ease soreness. Abrupt weaning may increase the risk of engorgement, mastitis, or emotional distress for both mother and child. Midwives should remind mothers that gradual change is nearly always more comfortable. Replacing one feeding at a time, every few days, allows both the body and child to adjust smoothly.

Emotional Aspects of Weaning

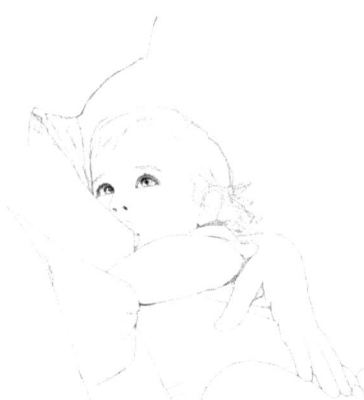

Weaning often brings mixed emotions. Some mothers feel ready and relieved, while others experience sadness or grief as breastfeeding ends. Hormonal shifts can intensify these emotions, and midwives can normalize this experience by explaining that emotional ups and downs are part of the body's adjustment process.

Children may show temporary clinginess, irritability, or disrupted sleep during weaning. Maintaining close physical contact and consistent routines helps ease the transition. Encouraging alternative forms of comfort—such as cuddling, reading together, or shared meals—preserves the connection as the nursing relationship changes. If emotional distress or guilt arise, midwives can offer reassurance and, when needed, refer mothers to counseling or peer support. Calm, informed guidance helps families navigate the transition with confidence and compassion.

Approaches to Weaning

Child-Led Weaning: in child-led weaning, the child naturally nurses less often and eventually stops on their own. This process tends to be slow and gentle, often unfolding over many months. The mother's body adjusts naturally to reduced demand, minimizing discomfort.

Parent-Led Weaning: parent-led weaning is guided by the mother's needs or circumstances, such as returning to work, medical concerns, or personal preference. Gradual change is most effective—replacing one feeding at a time with a snack, cup of milk, or comforting activity allows the child and body to adapt smoothly. Nighttime weaning may take longer, as many children nurse for comfort rather than hunger. Gentle methods, consistent routines, and partner involvement help maintain emotional connection while establishing new patterns.

Midwifery Guidance

The midwife's role is to provide steady support and reassurance through this transition.
- Emphasize that weaning is a personal decision and that extended breastfeeding remains safe and beneficial when mutually desired.
- Encourage gradual change and comfort measures to prevent engorgement.
- Suggest alternative bonding activities that maintain closeness and security.
- Normalize emotional fluctuations for both mother and child.
- Provide follow-up and referrals if physical or emotional challenges arise.

Weaning, when supported with patience and understanding, becomes not an end but a transformation—one that honors the shared journey and the evolving needs of both mother and child.

Exercise 14.6: Weaning and Extended Breastfeeding
Match each term with its definition.

1. ____Weaning
2. ____Extended breastfeeding
3. ____Child-led weaning
4. ____Parent-led weaning
5. ____Prolactin

A. Gradual process of reducing and ending breastfeeding
B. Hormone that supports milk production and declines with reduced feeding
C. Continuing to nurse beyond one year
D. Natural decrease in nursing initiated by the child
E. Gradual reduction initiated by the parent

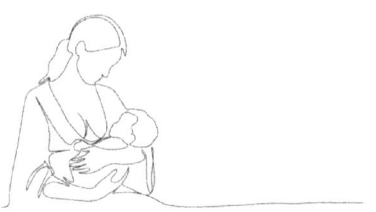

SPECIAL CIRCUMSTANCES AND MATERNAL HEALTH CONSIDERATIONS IN BREASTFEEDING

Maternal Health and Recovery

Most mothers can safely breastfeed regardless of delivery type, preexisting conditions, or postpartum challenges. Cesarean birth, perineal trauma, or exhaustion may temporarily affect positioning or frequency of feeding, but gentle support and comfort measures usually help establish normal patterns.

Encouraging skin-to-skin contact, rest, and pain management compatible with lactation allows recovery and bonding to progress together. Midwives can help mothers find positions that protect surgical sites, reduce strain, and maintain comfort.

Adequate nutrition, hydration, and emotional support remain essential for milk production and healing. Iron-rich foods, hydration, and rest aid recovery from blood loss and fatigue, while reassurance and calm presence help reduce stress hormones that can inhibit let-down.

Medications and Breastfeeding

Most medications prescribed in the postpartum period are compatible with breastfeeding. When medications are necessary, the goal is to balance maternal well-being with the baby's safety. Midwives should consult reliable resources such as *LactMed* or *Medications and Mothers' Milk* to verify safety and timing. In most cases, continuing to breastfeed while taking approved medications is safer and more beneficial than weaning prematurely.

If temporary interruption is required, hand expression or pumping can maintain supply until breastfeeding resumes. Reassure mothers that most treatments, including common antibiotics and pain medications, can be safely coordinated with lactation.

Breastfeeding After Complicated Births

Mothers who experience birth complications such as hemorrhage, retained placenta, or thyroid imbalance may face delayed lactogenesis or temporary low supply. These situations benefit from early support, frequent feeding, and close observation of infant intake and output.

With consistent midwifery follow-up, most women recover normal production within days to weeks. Emotional reassurance and individualized planning are key.

Special Feeding Situations

In cases of separation, illness, or maternal hospitalization, expressed milk remains the preferred nourishment. Safe storage, paced bottle feeding, and ongoing skin-to-skin contact help maintain the breastfeeding relationship during these challenges. Some babies require additional support due to prematurity, jaundice, or weak suck. Midwives can teach mothers how to combine direct breastfeeding with hand expression or pumping to protect supply until full feeding ability develops.

Developmental conditions may make breastfeeding challenging like:

- **Cleft Lip or Cleft Palate:** an opening in the lip or palate that affects suction and seal. Babies may breastfeed partially or fully depending on the type of cleft, often with positional adjustments and coordinated care from specialists.
- **Tongue-Tie (Ankyloglossia):** a short or restrictive lingual frenulum that limits tongue movement. It may cause shallow latch, nipple pain, or poor milk transfer. Assessment and referral for release may improve feeding.
- **Neurologic or Developmental Conditions:** conditions such as Down syndrome, congenital heart disease, birth injury, or seizures can affect feeding coordination. Gentle pacing, positioning support, and close weight monitoring guide safe breastfeeding.
- **Pierre Robin Sequence**
  A small lower jaw with airway concerns that can interfere with latch and breathing. These infants often require specialized positioning and multidisciplinary planning.

Supporting Emotional Health

Postpartum mood disorders can affect lactation by disrupting hormonal balance, appetite, and energy. Screening for depression or anxiety is an essential part of breastfeeding care. Gentle encouragement, regular meals, hydration, and rest all support recovery.

Midwives can help mothers understand that medication or therapy for postpartum depression is compatible with breastfeeding in most cases. Continuing to nurse can enhance oxytocin and endorphin release, offering emotional comfort for both mother and baby.

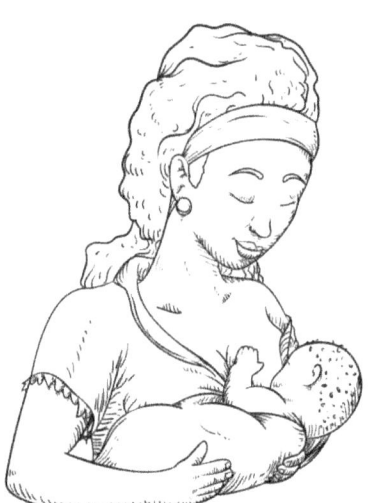

Holistic Midwifery Perspective

Breastfeeding occurs within the larger context of maternal recovery and family adaptation. Every mother's circumstances, health, and resources shape how lactation unfolds.

Midwives combine practical teaching with emotional and cultural awareness, helping mothers adapt to unique challenges while preserving connection and confidence. Whether the goal is exclusive breastfeeding, partial feeding, or gradual transition, informed support affirms that nourishing a baby is not defined by perfection but by presence, persistence, and care.

Midwifery Support and Cultural Considerations in Lactation

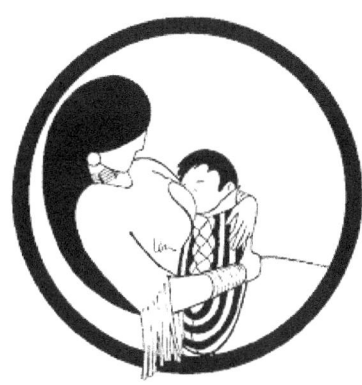

Cultural Beliefs and Practices

Feeding practices are deeply shaped by cultural, religious, and family traditions. In some communities, the first breastfeeding is considered sacred and begins immediately after birth. In others, rituals may delay the first feed or include prelacteal foods such as honey, herbal teas, or clarified butter.

Midwives can explore these traditions respectfully by asking open-ended questions about what is meaningful to the family. When traditional practices differ from evidence-based recommendations, discussion should focus on shared goals of infant health, bonding, and respect for heritage. Collaborative, culturally sensitive dialogue fosters trust and supports better outcomes than prescriptive advice.

Many cultures include foods, herbs, or rituals believed to enhance milk flow or postpartum recovery. While scientific evidence varies, these practices often hold deep emotional and social value. When safe, they can coexist with clinical care and strengthen the family's sense of belonging and confidence.

Global Perspectives and Lactation Equity

Worldwide, breastfeeding practices and support systems reflect the intersection of culture, economics, and access to healthcare. In some regions, the marketing of formula, limited maternity leave, or social stigma toward public breastfeeding creates barriers that shorten breastfeeding duration.

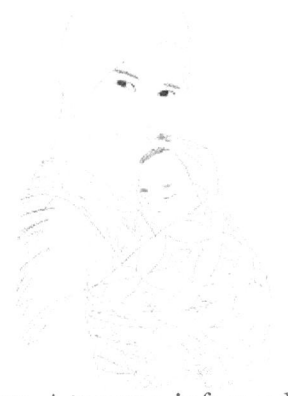

Lactation equity means ensuring that every family, regardless of race, income, or setting, has access to accurate information and compassionate care. Midwives play an important role in promoting equity by advocating for inclusive policies, supporting community programs, and amplifying cultural voices in maternal health.

Trauma-Informed Lactation Support

Some mothers may associate breastfeeding with discomfort, shame, or past trauma. A trauma-informed approach prioritizes autonomy, consent, and emotional safety throughout lactation care. Midwives should always ask permission before touching the breasts and explain each step of any procedure or assessment.

For mothers with a history of sexual trauma, modesty needs, or body dysphoria, adapting teaching methods to reduce exposure and increase choice helps create a sense of safety. Supportive positioning, privacy, and trusted companions can help rebuild comfort and confidence.

When breastfeeding is emotionally overwhelming, offering compassionate alternatives such as expressed milk, partial breastfeeding, or paced bottle feeding can help maintain connection while reducing guilt or distress. Midwives can remind families that nurturing and bonding come through many forms of loving care.

Inclusive Language and Family Structures

Midwives increasingly support diverse family structures, including single, adoptive, same-sex, and co-nursing families. Using clear and inclusive language such as *mother*, *baby*, or *family* demonstrates respect while recognizing individuality.

Some families share feeding responsibilities through milk sharing, donor milk, or supplemental nursing systems. When these practices are chosen, midwives can provide guidance on safe collection, storage, and hygiene while acknowledging their emotional and cultural importance.

Inclusive care emphasizes curiosity over assumption. Meeting each family where they are and honoring their values, roles, and relationships helps create trust and shared understanding.

Integrating Cultural Competence into Practice

Midwifery care blends science, empathy, and cultural humility. Asking families how feeding traditions are practiced in their community and what they hope for in their own experience opens the door to meaningful partnership.

Education works best as conversation, not correction. When conflicts arise between traditional practices and safety, midwives can help families find a respectful balance that preserves cultural integrity while protecting health. Providing materials in the family's preferred language, connecting them with peer counselors, and involving community leaders all strengthen lactation support.

Cultural humility, trauma awareness, and inclusive communication create an environment where every family feels seen, respected, and supported in their breastfeeding journey.

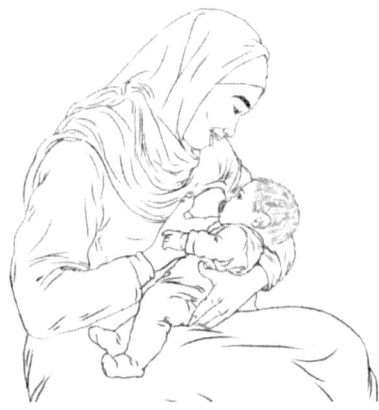

Cultural Traditions in Breastfeeding Around the World

- **Maori (Aotearoa/New Zealand):** breastfeeding is viewed as a sacred gift that connects generations. The first milk, or colostrum, is sometimes blessed by elders to honor ancestral strength passed through the mother's body.

- **India:** many families follow a ritual known as *annaprashan*, marking the baby's first solid food, but colostrum feeding is also celebrated as the first sacred nourishment. Some communities give the mother warm ghee, fennel, or fenugreek teas to encourage milk flow.

- **West Africa:** new mothers often receive intensive postpartum care called *lying-in*, during which female relatives prepare nutrient-rich foods such as groundnut soup or millet porridge to support lactation and healing.

- **Mexico and Central America:** traditional midwives (parteras) commonly use herbal infusions like anise, cinnamon, and atole (a warm corn drink) to promote milk flow. Breastfeeding in public is culturally accepted and often encouraged as a sign of maternal devotion.

- **Japan:** it is customary for new mothers to return to their parents' home for several weeks after birth (*satogaeri bunben*), where grandmothers provide rest and support for breastfeeding and recovery.

- **Scandinavia:** families emphasize prolonged skin-to-skin contact and shared parental leave, reflecting a social commitment to bonding and breastfeeding continuation for one to two years or more.

- **Indigenous North America:** many tribal communities view breastfeeding as a communal act of continuity and protection. Elders may bless the nursing mother or teach songs to calm the baby, reaffirming the spiritual bond between child, mother, and Earth.

Exercise 14.7: Choosing Effective Lactation Support
Answer the following questions.

1. The most effective first step when a mother expresses fear or discomfort during lactation teaching is:
   ☐ Give more instructions
   ☐ Ask permission before continuing and explain each step clearly
   ☐ Avoid discussing her concerns
   ☐ Encourage her to watch online videos instead

2. When cultural feeding traditions differ from recommendations, a midwife should:
   ☐ Require strict adherence to clinical guidelines
   ☐ Collaborate to find a safe adaptation that respects the tradition
   ☐ Ignore the practice to avoid conflict
   ☐ Ask another provider to handle the discussion

3. When maternal illness temporarily limits direct breastfeeding, the priority is to:
   ☐ Stop lactation until recovery
   ☐ Support hand expression and safe milk handling
   ☐ Switch directly to formula
   ☐ Wean the infant entirely

BREASTFEEDING PHYSIOLOGY AND PRACTICE ESSENTIAL TAKEAWAYS

Breastfeeding is a natural physiologic process sustained by hormonal coordination, emotional connection, and social support. Prolactin stimulates milk production, while oxytocin triggers milk ejection and deepens bonding between mother and baby. Understanding these mechanisms allows midwives to protect the delicate balance of rest, nutrition, and confidence that supports healthy lactation.

Successful breastfeeding depends on comfort, positioning, and trust. Early skin-to-skin contact, effective latch, and frequent feeding establish supply and prevent problems such as engorgement, blocked ducts, or nipple trauma. Teaching hand expression, proper pumping, and safe milk storage equips mothers to maintain breastfeeding through changing circumstances, including return to work or temporary separation.

Weaning and extended breastfeeding are both normal parts of the continuum of care. Midwives guide families through these transitions with reassurance, practical advice, and sensitivity to emotional changes. Gradual adaptation prevents discomfort and helps preserve the closeness formed through nursing.

Lactation support must also honor individual health, recovery, and diversity. Postpartum challenges, medication use, or emotional strain can influence milk supply and confidence, yet most situations can be managed safely with informed care. Culturally responsive and trauma-informed midwifery practice ensures that every family's values, beliefs, and experiences are respected.

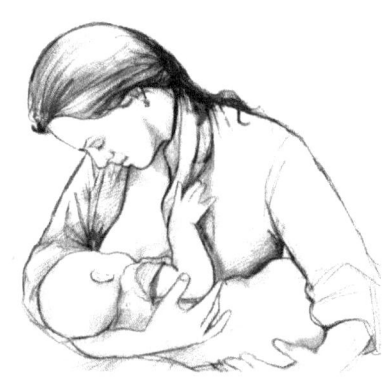

Through knowledge, empathy, and advocacy, midwives help families experience breastfeeding not only as nutrition, but as a foundation for lifelong connection, resilience, and health.

Chapter Fourteen Self-Assessment

Multiple Choice
1. Which hormone primarily stimulates milk synthesis?
    a) Oxytocin
    b) Prolactin
    c) Estrogen
    d) Cortisol

2. Which hormone causes milk ejection?
    a) Oxytocin
    b) Progesterone
    c) Estrogen
    d) Prolactin

3. The delivery of the placenta triggers which process?
    a) Lactogenesis I
    b) Lactogenesis II
    c) Mammogenesis
    d) Galactopoiesis

4. Which component is highest in colostrum?
    a) Fat
    b) Protein and antibodies
    c) Water
    d) Lactose

5. What factor most influences the balance between foremilk and hindmilk?
    a) Feeding length
    b) Breast fullness and milk removal
    c) Maternal diet
    d) Infant sleep cycle

6. Which position allows gravity to assist the baby's latch?
    a) Cradle hold
    b) Cross-cradle hold
    c) Laid-back position
    d) Side-lying position

7. What structure produces milk?
    a) Myoepithelial cells
    b) Montgomery glands
    c) Alveoli
    d) Lactiferous ducts

8. The main function of myoepithelial cells is to:
    a) Store milk
    b) Contract and push milk into ducts
    c) Produce lactose
    d) Support glandular tissue

9. Which position is often helpful after cesarean birth?
    a) Cradle
    b) Football
    c) Side-lying
    d) Laid-back

10. Which storage guideline is correct for milk kept in a refrigerator?
    a) Up to 24 hours
    b) Up to 4 days
    c) Up to 7 days
    d) Up to 10 days

11. When returning to work, most mothers should express milk:
    a) Once per day
    b) Every 3 hours
    c) Every 6 hours
    d) Only when breasts feel full

12. Which finding suggests mastitis rather than engorgement?
    a) Fullness only
    b) Fever and body aches
    c) Firmness without redness
    d) Brief tenderness

13. What is first-line management for a blocked duct?
    a) Ice only
    b) Massage and frequent feeding
    c) Hourly pumping
    d) Restrict fluids

14. What is the most reliable indicator of adequate milk intake?
    a) Pump output
    b) Feeding frequency
    c) Number of wet and dirty diapers
    d) Length of each feed

15. Which condition represents a primary cause of true low milk supply?
    a) Fatigue
    b) Hypothyroidism
    c) Long intervals between feeds
    d) Poor positioning

21. Which infant condition may require extra body support and breast compression during feeding?
    a) Colic
    b) Hypotonia
    c) Teething
    d) Jaundice

23. Which comfort measure helps during the physical phase of weaning?
    a) Wearing a tight bra for compression
    b) Applying warm compresses before feeding
    c) Using cold packs or gentle expression for relief
    d) Avoiding all breast stimulation

24. What can midwives do to promote lactation equity?
    a) Advocate for paid leave and access to lactation resources
    b) Focus care only on biological mothers
    c) Discourage traditional feeding practices
    d) Encourage formula feeding for working families

25. What is the best approach when a family's traditional feeding practice differs from standard recommendations?
    a) Insist on immediate adherence to clinical guidelines
    b) Explore the meaning of the practice and collaborate on safe adaptation
    c) Ignore the practice to avoid discomfort
    d) Report it to a higher authority

True or False
26. _____ Lactogenesis I begins during pregnancy with colostrum production.
27. _____ Delivery of the placenta triggers Lactogenesis II.
28. _____ Prolactin controls milk ejection while oxytocin stimulates milk synthesis.
29. _____ Milk "coming to volume" describes a gradual increase and compositional change.
30. _____ Stress and fatigue can temporarily suppress oxytocin release.
31. _____ Nighttime milk contains more melatonin than daytime milk.
32. _____ Covering the baby's hands or head can interfere with the breast crawl.
33. _____ A deep latch requires the baby to take most of the areola, not just the nipple.
34. _____ Engorgement is a normal, temporary phase when milk first comes to volume.
35. _____ Reverse pressure softening can improve areolar pliability and latch.
36. _____ Continued breastfeeding during mastitis can aid recovery.
37. _____ True low milk supply is more common than perceived low supply.
38. _____ Retained placenta can delay or prevent Lactogenesis II.
39. _____ Flat or inverted nipples always prevent breastfeeding success.

Fill in the Blank
40. Milk is produced in clusters called _____.
41. The glands in the areola that secrete oil are _____ glands.
42. The process of breast tissue growth during pregnancy is called _____.
43. Localized tenderness without fever suggests a _____.
44. Daytime milk is higher in _____, while nighttime milk contains more _____.
45. The resumption of milk production after a period of weaning is called _____.

Matching
46. Match each practice/support term with its definition.

    1. ____ Relactation
    2. ____ Double pumping
    3. ____ Flange fit
    4. ____ Hand expression
    5. ____ Cultural humility
    6. ____ Shared feeding
    7. ____ Lactation equity

    A. Cooperative feeding within a family or community
    B. Manual removal of milk using gentle compression
    D. Using a pump on both breasts simultaneously
    E. Correct size and comfort of pump breast shield
    F. Restarting milk production after little or no breastfeeding
    G. Equal access to lactation resources and support for all families
    H. Ongoing self-reflection and respect for diverse beliefs

Chapter Fourteen: Recommended Reading & References

Recommended Reading: Breastfeeding Physiology and Practice

- Geddes, Donna T., & Perrella, Sandra L. ***Breastfeeding and Human Lactation: Physiology, Research, and Clinical Practice.*** Academic Press, 2021. A comprehensive text exploring lactation science, anatomy, and physiology with an emphasis on current research and clinical applications.
- La Leche League International. ***The Womanly Art of Breastfeeding.*** 8th ed. Ballantine Books, 2010. A classic guide combining practical, emotional, and evidence-informed perspectives for mothers and caregivers.
- Lawrence, Ruth A., & Lawrence, Robert M. ***Breastfeeding: A Guide for the Medical Professional.*** 9th ed. Elsevier, 2022. The definitive medical reference on breastfeeding physiology, pathology, and clinical management.
- Mohrbacher, Nancy. ***Breastfeeding Answers Made Simple.*** Praeclarus Press, 2016. A practical and research-based guide offering clear solutions for common and complex breastfeeding challenges. Neifert, Marianne, & Bunik, Maya. ***Lactation and the Transition to Parenthood.*** Springer Publishing, 2020. Addresses both physiologic and psychosocial aspects of breastfeeding, emphasizing family-centered and trauma-informed care.
- Riordan, Jan, & Wambach, Karen. ***Breastfeeding and Human Lactation.*** 5th ed. Jones & Bartlett Learning, 2015. A foundational lactation consultant textbook combining research, anatomy, and applied techniques for clinical support.
- Walker, Marsha. ***Breastfeeding Management for the Clinician: Using the Evidence.*** 5th ed. Jones & Bartlett Learning, 2023. An evidence-based manual focused on assessment, management, and clinical problem-solving in lactation care.
- Wambach, Karen, & Spencer, Becky. ***Breastfeeding and Human Lactation.*** 6th ed. Jones & Bartlett Learning, 2021. An updated edition integrating modern evidence, cultural awareness, and global perspectives in lactation support.
- World Health Organization. ***Infant and Young Child Feeding: Model Chapter for Textbooks for Medical Students and Allied Health Professionals.*** WHO Press, 2009. An international teaching standard promoting consistent education and policy alignment in infant feeding and lactation care.

References

American Academy of Pediatrics. (2022). Policy statement: Breastfeeding and the use of human milk. *Pediatrics, 150*(1), e2022057988. https://doi.org/10.1542/peds.2022-057988

Binns, C., Lee, M., & Low, W. Y. (2016). The long-term public health benefits of breastfeeding. *Asia Pacific Journal of Public Health, 28*(1), 7–14. https://doi.org/10.1177/1010539515624964

Hinde, K. (2016, April 22). Breast milk: Liquid gold for infants, Hinde says. *NIH Record*. https://nihrecord.nih.gov/2016/04/22/breast-milk-liquid-gold-infants-hinde-says

Kent, J. C., Prime, D. K., & Geddes, D. T. (2013). Breastfeeding: Human milk composition and infant milk intake. *Pediatric Clinics of North America, 60*(1), 49–74. https://doi.org/10.1016/j.pcl.2012.10.002

La Leche League International. (2010). *The womanly art of breastfeeding* (8th ed.). Ballantine Books.

OhBaby!. (n.d.). Breastfeeding success. https://www.ohbaby.co.nz/baby/feeding/breastfeeding/breastfeeding-success

Victora, C. G., Bahl, R., Barros, A. J. D., França, G. V. A., Horton, S., Krasevec, J., ... Rollins, N. C. (2016). Breastfeeding in the 21st century: Epidemiology, mechanisms, and lifelong effect. *The Lancet, 387*(10017), 475–490. https://doi.org/10.1016/S0140-6736(15)01024-7

Woolridge, M. W., & Fischer, C. A. (2020). The neurobiology of breastfeeding: Hormonal, behavioral, and psychological perspectives. *Frontiers in Global Women's Health, 1*, 1–10. https://doi.org/10.3389/fgwh.2020.00001

World Health Organization, & UNICEF. (2018). *Implementation guidance: Protecting, promoting and supporting breastfeeding in facilities providing maternity and newborn services: The revised Baby-friendly Hospital Initiative.* World Health Organization

Answer Key

Please note: Answers are provided for the self-assessment questions at the end of each chapter. Answers for exercises are often discussed within the text, but some may vary based on individual circumstances. Suggested answers to exercise questions will be included in the *Birthsong Midwifery Workbook Instructor Manual*, scheduled for release in 2027.

Chapter One: Midwifery Yesterday & Today		
Multiple Choice 1. b) 2. b) 3. c) 4. c) 5. b) 6. a) 7. b) 8. d) 9. b) 10. a) 11. c) 12. a)	**Fill in the Blank** 13. holistic 14. physicians 15. individualized 16. informed	**True / False** 17. False 18. True 19. True 20. True 21. False

Chapter Two: Learning to Learn	
Multiple Choice 1. b) 2. c) 3. b) 4. a) 5. b) 6. a) 7. c) 8. d) 9. d) 10. c)	**Fill in the Blank** 11. science and art 12. Eisenhower 13. Kinesthetic 14. Survey, Question, Read, Reflect, Recite, Review 15. Prepare 16. andragogy; pedagogy 17. rubric 18. interpreting 19. paraphrase 20. critical thinking

Chapter Three: Terminology for Midwifery Practice			

Multiple Choice
1. b)
2. c)
3. b)
4. b)
5. d)
	Fill in the Blank
	6. hypoglycemia
	7. tachycardia
	8. hypotension
	9. last menstrual period
	10. induced abortion
	11. estimated date of delivery
	12. estimated date of confinement
	13. white blood cell
	14. within normal limits
	15. premature rupture of membranes
	16. four times a day
	17. spontaneous abortion
	18. temperature + pulse + respiration
	19. G 9 T 3 P 1 A 4 L 3
		True / False
		20. True
		21. True
		22. True
		23. False
		24. True
		25. True
		26. False
		27. True
		28. False
		29. True
			Matching
			30. Match the root with its meaning
			   1. E 2. B 3. C 4. A 5. D
			
			31. Match each anatomical plane with its description
			   1. A 2. B 3. C
			
			32. Match the abbreviation with its full term
			   1. B 2. D 3. F 4. C 5. H
			   6. A 7. G 8. E

Chapter Four: Reproductive Anatomy & Physiology

Multiple Choice	Number in Order	Matching	Fill in the Blank	True / False
1. d)	15.	16.	17. follicle-stimulating hormone (FSH)	27. True
2. b)	1. Mons pubis	1. D	18. luteinizing hormone (LH)	28. False
3. c)	2. Clitoris	2. C	19. progesterone	29. False
4. d)	3. Urethra	3. E	20. corpus luteum	30. False
5. d)	4. Introitus	4. B	21. fundus	31. False
6. b)	5. Fourchette	5. A	22. fimbriae	32. True
7. b)	6. Perineum		23. uterus	33. False
8. b)	7. Anus		24. perineum	34. False
9. c)			25. ampulla	35. False
10. c)			26. gynecoid	36. True
11. b)				37. False
12. b)				38. True
13. c)				39. True
14. b)				40. True
				41. False

Chapter Five: Biology for Midwives

Multiple Choice	Fill in the Blank	True / False
1. b)	11. nucleus	16. False
2. c)	12. transcription	17. True
3. b)	13. meiosis	18. False
4. b)	14. vernix caseosa	19. True
5. b)	15. polygenic	20. True
6. a)		21. False
7. c)		22. True
8. c)		23. False
9. b)		24. False
10. c)		25. True

Chapter Six: Biology for Midwives

Multiple Choice	True / False	Fill in the Blank
1. b)	14. False	26. ampulla
2. c)	15. True	27. five
3. c)	16. False	28. twelve to twenty-four
4. c)	17. True	29. ductus venosus, foramen ovale, ductus arteriosus
5. b)	18. False	30. Wharton's jelly
6. d)	19. False	
7. b)	20. True	
8. b)	21. True	
9. b)	22. False	
10. a)	23. True	
11. a)	24. True	
12. c)	25. True	

Chapter Seven: Physiology of Pregnancy

Multiple Choice	Matching	Fill in the Blank	True / False	Increase / Decrease
1. b)	**14.**	17. immunomodulation	22. True	36. Cardiovascular changes
2. d)	1. B	18. emotional lability	23. False	A. ↑
3. c)	2. C	19. pelvic congestion	24. True	B. ↑
4. b)	3. A	20. dilutional	25. True	C. ↓
5. c)	4. D	21. estrogen	26. True	D. ↑
6. b)	**15.**		27. True	E. ↑
7. b)	1. A		28. True	
8. b)	2. C		29. False	37. Other physiologic changes
9. b)	3. D		30. True	A. ↑
10. b)	4. B		31. True	B. ↓
11. b)	**16.**		32. True	C. ↑
12. c)	1. B		33. True	D. ↓
13. b)	2. D		34. False	E. ↑
	3. A		35. True	F. ↑
	4. C			G. ↓
				H. ↓
				I. ↑
				J. ↓

Chapter Eight: Health Promotion for Midwives

Multiple Choice	Fill in the Blank	True / False	Matching
1. b)	16. small, frequent	25. True	50. Nutrient and function
2. b)	17. upright	26. False	1. D
3. c)	18. peppermint	27. False	2. C
4. b)	19. counseling and domestic violence	28. True	3. A
5. b)	20. education and support	29. True	4. E
6. b)	21. 27	30. True	5. B
7. b)	22. brain; eggs	31. False	
8. c)	23. vitamin D	32. True	51. Discomfort and support
9. b)	24. vitamin B12	33. True	1. D
10. a)		34. True	2. C
11. c)		35. False	3. A
12. a)		36. True	4. B
13. b)		37. True	
14. b)		38. False	52. Activity and benefit
15. c)		39. True	1. A
		40. True	2. E
		41. False	3. C
		42. True	4. B
		43. False	5. D
		44. True	
		45. True	
		46. False	
		47. False	
		48. True	
		49. True	

Chapter Nine: Infection, Immunity, & Midwifery Practice

Multiple Choice	Matching	Fill in the Blank	True / False
1. b)	16. C	21. antibody screen	31. False
2. b)	17. A	22. MMR and varicella	32. True
3. c)	18. B	23. Group B Streptococcus	33. True
4. b)	19. D	24. fomite	34. True
5. c)	20. E	25. dried	35. False
6. b)		26. placenta	36. True
7. b)		27. regulatory T	37. False
8. b)		28. autoclave	38. True
9. b)		29. Lactobacilli	39. False
10. c)		30. Listeria	40. True
11. c)			41. False
12. a)			42. True
13. b)			43. False
14. c)			44. True
15. b)			45. True
			46. False
			47. False
			48. True
			49. False
			50. True

Chapter Ten: Prenatal Care

Multiple Choice	True / False	Fill in the Blank
1. c)	21. False	34. six-second
2. c)	22. True	35. fetoscope
3. b)	23. True	36. baseline fetal heart rate
4. b)	24. True	37. lie, presentation, position
5. b)	25. False	38. 110 to 160
6. c)	26. True	39. systolic and diastolic
7. c)	27. True	40. diagonal
8. b)	28. True	41. 90
9. c)	29. False	42. process
10. c)	30. True	43. refusals
11. c)	31. True	44. anticipatory
12. c)	32. True	45. guidelines and protocols
13. c)	33. True	46. staff
14. c)		
15. c)		
16. d)		
17. b)		
18. c)		
19. c)		
20. b)		

Chapter Eleven: Labor & Birth

Multiple Choice	Fill in the Blank	Matching	True / False
1. a)	15. dilation; baby	23.	25. False
2. a)	16. uterus	1. C	26. False
3. b)	17. head	2. D	27. False
4. b)	18. fetal heart rate	3. E	28. False
5. c)	19. fundus	4. B	29. True
6. c)	20. retraction	5. A	30. True
7. b)	21. physiologic (retraction) ring	**24.**	31. True
8. b)	22. thinning	1. A	32. False
9. c)		2. B	33. True
10. b)		3. C	34. True
11. b)		4. D	35. True
12. b)			36. True
13. c)			37. True
14. b)			38. True
			39. True
			40. False
			41. False
			42. True
			43. False
			44. True
			45. True
			46. True
			47. False
			48. True

Chapter Twelve: Placenta & Postpartum

Multiple Choice	True / False	Fill in the Blank	Matching
1. b)	21. True	31. involution	36.
2. c)	22. True	32. one	1. A
3. d)	23. False	33. vulvar or perineal	2. B
4. b)	24. True	34. one	3. C
5. b)	25. True	35. postpartum depression	4. D
6. b)	26. False		37.
7. b)	27. True		1. B
8. b)	28. True		2. A
9. b)	29. False		3. C
10. b)	30. True		38.
11. c)			1. A
12. b)			2. B
13. c)			3. C
14. b)			4. D
15. b)			
16. c)			
17. b)			
18. a)			
19. b)			
20. c)			

Chapter Thirteen: Midwifery Care of the Newborn			
Multiple Choice	**True / False**	**Fill in the Blank**	**Matching**
1. b)	21. True	33. one and five	43.
2. b)	22. True	34. thirty-four	1. D
3. b)	23. False	35. thirty to sixty	2. B
4. c)	24. True	36. lanugo	3. E
5. c)	25. False	37. thermoregulation	4. A
6. b)	26. True	38. oxygen, glucose, and warmth	5. C
7. b)	27. True	39. five to ten	44.
8. b)	28. True	40. vastus lateralis	1. E
9. b)	29. True	41. periosteum	2. B
10. a)	30. True	42. twenty-four to seventy-two	3. A
11. b)	31. True		4. D
12. b)	32. True		5. C
13. b)			
14. b)			
15. a)			
16. b)			
17. b)			

Chapter Fourteen: Breastfeeding Physiology & Practice			
Multiple Choice	**True / False**	**Fill in the Blank**	**Matching**
1. b)	26. True	40. alveoli	46.
2. a)	27. True	41. Montgomery	1. F
3. b)	28. False	42. mammogenesis	2. D
4. b)	29. True	43. blocked duct	3. E
5. b)	30. True	44. cortisol, melatonin	4. B
6. c)	31. True	45. relactation	5. H
7. c)	32. True		6. A
8. b)	33. True		7. G
9. b)	34. True		
10. b)	35. True		
11. b)	36. True		
12. b)	37. False		
13. b)	38. True		
14. c)	39. False		
15. b)			
16. b)			
17. c)			
18. a)			
19. b)			

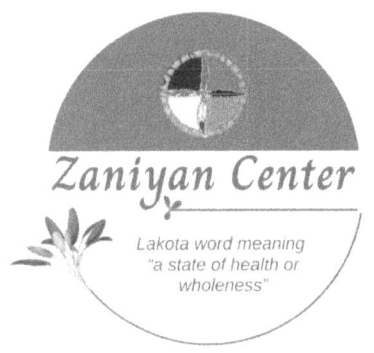

About Zaníyan Center

One hundred percent of the proceeds from this book support the Zaníyan Center, a 501(c)(3) nonprofit dedicated to promoting health through plants and connection with the earth. Our organization is rooted in Indigenous values and guided by the belief that community wellness begins with relationship — to land, to plants, to knowledge, and to one another.

At Zaníyan, we weave ancestral traditions with practical skills to strengthen personal and community resilience. Our work grows through many hands and takes many forms:

Community Projects

Our Free Herbal Tea Station brings connection and comfort to festivals, gatherings, and community events. We serve freshly brewed herbal teas while teaching people how to use bulk herbs, prepare simple remedies, and reconnect with everyday plant medicine.

Through our Growing Resilience Project, we offer a free food pantry open to all, along with a Little Free Library. We provide free seeds, plant starts, and food staples to anyone in need, believing that food sovereignty begins with access to land, to seeds, to skills, and to culturally meaningful foods.

We partner with **Seven Directions Neighborhood Farm** and the **Bethel School District Native American Youth Empowerment Program** to offer hands-on gardening experiences for children and their families. These programs teach planting, harvesting, seed-saving, and the deep relationships between earth and culture.

Our community library and learning garden offer a welcoming space for learning, rest, and reconnection. We maintain books and resources on herbalism, midwifery, permaculture, Indigenous knowledge, emergency preparedness, and sustainable living.

Education, Workshops, and Training

Zaníyan Center offers free and low-cost workshops throughout the year on herbal medicine, gardening, food preservation, midwifery topics, resilience skills, and earth-based ways of living. These classes are taught by experienced educators, midwives, herbalists, and cultural knowledge keepers.

Our books, both fiction and nonfiction, are part of this educational mission. The *Circle for the Earth* series explores themes of resilience, cultural continuity, herbal knowledge, birth, food sovereignty, and community survival in the face of disruption. The *Birthsong Midwifery Workbook* supports students and midwives with comprehensive, hands-on learning grounded in real-world practice.

Purchasing a book from Eagletree Press directly supports this work. Book sales help us provide free tea, distribute seeds and plant starts, offer youth programming, share supplies during emergencies, and maintain our community learning spaces.

Our Guiding Belief

At the heart of Zaníyan Center is a simple truth: **Connection to the land, reverence for life, and shared knowledge create a strong and sustainable future.**

To learn more about our programs or view our workshop schedule, visit **zaniyan.org**. Tax-deductible donations are always welcome and deeply appreciated.

www.ingramcontent.com/pod-product-compliance
Lightning Source LLC
Chambersburg PA
CBHW042357030426
42337CB00032B/5136